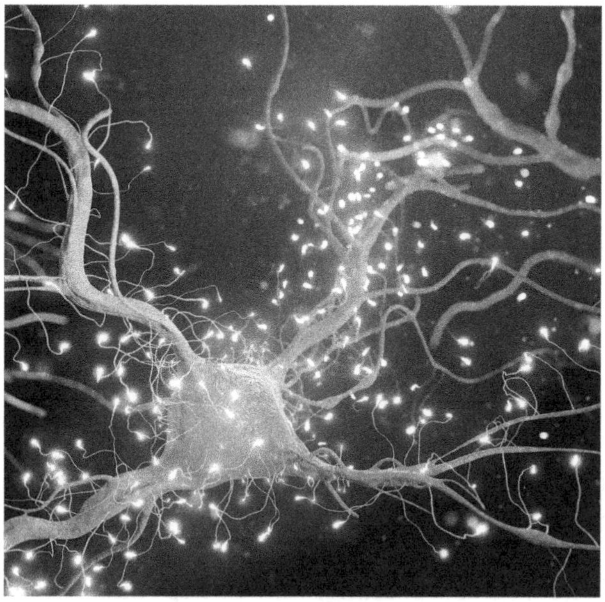

NEUROPATHIC PAIN:

A Clinical Guide to Diagnosis

Robert J. Schwartzman, MD

Publication date: February 27, 2024

ISBN Softback: 978-1-7345967-5-5
ISBN eBook: 978-1-7345967-4-8
Library of Congress Control Number: 2024904940
DOI: https://doi.org/10.17918/drexel-rjs-neuropathic-pain

NOTICE and DISCLAIMER

This book is the product of the author's personal and professional knowledge and experience regarding neuropathic pain. The author has consulted generally accepted reliable sources when compiling this work. The author and publisher provide this book as a reference and guide and make no representations or warranties of any kind concerning this book. Medical science changes rapidly and continuously. Neither the author or the publisher, nor any other party involved in the preparation of this book warrants or guarantees that the information contained in this book is accurate or complete. Practitioners should always rely on their own knowledge and experience in evaluating medical information. Patients should always consult the advice of their healthcare provider. The author, publisher, and any other party involved in the publication of this book disclaim responsibility for any injuries or damages of any kind claimed by any practitioner or patient arising from the use of this book. The use of this book demonstrates the acceptance of this disclaimer. The URLs listed in this book may contain typographical errors or other inaccuracies and are for reference and convenience only; they do not constitute medical advice. No warranties or guarantees of any kind are made with respect to the URLs, as with the rest of this book.

I Schwartzman, Robert J. MD II Neuropathic Pain: a Clinical Guide to Diagnosis

Cover and Interior Layout: Megan Leid
Publishing Advisor: Mel Cohen inspiredauthorspress@gmail.com
Contact Admin@rjsmedicalpress.com for reprints of specific chapters, the entire book, or Rights and Licensing Agreements
Publisher: RJS Medical Press LLC
Website: http://rjsmedicalpress.com

Printed in the United States of America

Neuropathic Pain: a Clinical Guide to Diagnosis is a practical volume written by a master clinician and pain specialist. Dr. Robert Schwarzman redefined Reflex Sympathetic Dystrophy (aka CRPS) with nuanced elaboration on other forms of neuropathic pain, from molecules to pain behavior. This book is a body of knowledge culminating in decades of experience diagnosing and treating neuropathic pain by an astute and compassionate observer. The book is equally valuable for all physicians who deal with pain, including physiatrists, neurologists, and general medicine physicians.

—Sayed Ausim Azizi, MD, PhD, FANA
Department of Neurology
Yale University School of Medicine

Dr. Robert Schwartzman stood at the forefront of the field of neurology. He was renowned for his unrivaled expertise in evaluating, treating, and diagnosing conditions associated with neuropathic pain. With a vast wealth of knowledge backed by years of experience, Dr. Schwartzman cemented his position as an indisputable leader in his field. This is another of his books that proves it. This book about neuropathic pain is a must-read by everybody interested in this subject matter.

—G. Peter Gliebus, MD FAAN,
Associate Professor, Academic Chair of Neurology
Drexel University College of Medicine

Over the years, I have had the opportunity to observe many examiners in Neurology, but no one has taught me more than Dr. Schwartzman, my chairman, for more than 25 years. With each Chairman's Rounds, there was something he taught me, along with the rest of the audience. Dr. Schwartzman was the consummate examiner and diagnostician; nowhere was this more evident than in his approach to neuropathic pain. His academic and thoughtful approach to the diagnosis and treatment of neuropathic pain is unparalleled. He has captured his decades of experience in writing this monumental work dedicated to diagnosing neuropathic pain. It is truly a gift to the medical community and will be an essential read for anyone caring for patients with neuropathic pain.

—Terry Heiman-Patterson, MD
Professor of Neurology
Director Center for Neurodegenerative Diseases
Temple University Lewis Katz School of Medicine

Dr. Schwartzman was the greatest clinical teacher I have ever met. His method, warmth, and vast knowledge were unparalleled. All of us still repeat his sayings or aphorisms, which were tremendously helpful as a teaching tool but also colorful and funny.

I had the privilege of being one of his Chief Residents. Six months that helped shape me and in which I learned and grew tremendously. Work was punctuated by our Friday evening meetings to debrief and talk about the previous week, the future, and life in general. I consider Dr. Schwartzman my principal mentor.

I will never forget him, and still tell my children about the great teacher who helped me become a neurologist and a better doctor.

—Victor C. Urrutia, MD, FAHA
Professor of Clinical Neurology
Director, The Johns Hopkins Hospital Comprehensive Stroke Center
Director, Sheikh Khalifa Stroke Institute
JHMI Medical Director
Director, Global Center for Organized Stroke Care

Dr. Schwartzman's teachings are exceptional pearls of wisdom: the knowledge and astute examination skills he taught, as well as his insights about life in general. He helped me become a good doctor and a good person.

He said medicine is a profession where you get to help people every day, and the added benefit is that you get paid for it!

—Rohini Bhole, MD
Associate Professor
Department of Neurology
University of Virginia
Drexel Neurology Residency Graduate 2014

I was privileged to serve under Dr. Schwartzman as a chief resident at Drexel Univ College of Medicine. The knowledge base he provided enabled me to open my own practice specializing in Complex Regional Pain Syndrome. His teachings carry me through my days as I often refer to his published papers and books. As a result, my patients benefit profoundly, and I am blessed with a very rewarding career. This book contains a treasure of knowledge that is an indispensable reference and a gift to all physicians.

—Lara Edinger, DO
Edinger Pain Management
10921 Wilshire Blvd., Suite 1109
Los Angeles, CA, 90024-4005

What a gift to have this manuscript left behind by such a highly respected neurologist and master diagnostician. Dr. Schwartzman taught me the wealth of information to be gleaned from the subtleties of a careful physical exam. *Neuropathic Pain: a Clinical Guide to Diagnosis* offers those seeking expert guidance a way to fill the void created by the passing of a generous scholar and tireless advocate of the patient suffering from neuropathic pain.

—Lynn Durmala, FNP-BC

Dr. Schwartzman had a brilliant gift of quickly assessing patients in a way that few others could because of his comprehensive understanding of the intricacies of the neurological system, yet in a compassionate and caring manner. Through my interactions with patients, I heard countless stories of his astounding ability to thoroughly diagnose conditions that puzzled patients' prior caregivers as they struggled with debilitating pain. He was always professional, knowledgeable, and kind—a rare physician with a blend of these admirable qualities.

I had the honor of knowing Dr. Robert Schwartzman as a patient initially, who, after a long search, was able to provide an accurate diagnosis and treatment. He became a wonderful mentor from whom I learned so much, attending his pain clinics for a decade. Through this mentorship, I then provided physical therapy for many of his patients with complex regional pain syndrome and brachial plexus traction injuries.

Finally, Dr. Schwartzman loved to share and teach what he discovered through decades of practice and research. I strongly believe that the insights conveyed in this book will continue to aid clinicians in diagnosing and understanding neurological pain disorders.

—Irene Connolly, PT, MS
Owner Cedars Therapy, LLC

"Standing on the shoulders of Giants"

Dr. Schwartzman was the most influential mentor I have had in my career. He had an encyclopedic knowledge of neurology (and everything else!), sage-like wisdom, and a great sense of humor! I am honored and privileged to be counted among his residents and chief residents. In the Winter of 2008, as I navigated the neurology residency interview trail, Drexel University/Hahnemann University Hospital was an interview I will never forget. I remember watching in awe and admiration as Dr. Schwartzman, the Neurology Maestro he was, masterfully conducted Neurology Grand Rounds. In this exact manner, every morning during Morning Report, Dr. Schwartzman, taught us how to use key pieces of the history and neurologic exam to precisely localize neurologic lesions as well as formulate a sophisticated differential diagnosis. "Age and Chief Complaint" became a statement all of his residents became familiar with. To this day, I continue to use the classical neurology teachings of Dr. Schwartzman in the evaluation of patients and in teaching my trainees. This book will be an invaluable resource to all who consult it, for it contains the distilled wisdom of an Academic Giant and one of the most talented Neurologists of our time, Dr. Robert J. Schwartzman.

—Gilbert Mbeo MD
Assistant Professor, University of Central Florida
Board Certified in Adult Neurology, American Board of Psychiatry and Neurology
Board Certified in Neurocritical Care, United Council of Neurologic Subspecialties
Board Certified in Interventional Pain Management, American Board of Psychiatry and Neurology
Neurologist, Neurointensivist and Interventional Pain Management Specialist

DEDICATION

For Sarah and Evan
because Pa promised

IN MEMORIAM

Robert Jay Schwartzman, MD

1939–2021

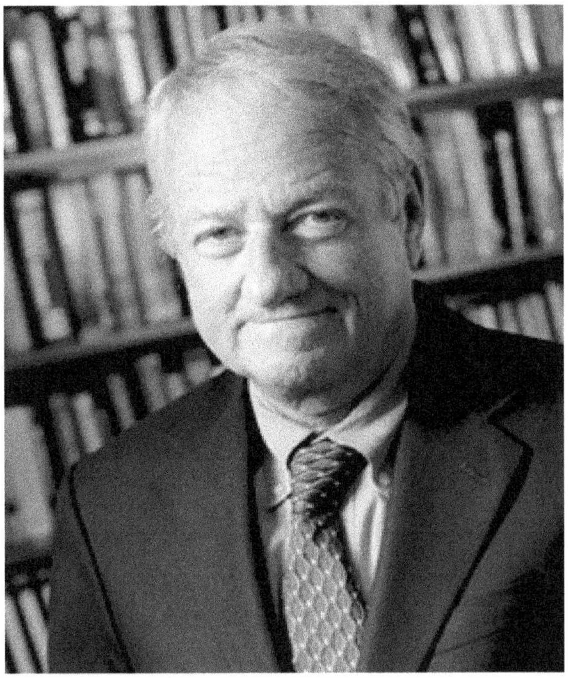

Dr. Robert J. Schwartzman was an Emeritus Professor and former Chairman of the Department of Neurology at Drexel University College of Medicine in Philadelphia, PA. At Drexel and his previous academic appointments, he always maintained a large clinical practice, treating patients for over 40 years.

He dedicated a major portion of his research and practice to treating chronic pain. Dr. Schwartzman taught students, residents, and colleagues that persistent pain was the symptom most likely to cause a patient to seek medical help, making pain a significant component of consultative neurology.

Dr. Schwartzman is best known for his groundbreaking work in the treatment of Complex Regional Pain Syndrome (CRPS), also known as Reflex Sympathetic Dystrophy (RSD). He founded the first CRPS clinic in the U.S. while at the ThomasJefferson University School of Medicine, pioneering the use of ketamine as a treatment for CRPS and other pain conditions.

After Dr. Schwartzman retired from academic responsibilities and clinical practice, he wrote this book. This book is the result of decades of clinical experience and research. It is intended as a guide for practitioners, presenting an organized approach to diagnosing neuropathic pain.

Marco Island, Florida
2023

ACKNOWLEDGEMENTS

I could not have completed the task of bringing this book to press after my husband's death without the support of my children, Jane (Bergman), Nancy, and David. A special thank-you must go to my son-in-law, Raymond Bergman, who tirelessly and patiently addressed my many and constant technical problems with electronics.

I would be extremely remiss if I did not thank Kirsten Erwin, whose dedication, editorial assistance, and expertise made this book possible. I also thank Dr. Helen Tuzio for her valuable insights and assistance in the preparation of this work.

Lastly, I thank my husband's many colleagues who offered comments, suggestions, and insights for this work. Unfortunately, I do not know their names, but luckily Dr. Schwartzman did.

Denise D. Schwartzman, 2023

CONTENTS

OVERVIEW OF PAIN

NEUROPATHIC SOMATIC PAIN

PAINFUL NEUROPATHIES

REFERRED PAIN

CHAPTER 1

OVERVIEW OF PAIN

Demographics

Pain is an unpleasant sensory and emotional experience associated with actual or potential tissue damage or described in terms of such damage (IASP definition). It is a subjective and highly personal experience. Due to the subjective nature of pain, its direct measurement is challenging and depends on the individual's self-report and behavior that provide an estimate of that individual's experience. There are a great number of factors unique to the individual that make the pain experience specific to each person. Between-person differences in the pain experience are independent of the pain-producing stimulus. It has been demonstrated experimentally that a painful stimulus of standard intensity is perceived differently between individuals. There are inter-individual differences in the cerebral activation evoked by the same painful stimulus that partly reflect differences in brain morphology. The experience of pain is associated with complex and dynamic biological, psychological, and social factors that vary among individuals.

Genetic Contribution to Pain

As noted above, there are great individual differences in the development of chronic pain syndromes among individuals as often demonstrated by the transition from acute to chronic pain. Most individuals do not develop chronic neuropathic pain after an injury to the somatosensory system. The intensity of pain cannot be predicted by the severity of an injury. Variability in pain ratings by individuals receiving the same noxious stimulus is associated with variability in pain-evoked cortical activations. There is also great individual variability to the analgesic responses for the same painful condition among patients.

Familial aggregation and twin studies are starting to give insight into these sources of variability noted in patients with neuropathic pain.

Single Gene Disorders of Pain

The inherited Mendelian disorders whereby a single mutated gene produces a specific disease includes:

1. Hereditary sensory and autonomic neuropathies (HSANs)
2. Familial hemiplegic migraine
3. Channelopathies (erythromelalgia, paroxysmal extreme pain disorder and familial episodic pain syndrome)

These genes encode a variety of ion channels, enzymes, transcription, and trophic factors. A common thread is the involvement of the SCN9A gene that encodes the NaV1.7 sodium channel.

Candidate Gene Association Studies

Recent work has demonstrated a wide variety of genes that are associated with clinical neuropathic pain. A meta-analysis of the A1180 polymorphism of the OPRM1 gene that encodes the μ-opioid receptor: while demonstrating concordant preclinical data, no statistical correlation was found between OPRM1 genotype and opioid requirement or pain levels in patients.

The heavily studied candidate genes for pain include:

1. COMT (Catechol-O-Methyltransferase) Val158Met allele:
   a. Associated with the musculoskeletal pain of temporal mandibular joint pain
   b. The biological effects of COMT polymorphism are modified by polymorphisms of estrogen receptor1 and guanosine 5-triphosphate cyclohydrolase 1 gene
2. Women with premenstrual syndrome and widespread pain
   a. Associated with S/S homozygous SLC6A4 transporter
3. Genes associated with the risk of generalized, widespread pain
   a. The rs13361160 and rs2386592 single nucleotide polymorphisms have been mapped to the CCT5 and FAM173 B genes on chromosome 5p15.2
4. Other genes that have been extensively studied in neuropathic pain states include:
   a. OPRM1
   b. HTR2A
   c. IL1A
   d. IL1B
   e. TRPV1
   f. TNF
   g. GCH1

Difficulties with this research have included:

1. Sample size of cohorts
2. Population substructure confound
3. Design of the studies
4. Selective publication bias

Epistasis, Gene and Environment Interactions, Small RNA's and Epi-

genetics

In addition to linkage and association studies that delineate the effect of DNA variants, trait variance is also determined by:

1. Gene x gene interaction (epistasis)
2. Gene x environmental interactions
3. Environmental factors which may also be impacted by epigenetic regulation

Some chronic pain states have been demonstrated to have DNA methylation and histone acetylation abnormalities.

The genetic contribution to the perception of pain has demonstrated biological mechanisms that contribute to individual pain responses. Catechol-o-methyltransferase (COMT), an enzyme that metabolizes catecholamines, is associated with pain-related mu-opioid receptor binding in the brain, which correlates with global pain sensitivity in some clinical circumstances. The mu-opioid receptor gene (OPRM1) A118G single nucleotide polymorphism (SNP) is correlated with pressure pain sensitivity and experimental pain responses. Genetic associations with pain vary by sex and ethnic group.

The genetic mechanisms that underpin the variability of pain responses are primarily reported in rare familial mutations that cause gain or loss of function of specific neurons and ion channels in pain pathways. Examples are severe pain disorders, such as erythromelalgia, and congenital insensitivity to pain. These conditions underscore the importance of ion channels such as sodium channel $Na_V1.7$, receptors (NTRK1), growth factors (NGF), and transcription factors, as illustrated by PRDM12. The heritability of pain is buttressed by twin studies. There is strong evidence that experimental pain perception, specific pain syndromes, and vulnerability to chronic pain are sculpted by genetic factors. It is estimated that 25% to 60% of pain conditions have some aspects of heritability depending on the specific condition. Candidate gene and genome-wide association studies (GWAS) are not as revealing as expected due to small sample sizes, low power, and inadequate phenotyping in many conditions. It has also been demonstrated that even large sample studies only detect SNPs in a given phenotype that explain heritability in a fraction of patients. The single whole exome sequencing study does not demonstrate a single variant that is associated at a genome wide level with pain perception. Gene interactions, epistasis, may be another cause of the inability to identify specific gene functions in the perception of pain.

Environmental and Demographic Factors Contributing to Pain

Many environmental factors contribute to the risk of developing chronic pain. These include age, gender, personality traits (catastrophizing), psychological stress, and a history of pain. Studies show that the level of pain prior to a surgical procedure may predict the degree of chronic post-operative pain. Post-physical injuries and pain during infancy may also be linked to the development of chronic pain. Stress is shown in prospective cohort studies to be important in the development of chronic widespread pain. The mechanism for stress effects may be mediated by dysregulation of the hypothalamic-pituitary-adrenal axis that has been associated with neonatal pain-related stress.

Epigenetics, stable molecular modifications exemplified by histone alterations and DNA methylation, are transmitted to daughter cells during mitosis and are essential for normal development and cell differentiation. Epigenetics is now defined as "the study of changes in gene function that are mitotically and/or meiotically heritable and that do not entail a change in the DNA sequence." Epigenetic modifications also have a crucial role in the silencing and expression of genes. The brain demonstrates hydroxymethylation and neurons are also methylated in a non-cytosine-guanine manner. The usual epigenetic modifications entail histone variants, posttranslational modifications of amino acids on the amino-terminal tail of histones, and covalent alterations of DNA bases. These epigenetic modifications are also important in the silencing and expression of noncoding DNA sequences. The methylation of cytosine bases followed by adenine and guanine methylation is the predominant modification in mammalian DNA: it occurs primarily in CpG dinucleotides but is also seen in non-CpG sequences. Methylation of cytosine in the promoter regions represses gene expression by preventing the binding of transcription factors or by recruiting mediators of chromatin remodeling (histone-modifying enzymes) as well as other repressors of gene expression. As noted above, neurons may be methylated in a non-cytosine (CH) manner which is typical of embryonic stem cells but is absent in differentiated cell lines. In the human brain, more than 80% of cytosine sites are methylated (less than 2% of CH sites are methylated). Methylation of CH sites coincides with synaptic development during childhood and adolescence. Active research is accumulating evidence that specific histone marks delineate transcriptional states. This gives an understanding of how a specific DNA sequence is utilized in different neuronal cell types. Recent experimental work demonstrates that the histone mark H3K4mel is associated with enhancers of pain-relevant genes.

Age-Related Factors and Pain

There are age-related differences in pain prevalence across the lifespan. Joint pain, lower extremity pain and neuropathic pain increase with age. Chronic pain increases until middle age and then plateaus. Headache, abdominal pain, back pain, and temporal mandibular disorder pain peak in the third to fifth decade and then decrease in prevalence. Older adults have lower acute pain intensity in some studies while age-related differences in the intensity of chronic pain are not consistently reported.

Experimental pain studies show that older subjects are less sensitive to brief cutaneous pain such as heat pain thresholds, but are more sensitive to sustained pain stimuli from deeper tissue. Older adults demonstrate increased temporal summation. Conditioned pain modulation decreases with age: the pattern of pain perception in older subjects shows enhanced pain facilitation and decreased pain inhibition.

Psychosocial Factors and Pain

The biopsychosocial factors that may contribute to age-related shifts in pain modulation include:

1. An increase in frequency of pain related illnesses
2. Systemic inflammation
3. The effects of oxidative stress
4. Altered autonomic function
5. Changes in neuronal structures and their function

An impact in perceived pain also occurs with impaired cognitive function, decreased sleep quality, and loss of social support, all commonly occurring with age.

There is strong evidence for the association between psychosocial factors and pain. Patients who suffer chronic pain have increased psychological distress, greater life stress, and more somatic symptomatology than individuals without pain. Several studies have demonstrated interactions between genetic and psychological factors in the risk of development of chronic pain.

Reward and Motivation

The multidimensional model of pain as proposed by Melzak and Casey, initiates the concept that there could be a partial separation of affective and motivational components of pain from its sensory discriminative qualities. These specific characteristics are subserved by different anatomical pathways, the medial ascending system for affective motivational features, and a lateral system for sensory discriminative aspects of pain. This model supports:

1. The concept that pain is a perception that involves the synthesis of sensory, affective, and cognitive dimensions
2. There is a distinction between pain and nociception
3. There may be a dissociation between the quality and intensity of pain and tissue damage.

Melzak also noted that nociceptive input is modulated by learning and memory. Later, descending bidirectional pain modulatory circuits, a major component of which is the rostral ventral nuclei of the medulla (RVM), are found to facilitate or inhibit nociceptive signaling depending on context, stress, expectation, motivation and learning. Clinical reports demonstrate specific multiple dimensions of pain by revealing dissociations between its affective, sensory, and cognitive components. The partial dissociation of affect from sensory discriminative features of pain are reaffirmed from cingulatomy surgeries in which pain is received as such but is not associated with suffering. The dissociation between affect and sensory discriminative aspects of pain is demonstrated by functional MRI studies that show pain unpleasantness can be altered independent of its intensity. Opioids are one of the most effective class of drugs used for both acute and chronic pain. They modulate the affective component of pain rather than its sensory-discriminative dimension. Experimental studies show that activation of cortical opioid receptors modulates pain aversiveness without altering evoked pain reflexes, which supports separate central mechanisms that mediate the affective dimension of pain. The aversive qualities of pain are essential for learning and for future decisions to avoid harmful situations.

The neural circuits that underlie aversive learning are thought to use a component of the mesolimbic reward valuation network, a major component of which is the ventral tegmental area and its projections to the nucleus accumbens (NAc). Experiments show that an unexpected reward increases phasic dopamine release in the NAc while the absence of an expected reward decreases it. The difference between an expected and an actual result is a prediction error that is an important component of reinforcement learning. Functional MRI studies demonstrate that pain prediction errors are encoded in the periaqueductal gray (PAG) that is an integrative nucleus for ascending nociceptive input and descending pain modulation. Expected value information is projected to the PAG from the ventromedial prefrontal cortex (PFC). Predictive error signals are relayed to prefrontal cortical regions that initiate behavioral alterations and include the orbitofrontal, anterior midcingulate and dorsomedial prefrontal cortices.

Pain Perception

Pain perception is also modulated by motivational, emotional, cognitive and the expectation of pain. Both the expectation of pain and its relief is shown to modulate the degree and quality of pain as well as the efficacy of opioids. Attention and distraction, as well as the emotional state of the patient, alter the perception of pain that is also reflected in the altered activity of pain related circuits as demonstrated by fMRI studies.

Positron emission tomography imaging studies show that placebo analgesia is concomitant with release of dopamine in brain reward nuclei. Functional MRI imaging demonstrates that cessation of a painful stimulation activates the NAc which is a critical component of reward-aversion pain processing. A series of experimental studies show that activation of dopaminergic neurons in the ventral tegmental area (VTA 10) and concomitant activation of dopaminergic receptors in the NAc may mediate the reinforcing effect of pain relief. Another series of experimental studies supports the concept that the mesolimbic motivational/reward circuitry is involved in both the perception and relief of pain. In an fMRI study of healthy subjects, the onset of a painful thermal stimulus is correlated with decreased activity in the NAc and is increased with its cessation.

As noted earlier, the opioid class of drugs is a principal agent for the relief of moderate to severe pain by suppressing its affective quality. The anterior cingulate cortex (ACC) expresses high levels of opioid receptors in humans that are consistent with its clinical efficacy. In experimentally induced pain, there is endogenous release of opioids in this region during pain and its relief. It is posited that relief of the aversive quality of pain is mediated by opioid signaling in the rostral ACC that induces dopamine release in the NAc. Recent imaging studies show that offset of a noxious stimulus activates the NAc in healthy subjects and increases self-reported pleasantness in concordance with activation of brain reward areas. There is also evidence that both decreased negative affect and increased positive affect to the emotion are associated with pain relief. Release of endogenous opioids in the rACC, concurrently with pain relief, support the concept that both positive and negative reinforcement learning participate in the motivation to seek pain relief.

The modulation of nociceptive input to the pain matrix is based on the interpretation of present experience, past pain history, emotional state and stress levels, as well as cognitive appraisal. The modulation of nociceptive signaling is primarily accomplished by "On" and "Off" cells located in the rostral ventral nucleus of the medulla. "On" cells in the nucleus facilitate pain transmission while "Off" cells mediate descending inhibition. Activation of these neurons is context dependent. Facilitation occurs when attention to a painful stimulus is required for an advantageous behavioral outcome and inhibition is predominant in the other contexts such as chronic neuropathic pain.

Reward Circuits

Reward circuits are shown to be important in the maintenance of chronic neuropathic pain. It is posited that rewards are a complex psychophysical construct that are composed of two major components. The first is hedonic pleasure, the liking of the emotion and the second is the motivation to obtain the reward. Hedonic qualities are posited to be encoded by the release of endogenous opioids in the orbitofrontal cortex, the ACC, the amygdala and the NAc. The motivation to attain rewards is posited to be driven by dopamine signaling in the mesolimbic circuitry. Both of these circuitries overlap with brain networks that are essential for motivational affective qualities of pain and its relief. Chronic pain alters behavioral goals by diverting attention from other motivations to those associated with pain relief. This shift in long lasting motivational drives and concomitant predominance of the affective qualities of pain are associated with pain chronification. Brain neuroimaging studies support this hypothesis by demonstrating anatomical alterations and molecular changes in gray matter density, white matter connectivity, glutamate, opioids and dopamine transmission. Furthermore, studies of signal changes in the NAc in patients with chronic back pain in response to an acute thermal stimulus differ from healthy controls. A positive phasic NAc signal at pain offset is posited to reflect prediction with the reward associated with pain relief. A negative signal is demonstrated in patients at pain offset that is posited to be due to return of attention to their persistent chronic pain after cessation of the acute stimulus. It is postulated that the motivational value of acute pain offset is altered in chronic pain conditions. A longitudinal study with fMRI of back pain patients demonstrates that intensity of functional connectivity between NAc and PFC predicts recovery or transition to chronic pain. This and other studies support the concept that the shift from sensory/discriminative qualities of pain (the lateral system) to emotional circuitry (medial system) may be a fundamental component of the chronification of acute pain.

CHAPTER 2

NEUROPATHIC SOMATIC PAIN

Overview of Neuropathic Somatic Pain Mechanisms

Pain problems are a major component of consultative neurology. The perception of pain is complex and is composed of a discriminative component (location, quality, and intensity), an affective component (unpleasantness), and a motivational and emotional component (anxiety, depression, coping maneuvers). Each component has its unique circuitry.

Pain itself may be characterized as:

1. Nociceptive, the physiologic alerting mechanism that protects the organism from further harm
2. Inflammatory pain that ceases when the inciting injury heals
3. Neuropathic pain, which is caused by injury to the somatosensory system that often continues after the injury has healed and is destructive to the organism.

Specific modalities of pain are expressed in pain states. Hyperalgesia is defined as heightened sensitivity to a painful stimulus. Allodynia is pain that is elicited from a non-painful stimulus. In neuropathic pain conditions mechanical and heat hyperalgesia are cardinal features. Dynamic mechanical allodynia refers to pain elicited by a moving cutaneous stimulus (a wisp of cotton stroked across the skin) whereas static allodynia refers to pain elicited by pressure at ordinarily non-painful thresholds. Mechano allodynia is carried by A-beta fibers (myelinated 8-12 μ fibers). Thermal hyperalgesia is associated with A-delta fibers that convey cold and polymodal C-fibers that respond to heat, tissue destruction, and chemical stimuli. Mechanical and thermal hyperalgesia (particularly cold) are major modalities of peripheral neuropathic pain. Radicular conditions (disc disease, spinal stenosis, trauma to nerve roots) are primary causes of peripheral neuropathic pain. Pain is a very dynamic and plastic process in that chronic pain afferences actually change the response characteristic of pain transmission neurons (PTNs). In general, they become more responsive. Pain is a very sensitive modality in that only one C-fiber when stimulated during microneurography can convey location, quality, and intensity of a stimulus. It is now clear that immune mechanisms are important at many levels of pain production and maintenance (microglia, astrocytes and satellite cells).

As a general chain of events, a tissue-modifying stimulus triggers the firing of transient receptor potential (TRPV1, TRPVIII, and TRPA1) receptors on primary pain afferents. In turn, they initiate action potentials in C-fibers and A-delta fiber nociceptive neurons (cell bodies are in the dorsal root ganglia) that synapse in different lamina of the dorsal horn. These second order neurons give rise to spinothalamic and other afferents that activate the pain matrix. Specific aspects of inputs into PTNs induce both central and peripheral sensitization of the pain matrix, which modifies anatomic, physiologic and gene expression of pain pathways at all levels.

Some Aspects of the Anatomy of Somatic Neuropathic Pain

The skin is a complex sensory organ that also serves homeostatic and immunologic barrier functions. It is a neuroimmune cutaneous system that signals the sensory modalities of touch, pressure, temperature, and pain. As noted earlier, these primary modalities are modified in pain states (hyperalgesia, allodynia, and hyperpathia). All chronic pain conditions induce plasticity in pain transmission neurons. It is poorly recognized that there is a descending facilitating and inhibitory pain control system, the diffuse nociceptive inhibitory control (DNIC) system in experimental animals and in the patients' conditioned pain modulation (CPM) system that modifies the transmission and physiology of pain transmission after a painful stimulus. This is a dynamic system that adjusts its sensitivity (thresholds) by complex mechanisms. Sensory transduction occurs following activation of primary intraepidermal nerve terminal C and A-delta nociceptive afferents. Activation of these primary intraepidermal nerve terminal C and A-delta nociceptive afferents is dependent on ligand activation of neuronal and non-neuronal skin cells of the neuroimmune cutaneous system (NICS). The epidermis is primarily composed of keratinocytes, melanocytes, Langerhans, and Merkel cells. These cells express sensor proteins and neuropeptides (substance P and calcitonin gene-related peptide) that are pivotal in nociception and neurogenic inflammation (vasodilation, plasma extravasation, and hypersensitivity). Keratinocytes comprise approximately 85% of dermal cells and form a tight junction with primary nociceptive nerve fibers. They express transient receptor potential vanilloid 1 (TRPV1) and transient receptor potential ankyrin (TRPA1) receptors. These channels are members of the transient receptor (TRP) superfamily of nonselective cation channels. TRPV1 channels are noxious heat-gated cation channels that are expressed on nociceptive primary afferents and also respond to protons, endogenous lipid ligands that include endocannabinoids, lipoxygenase, lysophosphatidic and linoleic acid metabolites as well as serotonin, bradykinins, prostanoids and reactive oxygen species (ROS) in the microenvironment following injury. These receptors (TRPV1 and TRPA1) are activated following injury or inflammation, depolarize nociceptive primary afferents in the skin whose central terminals project to the dorsal horn (DH) of the spinal cord. The dorsal root ganglia are composed of large diameter neurons that mediate mechanical modalities, small diameter neurons that mediate pain and temperature, as well as satellite cells that are similar to glial cells in the CNS. There are also blood vessels innervated by unmyelinated autonomic fibers in the DRG. Following injury, there is upregulation of various receptors on the neuronal elements of the DRG and under specific conditions cause sprouting of sympathetic fibers from the blood vessels. These fibers may form basket-like terminals around nociceptive and large mechanosensitive neurons. The spinal nerve-blood barrier and that of the DRG is not as tight as the blood-brain barrier. This is important in the pathophysiology of neuropathy caused by chemotherapy (direct toxic injury from cis-platinum and paclitaxel in the DRG) as well as autoimmune attack from activated lymphocytes and other cellular agents. In the skin, keratinocytes, macrophages, TRPV1-expressing nociceptors release nerve growth factor (NGF), prostaglandins (particularly E2), pro-inflammatory cytokines (IL-1, IL-6, and transforming growth factor beta 1 (TGFB1) as well as chemokines which sensitize (lower the threshold to fire) of primary afferent nociceptors. In many instances, after the nociceptors are exposed to the above noted "inflammatory soup," they fire spontaneously which is the origin of spontaneous pain in many chronic neuropathic pain syndromes.

Nociceptive afferents are principally unmyelinated (1μ C-fibers) and thinly myelinated (1-4μ) A-delta fibers. The A-delta fibers signal location, intensity, cold and the lancinating quality of pain (epicritic qualities or fast pain). C-fibers are slowly conducting, transmit a burning quality of pain, and are poorly localizing (second pain).

Peripheral Input and Central Sensitization

The transmission and processing of painful inputs to the pain matrix is critically dependent on the properties of ion channels that are expressed on A-delta and C-fiber afferents. These include voltage-gated ion channels and leak channels that in concert regulate resting membrane potential, set, and maintain the action potentials and firing properties of pain transmission neurons. A major cause of chronic neuropathic and inflammatory peripheral pain is due to dysregulation of ion channel expression caused by tissue and nerve injury that enhances pain transmission and neuronal excitability. Afferent nociceptive signals due to activation of specific receptors and ion channels on peripheral nerve endings of A-delta and C-fibers are propagated and synapse in the extremely complex circuitry of the spinal cord dorsal horn. These afferents release glutamate and substance P that activate second order neurons that ascend to CNS processing ensembles that process pain signals.

Physiological Properties of Pain Transmission Neurons

The physiological properties of pain transmission neurons are critically dependent on the expression density and function of their ion channels that define:

1. The resting membrane potential
2. The initiation of the action potential
3. Depolarization and repolarization kinetics
4. The refractory period
5. Transmitter release from their central terminals on second order neurons in the dorsal horn

Ion Channels

The relevant ion channels that determine these properties are:

1. Voltage-gated sodium, potassium and calcium channels
2. Leak channels
3. Ligand gated channels
4. Transient receptor potential channels

Sodium Channels

Particularly important for stimulus detection, initiation of action potentials in pain afferents and synaptic transmission are:

1. Na_v 1.7 and Na_v 1.8 isoforms of voltage-gated sodium channels
2. N-type calcium channels
3. Transient receptor potential channels

The sodium channel isoforms Na_v1.7, 1.8, and 1.9 that are essential for the physiologic properties of peripheral nerves do not interfere with CNS or cardiac function and have been extensively studied as targets for pain pharmacology. Mutations in the gene that code for the Na_v1.7 channel have demonstrated its role in human pain. It is expressed in peripheral neurons, the dorsal root ganglia (DRG), trigeminal and nodose ganglia as well as sympathetic ganglia neurons. It is activated by slow depolarizations that are close to resting membrane potential and sets the gain of nociceptor afferents. It is upregulated in inflammatory pain states, accumulates in neuromas, and is essential in ectopic impulse generation under these conditions. Genetic studies and functional profiling of mutant channels (from mutations in the SCN9A gene that encode the Na_v 1.7 channel) have demonstrated its function in inherited erythromelalgia. In this condition, patients experience severe pain (burning and aching) from innocuous warm stimuli. The missense mutations were shown to increase the activity of the channels and to increase their response to small depolarizing stimuli. Other gain of function mutations in the Na_v 1.7 channel impair channel inactivation and are associated with paroxysmal extreme pain disorder. These patients suffer rectal pain that in later life may be experienced in periorbital and perimandibular areas after a stimulus to the lower body. Autosomal recessive mutations of the Na_v 1.7 channel may demonstrate insensitivity to pain. In this condition, patients do not produce functional Na_v 1.7 channels. The exact role of the channel and its location in this deficit has not been determined. A polymorphism in the gene has been associated with hyperexcitability of DRG pain transmission neurons.

Gain of function variants of Na_v 1.7 channels enhance activity by: (1) impairing slow inactivation or (2) impairment of both fast and slow inactivation, (3) enhancing activation by producing a persistent (non-activating) current. These physiologic changes lower the action potential threshold of DRG pain transmission neurons, increase their firing frequency, and cause abnormal spontaneous firing that is also thought to be a mechanism for evoked and spontaneous pain in patients with peripheral neuropathies.

The Na_v 1.8 channel has been associated with painful peripheral neuropathies. It is expressed in DRG pain transmission neurons, their axons and in trigeminal and nodose ganglion neurons. It has depolarized voltage dependence, which renders it relatively resistant to inactivation during neuronal depolarization. It is a major component of the action potential upstroke (its inward current) and confers repetitive firing of depolarized neurons. It has a role in both inflammatory and neuropathic pain. Gain of function mutations in Na_v 1.8 channels have been associated with approximately 5% of patients with painful neuropathies by causing hyperexcitability and spontaneous discharge of DRG pain transmitting neurons (PTNs).

The Na_v 1.9 channel is expressed in DRG pain transmission neurons, the trigeminal ganglion neurons, and nociceptors of the myenteric plexus. It produces a non-inactivating current that is activated at hyperpolarized potentials close to the resting membrane potential. It prolongs and increases small depolarizations that increase DRG PTN excitability. It appears to be important in inflammatory pain as inflammatory mediators increase its current.

The Na_v 1.3 channel may be important for neuropathic pain, as it has been shown to:

1. Produce a persistent current that responds to small depolarizations
2. Is active close to the resting membrane potential
3. Is positioned to amplify small nociceptive afferences
4. Is rapidly inactivated which supports repetitive firing

Potassium Channels

Potassium channels regulate resting membrane potential and action potential repolarization in PTNs. They are divided into:

1. Voltage-gated ion-activated (sodium or calcium activated)
2. Two-pore channels
3. Inward rectifying channels
4. All of the above are important in the neuronal excitability of PTNs.

Decreased voltage-gated potassium channel function causes increased PTN firing and spike duration as well as decreased spike threshold. Experimental evidence in neuropathic pain models support a strong contribution of K_v channels as inhibitory to pain signaling in nociceptive afferents.

Two-pore potassium channels (K2P) support a hyperpolarized resting membrane potential through their effects on leak potassium currents. K2P channel subtypes that include TRESK, TRAAK, TASK and THIK channels are expressed in DRG PTNs. They are important regulators of primary nociceptive afferent fiber excitability often to mechanical and heat stimuli (hallmarks of neuropathic pain).

Calcium and sodium-activated potassium channels

Calcium activated potassium channels (Kca) are a determinant of after-hyperpolarization that follows an action potential and thus neuronal firing frequency and pattern. Kca channels include large (BK), intermediate (IK) and small (SK) channels: all of which when activated limit pain transmission neuronal discharge. There is decreased expression of SK and IK channels in human DRG PTNs after nerve injury that would increase their neuronal firing.

Recent experimental studies demonstrate decreased BK channel expression to brain derived neurotrophic factor (BDNF) – mediated down regulation at the transcriptional level. Microglia are activated after peripheral nerve injury and may be the source of the BDNF. Sodium activated potassium (KNa) channels are also involved in after-hyperpolarization and are important in the regulation of firing rate adaptation.

In summary, voltage-gated, ion-activated or leak potassium currents inhibit afferent pain signaling.

Voltage-gated calcium channels

Neurons express multiple types of voltage-gated calcium channels (Ca_v channels) that are the primary source of depolarization-induced calcium increase in PTNs. N-type calcium channels are high voltage-activated channels that trigger neurotransmitter release in the dorsal horn.

T type Ca_v channels regulate afferent pain signaling whose mechanisms include:

1. The support of rebound burst activity induced by increasing the activity of co-localized Na_v channels
2. An upregulation of Ca_v 3.2 channels in Aδ fibers (involved in mechano-transduction)
3. Interaction with the proteins of synaptic release which promote low threshold neurotransmitter release at specific dorsal horn synapses

Several gene families encode calcium-activated chloride currents that regulate neuronal excitability. Experimental studies of DRG neurons demonstrate that these chloride currents may be involved in after-depolarizations following neuronal discharge.

HCN channels

Hyperpolarization activated cyclic nucleotide-gated (HCN) channels are activated and open at negative membrane potentials and are a component of neuronal excitability and rhythm generation. Their four subtypes are expressed in DRG PTNs. Blockade of the channel decreases mechanical allodynia in both inflammatory and neuropathic pain models.

The Role of Endogenous Lipid Mediators in Peripheral Gating of Pain Signals

Nociceptive signals are modified prior to their arrival at the spinal cord dorsal horn. Primary sensory neurons (in the DRG), their terminals in the skin and peripheral tissues as well as adjacent host-defense cells (satellite cells) release a variety of proteins and peptides that effect nociceptive afference to the dorsal horn. Lipid-derived mediators are a major component of this peripheral gating mechanism by their interaction with nociceptor afferents, macrophages, mast cells, and keratinocytes. In general, most nociceptors are polymodal as they can signal different modalities of harmful stimuli. Nociceptor subclasses express distinctive membrane ion channels, receptors, and intracellular signaling proteins. After tissue and nerve terminal damage, these transduction molecules induce hyper-excitability in nociceptive afferents, which is called peripheral sensitization. As noted earlier, the clinical manifestations of this sensitization is mechanical and thermal allodynia in which innocuous mechanical and thermal stimuli are perceived as painful and hyperalgesia in which a mildly noxious stimulus is perceived as very painful. Peripheral sensitization is often accompanied by neurogenic inflammation. This vasodilatory response is caused by the release of substance P and calcitonin gene-related peptide (CGRP) from the activated C-fiber nociceptor primary terminals.

Nociceptors respond to endogenous proalgesic factors that are rapidly released following injury or are produced slowly during inflammatory states, tumor growth, or peripheral neuropathy. The first wave of proalgesic substances that may affect nociceptor terminals after injury are ATP and ADP leaked from damaged cells and bradykinin released from plasma globulin during blood clotting. Both activate excitatory receptors on primary nociceptive afferents. A later group of sensitizing and proinflammatory molecules includes substance P, CGRP, and lipid-derived mediators released by primary afferent nociceptor fibers and host-defense cells. Other proinflammatory mediators are prostaglandin E_2 (PGE_2) and prostacyclin (PGI_2). They activate specific G protein-coupled receptors on nociceptive afferents that increase membrane excitability and amplify the release of SP and CGRP. Essential components of this signaling cascade are the enzymes cyclooxygenase 1 (Cox)-1 and Cox-2 which convert arachidonic acid into PGH_2 the common precursor of all prostanoids.

Enzymatic and non-enzymatic conversions of membrane-derived polyunsaturated fatty acid (PUFA) oxidation form other lipid molecules that excite nociceptors and include:

1. Hydroxylated derivatives of linoleic acid
2. Hepoxilin A3
3. PGE2-glycerol ester
4. Prostamide F2α
5. Lysophosphatidic acid
6. Lysophosphatidyl inositol

A clear role of lipid-mediated signaling in the induction and maintenance of neuropathic pain is well established.

Recent experimental evidence demonstrates that bioactive lipids may also decrease and modulate pain initiation. These analgesic lipid mediators include:

1. Endogenous cannabinoids
2. Lipid-amide agonists of peroxisome proliferator-activated receptor–α (PPAR-α)
3. Products of oxidative PUFA metabolism.

Reactive Oxygen Species

Reactive oxygen species (ROS) are chemical species that contain oxygen and include peroxides, superoxides, hydroxyl radicals, and singlet oxygen. They are formed as a natural by-product of the normal metabolism of oxygen. They have major roles in cell signaling and homeostasis. If ROS increase dramatically they may damage cell structures and this process is known as oxidative stress.

Formation and Degradation

The reduction of molecular oxygen (O2) produces superoxide (.O2) which is the precursor of most other reactive oxygen species.

The hydroxyl radical is extremely reactive and removes electrons from molecules in its vicinity that produces a free radical from the affected molecule. This creates a propagating chain reaction. H2O2 is more damaging than the hydroxyl radical due to its lower reactivity which gives it more time to enter the nucleus of the cell and react with its DNA.

Production of Endogenous ROS

ROS are produced intracellularly primarily by:

1. NADPH oxidase (NOX) complexes that have 7 isoforms that are located in cell membranes
2. Mitochondria
3. Peroxisomes
4. Endoplasmic reticulum
5. Production of nitric oxide synthetase (NOS)

As noted, ROS are produced by multiple mechanisms that depend on the cell and tissue type.

The process of oxidative phosphorylation that creates ATP involves the transport of protons (hydrogen ions) across the inner mitochondrial membrane along the electron transport chain (ETC). Electrons undergo a series of oxidation-reduction reactions that occur in the proteins of the chain such that each acceptor protein along the chain has a greater reduction potential than the previous protein complex. The oxygen molecule is the final destination of electrons passing along the chain. Under normal conditions, oxygen is reduced to water. In approximately 0.1-2% of electrons that pass through the chain, oxygen is prematurely and incompletely reduced to make the superoxide radical. Electron leakage occurs primarily in complexes I and III. The superoxide molecule may inactivate enzymes or cause lipid peroxidation in its hydroperoxyl HO_2 form.

If mitochondria are severely damaged from environmental conditions (toxins, chemotherapeutic agents, anoxia) the cell undergoes apoptosis or programmed cell death. The surface of mitochondria contains layered Bcl-2 proteins that detect mitochondrial damage and activate BAX proteins that produce holes in the mitochondrial membrane. Cytochrome C leaks from the ruptured membranes and binds to APAF-1 (apoptotic protease activating factor 1) that is free in the cytoplasm. ATP in the mitochondrion provides the energy for the binding of APAF-1 and cytochrome C to form apoptosomes. Apoptosomes bind and activate caspase-9, also in the cytoplasm, which then cleaves the proteins of the mitochondrial membrane. The resulting protein denaturation ends in phagocytosis of the cell.

The interaction of $\cdot O_2$ with nitric oxide produces NO-peroxynitrate. Under physiologic conditions the antioxidant defense system primarily composed of manganese superoxide dismutase MnSOD, catalase, glutathione thioredoxin and glutathione peroxidase reduce superoxide to water and molecular oxygen. If the antioxidant defense system is over-whelmed by a large increase of ROS, formation of peroxynitrate and other ROS increases and causes oxidative stress. Peroxynitrate causes a bioenergetics failure of mitochondria by altering and disrupting metabolic enzymes, mitochondrial electron transport proteins (thus reducing the production of ATP), ATP synthase and membrane transport proteins. Its damage of MnSOD causes a feed-forward reaction that increases its own production, which further increases superoxide.

ROS and Cellular Respiration

1. There is leakage and loss of electrons (ē) primarily from mitochondrial complexes I and III
2. In neuropathic pain models:
    a. mtROS are elevated in spinal neurons, microglia and astrocytes.
    b. NOX-1, 2 (derived from NADPH oxidase) are expressed at the cellular membrane level and produce $\cdot O_2$ after phosphorylation of a cytosolic subunit
    c. NOX-1 derived from NADPH oxidase:
        i Translocates PKC_E to the membrane which enhances transient receptor potential vanilloid (TRPV1) activity in the DRG
    d. NOX-2 derived from NADPH oxidase:
        i Primarily expressed in phagocytic cells (macrophages and microglia) is upregulated after peripheral nerve injury (PNI) and induces $\cdot O_2$. Its expression may be initiated by Toll-like receptors (TLRs)
        ii Decreases TNF but induces IL-1β and demonstrates the expression of

the neuronal injury marker ATF3

iii In NOX-2 deficient mice there is decreased expression of Iba on peptidergic axons and a decrease of proinflammatory cytokines

iv Increases gene expression of proinflammatory cytokines in the DRG

e. NOX-4 (derived from nicotinamide dinucleotide phosphate, NADPH):

i Is expressed by DRG neurons on both myelinated (A-fibers) and C-fibers

ii It is also expressed by microglia, astrocytes and macrophages

iii Its expression in cellular organelles (endoplasmic reticulum, ER) produces the ROS H_2O_2

iv NOX-4 may decrease the neuronal proteins MPZ and PMP22 after nerve injury (shown in experimental sciatic nerve injury)

Effects of ROS

1. Positive effects:
   a. Induction of host defense genes
   b. Mobilization of ion transport systems
   c. Platelets that are involved in wound repair and blood homeostasis release ROS that recruit platelets to the site of injury. A link is established to the adaptive immune system by ROS recruitment of leukocytes
2. Damaging Effects of ROS:
   a. Damage of DNA and/or RNA
   b. Oxidation of polyunsaturated fatty acids in lipids (lipid peroxidation)
   c. Oxidation of amino acids in proteins
   d. Mediation of apoptosis
   e. Oxidative deactivation of specific enzymes via oxidation of cofactors
   f. Mitochondrial damage
3. In the pain state – ROS:
   a. Activate Ca/CaMKII in glutamatergic neurons
   b. Induce presynaptic inhibition of GABAergic neurons
   c. H_2O_2 increases action potentials of DRG neurons by activating cGK1α that increases neurotransmitter release from A-delta and C-fiber terminals of primary afferent neurons in the DH

Nitro-oxidative Species and Neuropathic Pain

Nitrosylation is the covalent incorporation of a nitric oxide moiety into another molecule. S-nitrosylation is the covalent attachment of NO to a cysteine residue that forms an S-nitrosothiol (SNO). S-nitrosylation is a post-translational protein modification that is a widespread signaling mechanism and is the primary driver of NO bioactivity. S-nitrosylation is targeted, reversible, spatio-temporally restricted and is important for a host of cellular functions. An important function is the allosteric regulation of proteins by both endogenous and exogenous sources of NO. It is the prototype redox-based signaling mechanism.

NO and Nociceptive transmission

NO action in regard to nociceptive transmission is complex and often opposing. In several pain models neuronal NO (neuronal) at high concentrations in the spinal cord increases pain sensitivity while pharmacologic inhibition and genetic deletion decrease it. Expression of neuronal nitric oxide synthase (nNOS) in sensory neurons is upregulated following peripheral nerve injury. Low concentrations of NO in the spinal cord have been shown to attenuate allodynia after nerve injury. NO may increase the anti-nociceptive effects of opioids, NSAIDs and the NO-releasing derivative of gabapentin (NCX8001) at peripheral transduction sites. NO-dependent activation of ATP-sensitive potassium channels may be a component of peripheral analgesia. These K_{ATP} channels are expressed in metabolically active tissues and are complex. They are hetero-octamers and have four regulatory SUR subunits (SUR1, SUR2A, or SUR2B) as well as four ATP-sensitive pore forming inwardly rectifying potassium channels (Kir6.x) with subunits (Kir6.1 or Kir6.2). The ratio of cellular ADP/ATP determines their opening that allows them to function as metabolic sensors thus linking cytosolic energetics with cellular functions. In both the central and peripheral nervous system K_{ATP} channels are a component of the regulation of neuronal excitability, neurotransmitter release and ligand effects. S-nitrosylation regulates Na^+ channels and acid-sensing channels in DRG neurons, the NMDA receptor channel complex. Ca^{2+} activated K^+ channels that are all-important in pathologic pain states. It has been demonstrated that nitric oxide activates ATP-sensitive potassium channels in sensory neurons by direct, S-nitrosylation.

Nitric oxide is a diffusible gas that is synthesized from L-arginine by NOS-1 (neuronal), NOS-2 (inducible), and NOS-3 (endothelial).

NOS-1

1. Constitutively expressed in the cytosolic compartment of post-synaptic terminals of neurons and stressed Schwann cells
2. Requires Ca2+ for activation (NMDA activation)
3. Decreased NOS-1 decreases chemotherapy and peripheral nerve injury pain

NOS-2 (Cytosolic Form)

1. Expressed in immune cells and glia
2. Toll-like receptor 2 activation initiates the transcription of NOS-2
3. Once translocated, NOS-2 is constitutively active; the process does not require Ca^{2+}

NOS-3

1. Increases in the DRG after administration of Freund's adjuvant
2. Requires Ca^{2+}/calmodulin activation

The activation of the NMDA receptor with its associated increased intracellular calcium induces the transcription of nitric oxide synthase.

Peroxynitrate Mechanisms of Disrupting Glutamate Homeostasis

1. Nitration and phosphorylation of NMDA subunits that increase intracellular calcium concentration
2. Decrease glutamate transporter (GLT-1) that increases its concentration at the synapse
3. Nitro-oxidative products decrease GAD-67 GABAergic DH neurons and decrease GABA release
4. Increase calcium influx and increase synaptic currents
5. Decreases glutamine synthesis

Mechanisms of Nitro-oxidative Species that Directly Modulate Neuroexcitability

1. TRP channel activation initiates the pain signal and concomitantly releases co-localized vasoactive neuropeptides (substance P (SP) and calcitonin gene related peptide (CGRP) to cause neurogenic inflammation
2. Induce post-translation modifications of proteins and lipids that drive pain
3. Mitochondrial DNA is a target for oxidation and nitration
4. Nitro-oxidative species trigger release of proapoptotic factors disrupting organelle dynamics in mitochondria
5. Toll-like receptors bind to a variety of endogenous danger signals that include those released from nitro-oxidative damaged mitrochondria. They also activate NF-kB and MAPKs pathways
6. NOX derived ROS (from NADPH-oxidase) are second messengers for NF-kB and p38MAPK
7. The Toll-like receptor 2-NOX-1 interaction:
    a. Upregulates adhesion molecules via the chemokine CCL3 which induces transendothelial cell migration
8. Mitochondrial derived ROS:
    a. Activate the NLRP3 inflammasome that proteolytically activates the inflammatory cytokine IL-1B

Nitro-oxidative Species Induce Mitochondrial Dysfunction – Mechanisms

1. Mitochondria are critically involved in energy production (ATP), lipid synthesis, apoptosis and cellular calcium homeostasis
2. NOX and NOS derived ROS disrupt mitochondrial homeostasis. There is increased metabolism during pain states that has been demonstrated to induce

a bioenergetics crisis with consequent degeneration of nociceptive primary afferent fibers

3. Mitochondria are a target of oxidation and nitration
4. Peroxidated lipid end-products:
    a. Form reactive aldehydes that induce covalent modifications (adducts) with an array of mitochondrial proteins that include mitochondrial antioxidants
5. Nitro-oxidant species:
    a. Release pro-apoptotic factors
    b. Nitric oxide decreases fusion and fission of mitochondria
    c. Decreased mitochondrial homeostasis is affected by:
        i Translocation of Bcl-2 associated x protein from the cytosol to the mitochondrial membrane that activates apoptotic pathways

Nitro-oxidative Species Induce Neuroinflammatory Signaling

1. In the course of tissue and/or nerve injury all forms of pain are induced that include:
    a. Nociceptive
    b. Inflammatory
    c. Neuropathic
        i Neuropathic pain states have a component of inflammatory pain that fades as the neuropathic pain states become predominant
2. At the site of tissue injury in addition to the release of hydrogen ion, serotonin, bradykinin, prostanoids – glia and immune cells release TNF alpha, IL-1B and BDNF (brain-derived neurotrophic factor)
3. Mechanisms for increased inflammation-induced neuronal hyperexcitability:
    a. Increased glutamate release from the terminals of nociceptive primary afferent fibers (A-delta and C-fibers)
    b. Increased AMPA post synaptic primary nociceptive fiber expression
    c. Phosphorylation of NMDA subunits that increase the receptor permeability to Ca^{2+} ions
    d. Down-regulation of astrocyte glutamate transporters
    e. Decreased GABA and glycine release from inhibitory interneurons
    f. Decreased K-Cl co-transporter KCC2 on postsynaptic terminals
    g. Nitro-oxidative species:
        i Regulate the production of proinflammatory mediators:
4. NF-kB and p38MAPK are induced and increase the transcription of proinflammatory cytokines
    a. Degrade NF-kB and p38MAPK phosphatases and thus maintain their concentration

b. Increase neuron to glia signals from released metalloproteinases
c. Increased TLR signaling:
   i Bind DAMP (damage-associated molecular pattern) that includes DNA and N-formyl peptides from damaged mitochondria
   ii ROS are second messengers for TLR signaling
   iii There is a rapid respiratory burst after activation of TLR2 and 4 from direct interaction of intracellular domain of NOX1,2 and 4 enzymes that is essential for NF-kB and p38MAPK dependent cytokine production
   iv Disruption of blood-brain barrier (BBB) tight junctions
   v TLR-NOX1 interaction via the chemokine CCL3 upregulates adhesion molecules
   vi Increase of lipid rafts by activation of NOX enzymes
   vii Increased transcription of TLRs
   viii ROS activate the inflammasome (protein complexes that cause proteolytic activation of the inflammatory cytokine IL-1B)
   ix Mitochondria are a source of ROS that activate inflammasomes (NLRP3). Nitro-oxidative species induce calcium influx that activates NLRP3 inflammasomes through the receptor TRMPM2
   x Transcription of NOX/NOS enzymes is upregulated by TLR4 and 9 as well as by NF-kB and p38MAPK
   xi ATP signaling via P2X7R (released from neurons) activate NOX2 in a calcium-p38 dependent manner

Type-specific Synaptic Plasticity Induced by ROS

A major component of central sensitization occurs in the spinal cord dorsal horn. Persistent and intense nociceptive afferent input from nociceptive afferents induces maladaptive neuroplasticity in the synapses of pain projecting neurons primarily of the spinothalamic tract. During the course of this maladaptive neuroplasticity, long-term potentiation (LTP) of excitatory postsynaptic currents is seen in spinothalamic pain projecting neurons while long-term depression (LTD) develops in GABAergic interneurons to the same nociceptive input.

Increasing experimental evidence supports a major role of reactive oxygen species in increasing pain transmission following peripheral nerve injury. A major effect of increased levels of reactive oxygen species (ROS) is the down regulation of GABA transmission in the dorsal horn following nerve and spinal cord injury. Lack of GABAergic inhibition of pain projecting neurons is a major factor in enhanced pain transmission in neuropathic pain states.

In the brain the development of LTP or LTD is posited to be caused by the frequency of stimulation. In the spinal cord cell type specific LTP develops in spinothalamic tract pain projecting neurons while LTD occurs in GABAergic dorsal horn neurons from the same nociceptive stimulus. Recent studies support the hypothesis that specific ROS subtypes are instrumental in cell type-specific synaptic plasticity. Superoxide radicals are posited to cause the induction and maintenance of spinothalamic pain projecting neuron LTP and DH GABAergic LTD, while hydroxyl radicals are essential for GABAergic DH LTD induction and maintenance.

ROS 'Activated' Receptors

1. TRPV1 (transient receptor potential family vanilloid 1:
   a. Expressed as C-fiber primary nociceptive afferents
   b. Linoleic acid metabolites that are created during production of eicosanoids are endogenous TRPV1 agonists when oxidized
   c. TRPV1 receptors are:
      i Are activated directly by modified proteins and lipids
      ii Are activated during thermal and mechanical hyperalgesia which are major components of neuropathic pain
2. TRPV2:
   a. Is a non-selective calcium permeable cation channel that is part of the Transient Receptor Potential ion channel superfamily of receptors
   b. It is physiologically activated by heat via free intracellular ADP-ribose acting in concert with free intracellular calcium. Oxidative stress (an accumulation of ROS that overwhelms anti-oxidant mechanisms) induces the enzyme PARP (Poly ADP-ribose polymerase) that activates the channel
3. TRPM2 is expressed by neurons, monocytes, macrophages, microglia and T cells. It is directly activated by nitro-oxidative species
   a. In turn, it activates MAPK and nuclear factor K light chain enhancer of activated B cell, (NF-kB) important for the production of proinflammatory cytokines
   b. The channel is directly activated by H_2O_2 and cytosolic ADP-ribose generated from damaged mitochondria
   c. The channel is vital for activation of spinal microglia and for macrophage infiltration into the spinal cord after peripheral nerve injury
   d. It activates ERK/MAPKs and induces nuclear translocation of NF-kB that is critical for the production of proinflammatory cytokines and chemokines
4. TRPA1:
   a. Is a member of the transient receptor potential channel family and contains 14N-terminal ankyrin repeats
   b. It is activated by both reactive and non-reactive compounds
   c. It is expressed by pepetidergic C-fibers and is activated by modified

proteins and lipids

d. A missense mutation of TRPA1 causes hereditary episodic pain syndrome

Carbonylation

1. Carbonylation are reactions that induce carbon monoxide into organic and inorganic substrates
2. Modifications of the side chains of histidine, cysteine and lysine in proteins to carbonyl derivatives (aldehydes and ketones) are caused by oxidative stress
3. Nitro-oxidative species induce protein carbonylation and membrane phospholipid peroxidation and nitration. These reactions produce reactive aldehydes exemplified by acrolein that directly activate TRPA1 receptors. After spinal cord injury, acrolein is elevated in both the dorsal root ganglia and the dorsal horn that may contribute to spinal cord injury pain.
4. At the site of injury the following compounds contribute to neuroexcitability:
   a. H_2O_2
   b. Peroxynitrate
   c. Carbonylated proteins
   d. Peroxidated and nitrated lipids
   e. Reactive aldehydes

Antioxidant Defense

An antioxidant is a molecule that inhibits the oxidation of other molecules. As noted earlier, oxidation is the loss of electrons during a reaction by a molecule, atom or ion. Oxidation occurs when the state of a molecule, atom, or ion is increased (loss of electrons).

Reduction is its opposite (gain of electrons) by a molecule, atom or ion. As noted above, the major producers of ROS during metabolism that occur in components of the pain matrix are:

1. NADPH oxidase (NOX)
2. Nitric oxide synthase (NOS)
3. Mitochondrial metabolism with loss of electrons from complex I and III

The ROS generated by these reactions in the course of energy production are damaging to multiple cellular functions and if not controlled may destroy the cell. The cell has evolved a complex network of antioxidant metabolites and enzymes that prevent oxidative damage to DNA, protein and lipids. In general, these systems prevent the ROS from being formed or assist in their removal prior to their causing cell damage. The major ROS generated that must be controlled are hydrogen peroxide (H_2O_2), the superoxide anion ($\cdot O_2$), nitrosative species and the hydroxyl radical.

The hydroxyl radical is very unstable and reacts rapidly and non-specifically with most biological molecules. The hydroxyl radical is derived from hydrogen peroxide by metal-catalyzed redox reactions such as the Fenton reaction. As noted above, ROS induce chemical chain reactions exemplified by lipid peroxidation, the oxidation of DNA, and proteins. Damage to proteins results in enzyme inhibition, denaturation and protein degradation.

The superoxide anion is a by-product of several steps in the mitochondrial electron transport chain. In particular, the reduction of coenzyme Q in complex III forms a highly reactive free radical as an intermediate $Q^{\cdot}$. This intermediate is unstable and leads to electron transfer directly to oxygen that forms the superoxide anion. Peroxide is produced from the oxidation of reduced flavoproteins in complex I.

Antioxidants are classified as hydrophilic (soluble in water) or lipophlic (soluble in lipids). Water-soluble antioxidants interact with oxidants in the cytosol and the blood plasma. Lipid-soluble antioxidants protect cell membranes from lipid peroxidation. Both species have a spectrum of concentrations in body fluids and tissues. Glutathione and ubiquinone are primarily confined within cells while uric acid is more evenly distributed. Interactions between antioxidants and their metabolites and enzyme systems may be both synergistic or independent. The effect of the antioxidant depends on its concentration, the reactivity of the specific reactive oxygen species and the state of other antioxidants with which it interacts.

1. Activation of Antioxidant Genes:
    a. Nuclear factor Nrf2 (erythroid-derived 2) –like 2 is a transcription factor that is encoded by the NFE2L2 gene. It is a basic leucine zipper (bzip) protein that regulates the expression of antioxidant proteins
    b. It is expressed in neurons, macrophages, astrocytes, Schwann cells and microglia
    c. Under homeostatic conditions Nrf2:
        i Nrf2 is anchored to the cytoplasm by binding to Kelch-like ECH-associated protein I (Keap1):
2. Keap1 sequesters cystosolic Nrf2 and ubiquinates it for degradation
    a. Under conditions of oxidative stress, Nrf2 is released and translocates to the nucleus where it binds to antioxidant response element (ARE) to elicit expression of more than 200 antioxidant genes
    b. The major antioxidants in pain states include:
        i Superoxide dismutase (SOD)
        ii Cytosolic SOD2 in mitochondria
        iii Catalase
        iv Glutathione
        v Heme oxygenase
    c. Another mechanism that contributes to antioxidant defense is the chelation of transition metals. This process prevents them from catalyzing the production of free radicals. The ability to sequester iron is particularly important and is effected by transferrin and ferritin

Glutathione

1. Glutathione is a cysteine-containing peptide synthesized in cells from its constituent amino acids. Its antioxidant properties derive from the thiol group in its cysteine moiety that is a reducing agent and is reversibly oxidized and reduced. It is maintained in its reduced form intracellularly by glutathione reductase. It has a central role in maintaining intracellular redox potential.

Antioxidant Enzyme Systems

1. A major defense against oxidative stress is an interacting network of antioxidant enzymes systems:
   a. Superoxide released from oxidative phosphorylation is converted to hydrogen peroxide and then water by further reduction. This pathway is first catalyzed by superoxide dismutase and then requires catalases and peroxidases

Superoxide dismutase, Catalase and Peroxiredoxins

1. Superoxide dismutases (SODs):
   a. Are a family of enzymes that catalyze the degradation of the superoxide anion into O_2 and H_2O_2
   b. In humans, the copper/zinc SOD is present in the cytosol. Manganese SOD is located in mitochondria
2. Catalase:
   a. Catalyzes the conversion of H_2O_2 to water and O_2 in concert with a manganese or iron cofactor
3. Peroxiredoxins:
   a. These are peroxidases that catalyze the reduction of peroxynitrate, organic hydroperoxides and hydrogen peroxide

Thioredoxin Systems

1. The thioredoxin system is composed of thioredoxin and thioredoxin reductase
2. Its active site has two closely located cysteines in its CXXC motif that cycle between an active dithiol form (its reduced state) and an oxidized disulfide form
3. It is an effective reducing agent and scavenges ROS and maintains other proteins in a reduced state
4. Active thioredoxin (after being oxidized) is regenerated by thioredoxin reductase utilizing NADPH as an electron donor

Glutathione System

1. This system includes glutathione, glutathione reductase, glutathione peroxidases and glutathione S-transferases:

   a. Glutathione peroxidase contains four selenium cofactors that catalyze the degradation of H_2O_2 and organic hydroperoxides
   b. There are four different glutathione peroxidase isoenzymes in animals with glutathione 1 peroxidase being the most abundant. It scavenges H_2O_2. Glutathione peroxidase 4 primarily acts upon lipid hydroperoxides. Glutathione S-transferase primarily affects lipid peroxides.

In cardiovascular disease, the oxidation of low-density lipoprotein (LDL) is particularly important in initiating atherogenesis. In both chronic and acute pain states, ROS are a major component of pain projection neuron hyperexcitability.

Anti-inflammatory Cytokines and Adenosine Signaling

1. IL-10 and TGF-B counter-regulate proinflammatory signaling in neuropathic pain states:
   a. IL-10 and TGF-B decrease NOX-2 activity and increase antioxidant production
   b. A2A/A3 (adenosine) decreases NOX activity and drives the production of anti-inflammatory cytokines and antioxidants

Opposition of Opioid Analgesia by Nitro-oxidative Species

1. NOX activity is increased by morphine:
   a. The downstream mediators are posited to be superoxide and peroxynitrate
   b. There is a possible interaction between mu-opioid receptors and TLRs which would increase the production of ROS
   c. Nitro-oxidative signaling disrupts endogenous opioid analgesia in supraspinal sites that are important for descending nociceptive inhibitory control (DNIC) and conditioned pain modulation (CPM)
   d. Nitration of metenkephalin in the RVM has been posited

As noted in this short overview of some aspects of somatic neuropathic pain, a great deal of information is known. Molecular mechanisms that control these basic cascades are rapidly being demonstrated and will undoubtedly lead to insights that will lead to better somatic neuropathic pain management.

Clinical diagnosis, experience, and judgment will be buttressed but will remain the cornerstone of treatment.

Antinociceptive Response to Injury

Endogenous Cannabinoids

Neuronal and non-neural cells in injured areas produce endocannabinoids (arachidonic acid derivatives) that suppress nociceptor sensitization and neurogenic inflammation. They activate CB_1 and CB_2 cannabinoid receptors that are Gi/o protein-coupled receptors.

CB1 expression is seen in nociceptive and non-nociceptive neurons in the DRG, trigeminal ganglion as well as macrophages, mast cells and epidermal keratinocytes.

Both CB_1 and CB_2 receptor activation have pleiotrophic effects that include:

1. Inhibition of voltage gated calcium and acid-sensing (ASIC) channels
2. Decrease of the calcium current evoked by capsaicin activation of TRPV1 channels
3. Block nerve growth factor induced TRPV1 sensitization

Peripheral CB_1 mediated mechanisms suppress nociceptive behavior in pain models and decrease CGRP release. The second cannabinoid receptor CB_2 has 40% homology with CB_1 and has receptors on cells of hematopoietic origin, which include those that interact with nociceptive afferents (macrophages and mast cells). In experimental pain models, CB_2 expression is upregulated in the DRG after nerve injury. CB_2 agonists attenuate calcium transients induced by capsaicin in human DRG neurons. Endocannabinoid lipids also interact with TRPV1 channels and G protein-coupled GPR55 receptors.

Anandamide and 2-arachidonyl-n-glycerol (2-AG) are well-characterized lipid mediators that are produced by enzyme-mediated hydrolysis of phospholipid precursors in cell membranes. Anandamide is active near its site of production and is inactivated by carrier-mediated endocytosis followed by the serine hydrolase fatty acid amide hydrolase cleavage to arachidonic acid and ethanolamine. Anandamide may also be transformed by Cox-2 to proalgesic prostamides. Increased anandamide is produced by calcium influx into nociceptors or to activation of Toll-like receptor-4 (TLR-4) in macrophages. Anandamide at the site of injury activates CB_1 receptors that modulate nociceptive input to the spinal dorsal horn (DH). In contradistinction to anandamide, 2AG is formed from the hydrolysis of phosphatidylinositol-4,5 biphosphate (PIP2). The B-isoform of Phospholipase C (PLC-B), activated by Gq-coupled receptors, hydrolyses PIP2 into 1,2-diacyglycerol (DAG) which in turn is converted by diacyl-glycerol lipase-α (DGL-α) to 2-AG.

2-AG mobilization in the brain and spinal cord is regulated by transducing Gq proteins and is essential in the descending modulation of pain that is associated with acute stress.

In summary, endocannabinoid lipids are rapidly recruited to areas of peripheral injury to dampen nociceptive afferent signaling.

Peroxisome Proliferator-Activated Receptor-α

PPAR-α is activated by ligand binding that produces the formation of a multi-protein complex comprised of the retinoid X receptor (RXR) and variable sets of protein activators. When activated it binds to responsive elements on DNA that enhance the transcription of anti-inflammatory proteins while concomitantly decreasing the activity of proinflammatory transcription factors by transrepression.

The transcriptional regulators that are modified by PPAR-α activation include:

1. Nuclear factor κB (NF-κB)

2. Signal transducers and activators of transcription (STATs)
3. Activator protein 1 (AP1)
4. Nuclear factor of activated T cells (NFAT).

These changes in gene expression occur over a matter of hours to days. PPAR-α is expressed in DRG PTNs, macrophages and other host defense cells which when activated suppress pain behaviors in neuropathic pain models. It appears to have a role in the tonic control of inflammatory and nociceptive pain. The rapid analgesic action of PPAR-α ligands (within minutes) and experimental studies suggest that it is involved in the regulation of calcium-activated potassium channels primarily BK_{Ca} ($K_{Ca}^{1.1}$) and intermediate-conduction IK_{Ca} ($K_{Ca}^{3.1}$) channels. Both channels modulate the excitability of primary sensory neurons.

Endogenous Agonists of PPAR-α

Oleoylethanolamide (OEA) and palmitoylethanolamides are produced by cleavage of distinct membrane phospholipids, N-oleoyl-PE and N-palmitoyl-phosphatidyl ethanolamine. The reaction is catalyzed by N-acyl PE-specific phospholipase D (NAPE-PLD) which is the same enzyme that induces anandamide release in neurons. Macrophages produce OEA, PEA and mono and polyunsaturated fatty acid amides (FAE) that inhibit inflammatory responses by activating PPAR-α. It has been posited that both in macrophages and pain transmission neurons, the cysteine hydrolase N-acylethanolamine acid amidase (NAAA) are converted into fatty acid and ethanolamine to limit their activity. OEA and PEA are tonically produced by DRG neurons and skin cells. Tissue damage has been shown to suppress FAE mobilization. It is possible that endogenouse FAE signaling at PPAR-α receptors is a tonic inhibitor of nociceptive and inflammatory responses to injury.

Nociceptive Homeostasis

An exudate at a site of injury evolves during the course of an inflammatory reaction. Initially there is a high concentration of proinflammatory lipid mediators that include: (1) prostanoids (PGE_2 and PGI_2) and (2) leukotrienes (LTB_4).

Over time, these mediators are supplanted by lipid molecules that:

1. Inhibit neutrophil infiltration
2. Clear cellular debris
3. Enhance antimicrobial activity of epithelial cells
4. Stimulate wound healing.

These bioactive lipids also are a component of the normalization of nociceptive signaling by binding to selective surface receptors on DRG PTNs and immune cells.

Epoxygenated Fatty Acids

Epoxygenated fatty acids derived from the enzymatic activity of the cytochrome P_{450} system catalyze the oxygenation of long-chain PUFAs that include arachidonic, eicosapentaenoic (EPA) and docosahexaenoic acids (DHA). Their oxygenation produces bioactive epoxide-containing fatty acids (EpFAs). They are active near their sites of synthesis and regulate vascular tone and inflammation. They are metabolized by enzyme-soluble epoxide hydrolase (sEH) into 1,2 hydroxy fatty acids, which have properties different from their substrate. Experimentally, they have been shown to modulate nociceptive signaling.

Lipoxins and Resolvins

Lipoxins are derived by enzyme-mediated oxygenation of arachidonic acid. They manifest transcellular biosynthesis that involves interaction among different cell types that make contact during an inflammatory response. A well-studied member of this class of mediators, LX4A4 may dampen nociceptive signaling by activating the ALX/FPR2 or CB_1 receptors on PTNs.

Resolvins and protectins are generated by complex multistep oxygenation of membrane PUFAs (EPA and DHA) rather than arachidonic acid. They demonstrate pro-resolving, immune-modulating and anti-nociceptive effects.

The Effects of Bioactive Lipid Mediators

Bioactive lipid mediators may modulate nociceptive input to the pain matrix in three stages:

1. Endogenous PPAR-α agonists (primarily OEA and PEA) may be involved in setting the threshold for nociceptive afferent activation by:
    a. Regulating transcriptional activity of the NF-κB complex
    b. Opening membrane ion channels of primary nociceptive afferents
2. During injury endocannabinoids are formed that suppress the effects of proalgesic molecules and attenuate nociceptor excitability
3. During healing, products of oxidized PUFA substrates that include lipoxins and resolvins help to return nociceptive thresholds to baseline.

Dorsal Horn Circuitry in Neuropathic Pain

As noted earlier, the transmission of pain involves subsets of thinly myelinated Aδ and unmyelinated C fiber afferent discharge from DRG pain transmission neurons (PTNs) that activate second-order DH spinothalamic and spinobulbar projection neurons.

The DH is a gating center that utilizes interacting excitatory and inhibitory ensembles of interneurons in its complex circuitry to process nociceptive inputs. Excitatory interneurons are essential for the physiologic and pathologic transmission of sensory input to projection neurons. Inhibitory neurons gate these afferents.

Anatomy of Dorsal Horn Circuitry

Lamina I and II comprise the superficial dorsal horn (DH). Lamina I is composed of heterogeneous types of spinothalamic and spinobulbar projection neurons. Lamina II, the substantia gelatinosa, has an outer and inner region that contains specific local excitatory or inhibitory interneurons. The deep dorsal horn, lamina III to V contains both interneurons and projection neurons (WDR, wide dynamic range neurons). Different subtypes of primary afferents from the DRG neurons project to lamina specific regions onto both projection and interneurons. There are descending projections from pain modulating areas of the brainstem and other CNS ensembles to pain projecting neurons.

Primary Nociceptor Innervation of the Skin

There are two primary nociceptor subtypes differentiated by their neurochemical profiles. Painful heat stimuli are transmitted by nociceptive C-fiber afferents that contain SP and calcitonin gene-related peptides (CGRP). They synapse on both projection and interneurons of lamina I and outer lamina II. These nociceptive afferents express TRPV1 (respond to heat, protons and capsaicin). TRPA1 (transient receptor potential ankyrin I) on C and A-delta fibers that are activated by irritant chemical stimuli. Non-peptidergic C nociceptive afferents transmit mechanical pain and synapse on interneurons of inner lamina II. The non-peptidergic afferents express lectin 1-B4. Both types of afferents have L-glutamate as their primary neurotransmitter. Co-localization of SP is particularly important in NMDA expressing pain-projecting neurons. Low-threshold C mechanoreceptors have been associated with a pleasant touch that primarily expresses tyrosine hydroxylase and the vesicular glutamate transporter subtype 3. Myelinated large diameter AB afferents from low mechanical threshold mechanoreceptors mediate discriminative touch exemplified by two point discrimination and stereognosis. These low threshold AB mechanoreceptors express δ-type opioid receptors and synapse on different neuronal populations from inner lamina II to V. Thermoreceptors comprise C and Aδ fibers. C-fibers terminate in layer I and II while Aδ fibers synapse in lamina I and V. Thermal sensation depends on temperature-dependent activation of specific TRP and cation channels. The projection neurons of the DH transmit sensory information by spinothalamic pathways and parallel tracts whose neurons are located in lamina I and III-V and receive afferences directly and by excitatory interneurons.

Lamina I

Lamina I contains the majority of spinothalamic projection neurons that include:

1. Nociceptive-specific neurons that transmit heat or mechanically evoked pain
2. Neurons that respond to innocuous cooling
3. Neurons that encode noxious heat, pinch, and cold.

These lamina I neurons are multipolar or fusiform in shape and express the neurokinin-1 receptor (NK1R) activated by substance P (important for central sensitization of PTNs). These neurons convey location, quality, and intensity of pain and contribute to its emotional valence via parallel spinothalamic pathways. They project primarily to thalamic ventral posterolateral, posteromedial, and posterior inferior nuclei that in turn relay to the primary (SI) and secondary (SII) somatosensory cortex. The posterior component of the ventral medial thalamic nucleus projects to the dorsal posterior insular cortex. NK1R lamina I neurons also project to the lateral parabrachial nucleus that connects with the amygdala and hypothalamus and the periaqueductal gray (PAG) an essential component of the circuitry involved in central pain processing. Other afferences that include glutamatergic projections from excitatory interneurons in lamina II modulate nociceptive lamina I projection neurons. Pyramidal neurons in lamina I synapse with non-nociceptive low-threshold C mechanoreceptors and with C afferents that express TRMP8 receptors that signal innocuous cooling. Peripheral inflammation induces upregulation of NK1R receptors on pyramidal neurons that may allow them to signal noxious sensation.

The Deep Dorsal Horn

The deep dorsal horn neurons are found in Rexed laminas III-V and are known as wide dynamic range neurons (WDR). They respond to both innocuous and tissue-damaging stimuli, have large receptive fields, and code stimulus intensity. The innocuous inputs to these projection neurons arise from large diameter (12-20μ) AB afferents. Lamina III WDR neurons have NK1R receptors and long dorsal dendrites that project into lamina I-II and are activated by peptidergic primary afferents. They also synapse with excitatory interneurons of deep lamina II that are nonpeptidergic nociceptive afferents. Lamina V neurons are a major component of the spinothalamic tract as well as projecting to the amygdala and hypothalamus that are involved in the affective component of pain processing.

Interneurons

Dorsal horn interneurons are located in lamina I-III with their major concentration in lamina II. They are heterogeneous in regard to morphology, neurochemical profile, physiologic properties, and connectivity.

The morphologic types include:

1. Islet cell (the predominant type)
1. Central
1. Radial
1. Vertical (which are excitatory or inhibitory)

Inhibitory interneuron neurotransmitters are GABAergic and glycinergic and in some instances, both. The majority of inhibitory interneurons have islet cell morphology. Radial, vertical, and central cells are primarily excitatory interneurons and utilize L-glutamate as their neurotransmitter.

Inhibitory neurons are comprised of subpopulations of GABAergic and glycinergic ensembles that make up approximately 1/3 of the neurons of the DH. GABAergic and glycinergic interneurons may coexpress parvalbumin, neuropeptide y, dynorphin, galanin or neuronal nitric oxide synthase. These different ensembles of interneurons have specific neurophysiological properties and afferent input.

Excitatory interneurons are divided into different groups dependent on differential expression of:

1. Vesicular glutamate transporters
2. Somatostatin
3. Somatostatin 2A
4. Opioid or glutamate receptors
5. Protein kinase Cv
6. Gastrin-releasing peptide
7. Calretinin

They receive specific primary afferents as exemplified by vertical interneurons that are the target of low-threshold AB and Aδ and C mechanoreceptors while interneurons that express vesicular glutamate transporter 3 or protein kinase Cv synapse with low-threshold AB mechanoreceptors. Excitatory interneurons have varied firing patterns primarily set by A-type Kv4 channels.

Specific Peptidergic and Nonpeptidergic Afferents

Nociceptors are modality specific. Peptidergic substance P, TRPV1 expressing nociceptors carry heat pain and synapse in the superficial dorsal horn on NK1R-expressing lamina I projecting neurons and neurons in outer lamina II. These afferences are also to either excitatory or inhibitory interneurons. Nonpeptidergic C afferents synapse with all types of excitatory interneurons and may not synapse with inhibitory interneurons directly. Mu-opioid receptors are expressed on peptidergic afferents and δ-opioid receptors are demonstrated on nonpeptidergic afferents.

The Functional Role of Interneurons in Dorsal Horn Circuitry

Nociceptive afferents synapse directly with spinothalamic projection neurons and form a feed-forward circuit by means of excitatory interneurons. This circuitry is extremely complex as exemplified by heat and mechanically induced pain. NK1R expressing nociceptive lamina I neurons synapse with peptidergic afferents that encode heat pain but also synapse with a polysynaptic nonpeptidergic pathway composed of mechanosensitive fibers that encode mechanical pain. The sequential activation of this pathway entails: (1) activation of excitatory interneurons of lamina II (central interneurons) that activate (2) vertical cells in outer lamina II that in turn (3) project to the NK1R spinothalamic neurons in lamina I. These pathways provide the anatomical basis of the polymodal response of lamina I spinothalamic projection neurons to mechanical and heat noxious stimuli. Vertical excitatory interneurons in outer layer II receive direct Aδ nociceptor projection and there is also a nociceptive projection to the neurons of the deep dorsal horn (WDR) in which lamina II excitatory interneurons relay nonpeptidergic C fibers to neurons in lateral lamina V (WDR neurons).

The Anatomy of Low-Threshold Mechanoreception to Noci-

ceptive Neurons

Low-threshold mechanoreception is able to activate pain-projecting neurons of the superficial dorsal horn to cause dynamic and static mechanoallodynia that are prominent features of neuropathic pain. Low threshold AB mechanoreceptors synapse with and activate excitatory interneurons in lamina III that express vesicular glutamate transporter-3 and project to protein kinase Cv-expressing interneurons of inner lamina II. There is then sequential activation of central interneurons in inner lamina II, vertical interneurons in outer lamina II and terminal projections to NK-1 expressing pain projecting neurons of lamina I. The direct Aδ and C-fiber mechanical input concomitant with excitatory interneuron mediated low threshold mechanoreceptor afference to the vertical excitatory interneurons of outer lamina II is posited to be the anatomical basis of mechanical allodynia. Another possible contributory pathway for mechanoallodynia is the C-fiber tactile low threshold C-mechanoreceptors that also project to inner lamina II and through excitatory interneurons may modulate the wide-dynamic nociceptive projection neurons of lamina I and V. During baseline conditions, low-threshold mechanoreceptors are blocked from activating nociceptive projection neurons by surround feed-forward inhibition.

Dorsal Horn Feed-forward Inhibitory Circuits

A gate control mechanism that reduces the transmission of mechanical, itch and nociceptive transmission to spinothalamic projection neurons is provided by local DH inhibitory interneurons.

The gate control theory of Melzack and Wall posits that large fibers that transmit innocuous stimuli synapse with and activate inhibitory neurons of the substantia gelatinosa that in turn inhibit the pain projecting neurons of the dorsal horn. It has been suggested that parv-albumin-expressing inhibitory GABA / glycinergic islet cells that are located in inner lamina II – IV are the anatomical basis for this pain dampening mechanism because they are the target of low-threshold primary afferents. Another contribution to this mechanism may be from islet cell interneurons that receive projections from low-threshold mechanosensitive C fibers. Dorsal horn inhibition may be effected both pre and postsynaptically. Inner lamina II and III GABAergic interneurons inhibit primary myelinated afferents that block low-threshold afferences to excitatory interneurons. Islet cell inhibitory interneurons modulate descending mono-aminergic input to pain transmission neurons. As noted in the gate control theory noxious stimuli may inhibit inhibitory neurons that would increase pain transmission. Compatible with this proposal has been the demonstration that direct projections from nociceptive substance P-containing fibers to inhibitory islet or central interneurons are activated by noxious stimuli enhance pain transmission by inhibiting a subset of other inhibitory islet cell interneurons.

Dorsal Horn Central Sensitization in the Context of Neuropathic Pain

The dorsal horn is a major gate in the CNS for the modulation and processing of nociception. In general, chronic neuropathic pain results from lesions of the somatosensory system that causes peripheral and central sensitization. Spinothalamic systems are primarily involved. Peripheral sensitization is a manifestation of maladaptive neuroplasticity caused by the expression and dysfunction of a wide spectrum of cation channels in nociceptors that include TRPV1 and voltage-gated sodium ($Na_v1.7$, 1.8, 1.9 and 1.3) channels in response to axon injury or different forms of tissue damage. Calcium channels control transmitter release in the dorsal horn as well as neuronal activity of pain projection neurons and plasticity in chronic pain states.

In the spinal cord during nociceptive afferent stimulation, there is co-release of substance P and calcitonin gene related peptides (CGRP) and glutamate on pain projecting neurons (PTNs). These neurotransmitters activate both neurokinin (NKR1) and N-methyl-D-aspartate (NMDA) receptors in chronic pain states which combined with loss of local DH and supraspinal inhibition causes hyper- excitability of pain transmission neurons. Major manifestations of central sensitization are windup (temporal summation) induced by specific Aδ and C-fiber discharge from tissue and nerve damage and long-term potentiation (LTP) from high-frequency stimulation. Homosynaptic LTP is the persistent increase in synaptic strength of excitatory glutamatergic synapses on dorsal horn projection neurons. Prolonged nociceptive stimulation may induce heterosynaptic LTP, long lasting facilitation of dorsal horn neurons to non-nociceptive AB or C-fiber afferences. Heterosynaptic LTP causes the change (facilitation) of adjacent non-activated synapses (by the nociceptive barrage) that: (1) expands the stimulus sensitive receptive fields beyond the area of the damaged tissue. LTP occurs both pre and post synaptically primarily by calcium mediated mechanisms.

In the post-synaptic pain transmission neuron there is calcium influx from:

1. L-type voltage-gated $Ca_v1.2$ channels
1. NMDA receptors (whose magnesium block has been lifted)
1. Ca^{2+} release from intracellular stores (primarily the endoplasmic reticulum)

The intracellular Ca^{2+} release may also be induced by metabotropic glutamate receptors or the tyrosine kinase B receptor that is activated by brain-derived neurotrophic factor (BDNF). The increased intracellular calcium activates enzymatic cascades mediated by protein kinases such as calcium calmodulin kinase II and extracellular signal-related kinase.

These enzymatic-mediated transformations cause:

1. Upregulation of α-amino-3-hydroxy-5-methyl-isoxazole propionic acid (AMPA) receptor expression and recruitment to the post synaptic membrane
1. Activation of transcription and local translation of synaptic proteins
1. Growth and structural changes of dendritic spines

Presynaptic mechanisms of central sensitization cause increased glutamate release from C afferents enhanced by nitric oxide that is generated from protein kinase G mediated activity.

Hyperexcitable spinal dorsal horn pain projection neurons demonstrate:

1. Reduced firing thresholds
1. Increased receptive field size
1. Spontaneous discharge
1. Greater evoked activity

Along with LTP, 'windup' is a major manifestation of central sensitization and is the increase in neuronal response to a constant stimulus. It is also known as temporal summation. It is induced by Aδ and C-fiber input to pain projecting neurons but once induced enhances responses to both nociceptive and low-threshold mechanical afferences (inputs). In general, if the nociceptive drive onto central pain projecting neurons is blocked, there is a slow return of pain projection neuronal response to baseline levels. Some degree of peripheral afference is needed to maintain central sensitization.

The characteristic properties of sensitized nociceptors are:

1. Spontaneous discharge (frequently termed ectopic)
1. A lowered activation threshold for thermal and mechanical stimuli (particularly in neuropathic pain states)
1. Increased discharge following suprathreshold stimulation.

The spontaneous barrage from sensitized nociceptors causes neuropathic central sensitization.

A subset of dorsal horn pain projecting neurons that contain the NK1 receptor (substance P) are responsible for windup of PTNs but also for activation of the brainstem projections of the rostral ventral medullary nucleus (RVM) and the PAG that modulate descending inhibition and facilitation of pain transmission. A loss or inadequate diffuse noxious inhibitory control (DNIC) modulation of pain transmission has been demonstrated in many chronic neuropathic pain conditions. Sensitized spinal circuits are restricted to the projection zones of the affected nerves. Descending nociceptive controls may be diffuse, bilateral, and nonsegmental.

Maladaptive Neuroplasticity in Primary Nociceptive Afferents and Excitatory Interneurons Following Nerve Injury

As noted earlier, experimental peripheral axotomy demonstrates sprouting of AB afferents into lamina I and outer lamina II. After a nerve injury, there may be a phenotype switch in which there is upregulation of expression of substance P on low threshold afferents. Still, evidence is lacking for substance P activation of NK1R receptors in nociceptive PTNs of lamina I. Prolonged noxious stimulation causes extracellular receptor-activated kinase (ERK1) mediated phosphorylation and downregulation of Kv4.2 channels in PTNs, increasing their excitability.

Loss of Inhibition in the DH with Central Sensitization

Loss of DH inhibition is one major mechanism underlying central sensitization. It also occurs at multiple levels of the pain matrix. Mechanisms that contribute to loss of GABAergic and glycinergic inhibition in the dorsal horn may follow axonal or nerve injury.

They include:

1. Excitotoxic damage
1. Long-term depression (LTD)
1. Reduced efficacy of $GABA_A$ or glycine receptor channels
1. Activation of TRPV1 receptors that induce LTD of excitatory input from myelinated afferents to inhibitory neurons.

In addition, peripheral axonal injury may initiate CA^{2+}-dependent signaling that causes a general down regulation of the excitatory projections of Aδ and C-fibers to GABAergic neurons.

Recent experimental studies have demonstrated a major role of spinal cord microglia in the induction and maintenance of chronic pain by release of mediators that modulate the plasticity of synaptic response in inhibitory and excitatory pain circuitry throughout the pain matrix. Microglia have been shown to reduce the efficacy of inhibition at the spinal cord level by secretion of BDNF that down regulates the potassium chloride exporter in lamina I neurons. This mechanism is based upon a depolarization shift in the equilibrium chloride potential such that chloride current flows from the PTN (depolarizing the cell) which reduces the efficacy of $GABA_A$ and glycine receptor-mediated inhibition.

The molecular mechanisms that lead to amplification of nociceptive signals at the level of afferent input and the central sensitization of pain transmission neurons are rapidly unfolding and are starting to unravel some of the questions in regard to pain vulnerability and resistance.

Dermatomes and Sclerotomes

A dermatome consists of the primary neurons of the DRG and their peripheral and central afferents that include cutaneous and visceral endings. Each dermatome is segregated as it enters the spinal cord: the medial fibers that are primarily myelinated and are mechanosensitive, and the lateral are pain and temperative fibers (segregation of the spinal roots at the dorsal root entry zone (DREZ)). Each dermatome maintains a specific topography throughout its projections in the CNS (brainstem, thalamus, and cortex).

A **sclerotome** refers to pain projection pathways from bones, ligaments, and fascia that project slightly differently from the dermatomal pattern. After traversing the dorsal root entry zone, C-fibers innervate the specific spinal segment, but also approximately two spinal segments rostrally and caudally by means of Lissauer's tract. There is thus overlap of sensory pain dermatomal innervations. There is a small contralateral segmental DH innervation through the anterior commissures.

The dorsal horn is cytoarchitecturally organized into Rexed layers (laminae).

A-delta fiber afferents synapse in lamina I and the outermost lamina II cells. There are also important synapses from A-delta fibers in lateral lamina V. Large mechanosensitive (heavily myelinated) fibers synapse in layers III and IV. The primary synaptic connections of C-fibers is in lamina I and the substantia gelatinosa (Rexed layer II). C-fiber collaterals project to the intermediolateral column (ILC) and the motor neurons of Rexed layers IX. Cells in lamina VII (primarily motor interneurons) and lamina VIII (autonomic neurons) also respond to painful stimuli. These neurons receive projections from the DNIC (descending pain-modulating system; principally from the rostral ventral medullary neurons). Rexed layer VII motor interneurons also synapse segmentally with C-fibers. Reflex connections from C-fiber afferents to motor neurons in IX and autonomic neurons of the intermediolateral column (ILC) are activated in pain states. There are sympathetic chemical connections at the site of injury, where released norepinephrine may excite upregulated sympathetic alpha-receptors on nociceptive afferents, as well as plastic sympathetic upregulations within the DRG. In addition to the secondary neurons (pain projecting neurons PTN) of Rexed layers I and II (the primary neurons are in the DRG), the neurons of lateral Rexed layers V and VI are pivotal for many of the secondary modalities of pain sensation seen in neuropathic pain states.

Neurons in these layers are wide dynamic in range:

1. They receive low threshold mechanoreceptive input (LTM; A-beta myelinated afferents)
1. Sympathetic afferents
1. Temperative (C-fiber; heat; A-delta cold fiber afferents) and nociceptive specific projections.

Integration of these afferent inputs determines if these neurons will depolarize.

Ascending Pain Pathways

The secondary axons of Rexed layers I, II (inner /outer layers), lateral V and VI form the major components of the lateral spinothalamic tract. The spinal thalamic tract (STT) decussates in the anterior spinal commissure and ascends contralaterally as the spinothalamic tract that synapses at brainstem and thalamic levels. Pain and temperature fibers decussate approximately at two segmental levels rostral to their level of entry. Therefore, there is a drop of pain and temperature sensations on the trunk of approximately two levels with spinal cord injury (often slightly higher posteriorly). Sacral fibers are outermost in the tract while those carrying cervical and arm pain are most medial. There is also segregation by modality.

The modalities may be segregated superiorly to inferiorly in the STT:

1. Temperature
1. Pain
1. Touch
1. Deep pressure

Medially placed anterolateral fascicular fibers comprise the spinoreticular thalamic pathway. It projects to the reticular core of the medulla and midbrain and synapses in the medial (DM) and intralaminar nuclei of the thalamus (centralis medialis, lateralis, and zona reticularis). This paleospinothalamic system synapses with the nucleus gigantocellularis, parabrachial nucleus, midbrain reticular formation, periaqueductal gray (PAG) and hypothalamic nuclei. Other fasciculi of the medial anterolateral pathway synapse with the brainstem reticular core by a series of short interneuronal projections. There is also a direct spinohypothalamic pathway.

The medial fasciculi of the spinothalamic pathway conduct pain from the gastrointestinal tract, periosteum, and peritoneum. There is some evidence that deep visceral pain may also be carried in a deep pathway in the posterior columns. It has been proposed that this primarily medial pathway (slowly conducting with widespread diffuse core and limbic projections) is for the affective components of pain. The direct fast conducting spinothalamic pathway projects to the ventroposterolateral (VPL) and ventroposterior medial (VPM) nuclei of the thalamic vertebrobasilar complex (VB). This system projects primarily to SI of the primary sensory cortex. This pathway mediates the discriminate aspects of pain (quality, localization, and intensity): it is generally referred to as the lateral pathway.

Visceral pain from the esophagus, stomach, small bowel, and proximal colon project via the vagus nerve that projects to the nucleus tractus solitaries (NTS).

The direct spinothalamic tract separates into two major divisions before synapsing in the thalamus (as noted above, it gives off collaterals to many nuclei in the brainstem as it ascends): the lateral division synapses in the VPL and some posterior nuclei, while the medial division synapses are in the intralaminar complex and submedius nucleus. As noted above, the spinoreticularothalamic pathway synapses with the parafascicular and centrolateral thalamic nuclei. Thus they overlap medial spinothalamic projections. The intralaminar fiber projections also overlap with direct spinothalamic projections.

Projections from the dorsal horn are widespread and overlapping. The lateral system, the discriminative pain pathway, is primarily composed of dorsal horn projections to the VB complex (VPM and VPL) of the thalamus and consequently to the primary sensory cortex. The affectual pain circuits comprise components of the reticular formation, the parabrachial nucleus, the amygdala, insular cortex, anterior cingulate gyrus, and SII. Both of these circuitries are commonly referred to as the pain matrix that encodes the discriminative, affective and motivational components of the perception of pain.

Neurotransmitters

The primary excitatory neurotransmitter in pain transmission neurons (PTNs) is glutamate. There is a contribution from aspartate and kainate. Na(V)1.7 sodium channels are pivotal for initiation of the action potential while a variety of potassium and HCN (hyperpolarization-activated cyclic nucleotide gated) channels return the membrane to its resting potential. HCN channels are activated with membrane hyperpolarization and conduct an inward excitatory current. Dorsal horn inhibitory interneurons utilize GABA-B and glycine, as their inhibitory neurotransmitters. The potassium chloride co-transporter is essential for inhibition in the DH. It functions under physiologic conditions to decrease intracellular chloride in pain transmission neurons. Thus if it is defective, afferents from inhibitory neurons that release GABA-B onto PTNs would depolarize (excite) PTNs as chloride would follow its electrochemical gradient (leave the cell) and the membrane potential would fall to threshold levels. The NMDA receptor (N-methyl-D-aspartate) is extremely important for plastic changes in the DH that occur in chronic pain states. They are a class of ionotropic glutamate receptors. NMDARs that have slow deactivation kinetics, are highly Ca^{2+} permeable, and require partial depolarization to relieve their external Mg^{2+} channel block. C-fibers coexpress substance P and calcitonin G-related peptide in addition to glutamate. Thus, a continual C-fiber input to NMDA receptors depolarizes these receptors due to the release of the neuromodulator SP, which depolarizes the receptor enough to release its Mg^{2+} channel block and allow sodium and calcium influx. Additionally, under conditions of a continuous C-fiber input lateral synaptic NMDA receptors move to the synapse and acquire more AMPA channels. The increased calcium concentration in the PTN activates calcium calmodulin II which in turn activates P38 mitogen-activated kinase (MAPK) and extracellular regulated kinase (ERK) 1/2 to effect gene expression through cyclic AMP response element (CREB transcription factor). The phosphorylation and dephosphorylation of intracellular enzymatic cascades determine PTN excitability. The induction of new protein synthesis by activation of CaMKII and ultimately the CREB transcription factor is a major cause of neuronal plasticity in chronic pain states.

Summary of Maladaptive Plasticity

Radicular trauma from disc and degenerative osteoarthritic conditions, as well as autoimmune disease, are major causes of chronic neuropathic pain. In the area of injury, the microenvironment that includes protons, bradykinin, leukocytes, serotonin, prostaglandin, and ROS (i.e. an "inflammatory soup") induces peripheral nociceptive afferent terminal sensitization. C-fiber activation (from the inflammatory milieu) induces phosphorylation of ERK in small DRG neurons (PTN). C-fiber stimulation also induces phosphorylation in MAPKs and extracellular signal-regulated kinases (ERKs) in neurons with myelinated fibers. These intracellular enzymatic cascades lower the firing threshold of the C-fiber and A-delta fiber nociceptors. Prolonged nociceptive afferent input from C-fibers (primarily the mechanical insensitive ones) induces central sensitization in the DH and other components of the pain matrix. Central sensitization refers to the increased synaptic efficacy in PTNs (pain transmission neurons at all levels of the pain matrix) that follows intense peripheral noxious stimuli from tissue injury or nerve damage.

Central sensitization is manifested by:

1. Reduction in pain thresholds
1. Enlarged peripheral receptive fields of PTNs
1. Amplification of pain

1. Decreased pain inhibition
1. After sensations (PTN firing is not stimulus bound)
1. Temporal summation ("wind-up)

This physiological state is similar in physiologic parameters to long-term potentiation (LTP) and depression (LTD) that are important for memory and learning.

In parallel with the molecular changes in pain transmission neurons is activation of segmental microglia. Chemokines released from activated neurons (fractalkine) as well as extracellular adenosine triphosphate (ATP) play pivotal roles in the physiology of PTNs. Microglia express several subtypes of P2XR (purine receptors) which contribute to pain signaling in the spinal cord under pathologic conditions such as neuropathic pain. Activated microglia secrete inflammatory cytokines which both induce and maintain neuropathic pain and contribute to central sensitization.

Microglia and Neuropathic Pain

As noted earlier, nociception is transmitted to the superficial lamina of the dorsal horn (lamina I and II) by thinly myelinated Aδ fibers and unmyelinated C-fibers. The former transmit sharp well-localized epicutic pain and the latter poorly localized and often delayed burning pain. AB larger myelinated fibers synapse in the deeper layers of the dorsal horn (primarily lamina III and IV) on projection neurons and excitatory and inhibitory interneurons. There is an anatomical link that is polysynaptic to pain projection neurons of the superficial dorsal horn that is strongly repressed by inhibitory interneurons (GABAergic and glycinergic) under normal circumstances. AB fibers carry mechanical sensation and proprioception and not pain. The complex neural networks of the dorsal horn are modulated and modified under pathological conditions of tissue inflammation and nerve injury. The loss of function of inhibitory neurons in the dorsal horn circuitry or reduced effectiveness of GABAergic and glycinergic inhibition is a major component of neuropathic pain.

Glial cells are astrocytes, oligodendrocytes and microglia and are approximately 70% of all cells in the CNS. Microglia, the resident macrophages of the CNS, are derived from macrophages of the yolk sac and are widely distributed throughout the central nervous system. They have small cell bodies with branched and motile processes that monitor their local milieu. They respond rapidly to stimuli that include inflammation and damage to both the peripheral and central nervous system. Activated microglia progress through a stereotypic series of changes in morphology, gene expression, function and number. They synthesize and release cytokines and other chemical mediators that induce immunologic responses and also alter the function of neurons. The morphological changes in microglia after activation are cell body hypertrophy, thickened and retracted processes, an increase in number and upregulation of their markers CD11b and Iba1 (ionized calcium-binding adapter molecule-1). Signaling neuronally derived molecules for microglial activation include:

1. Monocyte chemoattractant protein-1 (MCP-1 or CCL2), and
1. Metalloproteinase-9 (MMP-9)

These molecules are upregulated in the dorsal root ganglion after peripheral nerve injury and, when experimentally administered intrathecally in normal rats, induce microglial activation and allodynia. The substrates for MMP-9 are thought to include fractalkine, interleukin 1B and tumor necrosis factor-α. Microglia express a receptor for the cytokine interferon -γ (IFN-γ R) which when stimulated changes their morphology and increases their number. The source of IFN-γ has not been identified but appears to be important in transforming microglia into an activated state. The glycoprotein CSF 1 also has been demonstrated to activate microglia. Toll-like receptors, type I transmembrane signaling proteins that recognize pathogen associated molecular patterns are also a component of microglial activation.

Microglia are also important for the detection and removal of apoptotic neuronal debris. Following nerve injury, activated microglia are recruited to the dorsal horn (often to the specific segment of the spinal cord that supplies the injured dermatome) by chemokine and ATP signaling. They survey and modify sensory afferent input for damage by extension and movement of their processes. This is effected by ion channel activation, modulation of membrane potential, changes in cell volume and ion concentration and induces phagocytosis. The relevance of these mechanisms in neuropathic pain states has not been determined.

Peripheral nerve injury, and to a lesser degree inflammatory pathologies, cause dramatic upregulation of the ATP receptor P2X4 and the chemokine receptor CX3CR1 in spinal cord microglia. The signaling from activated microglia to dorsal horn neurons, both local circuit and pain projecting, is an essential component of both the induction and maintenance of neuropathic pain. A major mechanism for this effect is the activation of P2X4Rs that cause the synthesis and release of brain derived neurotrophic factor (BDNF) which causes an alteration of the transmembrane anion gradient in a subpopulation of dorsal horn lamina I neurons by down regulation of the neuronal chloride transporter KCC2. This causes an increase of Cl^- ion concentration within these neurons and when GABA or glycine is released onto these neurons Cl^- ion flows down its electrochemical gradient (less negative Cl^- intracellularly) which depolarizes the cell. The result is aberrant nociceptive output and a decrease of inhibitory tone that normally suppresses the polysynaptic pathways that connect AB input to lamina I pain-projecting neurons. This mechanism has been posited as a cause of the mechanical hyperalgesia and allodynia that is characteristic of neuropathic pain states. Recent experimental work has demonstrated that interferon regulatory factor-8 is an essential transcription factor for P2X4R upregulation. It is expressed in lymphocytes and dendritic cells. After peripheral nerve injury IRF-8 is selectively upregulated in microglia. Suppression of the upregulation of spinal IRF8 decreases PNI induced tactile allodynia. It has also been demonstrated that IRF8 induces the expression of genes associated with microglial activation including those involved in the upregulation of P2X4R. Other recently identified transcription factors that regulate microglial function include IF5, the E26-transformation-specific family transcription factor PV.1 which has been shown to control the function and phenotype of human brain microglia. Runt-related transcription factor 1 also regulates the activity state of microglia and is upregulated in spinal cord microglia after peripheral nerve injury. In order to effectively bind its ATP ligand, P2X4Rs need to be expressed on the cell surface. Trafficking of P2X4R receptors from intracellular compartments occurs when microglia are stimulated by Toll-like receptor 1 agonists lipopolysaccharide or the Ca^{2+} ionophore ionomycin. The chemokine CCL2 also increases P2X4R on the cell surface putatively by exocytosis of P2X4R-containing lysosomes. It is clear that microglial P24XRs are dynamically regulated and their increased expression on the cell surface may increase the responsiveness of microglia to extracellular ATP.

Activation of various cell surface receptors in spinal microglia induces intracellular signaling cascades. Activation of P38 MAPK (mitogen activated protein kinase) is an important component that leads to neuropathic pain after tissue and nerve injury. Cathepsin S through fractalkine and its receptor signaling and P2Y12R have been shown to be involved in P38 MAPK signaling. P38 MAPK is primarily activated in spinal cells that express the microglial markers CD11b / OX-42 and Iba1. P38 activation peaks in the first week after peripheral nerve, ventral root and spinal cord injury and remains elevated (after PN1) for three weeks. Minocycline, a nonselective microglial inhibitor, decreases neuropathic pain in animal models by inhibiting p38. MMP-9, ATP and the chemokines CCL2 and fractalkine which are released from DRG neurons from nerve injury-induced discharge, which activate spinal cord microglia. Studies have shown that both C-fiber activity and large myelinated AB fibers activate microglia after nerve injury. In addition to P38 MAPK extracellular signal-regulated protein kinase (ERK) is increased in the superficial dorsal horn following peripheral nerve injury. Upregulation of ERK 1 and 2 are seen first in dorsal horn neurons shortly after injury, then in microglia for several days and in astrocytes after 3 weeks.

The phosphorylation of p38 in microglia after activation of the P2X4 receptor increases the synthesis and release of BDNF and the cytokines IL-1B, IL-6, and TNFα in part by the activation of the transcription factor NF-kB. TLR4 activation by lipopolysaccharide also activates p38 MAPK and induces IL-1B release.

Experimentally blocking spinal p38 in pain models:

1. Decreases upregulation of IL-1B,
1. Decreases C-fiber-evoked responses, N-methyl-D-aspartate receptor mediated responses
1. Suppresses wind-up in wide-dynamic range dorsal horn neurons,
1. Decreases the inhibitory tone of the dorsal horn by decreasing $GABA_A$ receptor-mediated currents.

The released pro-inflammatory cytokines have a major modulatory role in excitatory or inhibitory synaptic transmission in the superficial dorsal horn circuitry. In experimental rat models of spinal cord injury, inhibition of ERK suppresses the hyperresponsiveness of pain projecting neurons by reducing the synthesis of prostaglandin E_2.

Recently, an ion channel of the TMEM 16 family (anoctamins) of transmembrane proteins have been described that have pleiotropic functions that include ion transport, phospholipid scrambling (translocation of phospholipids between the two monolayers of a lipid bilayer of a cell membrane) and regulation of other membrane proteins. TMEM16A (anoctamin-1) functions as a Ca^{2+}-activated Cl^- channel that has physiologic functions in transepithelial ion transport, smooth muscle contraction, olfaction, phototransduction, nociception and control of neuronal excitability. The Ca^{2+} activated channel has either anion or non-selective cation permeability.

In both in vivo and ex vivo preparations, microglia from TMEM16F conditional knockout mice demonstrate:

1. Absence of mechanical hypersensitivity after peripheral nerve injury
1. Decreased phagocytosis by spinal microglia
1. Altered morphology
1. Deficits of activation markers
1. Diminished branch motility and phagocytic ability

This evidence supports a role for phagocytic activity of microglia after nerve injury in the altered nociceptive processing that causes neuropathic pain.

Summary of Spinal Microglia in Neuropathic Pain

Activated microglia have altered expression of genes that upregulate cell-surface receptors (P2X4R being primary) and intracellular signaling molecules (p38 MAPK as primary) that produce and secrete diffusible factors that include BDNF and proinflammatory cytokines that modulate pain processing in the dorsal horn of the spinal cord.

Core Brain Regions Activated by Pain

The individual pain experience is extremely complicated and involves many brain areas, their reciprocal connectivity and modulation. The subjective experience of pain is modulated by cognitive, affective, and contextual factors which complicates the delineation of a primary core area for the perception of pain. Early imaging studies supported a major role of the insular cortex for encoding and processing nociception. Many studies have demonstrated that the neural correlate of pain is associated with the concomitant activation of the thalamus, primary and secondary somatosensory cortices (SI and SII), insula, anterior cingulate cortex (ACC) and the prefrontal (PFC) cortices.

In order to overcome the power deficits of many small imaging studies of various pain states and to capture 3 dimensional (3D) spatial information derived from voxel-based data the meta analytical method of activation likelihood estimation (ALE) was developed.

The method:

1. Provides statistical integration of voxel-based data across multiple studies

and

1. Allows an estimate of activation likelihood of a given area in a pain state

A quantitative assessment of brain regions involved in pain processing reveals that the insula, ACC, SII and the thalamus are activated by pain irrespective of modality and body part both in patients and healthy controls. The predominance of insular and anterior cingulate cortex (ACC) activations supports their essential role in pain processing and the experience of pain. The likelihood of activation includes the entire insular cortex with peaks in its anterior portions. The dorsal-posterior insula has been posited as the area of cortical representation of nociception, the anterior insula is associated with the integration of affective and interoceptive states. Present data supports the anterior insula as the essential cortex for the subjective experience of pain. It has been posited that the posterior insula is a non-specific relay for sensory information and codes its stimulus intensity. Neuroanatomical evidence suggests that the right anterior insula is a component of the afferent system for the interoceptive representation of pain. The anterior insula (AI) has been posited to code the homeostatic state of the body and to integrate it with the motivational drive to restore homeostasis and body protection. The anterior insula is activated during the perception of empathy for pain (watching pain in others). The anterior cingulate cortex is a limbic cortex that receives the same spinothalamic tract input as the anterior insula. The anterior insula and the ACC are frequently activated concomitantly and it has been suggested that AI is the site of pain awareness and the ACC is the site for the initiation of a behavioral response (pain avoidance). The ACC is associated with the emotional-motivational aspects of pain. ACC activation is associated with the unpleasantness of pain rather than its intensity. The AI, ACC and the thalamus are activated across pain modalities that suggest that they are components of a core network of brain areas involved in pain processing.

Pain Processing During Pathologic States

Chronic pain causes maladaptive neuroplasticity that is reflected by: 1) structural, 2) functional and 3) neurochemical brain alterations. Pain patients are less likely to activate the anterior insula and the thalamus than healthy control subjects. This has been posited to represent disrupted interoception that may be a cause for the absence of pain inhibitory activation during evoked pain. It has also been suggested that the less likelihood of a pain patient to activate AI and the cingulate gyrus may indicate a ceiling effect as the patient has continuing nociceptive input to nociceptive processing areas and is unable to increase the activation further (from experimental pain protocols). The above results, i.e. failure to activate AI, the cingulate cortex, and the thalamus support a proposed shift from the lateral discriminative pain system to the medial system that processes the affective-motivational aspects of pain during the process of pain chronification. The thalamus demonstrates structural changes, decreased activity during rest and attenuated pain-evoked activation during several categories of pain. These findings support the hypothesis that pain pathophysiology involves thalamocortical dysrhythmia.

The prefrontal cortex is an important brain region for inhibitory control of pain as demonstrated by its function during the reappraisal of pain and placebo analgesia. Recent studies have demonstrated a less likelihood to activate parts of the middle-frontal gyrus in pain states that may reflect decreased activation of the brain's inhibitory circuitry.

In summary: 1) functional brain mapping supports an essential rule for the insula and ACC in the perception of pain and 2) there is decreased activation in the anterior insula, cingulate cortex and thalamus in chronic pain patients when compared to healthy controls.

Neuropathic Pain Gain Control Mechanisms

Peripheral Sensitization and Fatigue

Peripheral nociceptors are more easily sensitized to thermal than mechanical stimuli. The manifestations of peripheral sensitization are:

1. Reduced thresholds
1. Increased suprathreshold responses
1. Spontaneous discharge

TRPV1 (transient receptor potential cation channel subfamily V member 1) is a transient receptor protein ion channel primarily responsive to heat and protons. After phosphorylation via multiple pathways, it is a major cause of peripheral sensitization to its ligands and heat. In inflammatory conditions, its activation threshold on C-fibers may be below body temperature causing them to discharge and producing spontaneous pain. If the receptor is repeatedly stimulated with mildly noxious heat stimuli it loses the phasic component of its response as well as its ability to generate action potentials due to a decrease of heat-induced inward currents. Nociceptors adapt with prolonged constant stimulation.

Peripheral sensitization and receptor fatigue are mechanisms of modulation of nociceptive input in the peripheral nervous system. Fatigue occurs with mild stimuli and sensitization with possible tissue damaging stimuli. Central sensitization in most instances requires a continuous afferent nociceptive drive to be maintained. Peripheral sensitization is a major mechanism of this nociceptive afference.

Pain modulation at the Spinal Cord Level

Lamina I-II neurons of the superficial dorsal horn respond to nociceptive specific afferent input. The pain projecting neurons of the deep dorsal horn respond to thermal, chemical and mechanical stimuli as well as to a broad range of intensities from the afferent input of peripheral nerves. The slow temporal summation of nociceptive neurons in the deep dorsal horn is termed "wind-up". During wind-up, repetitive stimulation at low frequencies (more than 1 impulse every three seconds), induces an increase of the wide dynamic range neuron (WDR) evoked response and post-discharge with each stimulus. "Wind-up" is induced by C-fiber input in WDR neurons and not high threshold or nociceptive specific neurons that only respond to nociceptive input. It is not induced by A-fiber afferences. "Wind-up" may be a mechanism to compensate for peripheral receptor fatigue. During prolonged low-frequency stimulation "wind-up" evolves into long-term depression in which synaptic efficacy is decreased. "Wind-up" is induced by activation of NMDA receptors after the magnesium block has been removed by depolarization of the neuron from C-fiber released substance P. There are no neuropeptides in AB fibers - which explains why low threshold afferences are unable to induce "wind-up". The major effect of NMDA activation is its permeability to calcium. After activation, the increased calcium concentration activates calcium calmodulin dependent kinases (CaMKI/II) and ERK that along with other intracellular cascades increase synaptic glutamate efficacy.

Descending Inhibition and Facilitation

Spinal nociceptive neurons are both tonically inhibited from local circuit GABAergic and glycinergic interneurons and also receive stimulus evoked inhibitory control projections (DNIC) from the rostral ventral medullary nucleus (RVM) located in the caudal medulla and the periaqueductal gray (PAG) nuclei of the midbrain. The RVM may also be excitatory to nociceptive DH neurons utilizing serotonin as the ligand for the 5HT3 receptor. The effects of DNIC are widespread and are a reflection of the wide dynamic range neurons that they target. They are also known as convergent neurons as they respond to all somatosensory modalities that includes thermal, chemical and mechanical. They may be projection neurons or interneurons for polysynaptic reflexes. The receptive fields of WDR neurons have a gradient of sensitivity, the center responding to any mechanical stimulus (including hair movement and light touch) while the periphery responds only to noxious stimuli. WDR neurons also receive afferences from viscera, muscles, and joints. This convergence of inputs allows them to monitor both the interface with the external environment and the internal milieu. WDR neurons have a dynamic physiology as the size of their peripheral fields and their output may change due to the evoked plasticity of both excitatory and inhibitory segmental processes. These WDR neurons are strongly inhibited when a nociceptive stimulus is applied to any part of the body that is beyond their excitatory receptive field. DNIC projections only modify convergent wide dynamic neurons and the inhibition is usually triggered only by a nociceptive conditioning stimulus. There is evidence that the level of pain induced by the conditioning stimulus may be associated with the degree of DNIC or conditioned pain modulation. A larger area for conditioning stimulation causes stronger pain inhibition posited to be due to spatial summation.

Recent experiments utilizing compression for conditioned pain modulation have been effective in inducing DNIC pain inhibition. The DNIC inhibition is potent, affects all of the physiological functions of the WDR neuron, and persists for some time after withdrawal of the test stimulus. A-delta and C-fibers are the primary afferences that trigger DNIC. DNIC anatomically is subserved by the parabrachial nucleus and the subnucleus reticularis dorsalis and possibly the nucleus raphe magnus via its on and off cells. The DNIC has been shown to modulate both "Off "and "On" cells in the RVM, the major component of the spino-bulbar-spinal inhibitory loop.

The posited function of this circuitry is to enhance spatial contrast of a pain signal by lateral inhibition that accentuates the most relevant and strongest nociceptive input for processing and response programming.

Pain Modulation from Higher Brain Levels

The brain can control its own ascending nociceptive afference. The RVM receives descending projections from the PAG that in turn is modulated by the hypothalamus, amygdala, and areas of the cerebral cortex. This allows cognitive and affective processes to modify pain processing at a spinal level. This is exemplified by the placebo affect in which expectation and conditioning can decrease dorsal horn excitability. As noted above, the posterior insular cortex is essential for coding the intensity of a painful stimulus while the anterior insula and anterior cingulate cortices are important for the integration of the affective and interoceptive aspects of the pain experience. The prefrontal cortex, the primary and secondary motor cortices are all components of the pain processing system and the programs to avoid tissue injury that reach the spinal level through dorsal lateral pathways of the spinal cord. Pain states activate the contralateral thalamus whose activity can be modified by transcranial cortical stimulation of the contralateral motor cortex. Maladaptive plasticity of the cortex has been clearly demonstrated in phantom limb pain. Cortical pain inhibition is primarily effected by modulation of the spino-bulbar-spinal loop of the caudal brainstem centered in the RVM.

Clinical Profiles Suggestive of Pain Mechanisms

Approximately 30% of patients with neuropathic pain respond to approved therapies. Presentation of sensory pain symptoms vary but patients can be characterized by different symptomatic pain profiles or phenotypes. A major goal of neuropathic pain management is to develop mechanism-based treatments. The differentiation of neuropathic pain from nociceptive pain is critical in this determination. Quantitative sensory testing combined with various screening questionnaires and the clinical evaluation are the platforms for the determination of sensory profiles in neuropathic pain patients.

The pain DETECT questionnaire is validated and consists of seven pain sensory symptom items, one pain course pattern item and one pain radiation item. The pain DETECT questionnaire has been shown to be effective in identifying neuropathic pain of varying etiologies and in determining pain intensity and its relationship to health status. It is also able to characterize specific symptom clusters by sensory symptoms.

Somatosensory abnormalities in patients with neuropathic pain syndromes utilizing quantitative sensory testing (QST) of the German Research Network in Neuropathic Pain protocol demonstrated:

1. A shift to hyperalgesia for nociceptive pain
1. Hypoesthesia for non-nociceptive parameters
1. Thermosensory or mechanical hypoesthesia was more frequent than

hypoalgesia

1. Mechanical hyperalgesia (blunt pressure, pinprick) was more frequent than thermal hyperalgesia, dynamic mechanical allodynia, paradoxical heat sensations or wind up
1. All sensory alterations were demonstrated in each neurological pathology but with different frequencies
1. Thermal and mechanical hyperalgesias occur most frequently with complex regional pain syndrome and peripheral nerve injury
1. Allodynia was frequent with postherpetic neuralgia
1. Postherpetic neuralgia and central pain had subgroups with either mechanical hyperalgesia or mechanical hypoalgesia
1. In central pain and polyneuropathy there were often combinations of gain and loss whose most frequent combination was thermal / mechanical loss without hyperalgesia
1. Mixed loss with mechanical hyperalgesia was noted in peripheral nerve pathology
1. Mechanical hyperalgesia without sensory loss is characteristic of trigeminal neuralgia

Clinical Expression of Pain Mechanisms

1. Persistent pain with hyperalgesia to heat that is restricted to the area of tissue injury supports the mechanism of peripheral sensitization:
   a. Nociceptors have lowered thresholds to heat and a low pH
   b. The pain persists for up to a day and is limited to the site of the injury
   c. Peripheral sensitization and fatigue are localized to the stimulated nociceptors and even to the stimulated part of the receptive field
1. Hyperalgesia to punctate stimuli (pinprick) and dynamic mechanical allodynia (light brushing) which may extend one or two segments above and below the area of tissue damage, is supportive of central sensitization. It may be long lasting and is frequently associated with spread. Receptive fields of central neurons expand and afferences that were not sufficient to discharge dorsal horn neurons are now capable of doing so. The loss of inhibition of local circuit DH GABAergic and glycinergic interneurons may no longer tonically inhibit AB polysynaptic pathways so that mechanical stimuli are able to drive pain projecting neurons of lamina I of the dorsal horn
1. Pain in a specific body region may be inhibited by AB large myelinated fiber activation only during the stimulation, is consistent with the gate control hypothesis
1. Pain inhibition from A-delta fiber activation is confined to the stimulated body part and is consistent with long-term depression (LTD). Synaptic efficacy of first order DH pain projecting neurons is attenuated due to decrease

of presynaptic neurotransmitter release or decrease in postsynaptic receptor density; LTD is induced by small, slow rises in postsynaptic calcium levels. The calcium concentration in the postsynaptic cell is a major determinant whether LTD or LTP is effected. LTD is a localized effect that can last for hours

1. Widespread pain that may involve the entire body associated with mechanical hyperalgesia is suggestive of deficits in descending inhibitory controls or supraspinal facilitation by modulation of the RVM nucleus. The duration of the effects outlasts the conditioning stimulus for a few minutes

Major advances have been made in an understanding of the molecular basis of neuropathic pain. In the future, there will be individualized mechanism based pain therapy.

The Neuroimaging of Neuropathic Pain

As noted above, chronic neuropathic pain is extremely complex at all levels and engages:

1. Sensory discriminative components
1. Affective motivational components
1. Cognitive components

It is a perception unique to each individual, dependent on genetics, a past pain history and present context. Acute pain activates different circuitry than chronic pain and there are many mechanisms leading to the chronification of acute pain. Central sensitization and pain modulation occur in the brainstem and spinal cord that are now starting to be imaged with high field 7 Tesla and MRI technology.

The neuroimaging modalities that are used to study the brain networks that underlie both acute and chronic pain include PET, EEG/ magnetoencephalography (concomitantly with imaging), single photon-emission computed tomography (SPECT/CT) and various MRI techniques, most recently including arterial spin labeling (ASL).

The major chronic pain states reported with these techniques include:

1. Chronic low back pain
1. Fibromyalgia
1. Osteoarthritis
1. Complex regional pain syndrome (CRPS)
1. Phantom limb pain
1. Chronic migraine
1. Chronic pelvic pain
1. Peripheral neuropathy

In addition, many experimental reports in rodents and healthy volunteers have allowed manipulations of the painful stimuli with neuroimaging and anatomical correlation. Neuroimaging has also given insight into the modulation of the pain experience, including attention, the anticipation of pain, empathy, placebo effects, meditation, emotional state (fear/anxiety), and reward aspects of pain relief.

Structural Changes in the Brain with Chronic Neuropathic Pain

Structural changes in the brain parenchyma occur with chronic neuropathic pain primarily demonstrated by voxel-based and cortical thickness analysis. CRPS, fibromyalgia, migraine, temporomandibular joint disorder, and chronic low back pain demonstrate regional increases and decreases in gray matter density and cortical thickness. These structural changes are demonstrated in the insular cortex, somatosensory cortices, motor cortex, and parietal cortices. Subcortical structural changes occur in the thalamus and basal ganglia. Possibly influencing the cognitive components of pain are alterations in the prefrontal cortex, hippocampus and amygdala (emotional regulation). Reversal of gray matter density in specific chronic pain entities are reported with effective therapy. The exact clinical correlation and meaning of these structural changes has not been elucidated. Gray matter changes are noted to increase over 3 years and to be correlated with increased low back pain in the face of minimal stress. Detailed evaluation of white matter connectivity between nodes of brain circuitries are obtained with the use of MRI tractography and fractional anisotrophy in various chronic neuropathic illnesses. Combined voxel-based morphometry and diffusion tensor imaging are utilized to evaluate the interactions between gray matter nodes and white matter alterations.

There is no specific brain area that solely encodes a painful stimulus. In the past, the dorsal posterior insular cortex was thought to be the major pain encoding cortical area. More recently, a core "pain matrix" that includes the thalamus, posterior and anterior insular cortex, SII, the ACC (anterior cingulate cortex), the PAG and central nucleus of the amygdala are thought to be the major pain encoding areas. The discriminatory components of acute pain are subserved by the lateral nuclei of the thalamic ventrobasal complex and project to SI and SII. The medial pain system of the pain matrix projects from the parabrachial nucleus and medial thalamic nuclei to the anterior cingulate area, which encode emotional aspects of pain, direct attention to the painful stimulus, the unpleasantness of pain and assigns response priorities. In chronic painful conditions there is a shift to the affective, emotional and reward circuitry which includes the mPFC (dorsal) - amygdala – nucleus accumbens. At a cellular level it has been shown that there is release of endogenous opioids in the rostral anterior cingulate region that is necessary for the release of dopamine in the NAc for relief of chronic pain. Functional studies have also demonstrated increased connectivity of the mPFC and the nucleus accumbens (NAc) in chronic neuropathic pain.

Intensity coding of pain is correlated with increased activity (fMRI) in the SI and posterior insular cortex in CRPS, low back pain and fibromyalgia when painful stimuli are applied to an affected area. Structural alterations during painful stimuli in chronic neuropathic pain disorders are also seen in SII and are thought to be a component of higher order sensory processing and integration. The primary motor, premotor, and supplementary motor cortices as well as the cerebellum are activated in fMRI studies in chronic neuropathic pain. Areas of the PFC that include the ventromedial PFC, the dorsolateral PFC and the orbitofrontal cortex are associated with alteration of cognitive processes and chronic pain. The temporo-parietal junction (a multimodal sensory area), precuneus, and posterior cingulate cortex demonstrate functional MRI alterations during chronic neuropathic pain. These are areas of the default mode network that is usually activated during mind wandering, introspection and self-referential thought (during the absence of a task). It is suggested that abnormalities in the DMN may be more apparent with chronic neuropathic pain.

Psychological Aspects of Pain Demonstrated by fMRI

Brain areas related to the affective and emotional components of pain – its unpleasantness and aversiveness include the anterior insular and anterior cingulate cortex that demonstrates altered function in chronic neuropathic pain states.

The psychological aspects of pain processing, which include fear and emotional states, demonstrate alterations in the central nucleus of the amygdala (fear processing) and alterations of the hippocampus that affect memory related circuitry.

Recent studies with high field MRI 7 Tesla technology demonstrate that brainstem components of the descending pain modulating system (DPMS) are active both during the development and during maintenance of central sensitization produced by the capsaicin model of experimentally produced neuropathic pain. Involvement of the DPMS is shown to be a mechanism in placebo anesthesia (its inhibitory action). This function (placebo anesthesia) can be blocked by naloxone.

A recent study demonstrates that the periaqueductal gray may integrate aversive prediction errors that may be important in aversive learning. Clearly, thalamic lesions are implicated clinically in central pain syndromes. Altered motor and general connectivity may be affected by changes in basal ganglia structure and function during chronic pain. The ventral tegmental area (dense projections to the nucleus accumbens) is gaining attention as alterations of the reward and affective components of the pain experience predominate in chronic neuropathic pain states.

Components of Neuropathic Pain

Static and dynamic mechanical allodynia and, to a lesser degree, thermal hyperalgesia and allodynia are major components of neuropathic pain. The most disturbing component of neuropathic pain, however, is spontaneous pain.

Patients with varying have lesions of the neuraxis that include spinal brainstem, thalamic and cortical lesions that developed mechanical allodynia on one side of the body, were evaluated with fMRI. Innocuous mechanical stimuli were delivered to the affected and normal side of the body. Brush and cold rubbing of the unaffected side of the body are not painful and activate the contralateral SI and SII somatosensory areas and the insular cortex. The same innocuous stimuli applied to the allodynic side of the patient's body evoke activity in similar parts of the somatosensory system, are extremely painful, and demonstrate lesser activation of SII and the insular cortices. There is increased activation of the contralateral SI and primary motor cortex (MI), and in the ipsilateral hemisphere (to the allodynic side), and increases of activation in the parietal operculum (SII), SI, and the insular cortex. There is additional activation of the premotor and motor areas, including MI, the supplementary motor area, the posterior parietal cortex, and the mid-anterior cingulate cortex of the ipsilateral hemisphere. It is postulated that the ipsilateral hemisphere may be a component of the shift from normal mechanical sensation to allodynia following deafferenting CNS lesions. The affected areas primarily link attention (posterior parietal cortices) and motor control (midanterior cingulate cortex). Under normal circumstances, the contralateral insular cortex and SII are activated by innocuous cold stimuli. The insular cortex receives spinothalamic afferences from the VMpo nucleus of the thalamus and from laminar I projecting neurons that are activated by cold.

A great deal of recent neuroimaging research in pain has focused on the inherent and altered connectivity between nodes and within brain circuitry. The advantage of resting state fMRI is that the acquisition of data can be acquired while chronic neuropathic pain patients are quietly resting in the MRI scanner. This data more closely reflects the natural state of brain activation during spontaneous pain (the most disturbing element of neuropathic pain). Resting state MRI investigates the degree of functional connectivity between nodes (nuclei of the "pain matrix") which is correlated with low frequency oscillations between these areas. The networks that are altered during chronic pain are:

1. The default mode network (DMN) that is active at rest (task free state)
1. The salience and sensorimotor networks that are active during various stimuli and are related to sensory and motor processing.

Different neuropathic pain conditions are shown to specifically activate components of the DMN. In patients with chronic low back pain there is decreased DMN connectivity within the medial PFC, posterior cingulate cortex and amygdala. In fibromyalgia there is greater connectivity between the DMN and the executive and salience circuitries. In addition, fibromyalgia patients demonstrate greater connectivity between the DMN and the insular cortex than that which is seen in healthy controls. Fibromyalgia also demonstrates a spectrum of alterations between the insular and other cortical areas. In chronic pain states, there are altered low-frequency oscillations that include the primary somatosensory cortex (SI), the supplementary motor area (SMA), the dorsolateral prefrontal cortex (DLPFC) and the amygdala. In CRPS, there is decreased resting state functional connectivity in the DMN and increased connectivity in sensory and motor areas with other pain processing areas.

Phantom Pain

Tracey reports unexpected findings in phantom pain, rather than loss of sensory input that would be characterized by structural and functional degeneration of the deprived sensorimotor cortex. If patients are asked to move the lost extremity rather than imagine its movement, there is preserved function of these areas. It is further shown that the lip area does not invade the adjacent hand area. It has been posited that phantom pain is associated with reduced integrational functional connectivity in the primary sensorimotor complex. In light of these findings, direct transcranial stimulation is utilized effectively to manipulate this aberrant functional connectivity to relieve pain in patients with phantom pain. This treatment effect buttresses the functional relevance between sensorimotor cortical plasticity and pain.

Neuroimaging of Chronic Neuropathic Pain

An extremely important aspect of neuroimaging in the study of chronic neuropathic pain is the demonstration (Balilhi) that both functional and structural (white matter properties) in cortico-limbic areas influence the risk for the development of chronic neuropathic pain. He demonstrated that increased connectivity between the mPFC (dorsal) and the amygdala and nucleus accumbens (NAc) differentiates persistent and recurrent back pain patients from patients who have less persistent back pain. Complicated fMRI studies show that relief from treatment interventions may be related to:

Increased activity of baseline reward circuits in response to evoked pain

Increased trait reward responsiveness.

This system (functional reward system) may also be a component of the mechanism of opioid analgesia and its activation may be necessary for the success of treatments that alleviate neuropathic pain. On a cellular level, it is shown experimentally that endogenous opioid release in the rostral anterior cingulate cortex is required for dopamine release in the NAc for analgesia of chronic neuropathic pain. Surprisingly, in another study focusing on the reward system in chronic pain, reports that only 20% of relief is needed for a significant benefit.

Tonic and slowly varying neural states are difficult to image. Neuroimaging with arterial spin labeling (ASL) may overcome this challenge and allow insight into long lasting perceptual experiences. The use of advanced acquisition ASL techniques recently demonstrates a major role of the contralateral dorsal posterior insular cortex in tracking ongoing pain. These studies demonstrate a brain region that is active over a continuous period and is correlated with the intensity of pain due to manipulation of the nociceptive stimulus.

Magnetic resonance spectroscopy is also used to define aspects of neuropathic pain. Its application in patients with fibromyalgia versus controls demonstrates increased glutamate/glutamine in the posterior insular cortex. Pressure pain thresholds are negatively correlated with the peaks of glutamate/glutamine. Furthermore, pregabalin, which is a partially effective treatment for FM, also lowers the concentration of glutamate/glutamine in the posterior insular cortex.

Intense research from worldwide laboratories has built an experimental and clinical base that is starting to unravel the underlying mechanisms of neuropathic pain. These studies will hopefully lead to a mechanism-based and personalized treatment options for neuropathic pain patients.

Clinical Aspects of Somatic Neuropathic Pain

The Nerve Root

Nerve roots exit and enter the spinal cord through the neural foramina. These are bony canals of varying length depending on the spinal segment. The contents of the neural foramina (canals) are the spinal nerve roots, recurrent meningeal nerves, and radicular blood vessels. The anatomical boundaries are the pedicles inferiorly and superiorly, anteriorly the intervertebral disc and vertebral body and posteriorly the facet joint. The superior and inferior facets are lined by synovium. The dorsal root ganglia (DRG) are in the foraminal canals.

The blood supply to a spinal nerve root derives from the corresponding radicular artery. At the root entry zone, blood vessels lie on the surface of rootlets and in inter-radicular spaces. Capillary density is high in the ventral root entry zone. In osteoarthritic degenerative conditions, facet joints are frequently remodeled by hypertrophic bone expansion. Tropism occurs whereby the facet rotates into the foraminal exit canals and the lateral recess. This process impinges on the exiting nerve root at its level. The facet joints are innervated by branches of the posterior primary ramus of the spinal nerve root. The clinical effect of degeneration of the annulus pulposus and the posterior longitudinal ligament are not well categorized. Both structures receive nociceptive innervations. Extruded disc material induces an inflammatory response around the nerve root eliciting the expression of IL-1, IL-6 and tumor necrosis factor-alpha that directly depolarize nociceptive C-fibers and A-delta afferents. Dorsal root ganglia have a less permeable blood-nerve barrier than the blood brain barrier. This is important in the context of chemotherapy-induced radiculopathy and autoimmune processes such as Sjogren's syndrome or paraneoplastic processes. The cell bodies in the DRG for PTNs may thus be directly affected in the course of these disorders.

Radicular pain is caused by depolarization of A-delta and C-fiber nociceptive afferents. A-delta primary nociceptive afferents (1-4 μ) cause lancinating well-localized pain in the expected dermatome. With root irritation, the lancinating pain is frequently followed by a deep aching pain that has a burning quality. This second pain is mediated by 1μ unmyelinated slowly conducting C-fibers. Sympathetic discharge elicited by somatic sympathetic reflexes may amplify and drive this pain in chronic conditions. The usual radicular pain radiates within its specific dermatome. However, it may be appreciated in only part of the anatomical confines of the dermatome. Thus, an L5 root injury may be felt just or predominately in the lateral thigh or great toe and not the lower back.

The pain is usually increased by mechanical maneuvers that increase intraspinal pressure or stretch the nerve root. The nervi nervorum that innervate the nerve sheath are sensitized so that a mechanical stimulus of the root rather than a tissue destructive one in the dermatome will depolarize them (basis for the straight leg-raising test and other provocative stretch maneuvers).

Dorsal Root Entry Zone

There is segregation of spinal root afferents at the dorsal root entry zone (DREZ). Medial dorsal root fibers carry proprioception, vibration, and light touch. Lateral dorsal root fibers (closest to the area dorsolaterally where discs extrude) carry lancinating pain (A-delta fiber mediated), cold (A-delta fiber), temperature and burning pain (C-fiber). Lesions that affect the dorsal root entry zone are, in general, painful. Lesions peripheral to the DRG in the neuronal exit canals cause numbness. Lesions of the medial branch of the posterior primary division of the dorsal root are associated with numbness and paresthesias (1½ inches laterally from the spinous process). Meningeal afferents from the dorsal root innervate the dura at each spinal segmental level. These are the recurrent branches of Spurling. The L5 branch is particularly relevant as its referred pain is to the top of the thigh when it is stimulated (often mistaken for L1, L2, L3 root pain).

Ventral Root Lesions

Ventral root lesions cause segmental weakness. If these axons are injured, there will be associated atrophy and fasciculation along with weakness of the innervated muscles. Early with compressive or irritative lesions, reflexes may be enhanced. This has been posited to result from the differential susceptibility of inhibitory afferents in the ventral root. In the lower extremity (if reflexes are increased), the examiner must always be aware of compressive or intrinsic spinal cord lesions that may injure the corticospinal tract and disinhibit neurons below the lesion level.

The Structural Bone and Ligamentous Anatomy of the Spine

The vertebral bodies are connected by intervening discs and partially supported by the anterior and posterior longitudinal ligaments. The posterior elements from the vertebral bodies are composed of the pedicles, laminae, and dorsal spine. The transverse dorsal spinous processes are the origin and insertions of the paraspinal musculature. The ligamentum flavum is on the ventral surface of the laminae, and the posterior longitudinal ligament runs dorsally on the vertebral body. The dentate ligament connects the spinal cord to the dura. The interspinous ligaments connect the spinous processes and facet joints. The facet and sacroiliac joints have a synovial lining. Spine stability depends on the integrity of its skeletal and ligamentous components as well as active muscular support from the paraspinal musculature. The L5 vertebral body is the load segment for the lower spine (subject to the weight of the upper body). The skeletal and ligamentous structures are most vulnerable at movement segments (C5-C6 cervically and L5-S1 in the lumbar spine). If a segment is fused, the next uppermost spinal segment becomes the movement segment. Stress on bone activates osteoblasts and molecular mechanisms that remodel bone. This is evidenced by endplate increased bone density (Modic's sclerosis). Transforming growth factor beta-1, osteoblast and osteoclast activation, and complicated bone metabolism are all important in this process. Voluntary and reflex activity of the paraspinal, sacrospinalis, abdominal, gluteus maximus and hamstring musculature not only support the spinal column but adjust their activity following pathologic processes. These adjustments change gait and posture, which in turn modify load and stress points in the vertebral column.

After the exit of the lumbar spinal roots from the cord, they course downward in the subarachnoid space prior to entering the exit foraminal canals. The area on the inner surface of the pedicle (area prior to the entrance of the foraminal canal) is known as the lateral recess. This area may be compromised by congenitally shortened pedicles (common in achondroplasias and other congenital bony dysostoses) or extruded disc fragments.

The lateral lumbar intervertebral canals are complex osteofibrous, neurovascular tunnels whose configuration is modified by degenerative change in the intervertebral disc and degenerative arthritic changes in the facet joints and the canal itself. Their shape and morphometric features are dependent on their level, vary individually, and change with age dependent degeneration.

In the epidural compartment that lies behind the vertebral bodies is a sagittal membrane that connects the deeper layer of the posterior longitudinal ligament (PLL) with the posterior midline of the vertebral body. This connection may be total or partial. Its clinical significance is that it prevents disc material (that has been extruded) from moving to the contralateral side. Meningovertebral ligaments connect the dura with the PPL, which prevents movement of the dura from the spinal canal. These ligaments vary in size from loose areolar structures to clear individual ligaments and may be midsagittal or more laterally placed. A double cross vault structure has been described between the PPL and the dura matter from L3 to the termination of the dural sac. Meningovertebral ligaments may also contain extruded disc material.

The subpedicular notch of the upper vertebra is the widest part of the canal (shaped like an inverted teardrop) and is often referred to as the neural foramen. The anterior wall of the intervertebral canal is composed of the posterolateral components of two articulating vertebrae and the intervening disc. The anterior inferior morphology of the intervertebral foramen depends on the apophyseal rings and the disc that often bulges physiologically at the lumbar level. The posterior wall of the nerve root canal is composed of the ligamentum flavum, the pars interarticularis of the dorsal vertebra and the superior articular facet of the ventral vertebra.

Nerve sleeve morphology is level dependent, has a variable oblique course from the thecal sac to the outer third of the intervertebral canal. Anomalous lumbosacral nerve roots have a variable course and often originate from an abnormal high or low position from the spinal cord. There may be conjoined roots (most often associated with an abnormal nerve root sleeve), a double set of nerve roots, or an anastomosis between nerve roots of adjacent levels. The dorsal root ganglion (DRG) may be variably placed in the intervertebral foramen. At L4 and L5 levels, the DRGs tend to be intraforaminal. The S1 DRG is intraspinal. An intraspinal position makes the ganglia more susceptible to compression from a superior articular facet or disc bulging. Extra-foraminal positions of the DRG have been reported at L4 and L5.

The sinuvertebral nerve has a recurrent course through the lateral neuro vertebral canal and supplies the laterodorsal outer annulus of the disc, the PLL, the anterior 2/3 of the dural sac and the anterior vascular plexus.

Other blood vessels that traverse the neurovertebral canal include:

1. Anterior and posterior spinal canal branches
1. Anterior and posterior radicular branches
1. Veins of the anterior and posterior internal vertebral venous plexus.

At each segment, there are one or two thick and one to four thin sinuvertebral nerves (SVNs) that originate close to the connection of the rami communicantes to the spinal nerve. The thin SVNs have extensive ramifications that form a network in the floor of the central lumbar canal that supplies the PLL. The PLL is posited to play a role in spinal proprioception and nociception and may be vulnerable to extruded proalgesic disc material. Adjacent to the semivertebral nerves, small branches from the rami communicates join the dorsal ramus in association with the segmental artery that enters the neural canal. The sympathetic nerve plexus and the SVNs inside the anterior longitudinal ligament are a network of nerve fibers that surround the intervertebral discs and the vertebral bodies. The dorsal ramus innervates the facet joints at the corresponding level and one below prior to its muscular and cutaneous innervations.

In summary, the principal innervation of the intervertebral disc is the sinuvertebral nerves. They are recurrent branches of the ventral spinal nerve rami that re-enter the intervertebral foramina and are formed by a somatic root from the ventral ramus and a sympathetic root from a grey ramus. The dorsal ramus, especially its medial branch innervates posterior structures that include the multifidus muscle and the facet joint.

The Innervation of the Lumbar Vertebra

The lumbar vertebral body is innervated primarily by nerves that enter through the basivertebral foramen on its posterior surface, are associated with blood vessels, and are concentrated in its center. The pattern of innervation closely follows that of the bone blood supply. Vertebral endplate nerves take origin from the basivertebral nerve trunk. The vertebral periosteum is lightly innervated but does not pierce the anterior or lateral cortices of the vertebral body. The sympathetic nerves that supply the vertebral body and accompany the nutrient artery through the BVF take their origin from semivertebral nerves that branch from the sympathetic trunk. They occupy the intervertebral canal and supply the posterior longitudinal ligament and the posterior annulus of the disc. The innervation of the posterior border of the endplate originates from the sinuvertebral nerves. The anterolateral periphery of the endplate is sparsely innervated. Immunohistochemical testing demonstrates that the sinuvertebral nerves of the vertebral body are CGRP positive (a nociceptive marker). Several reports have shown that elevated interosseous pressure causes pain in low back pain patients that can be relieved by vertebroplasty. This result has been posited to be associated with destruction of this innervation.

A detailed study of the sinuvertebral nerves at the craniovertebral junction undertaken because of their possible involvement in whiplash injury demonstrated that:

1. SVNs at C0-C1, C1-C2 and C2-C3 intervertebral levels arise from two roots, a somatic root from either the spinal nerve or ventral ramus and a sympathetic branch from the vertebral artery plexus or the superior cervical ganglion
1. C2 and C3 innervate the majority of structures of the cranio-vertebral junction and the basi-occiput, and that the C1 SVN supplied a small component of the atlanto-occipital joint.

All three SVNs followed an ascending and descending intraspinal course associated with the arterial supply of the cervical vertebral junction (CVJ).

The Anatomy and Innervation of the Intervertebral Disc

The intervertebral discs are located between vertebral bodies and are composed of a nucleus pulposus, annulus fibrosis, and cartilaginous endplates. Their blood supply is only to the cartilaginous end-plates. They are innervated only in the outer annulus fibrosus by branches of the sinuvertebral nerve from the ventral rami of the spinal nerve or from the grey rami communicantes. They are derived from the mesodermal notochord and a great deal of their metabolism is through the cartilaginous endplates. The constituents of a disc are collagen and elastin fibers and aggrecan. The annulus fibrosus is attached to the vertebral endplates. The cartilaginous endplate is a 0.1 – 1.6 mm hyaline cartilage layer. It is a semi-permeable membrane that allows diffusion between disc nuclear cells and the vertebral vasculature and restricts proteoglycan movement to the disc space. As a disc ages, it loses osmotic pressure in the nucleus, and with dehydration loses height which affects the ligamentum flavum, facet joints and the morphology of the neural foramina.

The pathology of disc disease with aging is:

1. "End-plate-driven" that involves endplate defects and inward collapse of the annulus fibrosus
1. "Annulus-driven" which involves a radial fissure of the annulus fibrosus with leakage of nucleus pulposus proteoglycans and or disc prolapse

A far lateral disc protrusion may just entrap the exiting nerve root that will affect the corresponding spinal segment. A more medial extrusion may compress the exiting nerve root and the next lower root as it descends prior to its exit.

General Features of Radicular Pain

Overview of Face and Body Root Innervations

All parts of the body surface are innervated by a nerve root and a peripheral nerve and have a specific pattern of referred pain. Thus, sensory complaints may be overlapping such that a particular pain distribution may be composed of a root, nerve, or plexus distribution as well as its referred pattern. The sensory patterns may be difficult to discern in the face and extremities. Further complicating sensory patterns are the radiations of sclerotomes and those of the posterior rami of the lower back. Each body part receives some overlapping root rostral and caudal innervations, and there is further overlap in the dorsal horn as noted above from Lissauer's tract.

Face

The V1-V3 divisions of the trigeminal nerve (V) are well demarcated. The C2-C3 roots comprise the preauricular nerve that innervates the side of the face overlapping V2 and V3. C2 involvement alone innervates an area just anterior to the ear. C2-C3 roots comprise the lesser occipital nerve which innervates the back of the head. C3-C4 comprises the post auricular nerve that innervates the ear and portions of the parietal skull. Cervical roots C3 primarily innervates the neck and C4 the trapezius ridge. C5 innervates the top of the shoulder. C6 innervates the thumb and index finger, C7 primarily the third and 4th finger and C8 the little finger. Thoracic roots T1 innervates the lower forearm and T2 the inner humerus. T4 innervates the nipples, T10 the umbilicus and L1 the groin. Lumbar roots L2 and L3 innervate the anterior thigh while L5 innervates it laterally. The cap of the knee is L3, the inner knee L4 and the outside of the knee are innervated by L5. A strip of the inner lower leg is innervated by L4. The outside of the lower leg and foot is innervated by S1. L5 innervates the great toe and top of the foot. The bottom of the foot medially is L5 and laterally is S1. The medial posterior thigh is L3 and more laterally S3. The anus is usually presented as being innervated by sacral roots S5 roots. Saddle areas are primarily S2-S4. A sclerotome is derived from an enlage somite. During development, the somite develops into a variety of different structures. These include disks, cartilage, joint capsules, and ligaments that refer pain to the body surface in specific patterns. In general, when a portion of a sclerotome is irritated by a mechanical or chemical stimulus (rupture of a disc, facet, and ligament irritation from disc material) pain may be experienced as originating from the dermatome innervated by a nerve although it originated from the facet. Sclerotogenous pain is often reported as a dull ache and is diffuse.

Referred Pain

A primary mechanism of referred pain is somatic and visceral convergence. The skin surface and a specific internal organ are innervated by the same DRG. In the instance of referred pain from the spine, pain may be projected to visceral or other structures in the territory innervated by lumbar and upper sacral roots. Pelvic and abdominal viscera may refer pain to the spine. Sclerotomal pain radiations from the upper part of the lumbar spine may be referred to the medial flank, groin, hip and anterior thigh. This occurs most often (my experience) from discogenic disease at L5-S1. The literature supports irritation of the superior cluneal nerves (that are derived from the posterior divisions of the first three spinal nerves) which innervate the upper buttocks as a source of referred pain. It has been proposed that pain radiations into the lower buttocks and posterior thigh originate from lower lumbar and upper sacral roots. As a general rule, referred pain: 1) has the same intensity as local pain; 2) stretch maneuvers that increase local pain similarly exacerbate referred pain.

Pain referred to the spine from visceral processes may be posturally related but are not influenced by back movement. A common functional relationship of root irritation and visceral activity is micturition and defecation initiated by L5-S1 root irritation.

Local Pain

Local pain in the spine is caused by pathological processes of the facet joint, ligaments, periosteum, capsule of apophyseal joints, and the annulus fibrosis. If there is pain from annulus fibrosis stretch or tear is debated. It is innervated by nociceptive fibers and disc contents initiate an immune response that may induce the release of inflammatory cytokines (IL-1, IL-6, and TNF-alpha among others) that theoretically could irritate nociceptive afferents.

Pain from these spinal structures is:

1. Steady and aching
1. Not lancinating
1. Usually is at the level of segmental involvement

Lumbar Radicular Pain

General Characteristics

1. Higher lumbar root pathology is usually caused by:
    a. Autoimmune Processes
    b. Connective tissue diseases
    c. Diabetes mellitus
    d. Vasculitides
    e. Congenital defects
    f. Metastases
    g. Meningeal disorders
1. Lower root involvement (L4-S1) is usually caused by:
    a. Degenerative disc disease
    b. Lumbar spondylosis
    c. Spondylolysis
    d. Lumbar spondylolisthesis
    e. Spinal stenosis
    f. Facet hypertrophy and tropism
    g. Lateral recess syndrome
    h. Surgical procedures
    i. Congenital lesions
    j. Ligamentous cysts
    k. Carcinomatosis of the meninges
    l. Metastatic disease (gastrointestinal tract)

Combined Lumbosacral root disease:

1. Tumor (metastatic and carcinomatosis of the meninges)

2. Trauma (lumbosacral junction)
3. Arachnoiditis
4. Congenital abnormalities
5. Diabetes mellitus
6. Collagen vascular and autoimmune processes

Congenital Defects of the Lumbar Spine

Lumbosacral Transition Vertebra

General Characteristics

1. Lumbosacral transitional vertebra (LSTV) is the most common congenital anomaly of the lumbosacral spine
2. Its prevalence has been estimated at 7% to 30% of the general population

Clinical Manifestations

1. The prevailing view is that there are no clinical consequences of the lesions
2. Some others describe:
   a. Pain may arise from the disc above the defect, from the contralateral facet or an anomalous articulation

Neuropathology

1. Sacralization of the lowest vertebral body or lumbarization of the upper-most sacral vertebra

Neuroimaging

1. MRI:
   a. Disc degeneration above the LSTV (reported)
   b. An association with spina-bifida
   c. Subtypes (Castellvi classification)
   d. A fusion of the fifth lumbar vertebral body to the sacrum or separation of the first sacral segment (creating 6 rather than 5 lumbar segments); importance is identification of the correct level for spinal surgery

Spina bifida

General Characteristics

1. Failure of the neural tube to close during the fourth week of embryogenesis creates the most common severe birth defect in the USA
2. Incidence of approximately 1 in 2000 births
3. Spina bifida:
   a. A neural tube malformation that involves the spinal cord and vertebral arches
   b. Severe forms:

i There is protrusion of the spinal cord and or the meninges through a defect in the vertebral arch

Clinical Manifestations

1. Clinical features depend on the level of the defect
2. Spinal cord clinical symptomatology starts at the defect level and usually includes:
   a. Leg paralysis
   b. Urinary and fecal incontinence
   c. Anesthesia of the affected segment and below this level
   d. Orthopedic anomalies of the hips, knees and feet
   e. Associated neurological complications:
      i Hydrocephalus
      ii Arnold-Chiari type II malformations

Neuropathology

1. Mutations in the 5, 10-methylenetetrahydrofolate reductase (MTHFR) and dihydrofolate reductase (DHFR) genes have been linked to the disease
2. Disturbance of the development of the embryonic tail bud
3. Spinal cord abnormalities may include:
   a. Overdistension of the central canal
   b. Duplication or splitting of the spinal cord
   c. Diplomyelia or diastematomyelia
   d. Tethering of the sacral end of the spinal cord
4. Associated defects:
   a. Sacral agenesis
   b. Anorectal and urogenital system anomalies

Neuroimaging

1. Associated rarely with a subcutaneous mass, cutaneous hyperpigmentation over the defect
2. Lack of fusion of the laminae of one lumbar or sacral vertebra
3. Facet joint or pedicle anomalies that include:
   a. Asymmetry of facet joints
   b. Narrow lateral recess
   c. Short pedicles

Articular Facet Joint Anomalies

General Characteristics

1. Congenital absence of the lumbosacral articular facet joint is rare; the L5-S1 is affected in approximately 80% of patients
2. May be associated with conjoined nerve roots

Clinical Manifestations

1. May cause spinal instability
2. Conjoined nerve roots may be associated with clinical signs and symptoms referable to the involved roots

Neuropathology

1. Possible defect in a neural arch ossification center has been posited

Neuroimaging

1. Approximately 0.25% of patients may have conjoined nerve roots in the normal population; most commonly at L5-S1
2. Conjoined nerve roots have been reported with anomalies of the vertebral arch, spondylosis, spondylolisthesis and bifid sacrum
3. Myelography with CT:
   a. Absence of the facet joint
4. 3D-CT evaluation:
   a. Demonstrates the articular process
5. Rare congenital absence of the posterior elements of the spinal column have been reported

Congenital Scoliosis

General Characteristics

1. Congenital scoliosis is the failure of normal vertebral development during the 4th to 6th week of gestation

Clinical Manifestations

1. Radicular pain from nerve root entrapment
2. Pain occurs both on the convexity and concavity of the curve
3. Concavity pain is posited to be generated by impingement of the facets. This frequently occurs at the apex of the lumbar curves at L3-L4 or L2-L3
4. Spinal stenosis pain:
   a. Usually, it is present with lumbar or lumbosacral deformity
   b. Patients develop postural change. They lean forward, develop a flat back and slightly bend their knees with walking
5. Patients may also have radicular pain from spondylolisthesis and degenerative disc disease

Neuropathology

1. Scoliosis is a developmental defect in the formation of the mesenchymal component of the vertebrae
2. Failure of formation:
   a. A normal fully segmented hemivertebra (normal disc space above and below

b. Semisegmental hemivertebra:
c. The hemivertebra is fused to the adjacent disc on one side
d. In segmented hemivertebra:
e. The hemivertebra is fused to the vertebra on each side
f. An incarcerated hemivertebra:
g. The affected vertebra is fused within the lateral margins of the vertebrae above and below
h. Unincarcerated hemivertebra:
i. Laterally positioned
j. Wedged vertebra

3. Failure of Segmentation:
   a. Block vertebra:
      i Bilateral bony bars
   b. Bar body:
      i A unilateral unsegmented bar is common
4. Mixed:
   a. A unilateral unsegmented bar with contralateral hemivertebra
   b. Progresses the most rapidly
5. Associated conditions with congenital scoliosis:
   a. May occur in isolation
   b. Occur with systemic anomalies in approximately 60% of patients which include:
      i Cardiac defects – 10%
      ii Genitourinary defects – 25%
      iii Spinal cord malformations
      iv Associated syndromes that include:
         0 Alagille syndrome
         0 VACTERL syndrome
         0 Jarcho-Levin Syndrome / spondylocostal dysostosis
         0 Klippel-Feil syndrome

Laboratory Evaluation

1. Renal ultrasound or MRI
2. Echocardiogram

Neuroimaging

1. MRI:
   a. All patients with congenital scoliosis need evaluation of the complete neuroaxis to rule out associated anomalies that occur in 20-40% of patients and include:
      i Chiari malformations
      ii Tethered cord

- iii Syringomyelia
- iv Diastematomyelia
- v Intradural lipoma

2. 3DCT
   a. Best delineates posterior bony anatomy

Adult Scoliosis

General Characteristics

1. Definition: a spinal deformity with a Cobb angle of more than 10° in the coronal plane in a skeletally mature patient
2. Separated into 3 major categories:
   a. Type I (primary degenerative scoliosis):
      i Disc or facet joint arthritis that affects the spinal column asymmetrically
   b. Type II (idiopathic adolescent scoliosis) which progresses into adulthood:
      i Combined with secondary degenerations
      ii Surgical or no surgical treatment
   c. Type III (secondary adult curves) in addition to:
      i Oblique pelvis due to leg length differences or hip pathology
      ii Idiopathic, neuromuscular or congenital scoliosis
      iii Lumbosacral junction asymmetry

Clinical Manifestations

1. Similar radicular pain that is seen with congenital scoliosis
2. Severe pain from spondylolisthesis, spinal stenosis, degenerative disc disease and facet syndrome

Neuropathology

1. Scoliosis will develop in approximately 30% of patients ages 50-54 that have a greater than 10° curve
2. Degenerative spine pathologies
3. Rare spinal cord tumors that differentially involve the spinal cord with asymmetric destruction of anterior horn cells that innervate paraspinal muscles (C shaped curve)
4. Osteoporosis and osteomalacia with fractures and remodeling of bone
5. Degenerative translational vertebral shift with pelvic obliquity

Laboratory Evaluation

1. Measurement of metabolic bone disease to evaluate osteoporosis
2. Sed rate and C-reactive protein

Neuroimaging

1. Radiographs determine:

a. The pelvic incidence:
   i The angle of incidence is the algebraic sum of the pelvic tilt (PT) and the sacral slope (SS)
   ii The pelvis does not change after adolescence and directly influences pelvic alignment that include the parameters of pelvic tilt and sacral slope, sagittal spinal balance and lumbar lordosis
b. Prognostic features for curve progression include:
   i Increasing intervertebral disc degeneration
   ii An intercrest line through L5
   iii Apical lateral vertebral translation >6mm

2. MRI:
   a. Excellent for evaluation of disc and soft tissue degenerative changes
   b. Excellent delineation of nerve root exit impingement, subluxation and canal parameters
3. CT / myelography:
   a. Delineation of the continuity of the contrast column
   b. Flexion and extension views delineate dynamic changes associated with spinal stenosis
   c. Delineation of the dural sac

Lordosis

General Characteristics

1. Increased angulation of the spine

Clinical Manifestations

1. Posturally-induced low back pain
2. Radiculopathy at the segmental level (usually L3-L5)
3. Signs of central or lateral spinal stenosis
4. Neural claudication symptoms

Neuropathology

1. Increased compression of the apophyseal joints
2. Increased anterior shear force at the lumbosacral junction
3. Possible precursor to spondylolisthesis
4. In the context of metabolic bone disease (primarily osteoporosis) it is combined with asymmetric arthritic disease or vertebral fracture
5. Asymmetric degeneration leads to spinal load imbalance with bone remodeling and further degenerative changes
6. Destruction of facet joints, joint capsules, disc and ligaments
7. There is frequent multisegmental instability

Laboratory Evaluation

1. MRI and CT evaluation:
    a. Facet joint degenerative changes (hypertrophy and tropism); thickened ligaments
    b. Central and lateral spinal stenosis
    c. Disc desiccation with degeneration and loss of disc height
2. Measurement of the lordosis angles in relation to the superior most vertebra
3. A sharp angle of L5 in relation to S1; the closer the angle is to the 180° plane > traction on L4, L5 and the S1 nerve roots

Achondroplasia

General Characteristics

1. The most common form of nonlethal skeletal dysplasia
2. Genetics:
    a. Mutation of the fibroblast growth factor receptor 3-gene (FGF-R3) that maps to chromosome 4p16.3 and is autosomal dominant
3. Prevalence is 0.36 to 0.6 per 10,000 live births

Clinical Manifestations

1. Short stature
2. Disproportionately shorter limb bones
3. Narrow trunk
4. Macrocephaly
5. Prominent forehead and flattened midface
6. Short broad hands; trident fingers
7. Neurological complications:
    a. Cervicomedullary spinal cord compression (foramen magnum stenosis)
    b. Sleep apnea
    c. Disordered respiration
    d. Myelopathy
    e. Hydrocephalus
    f. Ligament laxity
8. General medical complications:
    a. Musculoskeletal
    b. Cardiorespiratory
    c. Ear, nose and throat
9. 80% of individuals are symptomatic by age 60
10. Radiculopathy with claudication (often due to spinal stenosis at T12-L1)
11. Compressive cervical myelopathy

Neuropathology

1. Narrow spinal canal
2. Short pedicles

3. Narrowed exit foramina
4. Block vertebra
5. Abnormal chondrocyte proliferation in the growth plate

Laboratory Evaluation

1. Sleep studies to evaluate disordered respiration and sleep apnea
2. MRI:
    a. Evaluation of the foramen magnum and T11-L1 spinal stenosis
    b. Congenital canal stenosis

Congenital Spinal Stenosis

General Characteristics

1. Developmental lumbar spinal stenosis is a maldevelopment primarily of the dorsal spinal elements:
    a. Short pedicles
    b. Trefoil bony spinal canal

Clinical Manifestations

1. Similar clinical symptomatology as acquired stenosis with neurogenic cauda equina claudication
2. Cervical and lower lumbar radicular pain
3. Presentation is at an earlier age than acquired forms
4. Subtle clinical signs of spondylosis

Neuropathology:

1. Multilevel involvement with L3, L4 and L5 levels most severely involved
2. Severe stenosis at L1, L2 and S1 is rare

Neuroimaging

1. MRI:
    a. Shorter pedicle length
    b. Smaller cross sectional spinal canal area
    c. Block vertebra
    d. Narrowed exit foramina

Lateral Recess Syndrome

General Characteristics

1. The lateral recess may be the principal site of pathology in lumbar canal stenosis
2. Anatomy:
    a. Bordered laterally by the pedicles, posteriorly by the superior articular facet and ligamentum flavum and anteriorly by the vertebral body, end-plate margin and disc margin

b. It is funnel shaped and is narrowest in its cranial extent at the superior portion of the pedicle.

Clinical Manifestations

1. Radicular signs and symptoms
2. If the compression is in the intervertebral foramen, extension of the trunk in conjunction with ipsilateral side bending and rotation reproduces the symptoms

Neuropathology

1. Two morphologic forms cause root compression in the lateral recess:
   a. A congenital trefoil-shaped lateral recess becomes smaller; the superior articular facet hypertrophies or the disc margin enlarges from an endplate spur or a disc bulge
   b. Angular pinch-like encroachment of the lateral margin of the canal from facet endplate and disc margin alterations
   c. Composition of osteophytes that cause lateral recess encroachment:
      iv Fibrous and hyaline cartilage and cancellous bone
      v Intramembranous bone formation possibly due to segmental instability

Neuroimaging

1. CT measurement of the posterior edge of the vertebral body and the anterior part of the articular facet in the pedicular slice at the level of the upper vertebral platform:
   a. Lateral recess stenosis occurs when the nerve root is trapped in the bony margins of the lateral recess or exit foramen
   b. Narrowing is diagnosed when the anterior-posterior dimension is below 4mm

Tethered Cord

General Characteristics

1. Traction of the conus medullaris and cauda equina by a tight thickened filum terminale
2. Two clinical categories:
   a. Asymptomatic in childhood and presents for the first time in adult life
   b. Patients with pre-existing static skeletal/neurologic abnormalities that progress in adult life

Clinical Manifestations

1. Pes cavus (uni or bilateral)
2. Cutaneous stigmata (strawberry hemangioma; cutaneous dimple) over the sacrum

3. Back pain; may have anal and perianal pain; genital or diffuse leg pain
4. Motor and sensory radicular deficits of lumbar and sacral roots
5. Sphincter alterations
6. Symptomatic with specific positions; particularly the dorsal lithotomy position
7. Symptomatic following delivery or vaginal surgery (primarily due to the dorsal lithotomy position)
8. Urodynamic features:
    a. Hyperreflexia of the bladder (neurogenic bladder)
    b. Internal and external detrusor dyssynergia
    c. Decreased bladder sensation and compliance
    d. Hypocontractility of the detrusor muscle
9. General hyperreflexia of both upper and lower extremities
10. Associations with tethered cord:
    a. Terminal syringomyelia (caudal 1/3 of the spinal cord)
    b. Diastematomyelia
    c. Lipoma of the conus and lipomyeloschisis
    d. Unilateral pes cavus

Neuropathology

1. Combination of thickening of the filum terminale with:
    a. Low or dilated conus medullaris
    b. Spinal lipoma
    c. Dermoid cyst
    d. Diastematomyelia
    e. Hydromyelia
    f. Sacral agenesis

Neuroimaging

1. MRI:
    a. a. Tethered cord; tip of the conus medullaris is below the body of L2 instead of the L1-L2 disc space
    b. b. Most commonly associated with intra or extradural lipoma

Classification of Lumbosacral Nerve Root Anomalies with a Tethered Cord

1. Type I and II:
    a. One or more nerve roots exit the thecal sac at a more cranial (Type I) or caudal (Type II) level
2. Type III:
    a. Two or more nerve roots emerge from the thecal sac through a closely adjacent dural opening

3. Type IV:
   a. Two or more roots emerge from the dural sac as one nerve trunk
4. Type V:
   a. Two or more nerve roots are connected by an anastomotic branch after exiting the dural sac

Clinical Characteristics of Congenital Nerve Root Anomalies

1. Anomalies occur primarily at L4-L5
2. 20% of patients have other lumbosacral anomalies; rarely congenital absence of a facet joint on the side of the anomaly
3. They may be asymptomatic
4. May be associated with failure of back surgery for herniated disc or spondylosis as they are less mobile
5. In association with lumbar spondylosis and foraminal stenosis
   a. The affected roots are compressed between the transverse process of the last lumbar segment and sacral ala (S1) or in various relationships to the inner side of the pedicle and facet joint
6. Conjoined lumbosacral roots:
   a. Are found in approximately 1% of lumbar disc operations
   b. Most often at L5-S1
   c. Often not associated with a herniated disc

Conjoined Nerve Roots

General Characteristics

1. Two adjacent nerve roots that share a common dural envelope during their course from the dural sac
2. The incidence by CT, MRI and myelography vary widely 2-17% in patients studied with spine imaging

Clinical Manifestations

1. Straight leg raising test may be negative:
   a. A distinguishing clinical feature from disc herniation
2. Usual presentation is sciatic pain
3. The L5 and S1 roots are most frequently involved. L4 and L5 are next in frequency
4. Claudication pain rather than that of a fixed radiculopathy; radicular symptoms with rest pain are more common with disc herniation
5. Neurologic deficits (motor and sensory) are more common with disc disease

Neuropathology

1. The dorsal roots may be more commonly involved than the ventral roots
2. Bifurcation occurs close to the intervening pedicles; they then enter their

respective foramina

3. Abnormal root anastomosis is caused from a connection of a band of nerve fibers or a distal union in a common sheath
4. There is decreased mobility of the root which increases its risk of neuropractic or direct injury during neurosurgical procedures

Neuroimaging

1. 1. Features typical of conjoined roots include:
   a. a. MRI:
      i Equal density of the nerve root anomaly and the thecal sac
   b. Asymmetry of the subarachnoid space (pouching out) in the axial view at the level of the anomaly that may be above the intervertebral disc space
   c. Possible specific MRI signs:
      i Asymmetric morphology of the anterolateral corner of the dural sac
      ii Intervening extradural fat between the asymmetric dura and the nerve root
      iii Visualization of the entire course of the nerve root at the disc level
      iv Focal lateral recess and foraminal stenosis

Lumbar Synovial Cysts

General Characteristics

1. Lumbar synovial cysts arise from the zygapophyseal joint capsule
2. "Juxtafacet cysts" (also encompasses ganglion cyst) are similar clinically but differ histologically and may represent a spectrum of the same degenerative process
3. Possibly a cause of 1% of patients with low back pain
4. The greatest prevalence is in the seventh decade of life

Clinical Manifestations

1. The majority of spinal synovial cysts are at the L4-L5 level
2. Cysts may be asymptomatic
3. Present with radicular pain, neurogenic claudication or cauda equina syndrome
4. Back pain usually precedes compression symptoms
5. Myelopathy symptoms have been reported in cysts above L1-L2

Neuropathology

1. The synovial cysts have a lining of synovial cells and arise from the facet joint

Neuroimaging

1. MRI:
   a. The modality of choice; it has a 90% sensitivity compared to 70% with CT scanning

2. Low intensity signal on T1 weighted images and high-intensity signal on T2-weighted sequences. The signal varies depending on the concentration of proteinaceous material or blood in the cyst
3. Adhesion of a lumbar synovial cyst to the dura can cause a dural tear with a subsequent CSF fistula

Ligamentum Flavum Cyst

General Characteristics

1. Aging of the ligamentum flavum is associated with thickening and loss of elasticity
2. Most ligamentum flavum cysts are located laterally within the spinal canal
3. It is a well-defined elastic structure that is composed of 80% elastic and 20% collagen fibers rarely seen in other ligaments
4. Intraspinal ligamentum cysts primarily are found in the lower lumbar area at L4-L5 and may be associated with degenerative spondylolisthesis

Clinical Manifestations

1. The majority of symptomatic cysts present with radicular symptoms that mimic disc disease
2. Spinal stenosis

Neuropathology

1. Cysts of the ligamentum flavum are embedded in the inner surface of the ligament and are not related to the facet joint
2. Pathogenesis is posited to occur from ligamentous and fibro-collagenous degeneration
3. There are changes in proteoglycans, loss of elastic fibers, an increase in collagen tissue and mucinoid degeneration in the ligament
4. The cysts may hemorrhage due to mechanical stress

Neuroimaging

1. MRI:
    a. The modality of choice; on T1-weighted sequences they have variable signal intensity
    b. T2-weighted sequences demonstrate high signal intensity
2. Synovial cysts may have a calcified rim that does not occur with ligamentum flavum cysts
3. The CT characteristics of synovial cysts are:
    a. Cystic formation that may have a calcified wall
    b. They are located adjacent to facet joints
    c. Often demonstrate degeneration
4. CT characteristics:

a. The cysts are adjacent to the ligamentum flavum
b. Rarely demonstrate intraluminal hemorrhage
c. Calcium pyrophosphate crystals have been demonstrated in the ligament in patients with radicular pain

Differential diagnosis of intraspinal cysts

1. Juxta-articular cysts (ganglion and synovial cysts)
2. Ligamentum flavum cysts
3. Arachnoid cysts
4. Perineurial cysts
5. Dermoid cyst
6. Infectious cyst
7. Granuloma
8. Intraligamentous amyloid deposition
9. Ossification
10. Juxta facet joint cysts

Perineural Cysts (Tarlov cyst)

General Characteristics

1. Naba classification:
    a. The cysts are located in the perineural space between the endoneurium and perineurium
    b. Type I cyst:
        i Extradural meningeal cyst without spinal nerve root fibers
        ii Type II
            1. Spinal extradural meningeal cyst with spinal nerve roots
        iii Type III
            1. Spinal intradural meningeal cysts
2. Cystic dilatations of the lumbosacral roots at or distal to the junction of the posterior root or DRG
3. Incidence in adults is between 4-9%; there is no sex predilection
4. CSF filled

Clinical Manifestations

1. Most often, they are asymptomatic
2. A ball valve mechanism from hydrodynamic CSF forces causes the perineural cyst to fill with CSF and expand, which may cause:
    a. Back pain
    b. Radicular pain
    c. Rarely, bowel and bladder dysfunction
    d. Leg weakness
    e. Sexual dysfunction

f. Infertility

Neuropathology

1. The cysts are frequently multiple
2. Arachnoidal proliferation around the lumbosacral involved root
3. Putative absence of dura mater during development
4. Possible hemorrhage with hemosiderin deposition leading to venous drainage into the perineurium
5. Lining of the cyst contains nerve fibers and or ganglion cells; they have a synovial lining; pseudo-stratified columnar epithelium

Neuroimaging

1. MRI
   a. Fluid filled lesion with low signal on T1-weighted sequences and high signal in T2 weighted images
2. May erode bone; particularly prominent with sacral cysts
3. There may be communication of the cysts with the subarachnoid space

Disc Disease

L1-L2 Disc Space

General Characteristics

1. L5-S1 herniations is the most common level of herniation followed by L4-L5 > L3-L4 > L1- L2 (rare)
2. L5-S1 is the primary motion segment of the lumbosacral spine while L5 is the primary load segment. If there is fusion of L5-S1, then L4-L5 becomes the primary motion segment
3. Primary causes of disc herniation are not clear:
   a. Degeneration of the annulus, the nucleus pulposus, and the posterior longitudinal ligament has been posited. Rarely acute flexion injuries seem a likely cause of annulus pulposus tear.
4. Nucleus pulposus fragments generally extend through degenerated areas of the annulus most often dorsolaterally and asymmetrically. Central and medial protrusions may involve descending nerve roots prior to their entering the exit foramina. A far lateral protrusion compresses a single root at that level. Thus, a lateral protrusion at the interspace between L4-L5 will involve the L5 root. The L4 root is spared as it exits above the protrusion. A medial protrusion at L4-L5 may involve the L5 root as well as sacral roots S1-S2 prior to their exit
5. The affected interspace may be mechanically sensitive to pressure. There may be a slight decrease of sensation 1½ inch laterally from the corresponding spinous process. The dorsal rami syndrome (discussed below) may be

prominent

6. Mechanical stretch maneuvers are positive and exacerbated by Lasegue's maneuvers. This involves extension of the ankle with the leg extended
7. Tinel's signs are positive over the nerve that carries the affected roots. Tinel's sign (mechanical pressure on the nerve elicits pain) is positive in the sciatic notch and posterior popliteal fossa with L5-S1 root involvement
8. There is muscle tenderness of those muscles that are innervated by the sensitized roots (usually elicited by moderate squeezing). The root compression by the extruded disc material sensitizes the deep polymodal C-fiber and A-delta fiber afferent nociceptors such that mechanical pressure rather than tissue-destructive stimuli will depolarize them.
9. Pain radiations are consistent but most often consist of a combination of dermatome and sclerotome patterns. The latter (pain from structures of the embryonic somite-vertebrae, facet joints and their capsules, periosteum, ligaments) often activates structures not often thought of as emanating from the affected roots
10. Bilateral symptoms and sphincter (overwhelmingly bladder) dysfunction most often occur with large midline disc extrusion that compresses the cauda equina

L2-L3 Disc Space

1. L3 root affected
2. Pain:
    a. Anterior thigh
    b. Top of the knee
3. Weakness of thigh adductors, quadriceps and iliopsoas muscles
4. Decreased knee jerk

L3-L4 Disc Space

1. L4 root affected
2. Pain:
    a. Anterolateral thigh
    b. Medial leg below the knee
3. Weakness of the anterior tibialis; at times partial foot drop
4. 4. Knee jerk decreased

L4-L5 Disc Space

1. L5 root affected
2. Pain:
    a. Posterolateral gluteal area, lateral thigh, lateral leg below the knee, dorsal foot to the lateral malleolus, great toe and 2nd and 3rd toes
3. Extensor halluces longus; extensor digitorum, anterior tibialis, muscle

weakness

4. Reflex – decreased posterior tibial

Additional Radiations of L5 (Sclerotomal) and Signs

1. Hip
2. Top of the thigh:
   a. Somatic referred pain possibly from the innervations of the annulus fibrosis (controversial mechanism but the radiation is helpful)
3. Dural innervations at L5; the innervations of the recurrent nerve of Spurling at this level
4. Scrotum
5. Rarely the anterior lower abdominal wall
6. Weakness of the extensor hallucis longus, extensor digitorum brevis, and anterior tibialis that cause partial foot drop. There is also weakness of invertors of the foot which does not occur in the foot drop of peroneal palsy
7. Ankle jerk is unaffected
8. Straight leg raising test and its variants are positive. Irritation of nociceptive afferents in the affected root or its sleeve synapse with Rexed layer VII interneurons that then depolarize Rexed layer IX flexor motor neurons that elicit hamstring muscle contraction, which halts the further extension of the leg. This comprises a nocifensive reflex.
9. Chronic disc disease causes atrophy of the anterior tibialis and the extensor digitorum brevis
10. Tenderness with compression over the fourth lumbar lateral process and between the fourth and fifth spinous space, the ligaments and laterally in the sciatic notch

L5-S1 Disc Space

1. The S1 root is affected
2. Classic pain radiations:
   a. Mid gluteus maximus pain
   b. Tenderness in the sciatic notch, posterior thigh, posterolateral leg, lateral foot, heel and lateral toes.
   c. Especially helpful is the radiation to the little toe.
   d. Low calf dull pain to the heel.
3. Unusual pain radiations of S1 (components of the sclerotomal innervations):
   a. Groin
   b. Tip of the penis
   c. Ipsilateral vaginal wall
   d. Anus (controversial as there is evidence that this is an S5 root territory)
4. Weakness of plantar flexors, hamstring muscles, and flexion of the toes; abductor digiti (V^{th} metatarsal)

5. Depressed or absent ankle jerk
6. Positive straight leg raising test; tenderness of the sciatic notch, posterior popliteal fossa, and pain elicited by squeezing the gastrocnemius muscle; tenderness over the L5-S1 interspace; increased pain with walking on the heels but more difficulty walking on the toes due to plantar flexor muscle weakness.

Visceral Association with L4, L5, and S1 Root Disease

1. Increased frequency of micturition
2. Slight decrease of bladder emptying (30cc residual urine) with S1 disease
3. Increased pain during menstruation (sciatic radiations). Convergent innervations from the uterus, fallopian tubes and ovary to L5, S1 DRG (somatic-visceral convergence) cause pain in these distributions

Exacerbating Factors for L4-S1 Radicular Pain

1. Flexion and extension posture; sitting; driving a car
2. Valsalva maneuvers
3. Sleep (veins that overlie the root compress the sensitized root; patients awaken with back pain at 4-5 AM. Inability to lie down suggests intraspinal cord tumor (patients sleep upright in a chair). Awakening slightly earlier at night (3-4 AM) suggests a subarachnoid cyst that compresses the spinal cord.
4. The leg feels as if it will suddenly "give way" and will not support the patient's body weight when walking.

Relieving Factors for L5-S1 Disc Disease

1. Rest; supine position with flexed knees (pillow behind the knees)
2. Heat over the affected interspace
3. Some patients improve with exercise (heat may decrease conduction in sensitized pain nerve roots)

Extreme Lateral Disc Protrusion

1. Unremitting radicular pain without concomitant back pain (proximal portion of the intervertebral exit canal).
2. Pain is increased with extension and torsion toward the side of the extrusion
3. Intradural disc rupture with a free fragment may not cause sciatic pain, as it may not impinge upon the cauda equina roots.

Lower Sacral Radiculopathy

1. Usually, S2-S5 roots are involved concomitantly often from a large central disc herniation
2. Pain and sensory loss may be prominent in the perineal area:
   a. Usually asymmetrically
   b. "Saddle anesthesia."
   c. Prominent pain and numbness may also occur over the gluteus maximus,

posterior thigh and if S1 is involved the calf and heel
3. Urinary incontinence and retention; rarely fecal incontinence
4. Loss of ankle jerks
5. Varying degrees of paraparesis
6. Severe back pain
7. Reduced or absent anal sphincter tone; decreased bulbocavernosus and anal wink reflexes with S1-S5 lesions

High Lumbar Root Disease

In general, the L1-L3 roots are not affected by disc disease, as they are not motion segments.

They are involved by:

1. Diabetic plexopathy
2. Ilioinguinal neuropathy
3. Genitofemoral nerve injury from:
   a. Surgical procedures (hernia, catheterization of the femoral artery) and intra-abdominal surgical procedures
   b. Lymphoma
   c. Retroperitoneal hematoma
   d. Autoimmune processes.
4. Rarely the roots are involved in high impact injuries (MVA accidents, falls, and skiing injuries).
5. Differential diagnosis includes:
   a. Lumbosacral plexopathy and medical causes of radiculopathy:
      i Metastasis
      ii Autoimmune disorders
      iii Metabolic disorders (diabetes mellitus)
      iv Infectious diseases (HIV, CMV, and brucellosis)

Posterior Rami Syndrome

1. Also known as Maignes Syndrome or the dorsal ramus syndrome
2. Is due to activation or irritation of the primary division of a posterior ramus of a spinal nerve
3. Referred pain occurs in a tri-branched pattern at L5-S1:
   a. Innervation of the groin or pubic region
   b. Innervation of the lower back and upper gluteal region
   c. Anterolateral thigh or trochanteric area
   d. The affected posterior ramus ends cutaneously and may cause trophic skin changes:
      v Thickening or nodularity of the skin
      vi Hair loss

vii Neurogenic edema

e. These are sclerotomal radiations and thus can originate from several levels. Patients should have facet and spinous processes palpated over a wide area.

Sequestered Disc Fragments

General Characteristics

1. Sequestered intervertebral disc fragments are able to migrate both intra and extradurally within the spinal canal
2. Free disc fragments are often misinterpreted as a neoplastic mass
3. Unusual sequestered disc fragments have an incidence of 0.4%

Clinical Manifestations

1. Posterior epidural migration of a lumbar disc fragment:
    a. 78% male and 22% female; 37 and 10 patients respectively in one series
    b. Mean age 54 years
    c. Cauda equina compression in 46%
    d. Sciatic or anterior thigh pain in 40%
    e. 57% were localized to high lumbar areas

Neuropathology

1. Fibrocartilage with degenerative features that include:
    a. Increased chondrocyte density
    b. Mucoid degeneration
    c. Vascular proliferation and granular change
2. Anatomical barriers that limit disc fragment migration include:
    a. Sagittal midline septum (septum posticum) that is between the vertebral body and the posterior longitudinal ligaments (prevents the movement of the disc fragment across the midline)
    b. Peridural or lateral membrane which is posterolateral and attaches to the free edge of the PLL which restricts posterior migration of a free disc fragment

Neuroimaging (Disc Fragment)

1. MRI:
    a. Disc fragments may show different patterns of contrast enhancement
    b. There may be no disc space protrusion
    c. Peripheral enhancement of the disc fragment is due to the inflammatory response with vascular granulation tissue at the disc periphery

Neuropathology of Intervertebral Disc Disease

1. Factors involved in the initiation and progression of disc disease include:
    a. Age

   b. Abnormalities of load
   c. Decreased nutrient supply
   d. Hereditary
2. The change of the cellular microenvironment with disc degeneration includes:
   a. Loss of proteoglycan
   b. Loss of disc height
   c. Tears in the annulus fibrosus
   d. Associated spinal stenosis
   e. Neoinnervation
   f. Hypermobility of the affected segment
   g. Inflammation
3. Nerve fibers are found in the inner layers of the annulus fibrosus and nucleus pulposus in patients with low back pain. Innervation of the inner disc is only seen in painful discs and not normal discs
4. In patients disc lesions normally occur in the posterior portion of the disc
5. Recent studies in human prolapsed disc material have demonstrated upregulation in IL-2.
6. IL-2 promotes extracellular matrix degradation as well as:
   a. Increased expression of type I collagen
   b. It is a disintegrin
   c. Metalloproteinase with thrombospondin motifs and matrix metalloproteinases
   d. IL-2 decreases aggrecan and type II collagen expression levels
   e. It is posited that nucleus pulposus inflammatory cytokines are severely toxic to both disc cells and nerve fibers
   f. 759 proteins from the annulus fibrosus and 692 proteins from the nucleus pulposis have been identified in the proteome map of these tissues. 73 annulus proteins and 54 proteins from the nucleus pulposis are differentially regulated from normal discs and those that are degenerated
   g. The differentially expressed proteins are components of cell adhesion, cell migration and interleukin 13 signaling pathways

Neuroimaging

1. MRI:
   a. Delineates the herniated nucleus pulposis (HNP). It is a focal, asymmetric protrusion of disc material beyond the annulus. The HNP is most often hypointense
   b. High intensity signal may be seen in the posterior annulus on T2 weighted sequences
   c. Sagittal MRI delineates the relationship between the HNP, abnormal facets to exiting nerve roots within the neural foraminal exit canals

   d. Delineates sequestered disc fragments
2. CT:
   a. Is utilized in patients who are unable to undergo MRI due to a pacemaker or other internally implanted metal
   b. In subligamentous herniation, HNP is a smooth displacement of the disk margin into the neural foramen or the spinal canal. It effaces the epidural fat and displaces the dural sac
3. Myelography with CT delineates the relationship between the nerve root sleeve and the nerve itself to surrounding bony structures

Spondylolysis

General Characteristics

1. A congenital bony defect in the pars interarticularis (the junction of the pedicle with the lamina; often bound by cartilage)
2. Frequently encountered in young athletic patients but may be seen at all ages
3. A predisposition to fracture or disjunction with slight trauma or repetitive motion

Clinical Manifestations

1. May be asymptomatic in many patients
2. Spinal instability
3. Atrophy of the gluteal muscles if associated with spondylolisthesis
4. Local back pain at the level of involvement
5. Radiculopathy

Neuropathology

1. Developmental or acquired stress fracture often secondary to low-grade trauma
2. Classification:
   a. Type 1:
      i Congenital abnormality of L5 or the upper sacrum with displacement of the L5 vertebra on the sacrum
   b. Type 2 (isthmic):
      i A stress fracture of the pars interarticularis (fatigue fracture IIA); elongation IIB or acute fracture (IIC)
   c. Type 3 (degenerative)
      i Remodeling of the articular processes
   d. Type 4 (traumatic)
      i Acute fracture of the vertebral arch that may occur separately from the pars
   e. Type 5 (pathologic)
      i Generalized or focal bone disease that affects the vertebral arch

Neuroimaging

1. CT:
    a. Multislice CT with multiplanar reformatting is effective for detecting the bony defect. It is not sensitive for delineating early edema without a fracture line
2. MRI:
    a. Excellent for the detection of early bone marrow edema when a visible fracture line is not detected
    b. May identify associated nerve root compression

Spondylolisthesis

General Characteristics

1. Spondylolisthesis is the forward translation of one vertebral body over its inferior one
2. Bilateral spondylolysis predisposes to spondylolisthesis. The vertebral body, pedicles, and superior facets slip forward. The degree of slippage is usually graded by the percentage of displacement relative to the lower vertebra
3. Slippage in non-severe traumatic patients is L5 over S1 or L4 over L5
4. There may be progression of spondylolysis to spondylolisthesis occurs in adult patients
5. Low grade spondylolisthesis is less than or equal to 50% of the inferior vertebra; high grade spondylolisthesis is greater than 50% slippage (almost always requires surgical correction)
6. Average age of adult spondylolisthesis patients (>21 years of age) in a retrospective review with grade III, IV or V was 35 years (range 21 – 88 years)

Clinical Manifestations

1. Atrophy of the gluteal muscles innervated by L4, L5, S1
2. Weakness of the gluteus maximus, anterior tibialis, extensor hallucis longus is often prominent
3. Radicular pain occurs most often in L4-S1 distributions
4. Flexion and extension maneuvers are painful; patients have pain on standing rather than sitting (more common with discogenic disease) and are unable to wear high heels
5. Rare bladder involvement

Neuropathology

1. Types I-V (dependent on the degree of slippage)
2. Congenital hypoplasia of the pedicle
3. High grade dysplastic isthmic spondylolisthesis

Neuroimaging

1. Rare patients described with 2 DCT have congenital hypoplasia of the lumbosacral pedicles (pediatric)
2. Spondyloptosis:
   a. 100% subluxation of a superior vertebral body over its inferior one
   b. Spinal segment is lodged in the anterior or posterior space of the adjacent segment
   c. Complete disruption of structural elements of the vertebral column and the adjacent paravertebral soft tissues (associated with severe neurologic deficits)
   d. CT scan:
      i A horizontal oriented defect in the pars interarticularis that interrupts the complete bony ring of the posterior elements
      ii Demonstrates degenerative bony changes, congenital and dysplastic forms of the disease
   e. MRI scanning:
      i High signal intensity in the pars interarticularis on T2 weighted sequences that indicates fluid, a pseudoarthrosis or bone edema
      ii Lumbar paraspinal muscle morphometry in adult isthmic spondylolisthesis:
         1. Patients demonstrated higher cross-sectional areas (CSAs) of the erector spinae muscle; the multifidus (MF) had lower (dCSA) in patients than controls
         2. Posited that isthmic spondylolisthesis have selective atrophy of the multifidus muscle and compensatory hypertrophy of the erector spinae muscles

Spinal Stenosis

General Characteristics

1. Spinal stenosis refers to degenerative changes in bone, joints, and ligaments of the spine that narrow the spinal canal. These changes reach clinical significance more rapidly if there is congenital canal narrowing and small intervertebral foramina
2. Compression of lumbar and sacral roots are a consequence of these degenerative changes

Clinical Manifestations

1. Fluctuating aching and lancinating pain in the buttock, sciatic nerve distributions
2. Pain is exacerbated by prolonged sitting (>30-45 minutes) standing or walking (2-3 blocks). There is relief with rest. Severe patients have constant pain, but obtain some relief with a change in posture.

3. "Neurogenic claudication" causes:
    a. Gradual onset of weakness and heaviness of the legs associated with walking often associated with asymmetrical buttock and calf pain (neurogenic cramps" or "Charlie horse")
    b. Pain is relieved with rest. It is a deep ache rather than a squeezing burning sensation
    c. The numbness may begin in one leg, spread to the other and ascend if walking or exercise continues
    d. If the condition is severe patients may attain relief by squatting, lying flat with the legs flexed at the hips and knees (opens up the canal)
    e. Posture is forward flexed at the hip; the swing phase of gait may be restricted
    f. Rare urinary incontinence and impotence
    g. There are often concomitant cervical degenerative changes that compress the spinal cord such that knee and ankle reflexes are preserved. Ankle reflexes may be lost with exercise but return with rest
    h. Degenerative spondylolisthesis with pain radiating into the thighs with flexion and extension of the spine occurs if the slippage is at L4 over L5 or L5 over S1. The involved root compression causes paresthesia, sensory loss, weakness, and reflex loss.
    i. Lumbar stenosis has been associated with the syndrome of painful legs – moving toes which causes:
        i Burning lower leg pain
        ii Sinusoidal rhythmic toe movements that most often begin asymmetrically but may spread to the contralateral extremity

Neuropathology

1. The spinal roots are compressed by the vertebral body anteriorly, the facet joints laterally and the ligamentum flavum posteriorly
2. Spondylolisthesis increases the stenosis in the anteroposterior dimension
3. A spinal root may be compressed by "tropism" of a degenerated facet, overgrowth of an inferior or superior facet, against the floor of the intervertebral canal

Neuroimaging

1. MRI:
    a. Patients have a shorter pedicle length which causes a smaller cross-sectional spinal canal area (pedicle length of 6.5 mm and cross-sectional area of 213 mm)
    b. The canal stenosis is distributed uniformly throughout the lumbar spine in congenital spinal stenosis
    c. Degenerative spinal stenosis:

i Protrusion of discs at affected levels
ii Facet hypertrophy
iii Hypertrophy of the ligamentum flavum
iv CSA (cross-sectional area) of the dural sac is often less than 80 mm^2
v Associated degenerative spondylolisthesis
vi Narrowed nerve root foramina
vii Nerve root sedimentation sign:
1. A positive sign is the absence of nerve roots sinking to the dorsal portion of the dural sac

Coccydynia

General Characteristics

1. Coccydynia or coccygodynia definition:
    a. A painful syndrome in the region of the coccyx
2. The coccyx is composed of 3-5 vertebrae some of which may be fused
3. It attaches to the sacrum from two dorsal grooves being either a symphysis or as a true synovial joint
4. It has attachments to the gluteus maximus, the coccygeal muscle and the ano-coccygeal ligament

Clinical Manifestations

1. Pain at the end of the spine exacerbated by mechanical stimuli such as sitting, bicycling, rowing and riding
2. Patients may have L4-S1 root radiations (particularly in younger patients)
3. If roots are compromised, a pelvic tilt and atrophy of the gluteus muscle may be present

Neuropathology

1. Fracture, subluxation from mechanical trauma
2. Abnormal mobility
3. Disc degeneration at sacrococcygeal and intercoccygeal segments
4. Coccygeal spicule (bony excrescence)
5. Rare osteomyelitis or tumor
6. Extracoccygeal disorders that can cause coccygeal pain include:
    a. Pilonidal cysts
    b. Perianal abscess
    c. Hemorrhoids
    d. Radiations from nerve root involvement of the lumbosacral spine, sacro-iliac joints, piriformis muscle and involvement of the sacrum (metastasis)
    e. Visceral involvement of pelvic organs

Neuroimaging

1. Lateral x-ray of the coccyx in the standing and sitting position:
    a. Hypermobility
    b. Fracture
    c. Subluxation
    d. Metastasis
    e. Osteomyelitis
2. MRI:
    a. Disc abnormalities; extrusion of the nucleus pulposis or endplate abnormality
    b. Abnormalities of the coccyx tip that are located in the surrounding soft tissue and include:
        i Venous dilatations
        ii Soft tissue inflammation
        iii Vertebral bone edema

Facet Syndrome

General Characteristics

1. Lumbar zygapophyseal or "facet joint" pain is a major cause of chronic low back pain
2. Osteoarthritic degeneration causes irritation of the nociceptors that innervate the synovial membrane, hyaline cartilage, bone or fibrous capsule of the facet joint
3. Afferents from the facet joint are carried by the medial branch of the dorsal rami of the nerve root

Clinical Manifestations

1. Low back and radicular pain that is most often unilateral
2. Component of spinal stenosis pain
3. The pain is not relieved by position change
4. The pain is exacerbated by stress on the facet joint caused by retro- or lateral flexion of the spine; at the time the pain may be exacerbated by standing or walking

Neuropathology

1. Osteoarthritic degeneration of the joint with bony hypertrophy

Neuroimaging

1. It is controversial whether tropism, an asymmetry in orientation of a facet (rotates into or compresses the intervertebral foramen) is a preexisting developmental phenomenon or is secondary to progressive remodeling of the joint
2. Tropism may increase disc degeneration and degenerative spondylolisthesis

Lumbosacral Trauma

Acute Sprain and Strain

General Characteristics

1. Sprains are ligamentous injuries that are most often the result of a sudden extremely forceful muscle contraction or trauma
2. Strains are partial or complete tears of the muscle – tendon unit most often from a violent muscle contraction

Clinical Manifestations

1. When there is severe pain and paraspinal muscle spasm, the segmental nerve roots or their terminals may have been over stretched or otherwise injured
2. Recurrent aching pain in lumbar areas. Rarely there may be radiation into the buttocks and posterior thigh (never below the knee)
3. No weakness, sensory loss or reflex changes
4. Complaints of stiffness that are aggravated by specific movements
5. Range of motion particularly in flexion is decreased and painful

Neuropathology

1. Acute trauma does not cause degenerative disc or bony structural disease (in the course of repetitive movement, it may be by means of the molecular mechanisms that trigger bone remodeling). It may exacerbate pain by nerve root compression against osteophytes in foraminal canals, increasing the bulge of an annulus fibrosa or mechanically stimulating the nervi-nervorum of the nerve sheath and root sleeves or the A-delta and C-fibers within the nerve sheath.
2. The lumbar spine and the hips are extensively involved in spine mobility; L4 and L5-S1 bear the highest loads and are the primary motion segments. They are most often involved in sprain and strain spinal injury
3. Load-bearing sprain and strain injuries most often occur during the most forceful coupling patterns as exemplified by lateral bending with flexion-extension and axial rotation with lateral bending.
4. The translatory and rotary stability of the spine is maintained by the ligaments. Specific ligaments may contribute more to the translator or rotary component of spinal stability depending on loading characteristics
5. The strength of a ligament is proportional to its cross-sectional area; in general, a ligament with greater cross-sectional area provides a greater component of stability and is displaced less during physiological loading
6. All major ligaments may be involved either by severe direct trauma or repetitive motion. They include:
   a. The anterior and posterior longitudinal ligaments
   b. Ligamentum flavum

c. Intertransversal capsular ligaments
d. Capsula ligaments
e. Interspinous ligaments
f. Supraspinosus ligaments

7. The posterior ligaments are most frequently injured

Neuroimaging

1. CT and MRI:
   a. To rule out disc or nerve root involvement

Vertebral Fractures (Lumbar)

Overview

The lumbar spine is comprised of a mobile segment of five vertebrae between primarily immobile thoracic and sacral segments. The rib cage and intercostal musculature stabilize the thoracic spine, while the sacral segment is stabilized by its attachment to the ilium. Lumbar vertebrae are longer and heavier than those of the thoracic and cervical spine, and other distinguishing features from these spinal segments include:

1. Shorter and heavier pedicles
2. More laterally and ventrally projecting transverse processes, and
3. The spinous processes are broader and stronger.

During flexion, there is compression of the intervertebral disc anteriorly and the spinal canal is widened. Sliding occurs laterally in the articular process of the zygapophyseal joints. Flexion is restricted by the posterior ligamentous complex and the dorsal spinal musculature. Extension of the lumbar spine causes posterior compression of the disc and narrowing of the spinal canal associated with sliding movement of the zygapophyseal joint. Extension is limited by the anterior longitudinal ligament, ventral spinal musculature and the lamina and spinous processes.

Lateral bending compresses the disc on the concave side and separates the zygapophyseal joint associated with the over-riding of the joint on the concave side. Lateral bending is limited by the intertransverse ligaments.

Rotation of the lumbar spine compresses annulus fibrosus fibers of the intervertebral discs and is restricted by the facet joints and the iliolumbar ligaments.

Lumbar Vertebral Fractures

General Characteristics

1. The National Spinal Cord Injury Registry report shows that:
   a. 40% of spinal injuries are caused by motor vehicle accidents
   b. 20% by falls
   c. 40% by gunshot wounds, during contact sports, industrial and agricultural accidents

Clinical Manifestations

1. Patients present with severe pain, muscle spasm, deformity and neurologic deficits related to the level of injury
2. Fractures of the thoracolumbar junction frequently cause conus medullaris and lumbar nerve root damage.
3. Fractures that compress the conus medullaris cause:
   a. Paralysis of pelvic floor muscles
   b. Autonomous neurogenic bladder
   c. Constipation
   d. Impaired erectile and ejaculation function
   e. Asymmetric saddle anesthesia
4. Complete damage to the sacral spinal cord causes:
   a. Loss of bowel and bladder control
   b. Paralysis of sacrally innervated muscles of the lower extremity; often higher lumbar roots are concomitantly damaged that allows some flexion at the hip and partial flexion and extension at the knee with preserved knee reflexes. Sensation in lumbar dermatomes may be preserved.
5. Lower lumbar fractures cause solitary or multiple root deficits. A cauda equina syndrome may occur in the face of central disc herniation, fracture-dislocation and burst fractures.

Cauda Equina Syndrome Clinical Features

1. Compression of the lumbar and sacral roots below the L3 vertebral level
2. Radicular pain in lumbosacral root distributions; it is often asymmetric and unilateral and is increased with Valsalva maneuvers
3. There is flaccid, hypotonic and areflexic paralysis in:
   a. Glutei muscles
   b. Posterior thigh muscles
   c. Anterolateral muscles of the leg and foot
4. Asymmetric sensory loss in the saddle distribution. This involves the anal, perineal and genital regions and may extend to the anterolateral leg and lateral foot
5. The Achilles reflex (primarily S1-S2 segments) is lost and there is variable decrease of the patellar reflex (L2-L4).
6. Sphincter involvement is similar to that which occurs with conus medullaris lesions

Differential Points between Conus Medullaris and Cauda Equina Lesions

1. Cauda Equina:
   a. Early pain
   b. Late sphincter involvement

   c. Asymmetrical sensory examination
2. Conus Medullaris:
   a. Early and severe sphincter and sexual dysfunction
   b. Late pain
   c. More symmetrical sensory loss

Neuropathology

1. Specific fractures:
   a. "Burst" fracture of a vertebral body
   b. Pedicle, laminar or spinous process may be asymmetrically fractured
   c. Loss of height of a vertebral body by wedge or compression forces
2. If the patient falls and lands on his feet, calcaneal and hip fractures may be associated

Neuroimaging

1. Plain radiography determines:
   a. Alignment
   b. Identification of vertebral body margins
   c. The spinolaminar line
   d. Articular facet joints
   e. Interspinous distance
   f. Position of the transverse processes
   g. Oblique views for:
      i Pars interarticularis fractures
      ii Facet subluxation
   h. Abnormalities of alignment include:
      i Disruption of the anterior or posterior vertebral body lines
      ii Disruption of the spinolaminar line
      iii Rotary dislocation of facets
      iv Kyphotic angulation (misalignment and bony fractures)
      v Widening of the interpeduncular distance and disruption of the posterior margin of the vertebral body are signs of vertebral disruption
      vi Narrowing of a disc space
         1. A concomitant of a flexion injury
         2. Occurs at the level above the fractured vertebra
      vii A severe posterior ligament injury:
         1. Widening of a facet joint
         2. Complete baring of the facet
         3. Increase of the interspinous distance
2. Computed tomography:
   a. Best defines complex fractures and involvement of posterior elements
   b. Tridimensional reconstructions:

viii Define the extent of canal compromise
ix Define posterior element fractures

3. Magnetic resonance imaging:
    a. Excellent visualization of the spinal cord and ligamentous structures
    b. T2-weighted sequences have high signal intensity in the spinal cord in areas of injury and edema
    c. The anterior and posterior longitudinal ligaments may be identified on T1 and T2 weighted sequences

Lumbar Transverse Process Fracture

General Characteristics

1. The setting is almost always a high-impact rotary injury of the spine

Clinical Manifestations

1. Severe pain and muscle spasm at the site of injury
2. Associated paraspinal muscle injury with retroperitoneal hemorrhage causes:
    a. Severe pain at the injury site from sacrospinalis or paraspinal muscle hemorrhage
    b. Pain in the side, often with radiation to the groin
    c. A quiet patient whose position of comfort is often lying on the side with flexed legs
    d. Proximal > distal leg weakness
    e. Loss of the knee and ankle jerks on the affected side (depending on the level of the fracture and consequent retroperitoneal bleeding)
    f. Seven to 10 days following the injury there are signs of blood breakdown products in the skin and subcutaneous tissue of the affected flank (Grey Turner's sign)

Neuropathology

1. Fractured and displaced transverse processes at the affected level
2. Hemorrhage into the sacrospinalis, paraspinal and rarely the psoas muscle
3. Retroperitoneal hemorrhage

Neuroimaging

1. Radiographs and CT:
    a. Define the fractured and dislocated transverse process
    b. Define malalignment and associated vertebral structural damage
2. MRI:
    a. To evaluate disc, ligamentous and associated muscle hemorrhage and retroperitoneal blood

Pathologic Fractures

Osteoporosis

General Characteristics

1. Definition: a low bone mass with micro-architectural deterioration that leads to decreased bone strength with an increased susceptibility to fracture
2. Among insufficiency fractures associated with osteoporosis vertebral fractures are the earliest and most common
3. Approximately 20-25% of Caucasian women and men >50 years of age suffer a vertebral fracture
4. Vertebral fractures are a predictor of subsequent insufficiency fractures: one vertebral fracture confers a much higher risk of sustaining another

Clinical Manifestations

1. A bone mass density (BMDT-score) greater than 2.5 at the femoral neck is normal; many patients suffer vertebral fractures at this normal level
2. A large percentage of fragility fractures of the lumbar spine are missed clinically
3. Onset of sudden thoracic or lumbar pain, most often lancinating if a nerve root is involved
4. Multiple vertebral fractures lead to kyphosis, loss of height, chronic pain and loss of spine mobility

Neuropathology

1. There is an imbalance between bone resorption and formation
2. Remodeling of bone is constant with approximately 10% of bone mass undergoing the process at any time point
3. The activation of osteoclasts is regulated by molecular signals of which receptor activator of nuclear factor kappa – B ligand (RANK1) is prominent. It is secreted by osteoblasts
4. The interplay of molecular signaling of osteoprotegerin (OPG) and RANK1 are determinants of bone turnover
5. Trabecular bone has active turnover and develops decreased bone density and disrupted microarchitecture
6. Weak spicules of trabecular bone break ("microcracks") and are replaced by weaker bone

Neuroimaging

1. Radiography:
    a. Cortical thinning and increased radiolucency of bone
    b. Vertebral height decrease (vertical deformity (T4-L4))
2. Dual-energy x-ray:
    a. Dual-energy x-ray absorptiometry (DXA) is the present standard evaluation

 i Osteoporosis can be diagnosed if the bone mineral density is less than or equal to 2.5 standard deviations below that of a 30-40 year old healthy woman. This is computed as a T-score

3. MRI:
    a. Differentiation of benign from malignant fractures
    b. Benign fracture characteristics:
        i Maintenance of some normal marrow signal
        ii No involvement of posterior elements
    c. Fluid sign or gas within the vertebral body
    d. Low intensity band along the fractured end endplate (the fracture line)
    e. No tissue mass in the paravertebral or epidural space

Differential Diagnosis of Pathologic Fractures

1. Osteoporosis
2. Metastasis:
    i Pedicle involvement
    ii Vertebral body involvement
    iii Does not involve the disc
3. Corticosteroid use
4. Hyperparathyroidism (primary and more frequently associated with kidney disease)
5. Type-2 Diabetes
6. Myeloma (often multiple vertebrae are affected)
7. Hemangioma (often hemorrhage; trabecular pattern on radiographs)
8. Various bone cysts
9. Prolonged heparin use (fish mouth endplates)

Benign Bone Tumors Affecting Lumbosacral Nerve Roots

Osteoid Osteoma

General Characteristics

1. A primary benign bone lesion; it constitutes 10% of all primary benign bone tumors and 3% of all primary bone tumors

Clinical Manifestations

1. Most often they are seen in the first 3 decades; 3x more common in men
2. Predilection:
    a. Long bones; particularly of the lower extremities
3. Major symptom is pain:
    a. Localized and more severe at night

b. May be exacerbated or relieved by movement
c. Relieved by non-steroidal anti-inflammatory drugs (block prostaglandin activation of primary nociceptors in the lesion) and not by narcotics
d. Scoliosis occurs in 70% of patients when it involves the spine:
    i The most common cause of painful scoliosis in adolescents particularly if located in the thoracic or lumbar spine
e. If located in a pedicle, it may involve the exiting nerve root

Neuropathology

1. A highly vascularized nidus of connective tissue surrounded by sclerotic bone
2. The nidus is approximately 10 mm in diameter which is smaller than that seen in an osteoblastoma

Neuroimaging

1. CT is the best diagnostic modality to visualize the nidus
2. MRI:
    a. Increased signal intensity on T2-weighted sequences or enhanced T1-weighted sequences
        i Correlates with the degree of vascularity of the fibrovascular nidal stroma
        ii Correlates with the quantity of osteoid substance within the nidus
        iii Visualizes the soft tissue and bone marrow around the nidus

Differential Diagnosis

1. The major tumor to be differentiated is osteoblastoma

Osteoblastoma

General Characteristics

1. Rare benign osteoid-producing primary bone tumor
2. Affects the long bones
3. Males > females and most often seen in the second decade
4. 36% occur around the spine

Clinical Manifestations

1. Cervical vertebrae are rarely affected
2. Similar clinical signs and symptoms to osteoid osteoma
3. More aggressive than osteoid osteoma and erosion into the vertebral artery has been reported; blindness has been reported from occlusion of the posterior cerebral artery
4. May extend into the neuronal exit foramina

Neuroimaging

1. Similar to that of osteoid osteoma although a major differential point is these

lesions are usually larger than 2 cm whereas osteoid osteomas are less than 2 cm

Neuropathology

1. Histological features are similar to those of an osteoid osteoma except they are larger than 2 cm

Osteochondroma

General Characteristics

1. The most common benign bone tumor
2. 35% to 50% of benign bone neoplasms and 10% to 15% of all primary bone tumors

Clinical Manifestations

1. Involvement of the spine occurs in 2 to 5% of patients; male>female 2.5:1
2. Spine involvement is often seen in the setting of multiple osteochondromatosis
3. Usual occurrences are in long bones
4. Usual spine predilection is for cervical or upper thoracic levels
5. Patients described at L4 and L5 with radicular involvement
6. Often asymptomatic

Neuropathology

1. A developmental enchondromatous hyperplasia
2. Formation of cartilage-capped bony protrusions from a bony focus

Neuroimaging

1. CT:
   a. Differentiates the cartilaginous and bone components of the tumor
2. MRI:
   a. Demonstrates spinal cord or nerve root compression; a lobulated lesion
3. Conventional radiograph:
   a. Enchondromas present as oval shaped, linear and/or pyramidal osteolytic lesions
   b. Well defined margins
   c. Metaphysis and/or diaphysis of long tubular and flat bones

Differential Diagnosis

1. Atypical cartilage tumor
2. Chondroblastoma
3. Chondromyxoid fibroma
4. Ollier disease:
   a. Enchondromatosis

5. Maffucci Syndrome:
    a. Hereditary multiple exostoses
    b. Associated multiple cavernous hemangiomas

Hemangioma

General Characteristics

1. Occur primarily in the thoracic spine
2. Usually, they are asymptomatic
3. Symptoms may occur from:
    a. Epidural extension
    b. Expansion of the involved vertebra
    c. Spontaneous epidural extension
    d. Pathologic burst fracture

Clinical Manifestations

1. Thoracic hemangiomas produce more cord compression than lumbar ones
2. Intracanalicular root compression from extraosseous extension
3. Spinal stenosis from vertebral bone expansion

Neuropathology

1. Hamartomatous proliferation of vascular tissue of endothelial origin
2. Most often in the vertebral body of thoracic and lumbar vertebrae; they may be multiple

Neuroimaging

1. Reduced bone density between denser vertical trabeculae
2. MRI:
    a. Active lesions have low signal intensity on T1-weighted sequences with high signal intensity on T2-weighted sequences; quiescent lesions have high signal intensity in both sequences

Differential Diagnosis

1. Giant cell tumor
2. Aneurysmal bone cyst
3. Metastasis

Aneurysmal Bone Cyst

General Characteristics

1. A benign non-neoplastic expansible cystic bone lesion
2. Most common location is long bones but approximately 12-30% involve the spine
3. Lumbar spine is the most frequent location followed by the thoracic spine; 2% involve the cervical spine

4. Incidence is 114/100,000 people; age (1-59 years)

Clinical Manifestations

1. Most frequently encountered between 10-20 years of age
2. Most commonly found in the metaphyseal areas of long bones
3. Presenting symptoms:
    a. Well defined somatic pain, stiffness, and swelling
    b. Pathologic fracture may cause spinal cord compression and radiculopathy

Neuropathology

1. An expansible, tumor-like osteolytic lesion consisting of blood filled cavities separated by connective tissue septa; there is a surrounding thin cortical bone shell
2. May aggressively destroy and expand bone
3. Usually, a small lesion causes a pathologic fracture of a vertebra

Neuroimaging

1. Arise in the posterior elements of a vertebra and spreads to the pedicles and body
2. May involve the spinal canal
3. CT-3D reconstruction:
    a. Pedicle and vertebral body integrity
4. MRI:
    a. Multilocular cysts that are fluid filled; T2-weighted sequences have high-intensity signal
    b. Multiple cysts may have varying signal intensities on T1 and T2-weighted sequences due to different oxidation levels of blood and their breakdown products

Giant Cell Tumor (GCT)

General Characteristics

1. Comprise approximately 5% of primary bone tumors and approximately 20% of benign bone tumors
2. Slightly higher incidence in females
3. Majority are seen in patients older than 20 years
4. Primary location is the long bones of the extremities; a small proportion occurs in the pelvis, skull and spine

Clinical Manifestations

1. Pain and swelling at the lesion site are the most common symptoms
2. The tumor may be locally aggressive and impinge on a nerve root
3. Skull lesions (often sphenoid and temporal bones, rarely the occiput) produce

symptoms by their location

Neuropathology

1. Osteoclastic-like nuclear giant cells in a fibrohistiocytic stroma between osseous spicules
2. May also have foreign body-like giant cells
3. Histiocytes may be positive for CD68
4. Endochondral ossification

Neuroimaging

1. CT:
   a. Ground glass appearance; cytic lesion
   b. Expands bone
2. MRI:
   a. T1-weighted sequence equal intensity with muscle; T2-weighted sequence slightly intense signal

Differential Diagnosis

1. Chondroblastoma
2. Chondrosarcoma
3. Aneurysmal bone cyst
4. Dermoid cyst
5. Eosinophilic granuloma
6. Pigmented villonodular synovitis

Dermoid Cyst

General Characteristics

1. Congenital non-neoplastic lesions that originate from totipotent ectodermal cells which remain within the developing neural tube
2. Starts between the 3rd and 5th weeks of gestation
3. In approximately 50% of patients, there is a dermal sinus tract

Clinical Manifestations

1. Cysts are usually intradural in the lumbar and sacral spine
2. Symptoms may occur from tethering of the spinal cord in association with congenital nerve root abnormalities
3. Rupture causes chemical arachnoiditis
4. Infection of the cyst or sinus tract causes meningitis
5. May occur at the site of meningocele repair
6. Rarely they develop after a lumbar puncture or trauma

Neuroimaging

1. MRI:

   a. T1 and T2 weighted sequences demonstrate variable signal intensities according to the tissue in the cyst

Neuropathology

1. Contains epidermis, hair follicles and sebaceous glands, that are derived from residual embryonic cells

Eosinophilic Granuloma

General Characteristics

1. Eosinophilic granuloma (EG) is one of the Langerhans cell histiocytosis
2. Incidence of 1:150,000 people / year
3. The most common site is the skull; vertebral involvement is approximately 7%
4. EG is a self-limited disease

Clinical Manifestations

1. Most often patients are younger than 15 years of age
2. In addition to the skull and vertebrae, the pelvis, mandible and ribs may be involved
3. Thoracic vertebrae are most often affected followed by lumbar (35%) and cervical vertebrae (11%)
4. Male to female is 2-5:1
5. Usually, the neurologic deficits are rare:
   a. Pain may occur at the site
   b. Spinal cord compression may occur from cervical tumors
   c. Radiculopathy

Neuropathology

1. Single or multiple skeletal lesions
2. Lung involvement
3. Accumulation of pathologic Langerhans cells
4. Anti-CD1a immunolabeling

Neuroimaging

1. Lytic lesion often with osteoblastic activity on X-ray and CT
2. PET evaluation has 90% sensitivity and a specificity of 65%-80%
   a. False positive results occur from benign disease with an inflammatory component such as fibrous dysplasia or aneurismal bone cysts
   b. Low-grade tumors

Differential Diagnosis of Rare Benign Bone Lesions that can affect the Axial Skeleton with Consequent Radiculopathy

1. Neurofibroma

2. Leiomyoma
3. Chondromyxoid fibroma
4. Fibrous histiocytoma
5. Differential points for malignancy or benignity:
   a. Pedicle change with expansion is most often malignant
   b. Normal marrow preservation of a collapsed vertebral body on T1-weighted MRI sequences is most compatible with an osteoporotic fracture

Malignant Bone Tumors of the Lumbosacral Spine with Consequent Radiculopathy

Chordoma

General Characteristics

1. Rare tumors with an incidence of one/million people
2. Approximately 4% of primary malignant bone tumors and 20% of primary spine tumors
3. Divided into:
   a. Clival (skull base)
   b. Sacrococcygeal
   c. Cervical, thoracic and lumbar
   d. Almost equal distribution by site
4. Sacrococcygeal tumors have a male predominance of 2:1
5. Brachy gene in chordoma:
   a. A diagnostic marker that differentiates the tumor from myoepithelioma and chondrosarcoma
6. Classification:
   a. Notochordal hamartomas
      i Benign counterpart of chordoma
   b. Chondroid chordoma:
      i 5-15% of all chordomas
      ii Spheno-occipital areas of the skull base
   c. Differentiated chordoma:
      i Less than 10% of chordoma
   d. There is a correlation between the histological characteristic of a chordoma and its ability to metastasize:
      i Chondroid chordomas are the least aggressive while de-differentiated chordomas are the most aggressive

Clinical Manifestations

1. Sacral chordomas:
   a. May be associated with large exophytic soft tissue masses

    b. Bowel and bladder dysfunction (sacral roots)
    c. Severe back pain; painful sacral mass
    d. Intralesional surgery has a high rate of recurrence

Neuropathology

1. Physaliferous cells are characteristic; foamy appearance of the cytoplasm that contains multiple vacuoles which ultra-structurally are divided into smooth-walled and villous
2. Tumors stain for vimentin, the S-100 protein, epithelial membrane antigen and low molecular weight cytokeratins
3. Chondroid chordomas:
    a. Histological features of both chordoma and chondrosarcoma
        i Approximately 1/3 of cranial chordomas
        ii Express chordoma markers
4. De-differentiated chordoma:
    a. Sarcomatous regions comprised of spindle-shaped polygonal cells
    b. Metastasizes late

Neuroimaging

1. MRI:
    a. T2-weighted sequences demonstrate a hypointense, non-enhancing, interosseous lesion

Liposarcoma

General Characteristics

1. Liposarcoma is a common adult soft tissue sarcoma composed of three histologic subtypes:
    a. Well and de-differentiated
    b. Myxoid/round cell
    c. Pleomorphic
2. Z1C1 overexpression:
    a. A transcription factor important for neuronal development

Clinical Manifestations

1. Well-differentiated and de-differentiated liposarcomas occur:
    a. Retroperitoneum > extremities > para-testicular areas and trunk; invasion of the lumbosacral plexus and individual roots
    b. Motor and sensory loss in the plexi and roots that are involved.
2. De-differentiated tumors may metastasize (lungs primarily)
3. Retroperitoneal tumors may be >30 cm and invade viscera and the lumbosacral plexus; local reoccurrence is common
4. Myxoid/round cell tumors:

   a. Translocation of chromosome 12 and 16
   b. Interferes with adipocyte differentiation; abundant extracellular myxoid tissue
   c. Present in younger patients and its primary location is the proximal lower extremities
   d. Metastasizes to the skeleton, lumbosacral roots and pelvic plexi
5. Pleomorphic liposarcoma:
   a. Chromosomal gains, losses, duplications, and rearrangements have been described
   b. Usually, present with lower extremity involvement; rarely the retroperitoneum and mediastinum
   c. Resembles a non-adipocytic soft tissue sarcoma (malignant fibrous histiocytoma)
6. All types may involve lumbar and sacral roots

Neuropathology

1. Dependent on subtype
2. Pleomorphic liposarcoma resembles a non-adipocytic soft tissue sarcoma (malignant fibrous histiocytoma)
3. Myxoid/round cell liposarcoma:
   a. Abundant extracellular myxoid tissue
4. Well and de-differentiated tumors:
   a. Adipocytomas (WD Type)
   b. DD Types have an adipocyte-rich region that is demarcated from highly cellular spindle cell area

Neuroimaging

1. Intradural lesion that may diffusely invade the vertebral bodies and encase the cauda equina

Ewing Sarcoma

General Characteristics

1. Primitive neuroectodermal tumors (PNET) and Ewing sarcoma are in the same family of malignant small, round cell neoplasms whose origin is soft tissue or bone.
2. Usual sites for EWS-PNET are the chest wall, pelvis, and the extremities
3. Incidence rate is approximately 3 patients/1,000,000 people
4. Approximately 10% of EWS arise in extraskeletal soft tissue
5. Caused by rearrangements involving the EWS gene on chromosome 22q 12 and fusion partners from the ETS oncogene family; 95% of EW sarcoma family tumors have fusion of the central exons of the EWSR1 gene (Ewing Sarcoma Breakpoint Region 1)

Clinical Manifestations

1. The tumor may arise from the pedicles of L4-5, and L5 S1
2. 2. Primarily involves lumbar and sacral roots in the spine
3. 3. Cerebral and lung metastasis occur

Neuropathology

1. Poorly differentiated small round cell tumors
2. ES and PNET represent a single entity
3. Light microscopy reveals small round blue cells with hyperchromatic nuclei and minimal cytoplasm
4. EWS-PNETs co-express:
    a. CD99 (the glycoprotein MIC2) and vimentin

Neuroimaging

1. CT scan EWS-PNETs:
    a. Heterogeneous masses that invade surrounding tissue including bone
2. MRI:
    a. The mass is isointense to muscle on T1-weighted sequences and hyperintense on T2-weighted sequences

Osteosarcoma

General Characteristics

1. Osteosarcoma is the most common primary malignant bone tumor in children and young adults
2. Older adults are usually affected by sarcomatous transformation of Paget's disease of bone
3. Incidence of 1/100,000 people

Clinical Manifestations

1. A painful mass lesion
2. Pathologic fracture
3. Secondary causes include:
    a. Ionizing radiation
    b. Hereditary:
        iii Retinoblastoma
        iv Paget's disease of bone
        v Enchondromatosis
        vi Hereditary multiple exostoses
        vii Fibrous dysplasia
4. Presents between 5 and 30 years of age; a second peak occurs in the fifth and sixth decade
5. Pathologic fracture of vertebrae and compressive myelopathy and

radiculopathy

Neuropathology

1. A malignant spindle cell neoplasm that produces osteoid
2. Classified into 4 subtypes:
    a. Osteoblastic
    b. Fibroblastic
    c. Chondroblastic
    d. Telangiectatic
3. Classification is based on the predominant type of tumor matrix

Neuroimaging

1. Radiographs:
    a. An ill-defined mixed sclerotic and lytic lesion that arises in the metaphyseal region of the involved bone
    b. Destruction of the bone cortex
    c. Soft tissue mass with ossification
    d. Periosteal new bone formation with elevation of the cortex (Codman's triangle)
2. CT assessment is superior to MRI for assessment of new bone formation
3. MRI:
    a. T1 and T2 weighted sequences with fat suppression for the extent of bone and soft tissue involvement
    b. Macroscopic tumor emboli may be found in regional large vessels
    c. Telangiectatic osteosarcoma may present as a sacral mass

Chondrosarcoma

General Characteristics

1. Less than 10% of chondrosarcomas are in children; 0.5% of low-grade tumors arise from benign chondroid lesions
2. They are 27% of all primary bone tumors
3. Central tumors arise in the medullary cavity or periosteum

Clinical Manifestations

1. Most patients present between 40-70 years of age
2. Patients with Ollier disease, Maffucci syndrome, and hereditary multiple exostoses have a higher incidence
3. Insidious worsening pain that is most pronounced at night
4. Approximately 20% present as a pathologic fracture
5. Primary sites are the shoulder, pelvis or proximal femur
6. Rare spinal compression from pathologic fracture or radiculopathy

Neuropathology

1. Chondrocytes with small to slightly enlarged dense nuclei on a background of chondroid stroma
2. Neoplastic chondrocytes are arranged in lobar cords and clumps which cause endosteal scalloping

Neuroimaging

1. Radiograph:
   a. An expansile mixed sclerotic and centrally lucent lesion, with a narrow transitional zone and thin sclerotic margin
   b. Arcs and Wings calcifications
2. CT:
   a. Non-mineralized portion of the tumor is hypodense to muscle (high water content of hyaline cartilage)
3. MRI:
   a. Low to intermediate signal intensity on T1-weighted sequences; T2-weighted sequences, the lesion is hyperintense

Differential Diagnosis

1. May arise from an osteochondroma
2. Enchondroma (secondary chondrosarcoma)
3. Giant cell tumor
4. Bone cyst

Epidural and Vertebral Metastasis

General Characteristics

1. Metastatic tumors are the most common neoplasms of the intraspinal canal and nerve roots
2. Locations:
   a. Epidural > leptomeningeal > intraspinal
3. Epidural metastases occur primarily from direct extension of metastatic vertebral tumors; rarely a metastasis grows through the intervertebral foramina or directly metastasizes to the epidural space
4. Radiculopathy is secondary to direct compression by the tumor, metabolic and cytokine expression or a pathologic fracture that compresses the cauda equina
5. Differential diagnosis of common tumors that metastasize to vertebrae:
   a. Lung
   b. Breast
   c. Prostate
   d. Ovary
   e. Melanoma
   f. Renal cell

   g. Sarcoma
   h. Multiple myeloma
6. The most frequent sites of metastases are: thoracic > 70%; lumbosacral > 20%; cervical 10%

Clinical Manifestations

1. Local pain is the initial symptom. It is particularly evoked by mechanical stimuli (percussion over the involved vertebra)
2. Radicular pain:
   a. Thoracic metastasis usually present with bilateral radicular pain
   b. Lumbosacral roots most often have a unilateral presentation
   c. Cervical spine:
      viii C8-T1 (from Pancoast) tumor or metastasis may present with C8/T1 radicular pain, a Horner's syndrome and anhidrosis or hyperhidrosis.
      ix C8-T1 innervates the eye and T2 is the level for extremity sympathetic innervations (irritation or destruction)
   d. Herpes Zoster may be reactivated at the site of the lesion
   e. Deep boring pain that is worse at night
   f. Weakness, sensory loss, and atrophy with depressed or absent reflexes at the affected level

Neuroimaging

Solitary Vertebral Collapse

1. Malignant features by MRI:
   a. Ill-defined lesion margin
   b. Pedicle involvement
   c. Heterogeneous enhancement pattern
   d. Irregular nodular paravertebral soft tissue lesion
   e. Erosion of the end plate
   f. Star burst pattern of fracture is more likely traumatic

Benign CT Features of an Acute Vertebral Lesion

1. Cortical fractures of the vertebral body without cortical bone destruction
2. Retropulsion of a bone fragment of the posterior cortex of the vertebral body into the spinal canal
3. Fracture lines within the cancellous bone of the vertebral body
4. Intervertebral vacuum phenomena
5. Thin diffuse paraspinal soft tissue mass

Malignant Features of Spine Lesions by CT and SPECT

1. The posterior portion of the vertebral body is involved
2. Concomitant vertebral body and pedicle involvement
3. Extensive abnormalities that involve the vertebral body and vertebral arch,

but spare the pedicle are benign

4. Destruction of the anterolateral or posterior cortical bone of the vertebral body
5. Destruction of the cancellous bone of the vertebral body

Specific Patterns of Metastasis by Tumor Type (neuroimaging and some clinical correlations)

Lung cancer

1. Multiple vertebral levels are involved
2. The most common metastatic lesion
3. Thoracic vertebrae > lumbosacral > cervical spine
4. Cortical and cerebellar metastasis are often concomitant
5. A common cause of carcinomatosis of the meninges
6. Rarely anti-Yo antibodies with paraneoplastic cerebellar degeneration
7. Often bilateral lumbosacral roots are involved
8. Rarely anti-'Hu' antibodies and associated limbic encephalitis and anterior horn cell disease

Gastric and Colon Cancer

1. Colon cancer may destroy the sacrum and involve lower sacral roots
2. Kruckenberg metastasis (dropped metastases to the ovaries) from the stomach
3. Associated non-bacterial thrombotic emboli (NBTE) with stroke (mucinous adenocarcinoma is the most common tumor)
4. Extremely dense lesions on neuroimaging (mucin) with MRI
5. Hypercoagulable state may be associated
6. Pain in the lower abdomen and midlumbar areas
7. Belt-like pain radiations
8. Transverse colon or descending colon involvement:
   a. Central or left-sided abdominal pain
   b. Radiation to the second or third lumbar vertebrae

Metastatic Infiltration of the Pelvic Nerve Plexus

The Pelvic Nerve Plexus

1. Pain radiates to the low back usually diffusely but may have a dermatomal distribution

Iliopsoas Region Metastasis

1. Unilateral lumbar spine dull ache
2. Radiations to the groin, labia and testicles
3. Involvement is frequently of the upper lumbar roots
4. May be associated with a very dense vertebra

Breast Cancer

1. Multiple vertebral bodies are involved with radiculopathy
2. Has been associated with thoracic meningioma (only in women)
3. Carcinomatosis of the meninges is prominent and may be asymptomatic for long periods
4. May have delayed onset (years after a bilateral mastectomy)

Prostate Cancer

1. Osteoblastic and lytic bone destruction occur concomitantly
2. Multiple levels are involved
3. May metastasize through the paravertebral venous plexus (no valves; Batson's plexus communicates to the posterior fossa)
4. Most often radiculopathy and spinal cord compression are the neurological signs (lumbosacral roots)
5. Metastasizes to the petrous apex (Batson's plexus has no valves)
6. Midline vertebral pain

Ovarian Cancer

1. L1-L3 nerve roots > L4-S1 nerve roots
2. Associated with peritoneal implantation
3. L1-L3 > L5-S1 roots; the entire cauda equina may be involved
4. Rare associations:
    a. Paraneoplastic neuropathy
    b. Cerebellar degeneration
    c. Limbic encephalopathy
5. Gadolinium enhancement with MRI of the cauda equina
6. Dense marble vertebra (radiograph)

Melanoma

1. Usually multiple cerebral metastases
2. Unusual adhesive qualities of the tumor allow it to metastasize to the cardiac and intestinal surfaces
3. Almost never solitary
4. Cord compression rather than radicular presentation

Pancreatic Pain (Primary Cancer or Metastatic)

1. Straight through to the back. To the right of the spine if the pancreatic head is involved and left of the spine if the body and tail is the source of pathology

Uterosacral ligament metastasis

1. Metastasis from uterine or cervical cancer
2. Sacral radiations
3. Benign processes:

   a. Endometrial tissue may deposit on lumbosacral roots which causes pain with menstruation
   b. Fibroid tumors may cause traction on uterosacral ligaments

Posterior Gastric Wall Tumors

1. Pain radiates to the central thoracic spine

Retroperitoneal Metastasis

1. Thoracic or lumbar pain
2. Pain radiates to the lower abdomen, groin, anterior thigh, or flank
3. Characteristic tumors located retroperitoneally are lymphomas, renal cell carcinoma, and Schwannoma

Neuropathology

1. Malignant cells exit the primary tumor, attach to, degrade the proteins of the extracellular matrix, and metastasize via the bloodstream, the lymphatics or directly to adjacent tissue.
2. Specific cancers spread to particular tissues that may be mediated by chemokines and transforming growth factor beta
3. Critical mechanisms for growth of metastases include:
   a. Angiogenesis
   b. Endothelial progenitor cells incorporation into tumor vasculature
   c. Tumor cell mobility
   d. Epigenetic regulation:
      i Histone modifications
   e. Exosome factors

Neuroimaging (X-Ray, MRI and CT)

1. Destructive lesions of the vertebral body and particularly the pedicle and posterior elements; an osteoid osteoma (benign) may also affect the pedicle
2. The disc space is not involved
3. Multiple vertebral involvement suggests multiple myeloma, breast or lung metastasis
4. Involvement of the sacrum is characteristic of colon cancer
5. Multiple osteoblastic vertebral lesions suggest prostatic metastasis
6. A single dense vertebra on plain X-ray may occur with leukemia or lymphoma
7. Other MRI characteristics helpful in differentiating benign versus malignant vertebral fractures include:
   a. Posterior cortical bulging:
      ii 74% of malignant lesions versus 45% of benign lesions
      iii Epidural mass formation was seen in 77% of malignant lesions and 25% in benign lesions

iv Pedicle enhancement:
1. 93% of malignant lesions and 39% of benign lesions (may occur with osteoporotic fractures)

Lymphoma

1. Predilection for paravertebral lymph nodes
2. Intertwines with the lumbosacral roots of the cauda equina
3. Often arises in the epidural space with consequent spinal cord compression
4. May be associated with a very dense vertebra

Intrinsic Spinal Cord Tumors that Involve the Lumbosacral Roots

Differential Diagnosis

1. Ependymomas (myxopapillary)
2. Glioma of the filum terminale
3. Neurofibroma of the cauda equine
4. Cauda equina tumors:
    a. Hemangioblastoma
    b. Paraganglioma
    c. Ganglioneuroma
    d. Schwannomatosis
    e. Neurofibroma
5. Intraspinal pericytoma

Medical Conditions with Nerve Root Involvement

Vascular Claudication

General Characteristics

1. The mean annual incidence of peripheral arterial disease is increasing
2. Patients with critical limb ischemia (CLI) have a high risk of cardiovascular disease that includes myocardial infarction, stroke and death
3. Vascular insufficiency of peripheral nerves and nerve roots is grossly underestimated

Clinical Manifestations

1. Exercise induced (intermittent) or rest pain
2. Thigh and calf muscles are predominately involved
3. Burning and squeezing quality of the pain that improves with rest and recurs with further exercise
4. Hip and buttock pain with walking

5. Ischemic rest pain of the lower extremity:
    a. Primarily in the foot and toes
    b. Buerger's disease affects the medial foot
    c. The pain is worse at night
    d. Relieved by dependency
    e. Always in the context of severe peripheral vascular disease
6. Leriche syndrome:
    a. Atheromatous occlusive disease of the infrarenal aorta, common iliac arteries or both
    b. Hip and buttock claudication
    c. Impotence
    d. Decreased peripheral lower extremity pulses

Neuropathology

1. Atherosclerosis of large and medium sized lower extremity blood vessels
2. Coral reef aorta:
    a. Calcified plaques in the visceral part of the aorta; plaques cause decreased perfusion of the lower extremities, visceral ischemia and renovascular hypotension
3. Microembolization from the endoaortic calcified mass causes the "blue toe" syndrome
4. Critical limb ischemia is caused by:
    a. Severe atherosclerotic disease
    b. Thromboembolic disease
    c. Thromboangiitis obliterans
    d. Vasculitis
    e. Cystic adventitial disease
    f. Popliteal entrapment
    g. All processes may affect the nutrient supply to nerve roots

Neuroimaging

1. Arteriography to delineate the level and extent of arterial atherosclerosis

Adhesive Arachnoiditis

General Characteristics

1. Rarely occurs with the increased use of MRI and CT for the diagnosis of back pain rather than myelography with contrast
2. The use of water-soluble contrast material if myelography is necessary rarely causes adhesive arachnoiditis

Clinical Manifestations

1. Intractable low back and leg pain and paresthesia of the involved nerve roots

that is exacerbated by position

2. Burning pain, often encompassing several roots predominates over motor weakness

Neuropathology

1. The arachnoid membrane is thickened over the cauda equina
2. It has been described in the setting of:
   a. Lipid contrast use during myelopathy
   b. Repeated epidural blood patches
   c. Operative procedures
   d. Infections
   e. Subarachnoid hemorrhage
   f. Epidural anesthesia
3. Chronic inflammation of the arachnoid layer of the meninges
4. Possible immune features

Neuroimaging

1. MRI:
   a. Thickened meninges in the spinal canal with clumped nerve roots
2. CT / myelography:
   a. Clumping and adhesion of nerve roots

Ankylosing Spondylitis

General Characteristics

1. Is a chronic inflammatory disorder characterized by spondylitis, sacroiliitis, peripheral joint involvement
2. Extra-articular manifestations include:
   a. Uveitis
   b. Inflammatory bowel disease
   c. Psoriasis
   d. Cardiovascular disease
3. Approximately 95% of patients are histocompatibility antigen HLS-B27 positive

Clinical Manifestations

1. Low back pain is an early complaint. It often radiates to the posterior thigh and groin
2. Limitation of movement is constant and progressive; severe early morning stiffness or an increase in stiffness after periods of inactivity
3. In later stages, some patients develop cauda equina compression

4. Pain in the thorax and sternum with coughing or other Valsalva maneuvers
5. Progressive flexion at the hips and flexion spine deformity which may exacerbate gait difficulty

Neuropathology

1. Investigation of the IL-23 and Th17 axis that drives immune activation and chronic inflammation by the differentiation and activation of Th17 cells

Neuroimaging

1. X-ray:
   a. Destruction of the sacroiliac joint
   b. Bony bridging of the vertebral bodies ("bamboo spine")
   c. Dilatation of the lumbar thecal sac
   d. Fracture dislocation of the spine at all levels from minor trauma (flexion extension injuries are most common cervically)
   e. Destructive vertebral lesions; correlated with the return of pain after a period of quiescence or if the pain is localized

Aneurysm of the Abdominal Aorta

General Characteristics

1. Abdominal aortic aneurysms occur most commonly in patients over 50 years of age, men more commonly than women, who are hypertensive, smoke and have heart or blood vessel disease
2. Marfan and Ehlers-Danlos are the most common genetic illnesses in which they occur
3. Most, approximately 85%, occur below the kidney
4. AAA have an incidence of 2% in males over the age of 65
5. An aneurysm less than 5.5 cm have a one year rupture risk of less than 1%

Clinical Manifestations

1. The great majority of aneurysms are asymptomatic
2. As the aneurysm expands, there may be pain in the chest, lower back or scrotum
3. A pulsatile sensation in the abdomen
4. Pain may occur at lumbosacral root levels

Neuropathology

1. Aneurysms greater than 7 cm have a 33% chance of rupture with a mortality rate of 85-90%
2. Smoking is a major risk factor
3. In the tunica media and intima histologic analysis reveals:
   a. Accumulation of lipids in foam cells
   b. Extracellular free cholesterol uptake

   c. Calcification
   d. Adventitial inflammatory infiltrate
4. The basic mechanism has been posited to be proteolytic degradation of the tunica media by the increased expression and activity of matrix metalloproteinases
5. The serine protease granzyme B may also contribute to rupture by cleaving decorin that disrupts collagen and decreases the tensile strength of the adventitia

Neuroimaging

1. X-ray of the abdomen may reveal calcification in the walls of the aorta (approximately in 50% of patients)
2. Ultrasonography is the screen for AAA
3. CT scan has close to 100% sensitivity
4. Rarely plain x-ray or CT delineates erosion of vertebrae particularly at the T10-L1 level

Osteomyelitis of Vertebrae

General Characteristics

1. The usual organisms are staphylococci, mycobacteria, streptococcus equisimilis and rarely fungi
2. Vertebral osteomyelites are responsible for 2 – 4% of all bone infections
3. Infections may have a predilection for children and the elderly

Clinical Manifestations

1. Subacute or chronic back pain that is exacerbated by movement and is not relieved by rest
2. Mechanically sensitive area (percussion) over the spine in the involved segments or the patient has severe limitation of movement. Pain may be severe with slight motion
3. Radicular pain may occur if the nerve root is affected
4. General symptoms include fever, night sweats, difficulty moving from a standing to sitting position
5. Patients may be afebrile and may not have leukocytosis

Neuropathology

1. Destruction of bone trabeculae with inflammatory changes
2. Paravertebral mass (abscess)
3. Involvement of the vertebral body and the disc. Cancer does not breach the disc space. Fistula with drainage may be at a distance from the infected vertebrae which may occur with tuberculosis. Kyphosis (Pott's disease) is rare in the west but occurs in developing countries with spinal tuberculosis: the

usual sites are the lower thoracic and upper lumbar vertebrae.

Laboratory Evaluation

1. Elevated sed rate and C-reactive protein is the rule

Neuroimaging (MRI and CT)

1. Involvement of the disc space as well as the vertebral body
2. Trauma and postoperatively, the discs may be directly infected. In the case of vertebral osteomyelitis the bone infection is primary and then spreads to the disc
3. Subacute bacterial endocarditis (SBE) may be associated with severe back pain and demonstrate no changes on MRI

Epidural Abscess

General Characteristics

1. Usually a severe pyogenic infection of the epidural space that requires immediate neurosurgical intervention and antibiotic treatment
2. Spinal epidural abscesses occur in 0.2 to 2 patients per 10,000 hospital admissions
3. The most common cause is hematogenous spread from a septic focus or by extension from osteomyelitis
4. The most common organism is staphylococcal infection
5. Most infections occur in patients between 30 to 60 years of age
6. Risk factors include diabetes mellitus, trauma, intravenous drug abuse, lumbar puncture, epidural injections / catheters and following laminectomy

Clinical Manifestations

1. Low grade fever with severe localized pain over the involved segment that is mechanically sensitive (percussion)
2. Radicular component may supervene
3. Paraplegia, anesthesia below the affected level with sphincter dysfunction occur in later stages (spinal cord involvement)

Neuropathology

1. Pus and or inflammatory granulation tissue between the dura mater and the vertebral column
2. The infection is most frequent at the thoracolumbar levels (epidural space is larger); it is more frequently located posteriorly than anteriorly

Laboratory Evaluation

1. Leukocyte count (1,500-42,000 / mm^3)
2. Increased sed-rate and C-reactive protein

Neuroimaging

1. MRI yields the greatest diagnostic accuracy

Discitis

General Characteristics

1. May localize to the involved segment by hematogenous spread of a systemic infection (exemplified by urinary tract infection)
2. Following lumbosacral spinal procedures with concomitant osteomyelitis and spread into the disc space

Clinical Manifestations

1. Extreme mechanical and movement sensitivity that elicits radicular pain
2. Localized back pain from concomitant vertebral osteomyelitis

Neuropathology

1. Staphylococcus aureus is the most common organism; Escherichia coli and Proteus species are common in patients with urinary tract infections
2. Gram negative species are the most common organisms in i.v. drug abusing patients
3. Concomitant medical conditions are:
   a. Diabetes
   b. HIV infection
   c. Steroid use
   d. Cancer
   e. Chronic renal failure
4. The disc is nourished by direct diffusion from the adjacent vertebral body endplate. Septic emboli lodge in the metaphyseal arteries (end arteries) that causes infarctions of the endplates that is followed by infectious spread into the disc space
5. Spread may also occur through Batson's plexus

Laboratory Evaluation

1. Increased sed-rate and C-reactive protein
2. Leukocytosis
3. Following operative procedures, staphylococcus aureus and epidermidis as well as Streptococcus species are the most common causative species

Neuroimaging

1. MRI:
   a. Delineated characteristics include:
      i Location
      ii Osseous involvement
      iii Anterior versus posterior spinal location
      iv Soft tissue and iliopsoas involvement

b. Increased signal intensity on T2-weighted sequences with gadolinium enhancement noted in the disc space. Destructive enhancing bone lesions are demonstrated in patients with vertebral osteomyelitis

Inflammatory Processes that Affect the Cauda Equina

General Characteristics

1. Infectious, autoimmune, and carcinomatous meningitis all affect the nerves of the cauda equina

Clinical Manifestations

1. Clinical features depend on the specific underlying medical condition, whether the process is primarily demyelinating or axonal, the tempo of the underlying process and its extent
2. Most of the autoimmune processes are generalized while those due to infection are localized
3. Carcinomatous involvement affects the mental status and cranial nerves

Neuropathology

1. CMV in the later stages of a severe HIV infection
2. Lyme disease
3. Herpetic infection
4. Carcinomatosis of the meninges
5. Guillain-Barre syndrome and other autoimmune neuropathies
6. Lumbosacral plexitis
7. Sarcoidosis

Laboratory Evaluation

1. Sed rate and C-reactive protein are increased in both infective and autoimmune processes
2. Specific antigens for GBS and its variants

Neuroimaging

1. MRI:
   a. Hypertrophic nerve roots in many autoimmune illnesses
   b. Contrast enhancement of affected nerve roots
   c. Some congenital neuropathies manifest hypertrophic nerve roots (cauda equina) that cause a compressive neuropathy

Intraspinal Hemorrhage

General Characteristics

1. Most often occur with spinal cord malformations
2. The syndrome may be caused by subarachnoid, subdural, and epidural bleeding

Clinical Manifestations

1. Sudden severe midline back pain that often is associated with spinal cord compression and rapid progression of paraparesis, urinary retention, numbness and the onset of spinal shock

Neuropathology

1. Coagulopathy (Coumadin; newer anticoagulants may have a lesser incidence)
2. Arteriovenous and cavernous malformations
3. Rare spinal aneurysms
4. Rarely excruciating back and radicular pain with apoplectic onset occurs with:
   a. Spinal cord infarction
   b. Myelitis
   c. Compression fractures
   d. The Guillain-Barre syndrome

Laboratory Evaluation

1. Coagulation parameters
2. Sed rate and C-reactive protein
3. CSF evaluation if infection is suspected with PCR

Neuroimaging

1. MRI
   a. High signal intensity of the parenchymal spinal cord on T2-weighted sequences
      i Dorsal views if an AVM is etiologic
      ii Surround T1 hypointense ring (hemosiderin) suggests cavernous hemangioma

Differential Diagnosis of Infection Affecting Lumbosacral Roots

1. Herpes Zoster (thoracic; cervical and lumbosacral roots)
2. Brucellosis (L5 roots)
3. Lyme disease:
   a. Borrelia burgdorferi (spirochete) is the causative organism
   b. Radiculopathy occurs early in the course of the illness:
      i May be associated with cranial neuropathy (uni or bilateral VII, rarely other cranial nerves and meningitis)
      ii Single or asymmetric multiple root involvement
4. Chronic radiculopathy:
   a. Presents months after the initial infection
   b. Mild motor and sensory loss; not associated with meningitis or VIIth nerve palsy

    c. Distal paresthesia or radicular pain
5. CMV:
    a. General Characteristics:
        i Affects lumbar and sacral roots
        ii Most commonly encountered in severely affected HIV patients ($CD4^+$ count of < 50 mm^3)
    b. Clinical manifestations:
        i Rapidly progressive cauda equina syndrome
        ii Leg weakness, paresthesia and saddle region sensory loss, sphincter dysfunction, progressive weakness to flaccid paralysis
        iii Severe low back pain
        iv Polymorphonuclear pleocytosis with elevated protein and viral titers in the CSF; positive PCR
        v Gadolinium enhancement on MRI of involved roots in 50% of patients
        vi If acute neurologic symptoms and signs need to rule out:
            1. Infection or many other lesions of the cauda equina and conus medullaris
            2. Lymphomatous infiltration of the lumbosacral roots
            3. Syphilis (in an HIV-infected patient)
            4. Herpes simplex (type II with sacral root involvement)
            5. HIV-related polyradiculopathy
        vii Herpes virus 8 (lumbar and thoracic roots)
        viii EBV (isolated nerve roots)
        ix Tuberculosis (cold abscess):
            1. L1-L3 roots
            2. Some ethnicities have primarily cervical root involvement (Asian patients)
6. Syphilis:
    a. Dorsal root entry zone is the site of infection
    b. Pachymeningitis cervicalis > lumbosacral involvement
    c. Tabetic pain:
        i Thoracic > lumbosacral roots
        ii May simulate a thoracic or abdominal visceral emergency
7. HTLV1:
    a. Involvement is overwhelming in the cervical cord
    b. Isolated roots may be involved
8. HIV: L5; sacral roots
9. Spinal epidural abscess:
    a. General characteristics:
        i Occurs in the thoracic > lumbosacral > cervical cord
        ii Chronic lesions occur in the thoracic cord

- iii Infecting organisms:
  1. Staphylococcus aureus
  2. Gram-negative rods
  3. Anaerobes
  4. Skin flora (spinal operations)
  5. Mycobacterium
  6. Fungi

b. Risk factors:
- i IV drug abuse
- ii Spinal surgery
- iii Diabetes mellitus
- iv Epidural steroids:
  1. Recent fungal contaminant of steroid injections
- v Epidural catheters:
  1. Prolonged use for neuropathic pain patients
- vi Immunocompromised patients

c. Clinical Manifestations
- i Onset often occurs with severe back pain; delayed from the onset of the infection
- ii Spinal cord compression, infarction or parenchymal infection
- iii Deep boring midline pain in the spine with sudden radicular component
- iv Cauda equina involvement
- v Fever, leukocytosis and elevated sed rate
- vi MRI may demonstrate gadolinium enhancement of the involved roots

Differential Diagnosis of Systemic Disease Affecting Lumbosacral Nerve Roots that Cause Pain

1. Diabetes mellitus:
   a. Diabetic amyotrophy (femoral nerve or thoracolumbar plexitis from infarction)
   b. Vasculopathy of the vasa vasorum
   c. Clinical features:
   - i Patients > 60 years of age
   - ii Present with pain of neuropathic quality usually of the distal extremities
   - iii Prominent weakness
   - iv Concomitant weight loss
   - v Thoracoabdominal nerve root involvement
2. Sarcoid
3. Periarteritis nodosa:

   a. Proximal L1-L3 nerve root involvement; all roots may be affected
   b. Asymmetric involvement
4. Meningeal amyloid
5. Acute intermittent porphyria
6. Coproporphyrinuria
7. Variegate porphyria
8. Necrotizing arteritis
9. Hypertrophic pachymeningitis (IgG4)
10. All collagen vascular disease
11. Carcinomatosis of the meninges
12. Mixed collagen vascular disease

Differential Diagnosis of Immune Mediated Processes that Affect Lumbosacral Roots that May Be Painful

AIDP (Acute Inflammatory Demyelinating Polyneuropathy)

1. May affect proximal, distal and terminal somatosensory afferents
2. May present with apparent radiculopathy

CIDP (Chronic Inflammatory Demyelinating Polyneuropathy)

1. L5 S1 roots may be initially affected

Multiple Sclerosis

1. Affects the dorsal root entry zone at a junction of central and peripheral myelin; anterior horn cell damage
2. Amyotrophy of the affected extremity (several segment involvement as occurs with NMO); gray matter lesions are common in the hemispheres (acute and chronic autoimmune disease)
3. Some major autoimmune epitopes:
   a. GM1
   b. MAG
   c. GQ1b
   d. GAL-NAc-GDT/1a
4. Radiculopathy with increased sed rate (usually at L5)
5. Post-vaccination
6. Post viral infection
7. Acute disseminated encephalomyelitis (an overwhelmingly central demyelinating disease)

Miscellaneous Involvement of Lumbosacral Roots that May Be Painful

1. Endometriosis:
   a. Endometrial tissue is adherent to pelvic nerve roots (L5-S5)

   b. Catamenial cyclical pain with bleeds from the aberrant tissue and irritation of the lumbosacral roots
2. Laparoscopy for pelvic and abdominal processes with root injury:
   a. L1-L3 > involvement than L5-S1 roots
3. Epidural catheter trauma:
   a. Prolonged exposure to bupivacaine (directly toxic to the nerve root)
   b. Direct trauma to the root during catheter insertion
4. Arachnoiditis:
   a. General Characteristics:
      i Clumped scarred nerve roots in the dorsal sac (MRI evaluation)
      ii Occurs following multiple surgeries or hemorrhage during myelography with pantopague. Water-soluble contrast has eliminated this cause.
   b. Clinical Manifestations:
      i Severe burning pain in several root distributions > motor weakness
      ii No exacerbating or relieving factors
      iii Asymmetric reflex loss
5. Spina Bifida:
   a. May be associated with congenital defects of the pedicles, facets, and foraminal exit canals
   b. Conjoined nerve roots
6. Mxyopapillary Ependymoma:
   a. Asymmetric lumbosacral nerve root involvement
   b. Lower extremity weakness
   c. Bowel, bladder, and sexual dysfunction
7. Dropped Metastasis:
   a. Medulloblastoma
8. Traumatic nerve root avulsion:
   a. Severe trauma (often motorcycle accidents)
   b. Most often cervical nerve roots and the brachial plexus are injured
   c. MVA affect lumbosacral roots and the lumbosacral plexus
9. Plate fixation and pedicle screw displacement
10. Complications of epidural and spinal anesthesia:
   a. General Characteristics:
      i Toxic effects of anesthetic (usually 0.25% bupivacaine)
      ii Direct injury by needle or catheter
      iii Subarachnoid injection of anesthetic during epidural procedures
      iv Contamination of anesthetics with detergents, chemicals or organisms (bacteria or fungal)
      v Epidural abscess
      vi Risk of epidural anesthesia is increased with:

1. Lumbar spinal stenosis ("Pooling") of bupivacaine around nerve roots
2. Inadvertent subarachnoid injection of high volume of anesthetic
3. A combination of general and epidural anesthesia
4. Advanced age

b. Clinical Manifestations:
   i Radicular pain and weakness
   ii Lower extremity myoclonus and severe spasm
   iii Cauda equina syndrome
   iv May clear after days to weeks (the cauda equina are peripheral nerves and have regenerative capacity)

Cervical Nerve Root Disorders

General Characteristics

1. Cervical spine roots exit horizontally from the spinal cord to the neural exit foramina
2. The ventral and dorsal roots join just distal to the DRG (which most often is in the vertebral foraminal exit canal) and form a spinal nerve; the dorsal ramus supplies the paraspinal muscles (its origin is just distal to the DRG) as well as the cutaneous innervation of 1 – 1 ½ inches lateral to the spinous process

Clinical Manifestations of cervical root pathology

1. C1-C2 level:
   a. There is no disc between C1-C2
   b. Ligaments and joint capsules resist excessive motion at this level
   c. Cervical spinal nerve I only carries motor fibers
   d. It arises from the spinal column above the C1 vertebra
   e. It innervates:
      i Geniohyoid muscle (hypoglossal nerve)
      ii Thyrohyoid muscle (hypoglossal nerve)
      iii Omohyoid muscle (Ansa cervicalis)
      iv Sternohyoid (Ansa cervicalis)
      v Rectus capitis anterior muscle
      vi Partial innervation of the longus capitus muscle
      vii Rectus capitis lateralis muscle
      viii Partial innervation of the splenius cervicis muscle
      ix Rectus capitis posterior major muscle
2. C2 nerve root:
   a. Motor innervation:
      i Similar muscles innervated by C1 that move the head and neck and

include:
1. Longus capitis
2. Rectus capitis
3. Obliquis capitis
4. Longissimus capitis and cervicis
5. Rotatores
6. Semispinalis
7. Multifidi
8. Intertransversari

ii A small supply to the sternocleidomastoid muscle which is primarily innervated by the spinal accessory nerve

iii It innervates the skin of the scalp at the top of the head, over the top of the ear and the parotid gland

iv It forms part of the greater occipital nerve

3. C3 Nerve Root:
    a. Motor innervation:
        i Paresis of the scalene and levator scapulae
        ii Innervation to:
            1. Infrahyoid muscles
            2. Semispinalis capitis
            3. Cervicis
            4. Longissimus capitis and cervicis
            5. Intertransversari rotatores
            6. Multifidi
        iii Some innervation of the diaphragm
        iv Some innervation of the trapezius muscle that is primarily innervated by the spinal accessory nerve
    b. Sensory innervation of the lower occiput, the angle of the jaw and the upper neck
    c. In addition to motor and sensory symptoms, irritation of the root may cause the red ear syndrome. This represents neurogenic edema from the release of vasoactive neuropeptides (SP and GCRP).
    d. The red ear syndrome has also been described with temporomandibular joint syndrome and thalamic lesions
4. Cervical Root 4:
    a. Motor innervation:
        i Scalene and levator scapulae
        ii Rhomboid muscles
        iii Trapezius
        iv Sternocleidomastoid muscles
        v Diaphragm

b. Sensory innervation:
  i Innervation of the lower neck and parts of the trapezius ridge
  ii No reflex deficit
5. Cervical Root 5:
  a. Motor innervation:
    i Levator scapulae
    ii Rhomboids
    iii Serratus anterior
    iv Supraspinatus
    v Infraspinatus
    vi Deltoid
    vii Biceps and brachioradialis
    viii Some diaphragmatic innervation
  b. Sensory innervation:
    i Neck, shoulder and upper arm pain
    ii Cap of the shoulder
    iii Lateral arm
  c. Depressed biceps and brachioradialis reflex
6. Cervical Root 6:
  a. Motor innervation:
    i Serratus anterior
    ii Biceps
    iii Pronator teres
    iv Flexor carpi radialis
    v Brachioradialis
    vi Extensor carpi radialis longus
    vii Supinator
    viii Extensor carpi radialis brevis
  b. Sensory innervation:
    i Pain in the lateral arm and dorsal forearm
    ii Loss of sensation on the lateral forearm
    iii Loss of sensation in the first and second digits
  c. Depressed biceps and brachioradialis reflex; "inverted radial reflex"
7. Cervical root 7:
  a. Motor innervation:
    i Serratus anterior
    ii Pectoralis major
    iii Latissimus dorsi
    iv Pronator teres
    v Flexor carpi radialis
    vi Triceps

vii Extensor carpi radialis longus
viii Extensor carpi radialis brevis
ix Extensor digitorum

b. Sensory innervation:
   i Pain in the dorsal forearm; rarely a radiation to the middle digit
   ii Some sensory loss in the third and part of the fourth digits
c. Depressed triceps reflex:
   i Rarely, patients may have pseudomyotonia of the hand from misdirection of C7 fibers after root injury. The patient has normal muscle relaxation of the hand but on extension of the fingers, there is paradoxical flexion.

8. Cervical Root 8:
   a. Motor innervation:
      i Flexor digitorum superficialis
      ii Flexor pollicus longus
      iii Flexor digitorum profundus I-IV
      iv Pronator quadratus
      v Abductor pollicis brevis
      vi Opponens pollicis
      vii Flexor pollicis brevis
      viii Lumbricals
      ix Flexor carpi ulnaris
      x Abductor digiti minimi
      xi Opponens digiti minimi
      xii Flexor digiti minimi
      xiii Interossei (dorsal and ventral)
      xiv Abductor pollicis
      xv Extensor digiti minimi
      xvi Extensor carpi ulnaris
      xviiAbductor pollicis longis
      xviii Extensor pollicis longus and brevis
      xix Extensor indicis
   b. Sensory innervation:
      i Medial forearm and hand
      ii Fifth digit
   c. Depression of the finger flexor reflex

Cervical Disc Herniation

General Characteristics

1. Often there is an insidious onset of signs and symptoms at the segmental level
2. There are intradural communicating fibers between adjacent segments of the

posterior roots. The connections are densest between a specific cervical segment and the adjacent caudal root. Therefore a lesion may be one level higher than its actual location

3. Prefixed and postfixed brachial plexi may also alter root localization
4. Cervical root compression and syndromes are often incomplete
5. Lateral discs may cause weakness without pain particularly prominent with discs at the fifth and sixth segmental levels
6. All patients with pain have limitation of movement of the neck to all planes (particularly with hyperextension)
7. The pain is exacerbated with Valsalva maneuvers and with downward pressure on the head when it is in extension
8. Manual traction and abduction of the arm tend to relieve pain (opens the neural exit foramina)
9. Large and central disc herniations may compress the spinal cord:
    a. The central disc herniation may be painless
    b. Bilateral hand numbness and paresthesias may occur
    c. Paresthesias of the chest wall below the compression level may be appreciated
    d. Stiffness and hyperreflexia of the legs is produced by disinhibition of the corticospinal tracts
    e. The C7 nerve root is involved in approximately 70% of patients with HNP. The C6 root is involved in 20% and rarely the C5 and C8 roots are involved in the remaining 10% of patients

Clinical manifestations

1. C1-C2:
    a. There is no disc between C1-C2
2. C2-C3 intervertebral disc space:
    a. Rarely trauma induces C2-C3 disc extrusion
    b. Nonspecific neck and rarely shoulder pain most often; rarely radicular lancinating pain that radiates to preauricular areas and the lateral neck
    c. A retro-odontoid disc may result from an upper migrating disc fragment
    d. Concomitant cord injury may cause motor and sensory symptoms below the disc level
3. C3-C4 intervertebral disc space:
    a. Disc herniations at this level are rare
    b. May present with no or minimal pain
    c. May cause a myelopathy
    d. Hand numbness may be a prominent symptom
4. C4-C5 intervertebral disc space herniation:
    a. The C5 root is affected
    b. Pain is felt across the trapezius ridge to the shoulder

c. There is weakness of the supra and infraspinatus, deltoid and biceps manifested by:
   i Inability to abduct the arm (first 10-20°) and rotate it externally (supra and infraspinati) when the shoulder is adducted
   ii Slight biceps weakness
   iii Depressed biceps reflex
   iv Area of sensory loss over the deltoid muscle

5. C5-C6 intervertebral disc space herniation:
   a. The C6 root is affected from a laterally placed disc
   b. Pain in the trapezius ridge and cap of the shoulder
   c. Sensory radiations are to the anterior upper arm, radial forearm, thumb and index finger
      i Other sensory manifestations include:
         1. Tenderness above the scapular spine as well as the supraclavicular fossa and in the biceps muscle
   d. Motor manifestations:
      i Weakness of forearm flexion (biceps)
      ii Deltoid weakness manifested with poor arm abduction
   e. Diminished or absent biceps and supinator reflexes
6. C6-C7 intervertebral disc space herniation:
   a. The affected root is C7
   b. Pain radiates to the shoulder blade, scapular spine, posterolateral upper arm; less commonly to the elbow, dorsal forearm, index and middle fingers. Rarely, all fingers are numb
   c. Other radiations include:
      i Pectoral and axillary areas
      ii Tenderness is pronounced over the medial scapular border, the supraclavicular fossa and the triceps muscle
   d. There is weakness of the extensors of the forearm and often the wrist; the triceps is weak
   e. Decreased triceps reflex
7. C7-T1 intervertebral disc space herniation:
   a. The C8 root is affected
   b. Pain radiates along the medial side of the forearm; sensory loss is in the distribution of the medial cutaneous nerve of the forearm and of the ulnar nerve in the hand (half of the 4th finger and all of the 5th finger)
   c. Weakness is primarily in the intrinsic hand muscles supplied by the ulnar nerve that include:
      i Flexor digitorum profundus, third and fourth lumbrical, muscles of the hypothenar eminence, adductor pollicis, flexor pollicis brevis and the interossei
   d. The triceps reflex may be slightly depressed

Congenital Cervical Spine Defects with Root Involvement

Absent pedicle of the Cervical Spine

General Characteristics

1. Abnormalities of the cervical spine posterior arch are rare and are most often found incidentally
2. This defect may also occur in the thoracic, lumbar and sacral spine
3. The defect occurs on either side and is almost always unilateral
4. C6 is the most common level of occurrence (39%0 and C5 with 27%)

Clinical Manifestations

1. Most patients are asymptomatic
2. Headache and cervical pain
3. Radicular pain has been described in the upper extremities

Neuropathology

1. Failure of development of the ventral chondrification center during the sixth week of gestation
2. Absence of the pedicle and the lateral mass
3. Dysplasia of the inferior articulating facet at the adjacent level that causes anterior displacement

Neuroimaging

1. MRI:
    a. Useful to eliminate soft tissue injury associated with traumatic subluxations
2. Radiographs:
    a. An enlarged neural foramina due to the absence of the pedicle and posterior displacement of the articular mass of the affected vertebra
    b. Dysplastic posteriorly displaced articular facet and lamina
    c. Dysplastic transverse process
    d. Associated anomalies include:
        i Spina bifida occulta
        ii Vertebral body fusions
    e. Misdiagnoses include spinal tumor, bone tumor and fracture dislocation

Congenital absence of Posterior Elements of the C2 Vertebra

General Characteristics

1. Developmental anomalies of the axis are common

2. Anomalies of the posterior elements are rare and include:
   a. Invagination of the lamina of C2

Clinical Manifestations

1. Progressive myelopathy
2. Mechanical neck pain from cervical root irritation
3. A case report associating absence of C2 vertebra posterior elements with atlanto-axial dislocation and basilar invagination

Neuropathology

1. Failure of dorsal migration of cells from the second spinal sclerotome
2. Failure of chondrification that leads to failure of formation of the neural arch

Neuroimaging

1. Radiographs
   a. Anterolisthesis of C2 over C3
   b. Hypertrophied spinous process of C3

Apert Syndrome

General Characteristics

1. Prevalence is 1 in 65,000 live births
   a. Accounts for 4.5% of all patients with craniosynostosis
   b. Approximately 98% of patients have specific missense mutations in the linker between the second and third extracellular immunoglobulin domain of the FGFR2 gene that maps to chromosome 10q26

Clinical Manifestations

1. In early life:
   a. Headaches and vomiting due to increased intracranial pressure
   b. Stridor and sleep apnea
   c. Visual deficits due to corneal injury from exposure conjunctivitis
   d. Most patients have cognitive impairment although some have normal intelligence
2. Flattened asymmetrical face
3. Maxillary hypoplasia
4. Extremity and digit malformations that include:
   a. Coalition of distal phalanges with synychia of the hands
   b. Short humeri
5. Multiple CNS anomalies that include:
   a. Megalencephaly
   b. Absence of the corpus callosum
   c. Ventriculomegaly
   d. Gyral abnormalities and hypoplastic white matter among others

6. Dermatological features include:
   a. Hyperhydrosis
   b. Brittle nails
   c. Hypopigmentation
   d. Hyperkeratosis in the plantar surfaces among others
7. Cardiovascular defects include both atrial and ventricular defects:
   a. Tetralogy of Fallot
   b. Atrial and ventricular septal defects
   c. Dextrocardia among others
8. Gastrointestinal, genitourinary and respiratory features and anomalies are common

Neuropathology

1. Multiple CNS anomalies that include:
   a. Megalencephaly
   b. Absence of limbic structures and agenesis of the corpus callosum
   c. White matter, convolutional and gyral convolutional anomalies
2. Aplasia or ankylosis of shoulders, elbow and hip joints
3. Rhizomelia
4. During early infancy (< 3 months) there is premature closure of the coronal suture; the lamdoidal sutures are normal
5. The syndactyly is a keratinocyte growth factor receptor (KGFR) mutation

Laboratory Evaluation

1. 98% of patients have a missense substitution mutation in exon 7 of FGFR2

Neuroimaging

1. MRI:
   a. Delineates the cranial deficits that include:
      i Prominent convolutional markings,
      ii Enlarged ventricles
      iii Crowded foramen magnum
      iv Deficient septum pellucidum
      v Agenesis of the corpus callosum
   b. Spinal radiographs:
      i Spinal fusion at C3-C4 and C5-C6 is most common
      ii Multilevel fusion occurs in approximately 20% of patients
      iii Spina bifida occulta is seen in ~7% of patients
      iv Atlanto-axial subluxation occurs in 7% of patients

Differential Diagnosis

1. Beare-Stevenson syndrome (may have FGFR2 mutations)
2. Carpenter syndrome

3. FGFR3-associated coronal synostosis
4. Jackson-Weiss syndrome
5. Pfeiffer syndrome
6. Saethre-Chotzen syndrome

Klippel-Feil Syndrome

General Characteristics

1. There are several different classifications. Naquib classification:
   a. Type I: two sets of block vertebrae with open intervening spaces that can sublux gradually or with acute trauma
   b. Type II: craniocervical anomalies with occipitalization of the axis and basilar invagination; causes increased mobility at the craniocervical junction, possible foramen magnum encroachment; may also be associated with Arnold-Chiari malformation and syringomyelia
   c. Type III: Fusion of one or more levels with associated spinal stenosis
2. The usual presentation is in childhood but it can present in later life
3. Incidence is 2 patients per 1000 patients (Danish study); 0.71% incidence in 1400 skeletons (Washington University School of Medicine study)
4. Klippel-Feil syndrome-1 is caused by heterozygous mutations in the GDF6 gene on chromosome 8q22
5. Additional forms of Klippel-Feil syndrome include:
   a. AR mutation in the MEOX1 gene on chromosome 17q21
   b. AD mutation of the GDF3 gene on chromosome 12p13
   c. AR mutation due to mutation of the MYO18B gene that maps to chromosome 22q12

Clinical Manifestations

1. Upper cervical spine involvement tends to present earlier than lower cervical involvement
2. Short neck with decreased range of movement
3. A low hairline occurs in 40-50% of patients
4. Rotational loss is usually greater than loss of flexion and extension
5. May present with torticollis and facial asymmetry
6. Occipitocervical anomalies
7. Scoliosis may be seen in a significant proportion of patients
8. Cervical spinal stenosis
9. A Sprengel anomaly occurs in 20-30% of patients
   a. Omovertebral bone which is an osteocartilaginous connection that tethers the scapula to the spine
   b. Radicular pain primarily from midcervical root involvement

Neuropathology

1. The cross-sectional area of the spinal cord is smaller in KFS patients from C2-C7
2. In older patients complete fusion is more prevalent at C2-C7
3. Fusion of the posterior elements is more common than anterior element fusion
4. An arrest of normal vertebral development may affect appositional bone development
5. Associated deficits:
    a. Deafness
    b. Vocal cord impairment
    c. Cleft palate (AD pattern)
6. Defects of post-otic neural crest cells (PONC)

Laboratory Evaluation

1. Hearing evaluation

Neuroimaging

1. Radiographic features:
    a. Vertebral fusion at varying levels of the cervical spine
    b. Anterior-posterior narrowing of the vertebral bodies (Wasp-Waist sign)
    c. Focal canal stenosis C2-C7 (some patients)
    d. Hemivertebrae
    e. Spina bifida occulta
    f. Scoliosis
    g. Sprengel's deformity
2. CT:
    a. Better image features demonstrated than on plain radiography
    b. Delineates canal stenosis
3. MRI:
    a. Delineates canal stenosis and cord compression
    b. Rare anterior cervical meningomyelocele

Osteoarthritis of the Cervical Spine

Cervical Spondylosis

General Characteristics

1. Cervical spondylosis is a degenerative disease of the cervical spine that affects the:
    a. Vertebral bodies
    b. Intervertebral discs
    c. Nerve roots
    d. Spinal cord

e. Facet joints
f. Longitudinal ligaments
g. g. Ligamentum flavum

2. It is the most frequent cause of spinal cord pathology in patients older than 55 years of age; >80% of men and women over 50 years of age have some radiologic features of the disease
3. Possibly starts earlier in men than women
4. In young patients it may be secondary to an abnormality in a joint between the vertebrae

Clinical Manifestations

1. Chronic suboccipital headaches
2. Pain may be localized to the neck or radiate to the shoulder, scapular border (medial) or to the arm
3. Compression of the nerve roots causes radicular pain; the C6 root is the most commonly affected from degeneration at the C5-C6 interspace; the next most common roots affected are C7 and then C5
4. Cervical myelopathy:
   a. Has an insidious onset and is most common in 50-60 year old patients
   b. The sphincters are rarely involved at presentation
   c. Signs and symptoms occur from involvement of:
      i The corticospinal, posterior column, cerebellar and spinothalamic tracts
      ii Motor deficits from corticospinal and anterior horn cell dysfunction
      iii Central spinal cord syndrome
         1. Due to lamination of the corticospinal pathways the arms are more affected than the legs
      iv Brown-Sequard syndrome
      v Upper limb pain with a component of spinal cord compression
   d. Unusual manifestations:
      i Glove-like sensory loss
      ii Concomitant tandem cervical and lumbar stenosis. There are almost always degenerative changes at both levels
      iii Complex gait abnormalities; tandem gait is difficult in most patients from a combination of peripheral lower extremity proprioceptive loss and compression of the dorsal columns and spinocerebellar pathways
      iv Lhermitte's sign

The Neurological Examination

1. Forward flexed neck with limitation to all planes of movement; particularly severe in extension
2. Spurling's sign in which radicular pain is exaggerated by extension and lateral

bending of the neck toward the side of the lesion (further compromising the nerve root exit foramina)

3. Rarely Lhermitte's sign can be elicited
4. Atrophy of the C5-C6 innervated muscles, particularly the biceps; prominent trapezius muscle spasm and hypertrophy
5. Often atrophy of the median forearm musculature
6. Fasciculations that are spontaneous or mechanically induced in the shoulder girdle musculature
7. Weakness is more prominent proximally than distally
8. Sensory loss in affected dermatomes is less prominent than weakness
9. Inability to perform tandem gait
10. An inverted radial reflex with striking the biceps tendon. This requires two lesions:
    a. Compression above the C5-C6 level usually by a spondylitic bar at C4-C5
    b. Osteophytes that block the C5-C6 intervertebral foramen
    c. Sensation enters the disinhibited spinal cord (from compression at C4-C5) by higher C3-C4 and lower roots from vibration of the arm when eliciting the bicep's reflex
    d. There is no induction of the biceps reflex due to the osteophytes at C5-C6 but the disinhibited spinal cord fires at C8-T1 eliciting finger flexion
    e. Extremely rarely there is extension of the arm rather than flexion due to activation of C7 (triceps)
11. There are almost always concomitant signs of lumbosacral radiculopathy
12. Cortical spinal release phenomena in the form of Hoffman's and Babinski signs are present with spinal cord compression
13. Increased reflexes in the upper and lower extremities below the level of the lesion (disinhibited spinal cord)
14. Broad based and spastic gait

Neuropathology

1. Radicular arteries may be compressed in the dural sleeves
2. Contribution from a congenitally small canal
3. Intervertebral discs dehydrate and lose elasticity with age which leads to fissure formation
4. Ligaments become less elastic and develop traction spurs
5. The disc space narrows, the annulus bulges and the facets override which increases motion at that level which exacerbates the process
6. There may be concomitant disc herniation
7. Annulus bulging, facet hypertrophy and ligamentous thickening narrow the spinal canal
8. Overriding of the uncinate processes and their hypertrophy compresses the ventrolateral component of the nerve exit foramina. Facet hypertrophy and

degenerative changes narrow the dorsal component of the foramina:
   a. Thinning and fragmentation of the articular cartilage that leads to exposure of subchondral bone which leads to fibrosis, increased bone formation and cystic changes
   b. Loss of articular cartilage leads to new bone formation (osteophytes)

Laboratory Evaluation

1. EMG:
   a. Delineates the involved roots

Neuroimaging

1. Radiographs:
   a. Delineates uncovertebral and facet joint hypertrophy, the neural exit foramen, the intervertebral disc spaces and osteophytes
   b. Flexion-extension views are important in instances of instability
2. MRI:
   a. Excellent delineation of neural elements
   b. Better evaluation of any parenchymal spinal cord pathology
3. In selected patients myelography with CT delineates the relation of nerve roots to bone

Cervical Spinal Stenosis

General Characteristics

1. The AP diameter of the normal adult male cervical cord is 17-18 mm at levels C3-C5. The lower cervical levels measure 12-14 mm. Stenosis has a mean AP diameter of less than 10 mm and diameters of 10-13 mm are relatively stenotic in the upper cervical canal
2. The confines of the cervical spinal canal are:
   a. Laminae and ligamentum flavum posterolaterally
   b. The pedicles anterolaterallly
   c. Discs and the vertebral bodies anteriorly
   d. Extension of the neck reduces the overall canal area by 2-3 mm
   e. Central cervical spinal compression is due to bulging of the disc annulus, hypertrophy of the ligamentum flavum and spondylitic bony overgrowth
   f. Movement in congenital or acquired stenosis exacerbates the condition. The anterior roots are compressed between the annulus margins and spondylitic bony hypertrophic bars. In the posterior canal, hypertrophic facet joints and thickened infolded ligamentum flavum distort and compress dorsal roots.
   g. Neural elements are tethered anteriorly against the protruding disc annulus and spondylitic bony overgrowth in hyperflexion
   h. Lateral cervical stenosis is caused by encroachment of the lateral recess on

the neural exit foramina due to hypertrophy of the uncovertebral joints, the lateral disc margin and facet hypertrophy

Clinical Manifestations

1. If there is primary central spinal cord compression, there is minimal pain but weakness and sensory loss below the level of compression
2. Radicular pain at affected levels from concomitant nerve root compression
3. Often there are depressed biceps and brachioradialis reflexes. The inverted radial reflex is often present (due to concomitant spondylitic changes at C4 and C5-C6)
4. Poor tandem gait due to compression of the dorsal and ventral spinocerebellar tracts (both serve the legs while the cuneocerebellar tract provides coordinative functions for the arms and fingers and is not often affected to the same degree)
5. Minimal atrophy of C5-C6 innervated musculature
6. Neurogenic bladder may occur late in the course of the disease

Neuropathology

1. A congenitally small canal with short pedicles; acquired spondylosis
2. Disc degeneration, bulging and extrusion with concomitant facet and uncovertebral joint osteoarthritic overgrowth of bone
3. Hypertrophy and calcification of the posterior longitudinal ligament that is more common in Asian patients

Laboratory Evaluation

1. EMG:
2. Delineates the levels of radicular involvement

Neuroimaging

1. MRI:
   a. Grading system according to the T2-weighted sagittal images:
      i Grade 0: absence of canal stenosis
      ii Grade 1: subarachnoid space obliteration exceeding 50%
      iii Grade 2: spinal cord deformity
      iv Grade 3: spinal cord signal change
2. CT:
   a. Needed when there are complications and contraindications for MRI studies (metal implants and cardiac pacers)

Cervical Spondylolisthesis

General Characteristics

1. Degenerative lumbar spondylolisthesis is common in elderly patients
2. Cervical spondylolisthesis is most often caused by trauma

3. The injuries that lead to this condition include:
   a. Traumatic spondylolisthesis of the axis (hangman's fracture)
   b. Uni or bilateral facet dislocation and fracture subluxation
   c. Classification system for degenerative cervical spondylolisthesis:
      i Type 1: most common, occurs adjacent to relatively stiff spondylotic cervical levels
      ii Type II; occurs within spondylotic cervical segment

Clinical Manifestations

1. Decreased cervical range of motion
2. The affected levels are primarily C3-C4 and C4-C5
3. Neck pain is the initial symptom that may be associated with occipital radiations
4. Radicular symptoms
5. A combination of myeloradiculopathy

Neuropathology

1. Trauma with hangman's fracture of the axis
2. Bilateral or unilateral facet dislocation and fracture
3. Degenerative osteoarthritis with hypertrophic facet arthropathy that causes joint erosion, marginal osteophytes and subluxation; disc degeneration has been posited to be pivotal. Other evidence suggests that thinning of the facets and narrowing of the joint space is primary
4. Rare causes include:
   a. Renal osteodystrophy
   b. Congenital absence and hypoplasia of the C6 pedicles with C6-C7 spondylolisthesis

Neuroimaging

1. Radiographs:
   a. A large proportion of patients are demonstrated to be unstable with flexion and extension at involved levels
   b. Horizontal displacement (in 217 patients) averaged 3.9 mm
2. MRI:
   a. Delineates the location and extent of neurological compression at the level of the spondylolisthesis

Laboratory Evaluation

1. EMG:
   a. Delineates the affected roots

Cervical Perineural Cyst

General Characteristics

1. Tarlov (perineural) cysts are common and most often incidental findings in the lumbosacral spine
2. Rarely perineural cysts are symptomatic in the cervical roots
3. A Tarlov cyst is formed within the nerve root sheath at the dorsal root ganglion

Clinical Manifestations

1. Radicular pain at the affected level that is exacerbated by Valsalva maneuvers
2. Rarely, compressive cervical myelopathy

Neuropathology

1. The major histologic feature of the Tarlov cyst is the presence of nerve fibers in the cyst wall
2. The mechanisms posited for cyst formation include:
   a. Ball-valve formation from a hemosiderin deposition caused by blockage of venous drainage of the perineurium and epineurium (traumatic theory)
   b. Congenital arachnoid proliferation along existing nerve roots

Laboratory Evaluation

1. MRI:
   a. Isotense lesion on T1-weighted sequences; A hyperintense signal on T2 weighted images
   b. Displacement of the spinal cord

Neuralgic Amyotrophy

General Characteristics

1. Neuralgic amyotrophy is an acute painful multiple mononeuropathy that most often involves the upper brachial plexus
2. It may be restricted to one fascicle of one nerve, plexus or root
3. Hereditary neuralgic amyotrophy is primarily linked to chromosome 17q25.3. It is caused by heterozygous mutation in the SEPT9 gene.
4. It is AD.

Clinical Manifestations

1. Acute and recurrent episodes of brachial plexus weakness and atrophy most often preceded by severe pain in the affected arm
2. Usually it is asymmetric and involves plexi in a patchy distribution. It may involve the cervical and lumbar plexus as well as cranial nerves
3. There is amyotrophy and sensory loss
4. It is usually monophasic, autolimited and does not lead to a generalized polyneuropathy

Neuropathology

1. It may be restricted to one fascicle of one nerve or root
2. May be triggered by infection
3. Axonal neuropathy
4. Possibly episodic patients are affected on an autoimmune basis

Laboratory Evaluation

1. EMG:
    a. A severe axonal neuropathy

Neurogenic Thoracic Outlet Syndrome

General Characteristics

1. Most often affects the C8-T1 roots or the proximal trunk of the brachial plexus

Clinical Manifestations

1. Insidious onset of atrophy and weakness of the intrinsic hand muscles predominately in the muscles of the thenar eminence and radial digit flexors
2. Numbness and sensory loss occurs in the medial forearm but may be absent in some patients

Neuropathology

1. Most often the predominant root that is compressed is T1
2. The fibrous band extends from the first rib to either the tip of the elongated C7 transverse process or a rudimentary cervical rib

Laboratory Evaluation

1. EMG:
    a. Nerve conduction studies demonstrate attenuated compound muscle action potentials of the abductor policis brevis and often loss of sensory nerve action potential of the medial antebrachial cutaneous nerve

Neuroimaging

1. Radiographs:
    a. Cervical rib is demonstrated

Disputed Thoracic Outlet Syndrome

General Characteristics

1. Anatomy of the thoracic outlet:
    a. The sterno-costovertebral space:
        i The most proximal part of the thoracic outlet tunnel which is bounded
            1. Anteriorly by the sternum
            2. Posteriorly by the spine

3. Laterally by the first rib

ii The subclavian artery and vein as well as the C4-T1 roots of the plexus transverse the space

iii Nerve roots have exited the spine but have not formed trunks

iv Associated structures include:

1. The apex of the lung and the pleura
2. Sympathetic trunk
3. Jugular vein
4. Lymphatics of the neck
5. Rarely the space is congenitally narrowed

Scalene Triangle

1. Anatomy:
   a. Anterior scalene muscle anteriorly
   b. Middle scalene muscle posteriorly
   c. The first rib forms the base
2. Anterior scalene muscle:
   a. Origins are the transverse processes of C3-C6
   b. Insertion on the scalene tubercle of the first rib varies; tubercle insertion is between the subclavian artery and vein and pleural dome
   c. Variants of insertion:
      i Behind the artery
      ii Between the artery and the brachial plexus
      iii Entire base of the scalene triangle (traps the neurovascular bundle)
      iv Anterior insertion may merge with insertion of the middle scalene muscle (20% of patients)
      v The C5 and C6 roots may traverse the anterior scalene muscle rather than descend between the anterior and middle scalene muscles
3. Middle scalene muscles:
   a. Origin is the transverse processes of C2-C7
   b. Insertion is Chassaignac's retro arterial tubercle of the first rib
   c. May insert on the fibrous septum of the pleural dome; lateral fibers insert on the second rib
   d. The C8-T1 roots (individually or together is the lower trunk of the brachial plexus) are compressed by a more anterior or forward insertion of the middle scalene muscle (its sharp anterior edge)
4. First rib:
   a. Forms the floor of the scalene triangle
   b. T1 is closest to the rib
   c. Congenital rib anomalies bony ridge, hypoplasia and inward curvature may compress the neurovascular bundle

5. Scalene triangle congenital variations:
   a. The base of the triangle is 0.77 cm in men and 0.67 cm in women
   b. C5, C6, and C7 roots emerge from the apex of the triangle; the fibers of the middle and anterior scalene muscles also merge at the apex. Patients with C5, C6, and C7 root involvement have a greater incidence of roots that emerge from the apex:
      i Interdigitation of anterior and middle scalene muscles occurs in 70% of symptomatic patients
      ii Adherence of C5 and C6 roots to the middle scalene muscle may occur and places these roots under traction when the arm is moved
6. Costoclavicular space (compresses the brachial plexus)
7. Pectoralis minor space (compresses the lateral and medial cords of the brachial plexus)

Cervical Ribs that Compress Cervical Roots

General Characteristics

1. 0.17% to 0.74% (average 0.3%) of the general population (female > males, 2:1) have cervical ribs
2. Approximately 10% of patients with cervical ribs are symptomatic
3. Symptomatic patients often have suffered arm trauma or are in professions that require repetitive overhead arm movement
4. Aneurysmal dilatation or subclavian artery stenosis is most often associated with a rudimentary thoracic rib or a cervical rib

Clinical Manifestations

1. Neurological symptoms from cervical ribs are caused by nerve compression primarily of the lower trunk (composed of the C8, T1 roots)

Rib-Band Syndrome of Gilliat

1. A Roos type II band
2. Compression of the C8, T1 roots
3. Paresthesia of the 4th, 5th finger, medial forearm to the medial humerus
4. There is atrophy and wasting of intrinsic hand muscles

Neuropathology

1. Usual pathology in the sternocostovertebral space includes:
   a. Thyroid mass
   b. Enlarged thymus gland
   c. Parathyroid mass
   d. Lymph nodes
   e. Pancoast tumor (squamous or adenocarcinoma of the lung)

Other Structural Congenital Anomalies Affecting Cervical

Roots

1. Hypoglossal duct cyst (involvement of C3, C4 roots)
2. Branchial cleft cysts (involvement of C2-C5 roots)
3. Short pedicle and block vertebral bodies:
    a. Entrapment of the root under the pedicle and in the neural foraminal exit canal
    b. Achondroplasia (at all cervical levels) there are block vertebrae and often there is associated foramen magnum stenosis

Trauma of Cervical Nerve Roots

General Characteristics

1. The dorsal root of C2, C3 and C4 are frequently injured from flexion-extension injury (whiplash)
2. C8-T1 roots are most often involved from congenital anatomical predisposition
3. Damage to cervical roots occurs during transaxillary first rib resection:
    a. C8-T1 roots are most frequently involved
    b. C5, C6 roots are most often damaged with scalenectomy and neurolysis procedures (supraclavicular approach)
4. Surgical trauma:
    a. C5, C6 and C7 roots are most often affected with the repair of multi-level spondylosis, spondylolisthesis and disc decompression
    b. Instrumentation that requires plates and pedicle screws
5. High impact trauma (MVA, falls, contact athletics)
6. Injury by epidural catheterization with bupivacaine >0.25% or by trauma by the catheter itself

Clinical Manifestations

1. There is immediate pain that worsens over time and may spread extra-territorially (peripheral and central sensitization)
2. Pain radiations:
    a. Preauricular nerve territory (C2, C3 roots). The radiation overlaps with V2 and V3 radiations of the trigeminal nerve for which it may be confused
    b. Postauricular nerve territory (C2-C4 roots). This territory covers the ear, overlaps with C2 at the angle of the jaw and radiates to the parietal and occipital areas of the skull
    c. Specific radiations of C2 in isolation is to the base of the occiput, the angle of the jaw, parietal scalp and to the brow. The brow radiations are common with cough or Valsalva maneuvers with underlying Chiari malformations and with severe cervical spondylosis

   d. Greater and lesser occipital nerve distributions (C2, C3, C4) posterior root damage with radiation of pain to the basiocciput and occipital areas of the scalp that is associated with migraine headache
3. Motor manifestations:
   a. Flexion extension injury may damage the ansa hypoglossi:
      i Causes slight weakness of the sternocleidomastoid muscle as most of its innervation is derived from the spinal component of cranial nerve XI. Spasm of the muscle may be severe.
      ii Weakness of the suprahyoid muscles that are located above the hyoid bone in the neck and include the digastric, stylohyoid, geniohyoid and mylohyoid:
         1. Dysfunction of elevation of the hyoid and widening of the esophagus during swallowing
      iii Slight weakness of the scalene and trapezius muscles
4. Autonomic dysregulation occurs (usually adrenergic sympathetic overactivity) particularly with C8, T1 and T2 injury. The former causes sympathetic innervation to the face and eye while the T2 sympathetic ganglion is the primary innervation to the arm
5. Rotary subluxation of a facet joint presents with:
   a. Pain at the segmental level
   b. Torticollis (to the affected side)
   c. Segmental root weakness
6. Complex Regional Pain Syndrome I and II (CRPS)
   a. CRPS occurs most frequently after injury of small nociceptive afferents in soft tissue (type I) or injury of a specific nerve (type II)
   b. Hyperalgesia and thermal and mechanical allodynia; loss of sensation both may occur in a regional distribution
   c. Autonomic Dysregulation:
      i Temperature change (in general, in the early stages there is increased warmth and later there is coolness)
      ii Hyper or hypohidrosis
   d. Movement disorder:
      i Difficulty initiating movement
      ii Dystonia
      iii Weakness
      iv Tremor
      v Atrophy
   e. Severe spreading pain that involves multiple roots (regional)
   f. Dystrophic changes in the nails, hair and integument

Red Ear Syndrome

1. The C3 root is involved

2. Usually, one ear is involved but the process may be bilateral
3. The ear is beet red, slightly edematous and non-painful
4. 4. The face rather than the ear may show similar signs

Neuropathology of Cervical Nerve Root Disorder

a. Traumatic Injuries:
    - i Nerve root avulsion:
        1. High impact motor vehicle injury
        2. C5-C6 roots are the most often affected
    - ii Rotary subluxation of facet joints; jumped facet joints
    - iii Spondylolisthesis:
        1. Middle cervical segments are most often involved
    - iv Rare disc herniations (overwhelmingly disc disease is a degenerative process; trauma frequently exacerbates existing disease)

b. Traction injuries:
    - i Whiplash (severe flexion – extension injury)
    - ii Neuropraxis (Class I):
        1. Interruption of nerve conduction without disruption of axon continuity:
            a. A physiologic block of nerve conduction
            b. There are sensory and motor deficits distal to the injury
            c. The endoneurium, perineurium and epineurium are intact
            d. There is no Wallerian degeneration
            e. There is no conduction across the injured area
    - iii Axonotmesis (Class II)
        1. Loss of the continuity of both axon and its myelin sheath. The epineurium and perineurium are preserved:
            a. Wallerian degeneration occurs distal to the site of injury
            b. There are motor and sensory deficits distal to the injury
            c. EMG changes include:
            d. Lack of nerve conduction distal to the injury
            e. Fibrillation and sharp waves are detected 2 to 3 weeks following the injury in denervated muscles
    - iv Neurotmesis (Class III):
        1. Severance of the entire nerve fiber
        2. Wallerian degeneration occurs distal to the injury
        3. Severe sensory, motor and autonomic dysfunction of the innervated territory of affected fibers
        4. EMG and NCV parameters are similar to axonotmesis. There is no conduction distal to the injury
        5. Surgical injury to nerve roots during disc, spondylosis, spondylolisthesis and transaxillary and supraclavicular first rib resections

a. Congenital Anomalies that affect cervical roots:
   i Hypoglossal duct cysts
   ii Branchial cleft cysts
   iii Short and absent pedicles
   iv Achondroplasia
   v Basilar impression
   vi Platybasia
   vii Cervical syrinx
   viii Arnold Chiari malformations
   ix Cervical syringomyelia
   x Klippel-Feil Syndrome
   xi Rib-Band syndrome of Gilliat

Laboratory Evaluation

1. EMG

Neuroimaging

1. Ultrasound
2. MRI microneurography
3. CT evaluation if there is bony involvement

Lax Ligament Syndrome (that Attach the Odontoid Process to the Atlas)

General Characteristics

1. Four ligaments are involved:
   a. A cruciate posterior ligament that attaches the odontoid process to the axis
   b. Lateral ligaments that attach the odontoid process to the lateral mass of C1
   c. The alar ligament from the tip of the odontoid process to the rim of the foramen magnum
2. Normal posterior odontoid displacement with neck flexion is:
   i 3-5 mm in children
   ii 1-2 mm in adults
3. In abnormal displacement the C2 root is primarily involved with concomitant spinal cord compression

Clinical Manifestations

Differential Diagnosis of Cervical Ligament Disorders

1. Rheumatoid arthritis:
   a. Frequently there is tingling of all fingers, the arm and the hands most likely from cervical spinal cord compression

   b. Subluxation at high cervical levels with spinal cord compression
   c. The rheumatoid pannus erodes the cruciate ligament
2. Lax ligaments:
   a. Trisomy 21
   b. Ehlers-Danlos Syndrome (Type IV)
   c. Marfan's Syndrome
3. Trauma (flexion/extension) injury of the neck

Differential Diagnosis of Ligament Hypertrophy with Cervical Root Impingement

1. Acromegaly
2. Mucopolysaccharidosis:
   a. Morquio's Syndrome has concomitant absence or hypoplasia of the odontoid process
3. Posterior ligament ossification syndrome
4. IgG-4 syndrome - a form of pachymeningitis
5. Hirayama syndrome (ligament laxity at lower cervical levels with spinal cord compression)

Pachymeningitis with Cervical Root Compression

1. Syphilis:
   a. Dense fibrous dural thickening surrounding the roots and cervical cord
2. Sarcoid
3. Tuberculosis
4. IgG-4 syndrome and idiopathic pachymeningitis
5. Subarachnoid hemorrhage with consequent arachnoiditis
6. Hodgkin's and non-Hodgkin's lymphoma

Tumors of the Cervical Nerve Roots

General Characteristics

1. Schwannoma:
   a. Associated with neurofibromatosis (NFT) type I mutations on chromosome 17; Type II causes bilateral Schwannoma on the VIII nerve (the mutation is in chromosome 22)
   b. May affect multiple nerve roots concomitantly
   c. Root and plexiform involvement > in lumbosacral than brachial distributions
   d. A dumbbell tumor; characteristically it involves the nerve which enlarges the nerve exit foramen and occupies the intradural extramedullary space with slowly progressive cord compression
2. Neurofibroma

3. Meningioma:
   a. Intradural extramedullary growth; concomitant nerve root compression
   b. Plexiform (en-plaque growth)
4. Lymphoma (infiltration of nerve roots)
5. Leukemia:
   a. Hemorrhage into a nerve root (acute presentation)
   b. Infiltration of nerve roots (insidious presentation)
6. Carcinomatosis of the meninges:
   a. Primary tumors are lung, breast, GI tract and prostate
   b. Mental status alteration
   c. Asymmetric cranial nerve and radicular presentation
   d. Patients may be asymptomatic which has been seen with many tumors but primarily from the breast
7. Chordoma:
   a. Most common in the clivus and sacral vertebrae; rarely occur in the thoracic and cervical vertebrae (10%)
   b. Radicular signs and symptoms in the affected cervical roots
8. Osteogenic sarcoma is rare
9. Fibrosarcoma (degeneration of a neurofibroma):
   a. Exacerbation of radicular pain; spinal cord compression
10. Chondrosarcoma (rare):
    a. Radicular involvement
11. Ewing's sarcoma:
    a. Approximately 5% occur in the axial vertebrae
    b. Segmental radicular pain and dysfunction
    c. Pathologic fracture with spinal cord compression
12. Pancoast tumor:
    a. Occur at the apex of the lung
    b. Adeno or squamous carcinoma of the lung is most common:
       i Breast cancer
       ii Sarcoma following breast X-RT
    c. Involvement is primarily of the lower nerve roots (C8-T1) in the sterno-costovertebral space
    d. Pain (usually burning in quality) is along the medial forearm and into the 4th and 5th fingers
    e. Horner's syndrome occurs from involvement of the sympathetic innervation of C8, T1
13. Lymphomatous B-cell tumors:
    a. Diffuse radiculopathies
14. Post x-ray treatment sarcoma:
    a. Follows x-RT for breast cancer most frequently

   b. Involves roots of the brachial plexus C8, T1 >C5, C6
   c. May be delayed in onset from the last treatment by years
   d. Associated with myokymia in the irradiated arm
   e. Associated with skin changes that include hyperpigmentation, telangiectasia and proliferative endarteritis
   f. MRI reveals hypertrophy and swelling of the trunks and cords of the brachial plexus that enhance with contrast
15. Neuromyotonia with Hodgkin's disease:
   a. Rippling fasciculation in the innervated muscles of the affected nerve roots
   b. Anti-TA antibodies may be detected in the serum
16. Mixed salivary gland tumors:
   a. Infiltrate C1-C4 roots
   b. "Sugar coated" roots
17. Parotid gland tumors:
   a. VIIth nerve most frequently involved
   b. Cervical C2-C4 roots are involved less frequently
   c. Swollen parotid glands noted in diabetes mellitus, mumps, HIV, tumors, and uremia
18. Salivary gland cylindroma:
   a. Cervical C1-C4 roots are infiltrated
   b. May have concomitant cranial nerve involvement

Infection Involving Cervical Nerve Roots

Herpes Zoster

General Characteristics

1. Varicella zoster virus (VZV) is a human neurotropic alpha herpes virus
2. Primary infection causes varicella (chicken pox). After infection the virus becomes latent in cranial nerve ganglia, dorsal root ganglia and autonomic ganglia throughout the neuraxis
3. In older age as cell-mediated immunity to VZV declines or during immunosuppression that occurs with cancer, HIV or organ transplantation, the virus reactivates to cause shingles
4. VZV becomes latent in all ganglia and therefore can develop anywhere in the body
5. In general, resolution of the skin lesions is concomitant with decreased pain and its resolution in 4-6 weeks
6. Associated neurological complications include:
   a. Post herpetic neuralgia
   b. Meningitis or meningoencephalitis

c. Cerebellitis
d. Cranial nerve palsies:
   i Ophthalmoplegia (III)
   ii Ramsay Hunt syndrome (VII)
e. Multiple cranial nerve involvement
f. Vasculopathy (carotid / MCA stroke)
g. Myelopathy (T4 level often involved)
h. Inflammatory eye disorders:
   i Progressive outer retinal necrosis (PORN)
i. VZV reactivation may cause chronic radicular pain without rash (zoster sine herpete)
j. All neurological complications may occur without rash

Clinical Manifestations

1. C5, C6 > C4, C5 > C8, T1 are the most commonly involved roots (cervical)
2. Clinical symptomatology:
   a. Grouped vesicular eruption in a dermatomal distribution
   b. Sensory loss in a dermatomal pattern to all modalities; severe pain in the affected dermatome
   c. Atrophy, weakness much less than sensory alterations (subtle)
   d. May have dermatomal sensory alterations weeks to occasionally months prior to the vesicular eruption and there may be no eruption (herpes sine herpete); there is often burning pain in the affected dermatome

Post Herpetic Neuralgia

Clinical Manifestations

1. Spontaneous lancinating pain
2. Deep continuous ache with lancinating exacerbations in the involved dermatome
3. Decreased sensory threshold to pinprick, touch or temperature of the dermatome
4. Allodynia to both static and dynamic mechano and thermal stimuli of the neighboring dermatomes but at times of the affected dermatome

Neuropathology

1. During reactivation at the DRG, spinal root or cranial nerve levels
2. There is an inflammatory response that involves the leptomeninges with plasma cells and lymphocytes
3. DRG inflammation may be accompanied by hemorrhagic necrosis of nerve cells
4. The rash is concomitant with a VZV specific T-cell proliferation

Laboratory Evaluation

1. Anti-VZV IgM antibody in the serum or CSF
2. Anti-VZV IgG antibody in CSF
3. Detection of VZV DNA in blood mononuclear cells or CSF
4. VZV DNA is detected in CSF in blood MNCs during neurological involvement

Neuroimaging

1. MRI:
    a. Delineates parenchymal involvement in the brain, cerebellum and spinal cord

Herpes Simplex

General Characteristics

1. HSV is a ubiquitous virus; HSV-1 is usually acquired in childhood by contact with secretions that contain the virus
2. HSV-2 may be an indirect measure of sexual activity
3. Greater than 50% of the population are positive for the HSV-1 virus by age 30; HSV-2 correlates with the degree of sexual activity and starts to emerge at puberty
4. HSV-1 and HSV-2 can cause similar genital and orofacial primary infections after contact with infectious secretions:
    a. HSV-1 usually oral secretions
    b. HSV-2 most often from genital contact

Clinical Manifestations

1. Stimuli that trigger HSV reactivation include:
    a. Fever
    b. Local trauma
    c. Physical and severe emotional stress
    d. Exposure to ultraviolet light
    e. Hormonal deficits
    f. Immunosuppression
2. HSV is the most common identified viral focal encephalitis worldwide
3. Mutations in the UNC93B1 and TLR3 genes have been posited to cause susceptibility to HSV infection
4. Some primary infections are asymptomatic (mucocutaneous HSV infection)
5. The lesions may be painful, are manifest within several days of exposure and may erupt over 1 to 2 weeks
6. The mucosal lesions may present on the mucosal surface of the mouth or genitals and may be associated with malaise, myalgia and anorexia
7. Individual vesicles on mucosal surfaces rapidly collapse and form a shallow

painful ulcer less than 8 – 10 mm in diameter; they evolve to crusted ulcers that heal within 5 to 7 days

8. Recurrent mucocutaneous HSV infection can be subclinical (viral excretion without lesions) or mucosal and cutaneous lesions with shedding of the virus
9. Localized burning or paresthesias may precede recurrent lesions usually without constitutional symptoms. Recurrences may last 3 to 7 days and recur numerous times or only 1 to 2 times per year. Recurrences may last > 30 days in immunocompromised patients
10. Sacral HSV infection can be associated with meningeal inflammation as aseptic meningitis
11. The lesions have a painful erythematous base and may be dermatomal or can be regional that involve several roots
12. The encephalitis involves the medial temporal lobe most severely, the frontal and insular cortex less often:
    a. Seizures and mental status alterations are presenting signs and symptoms
    b. Aseptic meningitis is common

Neuropathology

1. In orofacial HSV the trigeminal ganglia is involved; in genital HSV infection the sacral (S2-S4) DRG are involved
2. Reactivation and replication of latent HSV is within the area supplied by the DRG in which latency was established
3. Dissemination can occur in patients with impaired T-cell immunity as seen with solid organ transplant and in HIV patients
4. There is a complex interaction between the host and HSV to control the micro RNA pathway that often favors viral infection and persistence. This is accomplished by decreasing immune detection, blocking apoptosis, promoting cell growth, or enhancing lytic or latent infection.
5. Encephalitis:
    a. An acute necrotizing encephalitis:
        i Widespread bilateral and asymmetrical necrosis in the temporal lobes
        ii Most often affected are the anterior parts of the parahippocampal, fusiform, inferior and middle temporal gyri
        iii Intense reactive inflammatory changes around the necrotic tissue

Laboratory Evaluation

1. Tzanck smear (does not distinguish between HSV-1 and HSV-2)
2. Polymerase chain reaction:
    a. Performed on the CSF
3. Antibody testing is able to demonstrate primary seroconversion

Neuroimaging

1. MRI

a. Delineates the brain temporal lobe parenchymal encephalitis

Lyme Disease

General Characteristics

1. Lyme disease is caused by infection with the spirochete Borrelia burgdorferi and the immune response that it elicits
2. The disease is transmitted to humans from infected ticks of the genus Ixodes

Clinical Manifestations

1. Stage I Lyme disease:
   a. Isolated erythema migrans with an undifferentiated febrile illness
   b. The stage occurs 1 to 30 days after the tick bite
   c. Erythema migrans develops in 2/3 of patients on average 7 days after the tick bite; the rash most often occurs at the site of the bite, expands over days. There may be concentric rings of erythema and clearing giving it a bull's-eye appearance. Approximately 80% of patients have only one episode of erythema migrans. Multiple lesions occur in 20% of patients from hematogenous dissemination
   d. Redness of the conjunctiva with tearing
   e. Co-infection from the same tick bite occurs with Ehrlichia species and Babesia microti in 15% of patients. They usually cause a high fever
2. Stage 2 Lyme Disease:
   a. Early dissemination develops 3-10 weeks following the initial bite in approximately 2/3 of patients
   b. Systemic manifestations include fever and malaise; other organ systems that become involved due to hematologic or lymphatic spread of organisms include:
      i Musculoskeletal system:
         1. Inflammatory arthritis that may begin as a polyarticular process that evolves into a large joint monarticular process
         2. Approximately 2/3 of patients have recurrences 2.5 months apart
      ii Neurologic complications include:
         1. Occurs in 5-20% of patients
         2. Cranial neuropathy most often uni or bilateral VIIth nerve paralysis (3% of patients)
         3. Meningitis and encephalopathy
      iii Cutaneous manifestations:
         1. Multiple erythema migrans lesions: erythematous macules (1-5 cm) that may be oval; they are evanescent and do not expand over days
         2. Borrelial lymphocytoma; a bluish red nodular lesion that occurs:

a. Ear lobe in children
b. In adults it is seen in the areola of the nipple, scrotum, nose and the extremities
c. The heart may be involved

4. Stage 3 Lyme Disease:
    a. This is a collection of signs and symptoms that occur months to years after the initial infection and remain controversial
    b. Lyme arthritis is the major manifestation of stage 3 disease
    c. Neurologic complications include:
        i Chronic progressive encephalomyelitis
        ii Unilateral or bilateral VIIth nerve palsy
        iii C5, C6 cervical roots are the most often affected
        iv Decreased cognitive function (controversial)

Neuropathology

1. Approximately 20,000 patients are reported annually in the USA; endemic areas are the coastal northeast, California and the Great Lakes region.
2. The disease is transmitted to humans by the bite of the Ixodes scapularis and pacificus ticks. It is posited that the tick has to feed for at least 36 hours for transmission to occur (for Borrelia burgdorferi).
3. Pathology in the knee joint may be prominent in stage 3
4. B. garini is the isolate in many cases of lymphocytic meningoradiculitis (Bannwarth syndrome) and white matter lesions. This is rare in North America.
5. A novel species of bacteria Borrelia mayonii has been isolated from patients in the upper Midwest. It has been associated with nausea and vomiting, diffuse rash and high spirochetemia

Laboratory Evaluation

1. Enzyme immunoassay (EIA) followed by Western blot testing
2. Polymerase Chain Reaction Testing:
    a. Can detect B burgdorferi DNA in the blood, CSF, urine or synovial fluid within weeks of inoculation. The test is positive in approximately 30% of patients with active disease
    b. There are disadvantages of PCR testing, the most notable of which is false-negative results due to the sparsity of spirochetes in the material that is tested

Spinal Infections Affecting Cervical Nerve Roots

General Characteristics

1. Upper cervical (occiput to C2) infection and abscess is rare (approximately 40 patients have been reported)
2. Long-term clinical sequelae are often due to proximity to the atlas and axis

3. Spinal epidural abscess has an incidence of approximately 2 to 25 patients per 100,000 hospital admissions
4. The cervical spine is divided into upper, subaxial and cervicothoracic areas. The upper cervical spine encompasses the occipitalocervical junction, C1 (atlas), and C2 the (axis). The subaxial spine is C3-C6 and C7-T1 is the cervicothoracic area.
5. The atlas lacks a vertebral body and forms a ring that articulates with the atlanto-occipital joint and the axis. The majority of head movement is provided by these two joints.
6. The odontoid process is an extension of the C2 vertebral body and with the posterior component of the anterior arch of the atlas.
7. The axis has pedicles and transverse processes that are (the transverse process) the attachment sites for muscles and ligaments. The atlantoaxial joint is stabilized by the transverse ligament of the atlantoaxial joint.
8. The apical and alar ligaments prevent posterior dislocation of the odontoid process.
9. The location of epidural abscesses is greatly determined by the presence of an epidural space. The dura mater is adherent to the foramen magnum superiorly and at the sacrococcygeal membrane caudally (inferiorly). There is very little anterior epidural space due to the dura, posterior longitudinal ligament and the periosteum all of which are adjacent to the vertebral body. Most spinal epidural abscesses are posterior. A true epidural space occurs at cervical, midthoracic and lumbosacral areas. Because the cervical area has a smaller epidural space, it is infected less frequently.
10. Spinal anatomy allows a bacterial infection to migrate to different vertebral levels.

Clinical Manifestations

1. Initial presentation is with neck pain and stiffness
2. Fever
3. Insidious onsets include disorientation, headache, sore throat and pain with swallowing
4. During evolution of the process patients develop quadriparesis and sensory loss as well as radicular pain at the involved segmental levels

Neuropathology

1. The source of the infection is most often hematogenous followed by ear, nose and throat infection, local skin and soft tissue infection and rarely upper respiratory tract, urinary, dental and meningeal infection
2. The most common pathogens are:
   a. Methicillin-sensitive Staphylococcus aureus in approximately 2/3 of patients; followed by Streptococcus pneumonia

   b. Rare reports of anaerobic organisms, fungi (actinomyces and candida)
3. The underlying diseases are most often an immunocompromised host and surgical procedures
4. Risk for infection include:
   a. Diabetes
   b. Immunosuppression
   c. Obesity
   d. Traumatic spinal cord injury
   e. Epidural catheter placement
   f. Intravenous drug use and chronic kidney disease

Laboratory Evaluation

1. Sedimentation rate, C-reactive protein and white blood count

Neuroimaging

1. Plain radiographs:
   a. To rule out cervical spondylosis, spondylolisthesis or fracture
   b. To delineate possible vertebral osteomyelitis, bony collapse or erosion
   c. If there are osseous changes in the upper cervical spine flexion-extension views to evaluate the odontoid stability are indicated
2. MRI:
   a. This is the modality of choice in suspected cervical epidural abscess with a sensitivity of 95% and specificity of >90%.
   b. T2 weighted sequences demonstrate high signal intensity of the abscess
3. CT:
   a. To evaluate vertebral end plates and facet erosion associated with osteomyelitis

Poliomyelitis

General Characteristics

1. Acute poliomyelitis is caused by small RNA viruses of the enterovirus genus Picornaviridae
2. The virus has a single-stranded RNA core that is surrounded by a protein capsid that has no lipid envelop thus making it resistant to lipid solvents and gives it stability at a low pH
3. Type 1 of its antigenic strains cause approximately 85% of patients that become paralyzed

Clinical Manifestations

1. The virus is spread by fecal-hand-oral secretions. The virus is shed in the feces for months
2. 1 to 3 days prior to the onset of paralysis patients may develop:

   a. Nausea, vomiting and abdominal cramps, pain and diarrhea
   b. Sore throat, fever, malaise and headache
   c. These symptoms may last for 2-3 weeks or up to 2 months
3. The major illness is comprised of:
   a. Aseptic meningitis (non-paralytic)
   b. Encephalitis
   c. Bulbar polio
   d. Paralytic polio
4. An acute attack is manifest by:
   a. Fever, nuchal rigidity
   b. Asymmetrical muscle weakness (may involve separate fingers in the hand)
   c. Rare transverse myelitis associated with paraparesis, urinary tract involvement
   d. Severe deep muscle and back pain may develop with paralysis
5. Hypo or hyperhidrosis and variation of extremity temperature

Neuropathology

1. Infection of the spinal cord and or the brainstem
2. The virus first multiplies in the oropharynx and then spreads to the mucosa of the ileum and Peyer's patches; most infections are enteric rather than neurotropic
3. Hemorrhagic necrosis of anterior horn cells of the spinal cord with atrophy of spinal nerve roots

Laboratory Evaluation

1. CSF:
   a. Lymphocytosis with slight elevation of protein
   b. Poliovirus may be recovered from a stool sample or pharyngeal swab
   c. Antibodies are detected in the blood early in the infection
   d. PCR amplification to demonstrate its strain
2. EMG:
   a. Delineates affected muscles

Post-Polio Syndrome

General Characteristics

1. Approximately 25 to 50% of patients that have recovered from paralytic polio develop new muscle weakness and pain several decades after the original illness

Clinical Manifestations

1. Pain in the originally affected muscles and the newly weak muscles

2. Weakness returns in formerly weak muscles; increased weakness may occur
3. Severe fatigue

Neuropathology

1. The mechanism and pathogenesis have not been completely determined. Possible mechanisms include:
    a. Metabolic failure in remaining anterior horn cells that have re-innervated the territory of lost neurons
    b. Accelerated effects of aging

Laboratory Evaluation

1. EMG:
2. To delineate involvement of new muscle groups

Neuroimaging

1. MRI:
    a. To exclude orthopedic, medical and neurologic conditions that may be causative of increased pain, fatigue and weakness

Parsonage-Turner Syndrome

General Characteristics

1. The illness may be sporadic or secondary to heterozygous mutations in the SEPT9 gene that maps to chromosome 17q25. It is an autosomal dominant condition
2. The disorder is classified as a brachial plexitis rather than a cervical root disorder

Clinical characteristics

1. The illness is also known as hereditary neurologic amyotrophy (HNA)
2. The sudden onset of severe lancinating pain in the upper trunk brachial plexus distributions (primarily C5, C6 and C7 root territory) is most characteristic
3. The painful episodes may be recurrent and are followed by weakness and atrophy of the affected muscles
4. In the SEPT9 hereditary form there may be associated dysmorphic features that include:
    a. Hypotelorism
    b. Long nasal bridge
    c. Facial asymmetry
    d. Cleft palate
5. Attacks have been described as triggered by infections, immunizations and increased use of the affected arm

Neuropathology

1. Primarily affects the upper trunk of the brachial plexus or one of the peripheral nerves that innervate the shoulder girdle. Rarely, it affects the middle cord and lower trunks and the suprascapular, long thoracic, and axillary nerves.
2. The etiology is controversial. Approximately 25% of patients have had a preceding viral infection and 15% a preceding immunization
3. The pathology is axonal

Laboratory Evaluation

1. Mutational analysis of the SEPT9 gene
2. EMG:
    a. An axonal process with positive sharp waves and fibrillation potentials in affected muscles
    b. NCV are usually normal but sensory amplitudes are decreased

Other Viral Illnesses that Primarily Affect Peripheral Nerves or the Spinal Cord

1. EBV
2. Hepatitis C
3. West Nile
4. Coxsackie (particularly serotype 6 and 9)
5. Adenovirus
6. Enterovirus
7. Zika virus

Differential Diagnosis of Systemic Diseases Affecting Cervical Nerve Roots

Diabetes Mellitus

1. Diabetic amyotrophy is much more common in L2-L4 roots
2. Putative involvement of the vasa vasorum in addition to axonopathy and demyelinating features of the polyneuropathy
3. May be bilateral; the second event occurs 6-8 weeks following the first

Acute Intermittent Porphyria

1. C5, C6 roots are most commonly involved
2. Overwhelming a motor neuropathy with severe atrophy and wasting of the involved muscles
3. Sensory symptoms > than signs may be patchy; often out of a dermatomal distribution

Variegate porphyria

1. Rare root involvement
2. May have associated skin rash

Post X-RT therapy

1. C5, C6 roots primarily are involved following cervical cord treatment
2. Myokymia may be prominent

IgG4 Pachymeningitis

1. May affect all cervical roots

Sicca Complex

1. Sicca complex:
   a. Autoimmune etiology
   b. May have patchy anhidrosis and sensory loss out of a dermatomal distribution
2. Probable dorsal root ganglionopathy
3. May involve definable cervical roots

Amyloidosis

1. Familial amyloid
2. FOLMA (familial oculoleptomeningeal amyloidosis):
   a. Meningeal involvement with nerve root compression

Isolated angiitis of the CNS/PNS

1. 1. Arteritis of the vasa vasorum that supply cervical nerve roots

Inflammatory Spondyloarthritis with Radiculopathy

1. Rheumatoid arthritis
2. Psoriasis
3. Ankylosing spondylitis
4. Crohn's disease
5. Ulcerative colitis
6. Behcet's disease

Vascular Malformations that May Involve Cervical Nerve Roots

Arteriovenous malformation

1. Nerve root (on the root itself)
2. Dural AVM with accompanying compression of the nerve root

Dilated vein compressing the nerve root

1. Venous congestion from severe cervical spondylosis or an extruded disc
2. Concomitant venous congestion of the spinal cord (myelomalacia) and the

nerve root:
  a. Postulated that veins over the nerve root cause mechanical pressure on the sensitized root that awakens patients with disc disease in the early morning

Foix-Alajouanine syndrome

1. Arteriovenous malformation involving the anterior spinal artery
2. Cervical nerve roots and the spinal cord may be compressed

Weber-Klippel-Trenaunay Syndrome

1. Arteriovenous malformation of an extremity
2. Enlargement of the bone and soft tissue components of the extremity
3. Enlarged epidural veins and their tributaries may compress segmental nerve roots

Superficial Siderosis

1. Hemosiderin deposits on nerve roots:
   a. Radiculopathy
   b. Cranial nerves I and VIII may be concomitantly involved
   c. Caused by repeat bleeding from aneurysms, cavernous hemangiomas or rarely telangiectasias
   d. Demonstrated by gradient ECHO or susceptibility weighted MRI sequences

Arachnoiditis

General Characteristics

1. Clumping together and scar formation of nerve roots:
   a. Secondary to:
      i Multiple surgeries
      ii No longer seen from myelography due to the use of water-soluble contrast media

Clinical Manifestations

1. Severe burning pain in several dermatomal distributions
2. Usually a regional rather than a clear radicular pattern
3. CT/myelography demonstrates clumping of nerve roots or a featureless dural sac
4. Minimal weakness; burning pain predominates
5. Asymmetric reflex loss
6. Rare bladder involvement
7. Rarely caused by aneurismal rupture of a vertebral or anterior spinal artery

Neuroimaging

1. MRI demonstrates gadolinium enhancement of the scar

Differential Diagnosis of Cancer vs X-RT Involvement of Cervical Nerve Roots

1. Usually X-RT treatment of head and neck cancer
2. Signs and symptoms are often delayed from six weeks to three months

Cancer

1. Painful (burning quality)
2. C8, T1 roots are primarily involved
3. Horner's syndrome
4. Pancoast tumor of the lung apex (adenoma or squamous cell carcinomas)

Cervical X-RT

1. Dysesthesias or paresthesias of the involved roots
2. C5, C6 roots are primarily involved
3. No Horner's Syndrome
4. Myokymia of the muscles in the involved dermatomes
5. X-RT of the breast, Hodgkin disease, head and neck cancers are the most common systemic illnesses treated
6. Often missed by conventional x-ray; MRI for diagnosis:
   a. Segmental radiculopathy
      i Pain is usually the most prominent symptom
   b. Burst fracture of the vertebral body:
      i Vertebral body star fracture (radiation of fracture lines from the center of the vertebral body)
      ii Bilateral radicular pain
      iii Fractured bone fragment may be displaced into the spinal canal or foraminal exit area
      iv Concomitant spinal cord direct injury and compression
   c. Lateral vertebral body translocation:
      i Severe high impact trauma (most often MVA)
      ii Bilateral radicular pain
      iii Associated severe spinal cord injury
7. Anterior vertebral body compression fracture:
   a. Middle-aged and elderly women
   b. Often occurs with minimal trauma in patients with osteoporosis
   c. Most often occurs in the thoracic spine but rarely effects cervical and lumbar vertebrae
   d. Lancinating radicular pain often exacerbated by Valsalva maneuvers and breathing

Thoracic Nerve Root Lesions (T1-T12)

General Characteristics

1. Lower thoracic and upper lumbar root lesions cause protrusion of the abdomen during inspiration
2. Abdominal muscle weakness causes difficulty in arising from recumbency. If the muscles are unilaterally paralyzed the umbilicus is pulled or deviates to the unaffected side during inspiration or when there is resistance to neck flexion against resistance (the patient is laying on his or her back)
3. Bilateral lower abdominal muscle weakness below or at the T10 level causes elevation of the umbilicus with neck flexion against resistance (Beevor's sign). The maneuver engages all abdominal rectus muscles and those above the umbilicus are stronger
4. The pain is usually lancinating with a burning paresthetic quality that radiates in a segmental distribution around the chest or abdomen
5. Pain is exacerbated or precipitated by any increase in intraspinal pressure or stretching of the dorsal root
6. There may be sensory loss in the affected root territory which is rarely complete due to the overlapping cutaneous innervation from adjacent nerve roots
7. Notalgia paresthetica is a condition in which there is paresthesia along the medial scapular border:
   a. There may be decreased pain sensitivity
   b. Possibly the territory of T2 to T6 roots or the upper trunk of the brachial plexus

Lesions that affect the T1 root

1. Muscle weakness occurs in:
   a. Abductor pollicis brevis
   b. Opponens pollicis
   c. Flexor pollicis brevis
   d. Lumbricals and dorsal and volar interossei
   e. Abductor digiti minimi
   f. Opponens digiti minimi
   g. Flexor digiti minimi
   h. Adductor pollicis
2. Sensory loss or paresthesia occurs in the medial arm
3. An ipsilateral Horner's syndrome (ptosis, meiosis and apparent enophthalmos) may be seen from loss of sympathetic innervation of the superior cervical ganglion
4. Depression of the finger flexion reflex

Thoracic Root Disease

Disc Disease

General Characteristics

1. Account for approximately 0.5% of disc protrusions
2. Thoracic discs are rare because they are not at motion segments which is thought to be a major mechanism for degenerative changes
3. The lower four thoracic discs are the most commonly affected

Clinical Manifestations

1. May occur suddenly from heavy lifting, high impact MVA and concomitantly with spinal cord injury
2. Dull boring midline ache with episodes of radicular lancinating pain
3. Intercostal or abdominal radiations
4. The pain is exacerbated by specific movements and Valsalva maneuvers
5. Radicular pain may be associated with signs of compressive myelopathy (paraparesis, sphincter disturbance and Babinski sign)
6. Upper thoracic disc herniations may radiate to the cervical spine and lower thoracic herniations to the lumbar spine
7. Pain may also be referred to the retrogastric, retrosternal and inguinal areas
8. Annular tears may have specific referral patterns:
    a. Anterior tears may refer to the ribs, chest wall, sternum and rarely viscera
    b. Lateral tears to musculoskeletal sites
    c. Posterior annulus tears local back pain
9. Sensory symptoms are the presenting complaint in approximately 25% of patients
10. Weakness is the presenting complaint in approximately 17% of patients
11. Incontinence of urine is the presenting symptom in 2% of patients. Rare bowel incontinence

Neuropathology

1. Degenerative changes similar to those of cervical and lumbar disc

Laboratory Evaluation

1. Medical evaluation of an underlying medical condition if clinically relevant (diabetes, amyloidosis, hereditary collagen disease)

Neuroimaging

1. Radiographs and CT:
    a. Jumped facet joint:
        i Overriding of the inferior over the superior facet joint
        ii Places traction on or directly injures the segmental root

   b. Rotary subluxation of the facet joint:
      i The facet joint is twisted; the synovial interfacet is breached
   c. MRI:
      i Delineates soft tissues, ligaments and parenchymal spinal cord pathology

Syrinx

General Characteristics

1. Syringomyelia is a fluid filled cavity within the spinal cord. It can occur with or without communication with the IVth ventricle

Clinical Manifestations

1. Atrophy at the segmental level
2. Early hyperhidrosis followed by anhidrosis of the affected segments
3. Severe lancinating radicular pain
4. Dissociated sensory loss at the segmental level (destruction of the spinothalamic fibers as they decussate in the anterior ventral commissure)
5. Long tract motor and sensory signs below the syrinx
6. Charcot joints of the shoulder, elbow or wrist
7. Scoliosis
8. Impaired sphincter function late in the course of the illness
9. Dysesthetic and radicular pain is most prominent in the neck and shoulders but also can affect thoracic roots

Neuropathology

1. Associated with Chiari malformations
2. Trauma
3. Small posterior fossa
4. Platybasia and basilar invagination
5. Arachnoid cysts, rhombic roof, vascularized membranes and post-inflammatory membranes
6. Cavitation of spinal cord gray matter; continuous with or adjacent to the central canal; an inner layer of gliosis

Neuroimaging

1. MRI:
   a. Imaging of the rostrocaudal extension of the spinal cord
   b. Gadolinium enhancement differentiates scar, disc material and tumor
2. CT:
   a. To assess the spinal canal particularly if the syrinx is traumatic
3. Myelography:
   a. Delineates widening of the spinal cord and subarachnoid block

4. Post traumatic syrinx:
    a. A further cystic degeneration of the spinal cord
    b. Usually there is a 2 to 3 segment loss of function above and below the level of injury
    c. Bilateral root involvement at the involved segmental level

Post thoracotomy Pain Syndrome

General Characteristics

1. Occurs in approximately 50% of patients after thoracotomy; approximately 30% of patients have pain 4 to 5 years following their procedure

Clinical Manifestations

1. Prolonged and often refractory and neuropathic pain of the involved roots or intercostal nerves

Neuropathology

1. Elements of both neuropathic and myofascial pathology
2. Retraction of muscle or direct radicular and nerve injury

Laboratory Evaluation

1. Sed rate and C-reactive protein (thoracic epidural catheters are utilized for pain relief and may cause an abscess or meningitis)

Neuroimaging

1. CT and MRI:
    a. To delineate infection or structural lesion that affects the intercostal nerve

Thoracic Nerve Root Involvement from Systemic Disease

Diabetic Thoracic Polyradiculopathy

General Characteristics

1. Affects predominantly elderly and middle-aged men with type 2 diabetes
2. In some series it affects the right side > than the left
3. It is often seen with cervical and lumbosacral radiculoplexus neuropathy

Clinical Manifestations

1. Most commonly occurs in elderly type II diabetics; median age range (32-83) for cervical radiculoplexus neuropathy approximately 20% also had thoracic involvement
2. Right side more often affected than the left (abdominal wall)
3. Usually involves 3-5 adjacent nerve roots between T6 and T12
4. It may be accompanied by profound weight loss

5. It may have an abrupt onset
6. Patients present with severe abdominal or chest radicular pain; at times the pain is out of a dermatomal distribution
7. The process is usually monophasic but in approximately 20% of patients it is recurrent
8. Weakness of affected intercostal and abdominal muscle

Neuropathology

1. Infarction or ischemia of the thoracic nerve roots (vasa vasorum); a microvasculitis
2. Nerve biopsy in patients with concomitant cervical radiculoplexus:
    a. Axonal degeneration, multifocal fiber loss
    b. Focal perineurial thickening
    c. Vessel wall inflammation
    d. Epineural perivascular inflammation
    e. Hemosiderin deposition
    f. Involves motor, sensory and autonomic fibers

Laboratory Evaluation

1. Type II diabetes with increased blood sugar
2. CSF:
    a. Mildly elevated protein (70 mg/dl)
3. EMG:
    a. Associated axonal neuropathy with paraspinal denervation
    b. Some patients had associated upper, medial and lower brachial plexus involvement

Neuroimaging

1. MRI:
    a. In those patients with concomitant upper extremity pain there may be bilateral brachial plexus involvement (contrast enhancement)
2. Ultrasound:
    a. Swelling of affected roots

Transthyretin Familial Amyloid Polyneuropathy (TTR-FAP)

General Characteristics

1. Is an autosomal dominant disorder due to mutations in the transthyretin gene that maps to the long arm of chromosome 18
2. It is characterized by extracellular deposition of transthyretin-derived amyloid fibrils in peripheral and autonomic nerves as well as the heart, gastrointestinal tract, kidneys, eyes and the connective tissue of the carpal and tarsal tunnels

3. TTR is a transport protein for thyroxine and retinol
4. It is primarily synthesized in the liver

Clinical Manifestations

1. Neuropathic involvement includes:
    a. Sensorimotor and autonomic neuropathy
    b. Lower and upper limb involvement
    c. Carpal tunnel syndrome (TTRL58H variant)
    d. TTR variants may cause CNS disease that includes:
        i Spastic paraparesis
        ii Nystagmus
        iii Leptomeningeal / cerebrovascular deposits that are associated with seizures, subarachnoid hemorrhages and dementia
    e. Late-onset patients have preservation of unmyelinated fibers that may be responsible for neuropathic pain
    f. Denervation of segmental thoracic discs may cause Charcot joints and radicular (thoracic) pain due to root irritation

Neuropathology

1. TTR mutations accelerate TTR amyloid formation by destabilizing the native tertiary and quaternary structure of the protein that induces conformational change. This process leads to dissociation of its tetramers into partially unfolded species that then self-assemble into amyloid fibrils.

Laboratory Evaluation

1. Congo red material in sural nerve biopsy or that of an affected organ
2. PCR molecular genetic testing to determine the specific variant

Ochronosis

General Characteristics

1. Alkaptonuria is an autosomal recessive disease caused by mutations in the HGO gene that maps to chromosome 3q1 which encodes homogentisic acid oxidase which catabolizes homogentisic acid (HGA)
2. The enzyme deficiency causes the accumulation and deposition of HGA in cartilage
3. Exogenous ochronosis is a bluish black pigmentation of the skin from phenol, trinitrophenol, benzene and hydroquinone

Clinical Manifestations

1. Dark urine in diapers, black cerumen and axillary pigmentation prior to age 10
2. Ear cartilage degeneration by the fourth decade
3. Gray-black scleral rings may be noted in the third decade

4. Arthropathy develops in the third and fourth decades
5. The knee, hip and shoulder joints develop the major arthropathy
6. The first manifestation may be the intervertebral disc degeneration of the lumbar spine which may also be seen in the thoracic spine
7. Degeneration of thoracic spine intervertebral discs may cause radicular pain

Neuropathology

1. Accumulation and deposition of HGA in cartilage causes its weakness and brittleness that leads to inflammation and degenerative changes
2. HGA undergoes oxidation / polymerization reactions that produces a melanin-like pigment
3. HGA induces oxidation of serum and chondrocyte proteins
4. Mechanisms of action include:
    a. HGA-induced proteome alterations
    b. Lipid peroxidation
    c. Thiol depletion
    d. Amyloid production
    e. Oxidative stress and protein oxidation

Laboratory Evaluation

1. Increased levels of homogentisic acid in the urine, blood and other tissues
2. Molecular genetic testing

Neuroimaging

1. Radiographs:
    a. Calcification and degeneration of multiple thoracic discs – "Rugger-Jersey" appearance
    b. MRI:
        i Evaluation of affected joints

Differential Diagnosis of Disorders that can Affect Thoracic Nerve Roots

Diabetic Dying Back Neuropathy

1. Shield sensory loss on the chest wall
2. Associated with distal dying back (length-dependent) dying back neuropathy of the extremities
3. Single or multiple dermatomal involvement of the chest wall or abdomen
4. Sensory loss or pain in the distribution of the ventral rami of the spinal nerve or the dorsal ramus of the spinal nerve, the paravertebral territory; the sensory loss may be in various combinations of these territories of the thoracic spinal nerves

Immune Mediated Disorders

1. Acute inflammatory demyelinating polyneuropathy (AIDP):

   a. Gd1b, Gal-Nac-GD1a antibodies
   b. Small fiber involvement may be associated with regional and focal severe pain
2. Chronic inflammatory demyelinating polyneuropathy (CIDP)
3. Sjogren's disease:
   a. May be primarily a dorsal root ganglionitis
   b. Involvement of the dorsal primary ramus or its medial or lateral divisions
4. Sicca complex:
   a. Dry eyes, mouth serous membranes
   b. Segmental and regional sensory loss and anhidrosis
5. Radiculopathy with increased sed rate:
   a. A poorly defined process
   b. Usually the lumbosacral roots are involved

Malignant and Benign Tumors that Affect Thoracic Nerve Roots

1. Malignancies:
   a. Leukemia:
      i Acute presentation from bleeding into a nerve root
      ii Hodgkin disease and non-Hodgkin disease lymphoma:
         1. Insidious and progressive nerve root involvement
         2. Paraneoplastic mechanisms
      iii Carcinomatosis of the meninges:
         1. Mental status alterations
         2. Cranial nerve involvement

Metastatic Cancers

1. Anterior mediastinal tumors (rarely involve thoracic roots):
   a. Thymoma and thymic carcinoma are usually locally invasive
   b. Thymic carcinoid (associated with multiple endocrinopathy syndrome type I (MEN)
   c. Thymic lipoma
   d. Hodgkin and non-Hodgkin lymphoma (NHL)
2. Primary mediastinal germ cell tumors:
   a. Mature teratoma
   b. Seminoma
   c. Nonseminomatous germ cell tumors
3. Posterior mediastinal tumors:
   a. Peripheral nervous system benign and malignant neoplasms are more frequent in the posterior mediastinum
   b. They develop from peripheral nerves, sympathetic and parasympathetic ganglia as well as neural tube embryonic remnants and include:
      1. Schwannoma

    2. Neurofibroma
    3. Melanotic Schwannoma
    4. Ganglioneuroma
    5. Granular cell tumor
    6. Malignant melanocytic nerve sheath tumor
    7. Neuroblastoma
    8. Neurofibrosarcoma (non-Recklinghausen disease)
4. Metastatic disease (similar to those that affect cervical roots)
5. Multiple myeloma (primarily affect roots by vertebral collapse and compression of the neural root exit foramina)
6. Osteoclastic myeloma
7. Plasmacytoma
8. Paget's disease (sarcomatous degeneration)
9. GI cancer (sacral bone involvement with colon cancer); lumbar and sacral roots > thoracic root involvement
10. Giant articular bone cyst (vertebral fracture)
11. Osteoid osteoma:
    a. Refractory to narcotics but responsive to prostaglandin inhibitors
    b. Involves the posterior elements of the vertebral body (pedicles and facets)
    c. Radicular symptoms
12. Vertebral body sarcoma
13. Chondrosarcoma
14. Enchondroma:
    a. Involve the nerve root exit foramina
    b. Approximately 4% involve thoracic vertebrae
15. Brown bone cyst:
    a. Occurs with hyperparathyroidism
    b. Bone resorption, fractures and radicular pain
16. Hemangioma of the vertebral body:
    a. Most often they are incidental findings (on MRI T2-weighted sequences)
    b. May weaken the vertebral body
    c. The lesions are extremely vascular
    d. May compress the exiting nerve root
17. Thoracic meningioma in women:
    a. Extremely rare location for a meningioma in men
    b. Increased growth of the tumor in pregnancy and with breast cancer
18. Schwannoma:
    a. Typically enlarges the foraminal nerve root exit canal
    b. Scalloping of the affected vertebral body (a sign of chronic pressure)
    c. A dumbbell tumor (both enlarging the nerve root and expanding in the intradural extramedullary space)

19. Neurofibroma
20. Melanotic Schwannoma:
    a. Some tumors are part of the Carney syndrome
    b. May have dumb-bell characteristics on MRI
    c. Melanin granules in tumor cells
21. Hemangiopericytoma of the thoracic spine
    a. Most often found in the cranial cavity
    b. Very rare in the spine but when they occur they are intradural extramedullary in location
    c. They invade nerve roots and cause radicular pain

Infections Involving Thoracic Roots

1. HZ (Herpes Zoster):
    a. Thoracic dermatomes are most commonly involved
    b. Clinical symptoms (similar to that of cervical roots)
    c. A dorsal root ganglionitis
    d. Rarely a hemorrhagic spinal cord infarction is associated (paraparesis is most often at the T4-T6 level)
2. HIV:
    a. Usually, the cervical cord is involved
    b. Vascular degeneration of the cord
    c. Rare radicular complaints
3. Staphylococcus aureus:
    a. Young IV drug abusers; there are end arteries to the disc
    b. The disc space is infected:
        i Enhancement of the disc with contrast on MRI
        ii The vertebral body is spared: there is often pre and postvertebral ligament inflammation (enhancement with gadolinium on T1 weighted sequences)
        iii Disc space infection causes severe lancinating radicular pain; minimal movement initiates pain (touching the patient's bed)
        iv Spinal cord involvement by contiguous spread or by venous infarction
        v Gram-negative disc space infection following surgery:
            1. Involvement and signs of infection may be delayed for up to six weeks from the procedure
            2. Pain, swelling, erythema and edema at the operative site
                a. Invariably high sed rate and C-reactive proteins
2. Tuberculosis:
    a. T4-T6, T11-T12, L1-L2, the usual location of the infection
    b. The infection is more common in the cervical spine in Asian patients

   c. Disc space is infected > than the vertebrae; bony sclerosis of the vertebral body and endplates on neuroimaging is common
   d. Pott's disease:
      i Acute kyphotic angulation
      ii Occurs from vertebral body collapse and loss of disc integrity
      iii May cause spastic paraparesis
   e. Cold abscess may occur along the iliopsoas muscle; T10-T11 root may be involved; blurring of the proas stripe on x-ray of the abdomen
3. Actinomycosis:
   a. Extension of active lung infections into thoracic vertebrae
   b. Abscess with radicular symptoms
   c. Characteristic sulfur granules in the abscess
   d. Rural population
4. Nocardia:
   a. Occurs in immunocompromised patients
   b. Epidural vein involvement
   c. The fungus is often in a lung abscess
   d. Associated with osteomyelitis

Unusual Causes of Thoracic Nerve Root Involvement

1. Paravertebral mesothelial cyst
2. Thoracic root entrapment from intrathecal coiling:
   a. Catheters are placed for the treatment of intractable thoracic pain (most often after thoracic surgery)
   b. Nerve root irritation is caused by loops in the catheter

Cervical Plexus

Overview

The cervical plexus is composed of the anterior rami of C1-C4 that are derived from the C1-C4 cervical segments of the spinal cord. It lies behind the sternocleidomastoid muscle and anteriorly to the scalenus medius and levator scapulae muscles. The plexus anastomoses with the accessory nerve (XI), the hypoglossal nerve (XII) and the sympathetic trunk. The nerves derived from the cervical plexus innervate the back of the head, overlap with the cutaneous territory of the Vth nerve and are synergistic in head flexion and swallowing physiology. The branches of the cervical plexus emerge from the posterior triangle of the neck midway on the posterior border of the sternocleidomastoid muscle.

The terminal cutaneous branches of the cervical plexus are:

1. The greater occipital nerve, which innervates the skin of the posterior scalp, is the terminal branch of the dorsal ramus of C2 with a contribution from C3.
2. The lesser occipital nerve is derived from the anterior divisions of C2 and C3

and innervates the mastoid process and lateral head; the mastoid innervations overlap that of the sensory innervation from cranial nerve VII.

3. The greater auricular nerve (C2-C3) which innervates:
   a. The skin of the lower cheek and the mandible (overlaps V2, V3)
   b. The auriculotemporal and buccinator terminal nerves of cranial nerve V (overlaps).
   c. It also innervates the neck below the external ear.
4. The cutaneous branches of the transverse colli nerves (C2-C3) which innervate the neck (primarily anteriorly).
5. The supraclavicular nerve (C3-C4) which innervate the skin of the supraclavicular fossa (immediately above the clavicle). May cause misdiagnosis with localizations of spinal cord injury levels.
6. C1 is a purely motor root.
7. Anatomical variants include:
   a. Great auricular nerve communication with the mandibular nerve
   b. Spinal accessory nerve communication with C2.

The innervations of the muscular branches of the cervical plexus is derived from the ansa hypoglossi:

1. A loop formed by C1 which curves with the hypoglossal nerve and joins the fibers from C2 and C3 roots that innervate infrahyoid muscles:
   a. Sternohyoid
   b. Omohyoid
   c. Sternothyroid
   d. Thyrohyoid
   e. Geniohyoid

These muscles are synergistic in head flexion and swallowing physiology:

1. The phrenic nerve which innervates the diaphragm (C3- C5); C4 is the dominant root.
2. Branches to the middle scalene (C3-C4) that affects:
   a. Lateral neck flexion
   b. Levator scapulae muscles (C3-C4); rotation of the scapula.
3. Branches to the spinal accessory nerve that include:
   a. C2 to the sternocleidomastoid muscle.
   b. C3-C4 to the trapezius muscle.
   c. These branches course with CNXI.
4. Swallowing function
   a. Hyolaryngeal complex

Hyolaryngeal Complex

An important component of the pharyngeal phase of swallowing is the elevation of the hyolaryngeal complex. This is accomplished by the submental muscles (mylohyoid, geniohyoid and anterior digastric and the thyrohyoid muscles). Hyolaryngeal elevation displaces the larynx above the food bolus, shortens the pharynx, and opens the upper esophageal sphincter. The hyolaryngeal complex is comprised of the hyoid bone, thyrohyoid membrane and the laryngeal cartilages that are the attachment site for the cricopharyngeus muscle; the cricopharyngeus muscle forms the upper esophageal sphincter. Other muscles that may contribute to the elevation of the hyolaryngeal complex are the posterior digastric, stylohyoid, and long pharyngeal muscles.

Anatomically, an anterior and posterior sling of muscles suspends the hyolaryngeal complex and along with the thyrohyoid muscle, elevates it during swallowing. The anterior component of the sling is composed of the mylohyoid, geniohyoid, and anterior digastric muscles that insert on the hyoid bone. The posterior digastricus and stylohyoid may also contribute to the anterior sling. The posterior ring is composed of the long pharyngeal muscles that include the stylopharyngeus, salpingopharyngeus and palatopharyngeus muscles that are stabilized by the levator veli palatini. The distal posterior ring muscles insert on the posterior edge of the thyroid cartilage and lateral pharyngeal walls proximal to the upper esophageal sphincter. The thyrohyoid muscle is intrinsic to the hyolaryngeal complex and approximates the thyroid and hyoid bone.

In summary, the submental muscles (mylohyoid, geniohyoid, and anterior digastric) and the thyrohyoid muscle primarily elevate the hyolaryngeal complex that opens the upper esophageal sphincter during the pharyngeal phase of swallowing. The ansa hypoglossi of the cervical plexus is pivotal in the innervations of many of the muscles required for the pharyngeal phase of swallowing.

Lesions of the Cervical Plexus and the Sensory Components of the C2-C4 Branches

Cervical Plexus

General Characteristics

1. The sensory component of the cervical plexus is frequently injured by "whiplash" traction injuries that are often misdiagnosed. The sensory components, particularly C2 and C3 are most often involved although the motor components of the ansa hypoglossi may also be injured

Clinical Manifestations

1. Sensory loss primarily in the territories of the greater and lesser occipital nerves and the great auricular nerve
2. Complex regional pain syndrome type I and II of the face and ear with associated:
   a. Neurogenic edema and autonomic dysregulation:
      i Swelling
      ii Erythema

iii Hyperhidrosis

3. Dysfunction of the external esophageal sphincter and the muscles innervated by the ansa hypoglossi

Neuropathology

1. Trauma usually causes a neuropractic injury
2. The cervical plexus may also be injured by:
   a. Penetrating injuries
   b. Carotid endarterectomy or radical neck dissection for malignancy
   c. Tumors

Neuroimaging

1. MRI:
   a. To delineate specific pathologies in the neck
2. Ultrasound:
   a. Delineates the anatomy of the plexus

The Greater Occipital Nerve (GON)

General Characteristics

1. Innervates the skin of the occiput (posterior scalp)
2. The greater occipital nerve (GON) is the medial branch of the dorsal ramus of the C2 spinal nerve. The GON takes a downward lateral course and is covered by the splenius capitis, the longissimus, and the semispinalis muscles. Rarely, it may course within the inferior oblique muscle. It pierces the semispinalis capitis muscle and emerges into the scalp through the aponeurotic fibrous attachment of the trapezius muscle and the sternocleidomastoid muscle to reach the superior nuchal line
3. The nerve splits and its medial branch innervates the occipital skin while its lateral branch innervates the area behind the pinna below the superior nuchal line.
4. The GON emerges through the semispinalis muscle 3 cm below the occipital protuberance and 1.5 cm lateral to the midline. The nerve is rarely compressed between the posterior arch of C1 and the lamina of C2. Variations of GON are usually in the vertical axis.

Clinical Manifestations

1. Pain and paresthesias in the cutaneous territory it innervates
2. Severe C2 irritation:
   a. Pain projected to the brow and behind the eyes
   b. A frequent trigger of unilateral migraine headaches

Neuropathology

1. The six major compression points along the course of the nerve:

   a. The most proximal (deepest point) is between the semispinalis and the obliquus capitis inferior adjacent to the spinous process
   b. At the entrance into the semispinalis muscle
   c. At the nerve exit from the semispinalis muscle
   d. At the entrance of the nerve into the trapezius muscle
   e. Where the nerve exits the trapezius fascia insertion into the nuchal line
   f. The area where the occipital artery crosses the nerve at the distal region of the trapezius fascia
2. Neurofibroma
3. Direct trauma

Neuroimaging

1. Ultrasound:
   a. Delineation of the nerve
1. MRI
   a. To delineate a structural lesion

The Lesser Occipital Nerve (LON)

General Characteristics

1. The LON takes origin from the dorsal ramus of C2 and rarely from C3
2. It ascends along the posterior border of the SCM muscle, near the cranium it perforates the deep fascia to ascend over the occiput to innervate the skin and communicates medially with GON. The nerve usually exits the posterior border of the SCM superior to the exit of the great auricular nerve, 6 to 7 cm lateral to the midline and 4 to 6 cm caudal to a line that connects the lowest points of the external auditory canal.
3. The upper back muscles of the cervical region are innervated by:
   a. Branches from the dorsal rami of the second and third cervical nerves
   b. Branches that arise from the posterior cervical plexus, a series of loops between the first and second and the second and third dorsal rami. Rarely there is a loop to the fourth dorsal rami.
4. There are articular branches of the C2-C3 facet joints that arise from communicating branches between the third occipital nerve and the C2 dorsal ramus

Clinical Manifestations

1. Pain and paresthesias of the mastoid, lateral and posterior head and lower portion of the occiput
2. The symptoms are most often in the C2 distribution

Neuropathology

1. Associated with flexion-extension or rotary injury of the neck (motor vehicle accidents, falls, and athletic injuries).

2. Very frequently associated with upper trunk (C5-C6) brachial plexus traction injuries.
3. Lacerations
4. Surgical procedures of the posterior triangle of the neck.
5. It is most often a neuropractic injury
6. Areas of nerve compression:
    a. Zone 1:
        i Emergence of the LON from deep to or behind the SCM muscle
    b. Zone 2:
        i The cephalic ascent of the LON along or posterior to the SCM
    c. Zone 3:
        i Caudal to the nuchal line

Neuroimaging

1. Ultrasonography for delineation of the anatomy (areas of compression) and pathology of the nerve
2. MRI:
    a. To delineate underlying pathologies that include:
        i Trauma
        ii Fibrositis
        iii Myositis
        iv Fracture of the atlas
        v Compression of the C2 nerve root
        vi C1-C2 arthrosis syndrome
        vii Atlantoaxial lateral mass osteoarthritis
        viii Hypertrophic cervical pachymeningitis
        ix Cervical cord tumors
        x Chiari malformation
        xi Neurosyphilis

The Third Occipital Nerve

General Characteristics

1. The medial branch of the posterior division of the third cervical nerve gives off the third occipital nerve while coursing under the trapezius muscle
2. The nerve pierces the trapezius muscle, lies medial to the greater occipital nerve with which it communicates

Clinical Manifestations

1. Pain in the skin of the lower part of the occiput
2. A trigger for migraine headaches

Neuropathology

1. Neuropractic injury from self-retaining retractors in the midline
2. Similar pathologies as those that affect C2

Laboratory Evaluation

1. Medical evaluation of underlying pathologies

Neuroimaging:

1. Ultrasonography to delineate the anatomy of the nerve and possible zones of compression
2. MRI:
    a. To delineate underlying pathologies

The Great Auricular Nerve

General Characteristics

1. Originates from the cervical plexus. It is composed of branches of spinal nerves C2 and C3
2. It winds around the posterior border of the SCM, perforates the deep fascia, ascends beneath the platysma muscle to reach the parotid gland to divide into anterior and posterior branches
3. The anterior branch innervates the skin over the parotid gland and communicates with the VIIth nerve within the gland
4. The posterior branch innervates:
    a. The skin over the mastoid and the back of the ear (except its upper part)
    b. Lobule and lower concha of the ear
    c. Communicates with the auricular branch of the vagus and the posterior auricular branch of VII

Clinical Manifestations

1. Paresthesias and pain in the lower cheek, lower pinna of the external ear (overlaps the auriculotemporal nerve of the Vth cranial nerve)
    a. Irritation of this nerve causes:
        i Neurogenic inflammation and vasodilation of the pinna; the probable genesis of the "red ear" syndrome (C3 root is involved).
        ii C-fibers within the nerve release substance P (which interacts with mast cells that release histamine) and calcitonin gene-related peptide. The former (SP) causes endothelial plasma leakage and the latter (CGRP) vasodilation of the affected vessels

Neuropathology

1. Damaged during surgical procedures to the neck or face:
    a. Facelift
    b. Parotid surgery
    c. Carotid endarterectomy

   d. Traction injury from MVA and falls (neuropractic pathology)
   e. Lacerations and gunshot wounds

Neuroimaging

1. Ultrasound guided

Transverse Colli Nerves

General Characteristics

1. Innervation of the anterior and upper neck (C2-C3 roots)

Clinical Manifestations

1. Pain in the anterior and upper neck

Neuropathology

1. Trauma (flexion, extension, and rotary neck injuries)
2. Surgical procedures in the neck

Neuroimaging

1. Ultrasonography
2. MRI:
   a. To delineate specific underlying pathologies

Supraclavicular Nerves

General Characteristics

1. Innervate the supraclavicular fossa and clavicle
2. May innervate the anterior chest wall to T2

Clinical Manifestations

1. Paresthesia and pain in its innervation territory
2. May give a false level following spinal cord injury (a lower sensory level than expected)

Neuropathology

1. Flexion-extension and rotary neck injuries (MVA and falls)
2. Biopsy of lymph nodes
3. Supraclavicular approach for first rib removal or neurolysis of the upper trunk of the brachial plexus in thoracic outlet surgery for thoracic outlet syndrome

Neuroimaging

1. Ultrasonography

Detailed Innervation of the C1, C2 and C3 Nerves

1. C1 nerve:
   a. The C1 nerve does not innervate cutaneous tissue on the body surface
2. It supplies deep somatic tissue in the suboccipital area that includes:

- i The short muscles of the occipital triangle (through its dorsal ramus)
- ii The SCM and trapezius muscle
- iii Atlanto-occipital joint (by its ventral ramus)
- iv The sinuvertebral nerve of C1 innervates:
  1. Median atlantoaxial joint
  2. Dura matter of the posterior fossa
  3. Vertebral artery
  4. This innervation is in conjunction with the sinuvertebral nerves of C2 and C3

3. C2 nerve:
   a. The dorsal ramus of C2 innervates the splenius capitis and semispinalis capitis to become the greater occipital nerve
   b. The ventral ramus supplies:
      - i Articular branches to the lateral C 1 / 2 joint
      - ii Prevertebral muscles, SCM and trapezius
4. C3 nerve:
   a. The dorsal ramus of the C3 nerve divides into 3 major branches:
      - i The lateral branch:
        1. Innervates the splenius capitis, cervicis and longissimus capitis
      - ii Deep medial branch:
        1. Innervates the semispinalis cervicis and multifidus
      - iii The superficial medial branch:
        1. Also known as the third occipital nerve
        2. Innervates the C2-C3 zygapophyseal joint
        3. Suboccipital cutaneous innervation

Injury of the Motor Roots of the Cervical Plexus (Ansa Hypoglosossi)

Ventral root of C2

Clinical Manifestations

1. Inability to elevate the hyolaryngeal complex during the pharyngeal component of swallowing:
   a. Failure to adequately open the upper esophageal sphincter
   b. Aspiration pneumonia
   c. Weakness of infrahyoid muscles
2. Middle scalene muscle weakness
   a. Decreased anterior and lateral head flexion
3. Slight weakness of the sternocleidomastoid muscle:
   a. Depressed rotation of the head contralaterally

4. Slight weakness of the trapezius muscle:
   a. Depressed shoulder elevation

The Phrenic Nerve

General Characteristics

1. Spinal accessory component (C2 innervation) involvement weakens the lateral half of the diaphragm.
2. An anastomotic variant in which the phrenic nerve receives an anatomic branch from the subclavian nerve; the diaphragm may be normal in this instance with a proximal phrenic nerve lesion.

Clinical Manifestations

1. Unilateral paralysis causes dyspnea on exertion but not at rest.
2. Bilateral phrenic nerve paralysis causes severe dyspnea on exertion and may lead to alveolar hypoventilation and hypercarbia.

Neuropathology

1. May be involved with viral infections that include Parsonage –Turner syndrome or neuralgia amyotrophica.
2. Rarely involved with traction injury but not infrequently damaged with scalenectomy and neurolysis procedures in thoracic outlet surgery (lies adjacent to the middle scalene muscle).
3. Aortic aneurysm (compression)
4. Intrathoracic neoplasm (infiltration)
5. Enlarged mediastinal lymph nodes
6. Subclavian vein or internal jugular vein catheterization (direct trauma)
7. Central vein catheter placement
8. Breast cancer (neck metastasis); if associated with damage to the sympathetic chain and recurrent laryngeal nerve it is Payne Syndrome.
9. Injured during coronary by-pass surgery (neuropraxis or dissection of the internal mammary artery)
10. Clipped in association with the inferior vena cava during liver transplantation
11. Amyotrophic lateral sclerosis
12. Diabetes mellitus
13. Critical care neuropathy (difficulty removing a patient from mechanical ventilation)
14. Mediastinal X-RT
15. Herpes Zoster
16. AIDP
17. Injury after radio-frequency denervation of cervical medial branches

Neuroimaging

1. X-ray:
2. Elevated diaphragm on the affected site
3. Multislice spiral computed tomography:
   a. Delineates pericardiophrenic bundles
4. The diaphragm paradoxically moves upward with inspiration (fluoroscopy)

Pharyngeal Plexus

General Characteristics

1. Lies in the retropharyngeal space between:
   a. Anteriorly:
      i Superior and middle pharyngeal constrictor muscles
   b. Posteriorly:
      i Longus capitis and colli muscles
      ii Prevertebral fascia
      iii Second and third cervical vertebrae
2. Composed of:
   a. Sensory fibers of IX and X
   b. Motor fibers of IX and X
3. Experimental information suggests:
   a. Stimulation of the pharyngeal plexus elicits vocal cord adduction
   b. Glottic closure reflex is affected (in porcine model) by the interior superior laryngeal nerve. Some studies reveal that the external branch of the superior laryngeal nerve, the communicating nerve of Galen and the recurrent laryngeal nerve also may play a role in the innervations of the thyroarytenoid muscle (pivotal in the gliotic closure reflex).
   c. The lingual branches of the glossopharyngeal nerves are thickened and course through a slit between the constrictor pharyngis superior and medius muscles, where they may be compressed.

Clinical Manifestations

1. Failure of the glottic closure reflex affected by the thyroarytenoid muscle (reflex).
2. Complaints that food gets stuck in the back of the throat and difficulty initiating deglutition.

Neuropathology

1. Direct injury from surgical and dental procedures
2. Head and neck X-RT for malignancy
3. Associated with brachial plexus and cervical plexus neuropractic injuries.

Neuroimaging

1. MRI (primarily utilizing defined landmarks rather than direct visualization of the plexus).

The Brachial Plexus

Overview

The brachial plexus derives from the anterior primary rami of spinal segments C5, C6, C7, and T1. It is approximately 0.5 cm long in adults and extends from the spinal column to the axilla. Its detailed anatomy in this course is important as to which of its components are injured or affected by its varied pathologies. It is divided into roots, trunks, divisions, cords, and branches. The C5-C6 roots coalesce to form the upper trunk; the C7 primary anterior ramus forms the middle trunk and the anterior primary rami of C8-T1 the lower trunk. In approximately 60% of patients, the C4 spinal root is a component of the upper trunk. In this instance, the plexus is prefixed, as all of the spinal root contributions are placed up one level. In this situation, the T1 spinal root of the lower trunk is less prominent. In approximately 7% of patients, C5 contributes minimally to the plexus and spinal roots are shifted down one level. If this occurs, T2 contributes to the lower trunk and C7 to the upper trunk.

The C5-C6 roots course downward and coalesce to form the upper trunk between the scalenus medius and scalenus anterior muscles. The anterior division of the upper and middle trunk fuses and forms the lateral cord, while the anterior division of the lower trunk becomes the medial cord. The three posterior divisions of the upper, middle, and lower trunks form the posterior cord.

The brachial plexus is in close proximity to mobile components of the neck and shoulder that make it susceptible to traction injuries. The trunks are superficial in the supraclavicular fossa. The lower trunk is adjacent to the subclavian artery and the apex of the lung. The divisions of the plexus are retroclavicular and lie between the clavicle and the first rib. Infraclavicularly, the cords surround the axillary artery and are close to the proximal humerus and the glenohumeral joint. Cords are situated below the clavicle in the axilla and are the longest components of the plexus. There are anatomic variations between the cords.

The spinal nerves derived from the cords and trunks may be purely sensory, motor or mixed sensory motor. The nerves that arise directly from spinal roots include the dorsal scapular nerve, the long thoracic nerve, and a branch to the phrenic nerve. The subclavian and suprascapular nerves arise from the upper trunk. The subscapular and thoracodorsal nerves arise from the posterior cord that terminates as the axillary and radial nerves. The proximal medial cord gives rise to the motor branch that innervates the medial pectoral muscle. The distal medial cord gives rise to the medial brachial and medial antebrachial cutaneous nerves. The medial cord gives a small branch to the median nerve and makes up the ulnar nerve. The proximal portion of the lateral cord gives rise to the lateral pectoral nerve. The termination of the lateral cord is the musculocutaneous nerve. It also gives off a lateral branch that joins the branch from the medial cord to form the median nerve.

The median, ulnar, radial, axillary nerves take origin in the peripheral axilla. The proximal portions of the median, ulnar, and radial nerves are adjacent to the proximal humerus and the axillary artery. Plexus trunks form at the lateral border of the anterior and middle scalene muscles.

The major blood supply of the brachial plexus derives from the subclavian artery. The supraclavicular components of the plexus are supplied by the ascending cervical, deep cervical and the superior intercostal arteries. The roots are supplied by branches from the vertebral artery. The infraclavicular plexus and cords are supplied by the subclavian, axillary, and subscapular vessels.

Terminal Nerves that Arise from the Cervical Roots

1. The phrenic nerve:
    a. As noted earlier, the major root that innervates the diaphragm is C4.
    b. It receives contributions from C3 and C5.
    c. The phrenic nerve crosses the anterior scalene muscle to enter the thorax.
2. Dorsal scapular nerve: arises from the C5 nerve root immediately after it emerges from the intervertebral foramen, courses between the middle and posterior scalene muscle to innervate the levator scapular and the major and minor rhomboid muscles.
3. The long thoracic nerve arises from the C5, C6 and C7 roots, descends along the lateral chest wall to innervate the serratus anterior muscle

Nerves that Arise from Brachial Plexus Trunks

Suprascapular Nerve

1. The suprascapular nerve arises from the upper trunk, descends posteriorly between the omohyoid and the trapezius muscle, through the scapular notch to innervate the supra and infraspinatus muscles.
2. Nerve to the subclavius muscle: May arise from the C5 root or the upper trunk to innervate the subclavius muscle that lies between the clavicle and the first rib.
3. Medial pectoral nerve: Arises from the medial trunk whose major roots are C8 and T1. It innervates the pectoralis major and minor muscles.

Nerves that Arise from the Brachial Plexus Cords

Lateral Pectoral Nerves

The major roots contributing to the nerve are C5, C6, and C7. The nerve usually arises from the lateral cord.

Anatomic variations occur and include the origin from the anterior division of the upper and middle trunks.

Subscapular nerves

The primary roots of the nerves are C5 and C6. The upper and lower subscapular nerves arise from the posterior cord in the axilla. The subscapularis nerve innervates the subscapularis muscle; the lower subscapular nerve innervates both the subscapularis and the teres major muscles.

Thoracodorsal nerve

The major roots comprising the nerve are from C5-C7. The primary root is C7. The nerve takes origin from the posterior cord to innervate the latissimus dorsi muscle.

Anatomic variants include origins from:

1. The radial nerve
2. The axillary nerve

Medial Cutaneous Nerve of the Arm

The nerve originates from the medial cord to innervate the medial upper arm above the elbow.

Medial cutaneous nerve of the forearm usually arises from the medial cord. An anatomic variant is an origin from the medial cutaneous nerve of the arm. It innervates the medial forearm to the wrist.

Musculocutaneous Nerve

The musculocutaneous nerve is the termination of the lateral cord. It innervates the coracobrachialis, biceps brachii, and the brachialis muscles. Its major contributing roots are C5 and C6. In some patients, there is a contribution from C7. It terminates as the lateral cutaneous nerve of the lateral forearm from the elbow to the wrist.

A lateral branch fuses with a branch from the medial cord to form the median nerve.

An anatomic variant in a small number of patients includes:

1. An origin of the nerve from the anterior division of the upper trunk.
   a. In this instance, the lateral branch to the median nerve arises from the middle trunk.

Axillary Nerve

The axillary nerve is one of the terminal branches of the posterior cord and is primarily composed of the C5 and C6 spinal nerves. It traverses the quadrilateral space (teres major inferiorly, triceps laterally, the humerus medially, and the teres minor superiorly). It innervates the teres minor and deltoid muscles. Its cutaneous branches innervate the lateral proximal arm over the deltoid muscle.

Radial Nerve

The spinal nerves that comprise the radial nerve are from C5-C8. T1 contributes in approximately 10% of patients. It is the termination of the posterior cord. A branch arises in the axilla, the posterior cutaneous nerve, which innervates the posterior upper arm to the elbow. In the upper arm, it descends medially to the humerus between the medial and long heads of the biceps muscle in the spinal groove. Its branches in the upper arm innervate the medial, lateral, and long heads of the triceps brachii and the anconeus muscle. At the lateral aspect of the upper arm (after exiting the spinal groove), it innervates the brachioradialis, extensor carpi radialis longus and a small component of the brachialis muscle (whose main innervation is the musculocutaneous nerve). It gives off the posterior antebrachial cutaneous nerve that innervates the posterior forearm. At the elbow, it divides into the sensory superficial radial nerve and the motor posterior interosseous nerve. The posterior interosseous nerve traverses the radial tunnel at the elbow that is composed of the radius, the capsule of the radiocapitular joint and the tendons of the biceps brachii and brachialis muscles medially and the brachioradialis, extensor carpi radialis and the extensor carpi ulnaris that form the anterior and lateral walls. A fibrous band around the superficial head of the supinator muscle forms the Arcade of Frohse that is the end of the radial tunnel. The superficial radial nerve travels into the forearm underneath the brachioradialis muscle outside of the radial tunnel. The nerve innervates the extensor surfaces of the hand and fingers (with the exception of the fingertips that are innervated by the median and ulnar nerves) as well as the medial dorsal hand and medial fingers that are innervated by the dorsal ulnar cutaneous nerve. The posterior interosseous nerve courses through the radial tunnel and descends under the Arcade of Frohse. It innervates the supinator, extensor digitorum communis, extensor digiti minimi, extensor carpi ulnaris, abductor pollicis longus, extensor pollicis longus and brevis and the extensor indicis proprius.

Median Nerve

The median nerve is composed of spinal nerves C5 - T1 and is formed from the fusion of branches of the medial and lateral cords. Its sensory components are primarily derived from spinal segments C6 and C7. Rarely the C5 spinal segment is a component of the nerve. Sensory fibers arise from the upper and middle trunks to the lateral cord. Motor fibers course through all of the trunks and the medial and lateral cords. The median nerve reaches the antecubital fossa through the anterior compartment of the upper arm. It passes through the two heads of the pronator teres muscle and between the flexor digitorum superficialis and profundus muscles to reach the wrist. It innervates the pronator teres, flexor carpi radialis, palmaris longus, and flexor digitorum superficialis from branches given off in the forearm. It gives of the purely motor anterior interosseous nerve that innervates the flexor digitorum profundus 1 and 2, flexor pollicis longus and the pronator quadrates muscle. Prior to entering the carpal tunnel at the wrist, it gives off the palmar cutaneous nerve that innervates the thenar eminence. The nerve then enters the carpal tunnel that is composed of the carpal bones and a dorsal transverse ligament. It also contains nine flexor tendons to the fingers as well as the median nerve. Either within or just distal to the tunnel the recurrent branch of the nerve arises to innervate the abductor pollicis brevis, opponens pollicis, and the superficial head of the flexor pollicis brevis. The nerve supplies the first and second lumbrical muscles and digital branches to the volar and dorsal tips of the thumb index and long finger as well as the medial one-half of the ring finger.

Ulnar Nerve

The ulnar nerve is comprised primarily of spinal nerves C8 and T1, but in over 50% of patients, there is a contribution from the C7 spinal nerve that innervates the flexor carpi ulnaris muscle. This innervation derives from a branch of the lateral cord. The nerve is the termination and then continuation of the medial cord. It descends anteriorly to the teres major and latussimus dorsi muscles to enter the upper arm. It courses down the posterior compartment of the upper arm to the ulnar groove at the elbow. The ulnar groove comprises the medial epicondyle of the humerus and the olecranon process of the ulna. The ulnar collateral ligament bounds it inferiorly. Distal to the ulnar groove (1-2.5 cm), the nerve courses under a fibrous aponeurosis that connects the humeral and ulnar heads of the flexor carpi ulnaris muscle. The ulnar groove and the aponeurosis form the cubital tunnel. There are no branches from the ulnar nerve in the upper arm. The nerve traverses between the flexor carpi ulnaris and flexor digitorum profundus to the wrist. Its forearm branches innervate the flexor carpi ulnaris and the flexor digitorum profundus III and IV. The dorsal ulnar cutaneous nerve innervates the dorsum of the medial hand and fourth and fifth fingers. Prior to entering Guyon's canal at the wrist, it gives off the palmar branch that gives sensory innervation to the hypothenar eminence and innervates the palmaris brevis muscle. Guyon's canal is formed radially by the hook of the hamate bone and the pisiform bone on its ulnar side, the pisohamate ligament inferiorly and the transverse carpal ligament superiorly. Either within or immediately distal to Guyon's canal the ulnar nerve gives off its terminal branches. The superficial sensory branch innervate the volar components of the fifth finger and the ulnar half of the fourth finger as well as the dorsal distal aspects of these digits. The deep motor branch of the ulnar nerve innervates the hypothenar muscles, the third and fourth lumbricals, the interossei, adductor pollicis and the deep head of the flexor pollicis brevis muscle.

Clinical Manifestations of Brachial Plexus Disorders

Supraclavicular Level

1. Supraclavicular lesions present in myotomal and dermatomal distributions
2. Cervical root derived terminal nerves:
    a. Phrenic nerve (C3-C5); C4 is the predominant root
    b. Dorsal scapular nerve:
        i Arises from the C5 root as it exits the intervertebral foramen
        ii Innervates the major and minor rhomboid muscles and the levator scapuli.
        iii The muscles pull the scapulae medially, rotate it and hold it against the chest wall.
    c. Long thoracic nerve:
        i Arises from C5, C6 and C7 spinal nerves
        ii Innervates the serratus anterior muscle
        iii Function:
            1. Pulls the scapula forward around the thorax to achieve anteversion of the arm.
            2. Compresses the scapula against the wall of the thorax
            3. Assists with elevation of the ribs with respiration
            4. A component of arm elevation
            5. Protraction of the scapula
            6. Role in upward rotation of the scapula in synchrony with the trapezius muscle.

Upper Trunk Lesions

1. Suprascapular nerve:
    a. Arises from the upper trunk immediately after it forms
    b. Function:
        i Abducts the arm at the shoulders, it is the main agonist of this movement for the first 10-15 degrees of its arc. Beyond 30 degrees, the deltoid muscle is the primary arm abductor.
        ii Stabilizes the shoulder joint by effecting pressure medially that helps to hold the humeral head in the glenoid fossa.
        iii Provides sensory innervations to the acromiocalvicular and glenohumeral joints.
        iv The infraspinatus muscle:
            1. Externally rotates the humerus
            2. Stabilizes the shoulder joint
    c. Diagnostic points:
        i Lesions at the level of the formation of the trunks:
            1. The serratus anterior and the rhomboids are normal
            2. Lesions at mid or upper trunk segments:
                a. The supra and infraspinatus muscles are normal.

Lateral Cord Lesions

1. Lateral pectoral nerves:
   a. Most often arise from the lateral cord. Anatomic variants are its origin from the anterior division of the upper and middle trunks
   b. Function:
      i Innervates the pectoralis major muscle that is also innervated from the medial pectoral nerve.
      ii Flexion and adduction of the humerus
      iii Rotates the humerus medially
      iv Sensory innervations of the anterior chest wall

Musculocutaneous Nerve

1. Most often is the termination of the lateral cord:
   a. Gives off a branch that combines with a branch from the medial cord that forms the median nerve
   b. Its major spinal nerves are C5 and C6 although there is a contribution from C7 in greater than 50% of patients.
2. It innervates:
   a. Coracobrachialis
   b. Biceps brachii
   c. Brachialis
   d. Forms the lateral cutaneous nerve of the forearm
3. Function:
   a. Coracobrachialis:
      i Flexes and adducts the arm
      ii Medial rotation of the humerus
      iii Stabilization of the humeral head within the glenoid fossa
   b. Biceps brachii:
      i Supination of the forearm
      ii Flexion of the forearm
      iii Minor functions:
         1. Forward flexion of the shoulder
         2. Aids abduction of the arm
         3. Short head contributes to adduction of the arm
         4. Stabilization of the shoulder
      iv Lateral cutaneous nerve of the forearm
         1. Sensation from the lateral elbow to the wrist (laterally)

Medial Cord

1. Medial pectoral nerve:
   a. Innervates both the pectoralis major and minor muscles
   b. Function:

- i Adduction and medial rotation of the arm
- ii Poland Syndrome (congenital absence of the muscle) may be asymptomatic

2. Medial cutaneous nerve of the arm
   a. Provides sensation to the medial upper arm to the elbow
3. Medial cutaneous nerve of the forearm:
   a. May arise from the medial cutaneous nerve of the arm
   b. Function:
      iii Sensory innervation of the medial forearm to the wrist

Posterior Cord

1. Thoracodorsal nerve:
   a. Most often arises from the posterior cord. Rarely its origin is the radial or axillary nerves
   b. Its major spinal nerve is C7, but it receives contributions from C5 and C6
   c. Function:
      - i Extension and adduction of the arm
      - ii Horizontal abduction of the arm
      - iii Internal rotation
      - iv Flexion from an extended position
      - v Synergistic for extension and lateral flexion of the lumbar spine
2. Subscapular nerves:
   a. The upper subscapular nerve innervates the subscapularis muscle. Derived from C5, C6 spinal nerves
   b. Function:
      - i Rotates the head of the humerus medially
      - ii Draws the humerus forward and downward if the arm is raised
      - iii Prevents displacement of the humerus

Lower Subscapular Nerve

1. Supplies the lower part of the subscapularis muscle as well as the teres major
2. Its spinal nerves are C5 and C6
3. Function:
   a. The subscapularis is the major and most powerful muscle of the rotator cuff
   b. Stabilizes the glenohumeral joint

Axillary Nerve

1. One of the terminal branches of the posterior cord. Its spinal nerves are C5 and C6. It innervates the teres minor and deltoid muscles. Its sensory innervation is the lateral proximal arm over the deltoid muscle.
2. Function of the deltoid muscle:

   a. Anterior fibers:
      i Shoulder abduction
      ii Medial rotation of the humerus
   b. Posterior fibers:
      i Transverse extension
      ii Lateral rotation
   c. Lateral fibers:
      i Shoulder abduction
      ii Stabilizes the humeral head
3. Teres minor muscle:
   a. Part of the rotator cuff that stabilizes the humeral head in the glenoid fossa
   b. Is synergistic with the posterior fibers of the deltoid to laterally rotate the humerus
   c. Transverse adduction and extension of the arm

Radial Nerve

1. The continuation of the posterior cord following branching of the axillary nerve. Its major spinal nerves are C5-C8 although approximately 10% of patients have a contribution from T1
2. Innervates:
   a. The long, medial and lateral head of the triceps and the anconeus muscle
   b. Brachioradialis, extensor carpi radialis longus and the brachialis (major innervations is from the lateral cord)
   c. In the axilla, it gives off the posterior cutaneous nerve that innervates the posterior arm to the elbow. The posterior antebrachial cutaneous nerve innervates the posterior forearm. The superficial radial nerve innervates the extensor surface of the hand and fingers except for the distal fingertips. The dorsal ulnar cutaneous nerve supplies the dorsal medial hand and medial fingers
   d. In the forearm, it innervates the extensor carpi radialis brevis, supinator, extensor digitorum communis, extensor digiti quinti, and extensor carpi ulnaris.
   e. Above the wrist branches innervate the abductor pollicis longus, extensor pollicis longus and brevis and the extensor indicis
   f. In the hand, it gives off dorsal digital nerves
   g. At the elbow the motor posterior interosseous nerve arises

Function of the Radial Nerve

Triceps Muscle

1. Primary extensor of the elbow joint

2. Fixates the elbow when the hand is used
3. Long head:
   a. Used for sustained force
   b. Synergistic for control of the shoulder and elbow
   c. Retroversion and adduction
4. Lateral head
   a. High-intensity force movements
5. Medial head:
   a. Used during low force precise hand movements

Anconeus Muscle

1. Assists in elbow extension and supports the elbow in full extension
2. Protects the elbow joint capsule in the olecranon fossa during extension of the elbow
3. Abducts the ulna

Brachioradialis Muscle

1. One of the few muscles that receives innervations directly from the radial nerve (the triceps, anconeus, and extensor carpi radialis are the others). The other radial nerve innervated muscles receive their innervations from a deep branch of the nerve.
2. Function:
   a. Flexes the forearm at the elbow
   b. Stabilizes the elbow during rapid flexion and extension
   c. Synergistic with the brachialis and biceps muscles

Supinator Muscle

1. Curved around the upper 1/3 of the radius and innervated by the deep branch of the radial nerve
2. Function:
   a. Supinates the forearm

Extensor Carpi Radialis Longus

1. Innervated by the radial nerve. All other major extensor muscles in the superficial layer of the posterior compartment of the forearm are innervated by the posterior interosseus nerve and include:
   a. Extensor digitorum
   b. Extensor carpi radialis brevis
   c. Extensor carpi ulnaris
   d. Extensor digiti minimi
2. Function:
   a. Extension of the wrist
   b. Radial abduction of the hand at the wrist

Extensor Carpi Radialis Brevis

1. Innervated by the posterior interosseous nerve
2. Function:
    a. An extensor and abductor of the hand at the wrist

Extensor Digitorum Communis

1. Innervated by the posterior interosseous nerve
2. Function:
    a. Principal action is extension of the proximal phalanges, the middle and terminal phalanges are extended by the interrossei and lumbricals
    b. Extends the phalanges, the wrist and the elbow (weak).

Extensor Carpi Ulnaris

1. Innervated by a deep branch of the radial nerve (C7, C8 spinal segments)
2. Function:
    a. Extends and adducts the wrist

Extensor Indicis, Extensor Pollicis Longus and Brevis, Extensor Digiti Quinti

1. Innervated by the posterior interosseous nerve
2. Function:
    a. Extension of the thumb (metacarpophalangeal and interphalangeal joints)
    b. Extension of the index finger and wrist (extensor indicis) and extension of the little finger at all joints (extensor digiti quinti)

Median Nerve

1. Formed by fusion of branches from the medial and lateral cords (spinal segments C6-T1):
    a. Motor fibers arise primarily from C6-T1 spinal segments
    b. Sensory fibers from C6-C7 spinal segments
    c. The sensory fibers transverse the upper and middle trunks to the lateral cord
    d. Motor fibers traverse all of the trunks to both the medial and lateral cords
    e. In the forearm the median nerve innervates:
        i Pronator teres
        ii Flexor carpi radialis
        iii Palmaris longus
        iv Flexor digitorum supeficialis
2. Pronator Teres:
    a. A forearm pronator (C6-C7)
3. Flexor carpi radialis (C6-C7)
    a. A radial flexor of the hand
4. Palmaris longus (C7-T1)

5. Flexor digitorum superficialis (C7-T1)

In its descent and after it passes between the two heads of the pronator teres the purely motor anterior osseous nerve takes origin to innervate:

1. Flexor pollicis longus (C7-C8)
2. A flexor of the terminal phalanx of the thumb
3. Flexor digitorum profundus and (C7-C8)
    a. A flexor of the terminal phalanges of the second and third fingers
4. Pronator quadrates (C7-C8)
    a. A forearm pronator

The median nerve divides into its terminal branches at the distal end of the carpal tunnel. The motor branches innervate the first and second lumbricals and the thenar muscles.

1. First and second lumbricals (C8-T1):
    a. Flexors of the proximal and extensors of the two distal phalanges of the second and third fingers
2. Abductor pollicis brevis (C8-T1):
    a. An abductor of the metacarpal of the thumb (possibly the best muscle to test for median nerve weakness)
3. Oppenens pollicis (C8-T1)
    a. Brings the metacarpal of the thumb into opposition
4. Superficial head of the flexor pollicis brevis (C8-T1)
    a. Flexes the proximal phalanx of the thumb

Variations in the Innervation of Intrinsic Hand Muscles

1. Riche-Cannieu Anastomosis:
    a. Anastomosis between the motor branch of the median nerve and the deep ulnar nerve branch in the radial aspect of the hand.
2. Adductor pollicus and first dorsal interosseous muscles may be exclusively supplied by the median nerve in 2% of patients.
3. The abductor pollicius brevis and flexor pollicis brevis may be supplied exclusively by the ulnar nerve in 2% of individuals.

Ulnar Nerve

The ulnar nerve derives from the C7, C8, and T1 spinal nerves and is the main branch of the medial cord. In its descent into the arm, it traverses the axilla beneath the pectoralis minor muscle and lies medial to the brachial artery in the upper arm. The C7 component arises from a branch of the lateral cord to innervate the flexor carpi ulnaris muscle. It enters a groove in the distal arm between the medial humeral epicondyle and the olecranon process. The dorsal component of this osseous fibrous canal is an aponeurosis between the olecranon and medial epicondyle. It is bound inferiorly by the medial ligament of the elbow joint. This canal is the cubital tunnel. Distal to the elbow joint originate its first two muscular branches.

1. The flexor carpi ulnaris (C7-T1):
    a. Flexor of the wrist
2. Flexor digitorum profundus III and IV (C7-C8):
    a. A flexor of the terminal phalanges of the fourth and fifth fingers

In the distal forearm, it gives off the palmar cutaneous branch that innervates the skin of the hypothenar eminence. Shortly thereafter, it gives off the dorsal cutaneous branch that innervates the dorsal ulnar hand and the dorsal components of the fifth finger and one-half of the fourth finger. The ulnar nerve proper enters the wrist lateral to the tendon of the flexor carpi ulnaris muscle and gives off the superficial terminal branch. This sensory branch innervates the distal ulnar palm and the volar aspect of the fifth and one-half of the fourth finger. The nerve then traverses Guyon's canal whose medial component is the piriform carpal bone and the hook of the hamate carpal bone laterally to become the deep muscular branch.

1. It innervates intrinsic muscles of the hand that includes:
2. Palmaris brevis (C8-T1):
    a. Tenses the skin of the palm on the ulnar side of the hand to deepen the hollow of the palm
3. Abductor digiti minimi (C8-T1):
    a. An abductor of the fifth finger
4. Opponens digiti minimi (C8-T1):
    a. An opposer of the fifth finger
5. Flexor digiti minimi (C8-T1):
    a. A flexor of the fifth finger at the metacarpophalangeal joint
6. Lumbricals III and IV (C8-T1):
    a. Flexors of the metacarpal phalangeal joints and extensors of the proximal interphalangeal joints of the fourth and fifth fingers
7. Interosseous muscles:
    a. Flexors of the metacarpophalangeal joints and extensors of the proximal interphalangeal joints. The four dorsal interossei muscles are finger abductors. The three palmar interossei muscles are finger adductors:
        i Variants are:
            1. Innervation of the first dorsal interosseous by the median nerve (1% of individuals)
            2. First dorsal interosseous is innervated by the radial nerve (Froment-Rauber nerve)
8. Adductor pollicis (C8-T1):
    a. An adductor of the thumb
    b. It receives median nerve innervations in approximately 2% of individuals
9. Deep head of the flexor pollicis brevis (C8-T1):
    a. A flexor of the first phalanx of the thumb

Clinical Manifestations

1. Total Brachial Plexus Paralysis:
    a. There is paralysis of the entire arm that hangs limply at the patient's side. There is severe atrophy of all muscle groups
2. Anesthesia of the arm distal to a line extending obliquely from the tip of the shoulder to the medial arm approximately ½ way to the elbow.
3. Areflexia of the upper extremity

Upper Plexus Lesions

Most commonly involve the C5 and C6 spinal nerves of the upper trunk of the plexus.

1. Motor signs:
    a. C5-C6 spinal nerve innervated muscles are paretic or paralyzed and atrophic. These muscles include:
        i Deltoid
        ii Biceps
        iii Brachioradialis
        iv Brachialis
2. If the lesion is very proximal the supraspinatus, infraspinatus, and subscapularis may be involved. The arm is internally rotated and adducted and the forearm is extended and pronated. The palm faces out and backward:
    a. There is weakness of:
        i Shoulder abduction: deltoid and supraspinatus
        ii Elbow flexion: biceps brachioradialis and brachialis
        iii External rotation of the arm: infraspinatus
        iv Forearm supination: biceps
    b. Very proximal lesions involve the rhomboids, levator scapulae, serratus anterior, and scalene muscles.
3. Sensory signs:
    a. Sensation is often intact
    b. Sensory loss does occur over the lateral/upper arm and the deltoid muscle in some patients
4. Reflex signs:
    a. Depression of the biceps and brachioradialis reflexes

Middle Plexus Lesions

1. Lesions of the middle trunk or the individual anterior primary ramus of C7 are involved
    a. Motor signs:
    b. Involvement of C7 innervation to the radial nerve is primarily involved which causes weakness or paralysis of extension of the forearm, hand, and fingers

c. The paretic or paralyzed muscles are:
    i Triceps
    ii Anconeus
    iii Extensor carpi radialis and ulnaris
    iv Extensor digitorum
    v Extensor digiti minimi
    vi Extensor policis longus and brevis
    vii Abductor pollicis longus
    viii Extensor indicis
d. Forearm flexion is maintained by the brachioradialis and brachialis (C5-C6 spinal nerves)

2. Sensory signs:
    a. Patchy sensory deficit over the extensor surface of the forearm and the dorsum of the hand
3. Reflexes:
    a. Triceps reflex is depressed or absent

Lower Plexus Lesion

1. Primary injury involves the C8-T1 spinal nerves or the lower trunk of the plexus
2. Motor signs:
    a. Musculature supplied by the C8-T1 spinal nerves is affected. There is weakness of wrist and finger flexion and in the intrinsic hand muscles. There is usually severe hand atrophy leading to the "claw" hand deformity
3. Sensory signs:
    a. Decreased sensation of the medial arm and forearm and the ulnar side of the hand.
4. Reflex signs:
    a. Loss of finger flexion
5. If T1 is damaged, sympathetic fibers to the superior cervical ganglia are interrupted which causes a Horner's syndrome. If T2 is damaged, there is an interruption of the sympathetic innervation of the arm.

Lesions of the Lateral Cord

Usually, result in weakness of the muscles innervated by the musculocutaneous and lateral head of the median nerve.

1. Motor signs:
    a. Weakness of the biceps brachii and brachialis:
        i Flexion of the elbow
    b. Coracobrachialis:
        i Supination of the forearm

c. Median nerve innervated muscles:
   i Pronator teres:
      1. Pronation of the forearm
   ii Flexor carpi radialis:
      1. Radial wrist flexion
   iii Palmaris longus:
      1. Flexion of the wrist
   iv Flexor digitorum superficialis:
      1. Flexion of the middle phalangeal joints (second through fourth digits)
   v Flexor digitorum profundus I and II:
      1. Flexion of the distal phalanges of the second and third fingers
   vi Pronator quadratus:
      1. Pronation of the forearm

2. Sensory signs:
   a. Loss of sensation in the distribution of the lateral cutaneous nerve of the forearm:
      i Sensory loss in the lateral forearm
      ii Branch of the musculocutaneous nerve
3. Reflexes:
   a. Depression or absence of the biceps reflex

Lesions of the Medial Cord

1. Cause weakness of the muscles innervated by the ulnar nerve and the medial component of the median nerve
2. Ulnar innervated muscles that are weak include:
   a. Flexor carpi ulnaris:
      i Ulnar flexion of the wrist
   b. Flexor digitorum III and IV:
      i Flexion of the terminal digits of the fourth and fifth fingers
   c. All of the ulnar innervated small intrinsic hand muscles
3. Median innervated muscles include:
   a. Abductor pollicis brevis
      i Metacarpal abduction of the thumb
   b. Opponens pollicis:
      i Opposition of the thumb
   c. Superficial head of the flexor pollicis brevis:
      i Flexion of the proximal phalanx of the thumb
   d. Lumbricals I and II:
      i Flex the first two metacarpophalangeal joints and extend the digits of the second and third fingers

4. Sensory Signs:
    a. Loss of sensation of the medial arm and forearm due to injury of the medial cutaneous nerves of the arm and forearm.
5. Reflexes:
    a. Loss of the finger flexor reflex

Proximal Lesions of the Medial Cord

1. Injury of the medial anterior thoracic nerve:
    a. Weakness of the lower sternocostal portion of the pectoralis major muscle and the pectoralis minor muscle.

Lesions of the Posterior Cord

Posterior cord lesions cause weakness in the muscles innervated between the subscapular and thoracodorsal, axillary and radial nerves.

1. Motor signs:
    a. Subscapular nerve innervated muscles:
        i Weakness of the teres major and subscapularis muscles:
            1. Internal rotation of the humerus
    b. Thoracodorsal innervated muscles:
        i Latissimus dorsi weakness:
            1. Extension, adduction, transverse extension (horizontal abduction), flexion from an extended position and internal rotation of the cap of the shoulder joint
            2. Synergistic role (therefore weakness) in extension and lateral flexion of the lumbar spine
    c. Axillary nerve innervated muscles:
        i Deltoid:
            1. Arm abduction
        ii Teres minor:
            1. Lateral rotation of the shoulder joint
        iii Sensory loss:
            1. Distribution of the lateral cutaneous nerve of the arm that includes a diminished sensation of the lateral arm.

Radial Nerve

1. Weakness of elbow extension, wrist extension, supination of the forearm and finger extension. There is a minimal contribution to elbow flexion. Proximal lesions cause triceps reflex loss.
2. Sensory signs: sensory loss in the extensor surface of the arm and forearm, dorsum of the hand and first four fingers distribution
3. Reflexes: depression of triceps and radial reflexes

Neuropathology of Nerve Injuries

Neuropraxis

1. Neuronal dysfunction due to transient conduction block.
2. Compression of a nerve may cause segmental ischemia. If of short duration there may only be a reversible physiologic conduction block that lasts for minutes to hours. There may also be paranodal and then segmental demyelination. In this instance, recovery may take several weeks and is effected by remyelination

Axonotmesis

In this instance, the axon is interrupted, but the epineurium is preserved. The axon distal to the lesion degenerates over 7-10 days. Regenerating nerve sprouts from the proximal portion of the injured nerve attempt regeneration. The intact epineurium enhances the chance of reinnervation. Axons grow at a rate of 1 mm/day, so this process may require months to over a year.

Neurotmesis

1. The axon and epineurium are interrupted. The difference between axonotmesis and neurotmesis can only be determined by direct vision (surgery). Scarring from overlying tissue damage often prevents reinnervation.

Neuropathology

1. Dependent on the particular process affecting the plexus

Neuroimaging

1. Primarily high-resolution MRI (microneurography)
2. Ultrasound is useful for focal neuropathies and lesions

Laboratory Evaluation

1. EMG:
    a. The EMG is essential in evaluating radiculopathy, plexopathy, and mononeuropathy.
    b. Combined with motor and sensory NCVs, it supports the localization determined by the clinical examination

Traumatic Brachial Plexus Injury

Overview

1. The longitudinal excursion of the brachial plexus is 15.3 mm.
2. The greater the traction on the plexus, the greater the injury (between

neuropraxia, axonotmesis to neurotmesis).

3. The primary roots are the most susceptible to traction injury since they are arranged in parallel bundles rather than a lattice structure and therefore have decreased tensile strength.
4. Shoulder depression and lateral head flexion contralaterally injure the upper and middle trunk.
5. Traction on the hyper-abducted arm causes traction on the lower > middle > upper trunk.
6. Preganglionic injuries are usually caused by avulsion of the root.
7. Traction injuries may affect all or a portion of the plexus to a varying degree.
8. C5 and C6 rupture occur close to the exit foramina. C8-T1 rupture is often closer to the spinal cord.
9. The pathology is categorized as neuropraxic axonotmesis and neurotmesis.
10. Treatment (surgical intervention) is dependent on the type and severity of the injury:
    a. Most closed injuries are neuropraxic or axonometric that may recover spontaneously:
        i Upper trunk lesions usually demonstrate signs of recovery in 2-3 months
        ii Four to five months are required for recovery in middle and lower trunk lesions
    b. High impact injuries and those causing near total paralysis need to be evaluated earlier for possible surgery (3 weeks to 3 months)
    c. Injuries that more likely sever nerves such as lacerations or gunshot wounds need to be evaluated for possible surgical repair within 72 hours.
    d. Associated conditions that cause neurological worsening after injury:
        i Hematoma
        ii Concomitant bone and vascular injury
        iii Compartment syndromes

Avulsion Injury

General Characteristics

1. C5-C6 root lesions after severe trauma:
    a. 27% avulsions; 33% ruptures
2. Most often are caused by high impact trauma:
    a. MVA (motorcycle injuries are the most common)
    b. Football, skiing, mountain climbing accidents and falls.
3. C8-T1 root lesions:
    a. 98% are avulsion, and 1-2% are ruptures

Clinical Manifestations

1. Total plexopathy may occur with high impact trauma:
    a. Avulsion is greater in C8-T1 roots > C5, C6 and C7 roots
2. Early severe burning pain in an otherwise anesthetic hand; most severe proprioceptive loss if any sensation is proximal
3. Horner's syndrome is present in (C8-T1 avulsion)
4. Paralysis of the serratus anterior, rhomboids, infra and supra spinatus muscles
5. Negative supraclavicular Tinel's sign
6. May have associated spinal cord symptoms and signs

Neuropathology

1. 1. Neurotmesis of the roots

Neuroimaging

1. Traumatic meningocele
2. Fracture of a transverse process
3. Flattening of the root sleeve
4. Extravasation of contrast through the torn root sleeve during myelography
5. High-resolution MRI may demonstrate the lesions and is now more commonly used than myelography
6. Ultrasound is used for focally associated neuropathies

Laboratory Evaluation

1. EMG:
    a. Sensory, motor, and mixed sensorimotor nerve conduction studies
    b. SNAP (sensory nerve action potentials) are normal if the lesion is distal to the dorsal root ganglion
        i It requires 7-10 days for SNAPs to disappear with a completely severed nerve
    c. Positive sharp-wave and fibrillation potentials in affected muscles and paraspinal muscles:
        i May require one week to appear in paraspinal muscles and three weeks following axonal injury
        ii The Motor Unit Action Potentials (MUAPs) voluntarily recruited are immediately affected

Obstetric Complications

General Characteristics

1. Incidence ranges from 0.38 to 2% per 1000 live births
2. Three types of injury occur:
    a. Diffuse plexopathy
    b. Upper trunk plexopathy (Erb's)
    c. Lower trunk plexopathy (Klumpe's)

3. Risks for brachial plexus injury during childbirth:
    a. Diabetic, multiparous, obese mothers
    b. Greater than 4500 gram fetuses
    c. Mothers that are short
    d. Breech presentation
    e. Long and difficult labor
    f. Forceful downward traction of the head

Clinical Manifestations

1. Erb's palsy (C5-C6 roots; upper trunk)
2. The most common obstetrical brachial plexus injury:
    a. Stretch of the upper trunk
    b. Severe traction may avulse the C5 and C6 spinal nerves
    c. Occurs with shoulder dystocia in a vertex presentation or the aftercoming head in a breech presentation
    d. Upper trunk lesions cause weakness of muscles that include:
        i Supra and infraspinatus
        ii Deltoid
        iii Biceps brachii
        iv Teres minor
        v Brachioradialis
        vi Extensor carpi radialis/longus/brevis
        vii Supinator
    e. Weakness of the diaphragm or serratus anterior suggests root avulsion (proximal to the upper trunk)
    f. Sensory loss < motor deficit

Klumpke's Paralysis (C8, T1 roots)

1. Face presentation with hyperextension of the neck or with a breech delivery with hyperabduction of the arm
2. Weakness of hand muscles
3. Sensory loss < motor deficit

Neuropathology

1. Primarily axonotmesis and neurotmesis (with avulsion)

Neuroimaging

1. To assess for associated humeral or clavicular fracture; diaphragmatic paralysis.
2. MRI:
    a. To assess for nerve root avulsion

Laboratory Evaluation

1. EMG:
    a. Determines the site and severity of the lesion.

Thoracic Outlet Syndrome

Overview

The major components of the thoracic outlet are the sternocostovertebral space that forms the most proximal part of the thoracic outlet tunnel and is bound:

1. Anteriorly by the sternum
2. Posteriorly by the spine
3. Laterally by the first rib

The subclavian artery, subclavian vein, and C4 to T1 spinal nerves traverse this space. Associated structures include the apex of the lung and pleura, sympathetic trunk, jugular vein and lymphatics of the neck. It may be congenitally narrowed.

The usual pathology of the sternocostovertebral space includes:

1. Thyroid masses
2. An enlarged thymus
3. Parathyroid Mass
4. Lymph nodes or lung tumors that cause the Pancoast Syndrome (squamous or adenocarcinoma of the lung)

The scalene triangle is bound by the anterior scalene muscle anteriorly, the middle scalene posteriorly with the first rib forming its base. The origins of the anterior scalene muscle are the transverse processes of C3-C6.

The insertion of the anterior scalene muscles on the scalene tubercle of the first rib varies between the subclavian artery and vein and the pleural dome.

Variants of this insertion include:

1. Behind the artery
2. Between the artery and the brachial plexus
3. The entire base of the scalene triangle (which traps the neurovascular bundle). The anterior insertion may merge with the insertion of the middle scalene muscle in 20% of patients. The C5-C6 spinal nerves may traverse the anterior scalene muscle rather than descend between the anterior and middle scalene muscles.

The origin of the middle scalene muscle is the transverse processes of C2-C7. It inserts on the retro arterial tubercle of the first rib (Chassaignac's tubercle). It may insert on the fibrous septum of the pleural dome in which case its lateral fibers insert on the second rib. The C8-T1 spinal nerves as the lower trunk of the plexus may be compressed by a more anterior or forward insertion (its sharp anterior edge). Rarely, congenital fibromuscular bands are noted along the anterior edge of the muscle that may also compress the C8-T1 spinal nerves.

The first rib forms the floor of the scalene triangle. The T1 spinal nerve is closest to the rib. Congenital rib anomalies, bony ridges, hypoplasia, or inward curvature may compress the neurovascular bundle. There are congenital variations in the size of the base of the scalene triangle that may cause compression of components of the plexus. Its usual size is approximately 0.77 cm in men and 0.67 cm in women. The C5-C7 spinal nerves emerge from the apex of the triangle in association with interdigitation of the anterior and middle scalene muscles. This anatomical feature is noted in a large percentage of patients with neurogenic thoracic outlet syndrome. Adherence of the C5-C6 spinal nerves to the middle scalene muscle may also irritate these nerves and cause pain. Pathology in the costoclavicular and pectoralis minor space compresses the brachial plexus with various arm positions.

Anatomical Variations of the Thoracic Outlet

1. Bone defects:
   a. Cervical rib
   b. Abnormal or rudimentary first rib
2. Congenital bands or ligaments
3. Pectoralis minor insertion variations (hyperabduction syndrome)
4. Large subclavius muscle
5. Tight thoracic inlet
6. Scalene triangle congenital defects:
   a. Narrow scalene triangle
   b. Proximity of anterior and middle scalene muscles
   c. High emergence of spinal nerves from the triangle
   d. Interdigitated muscle fibers between the middle and anterior scalene muscles.
   e. Adherence of spinal nerves C5-C6 to the anterior scalene muscle
7. Congenital narrowness of the costoclavicular space
8. Clavicle anomalies (acromial head depression compresses the costoclavicular space)
9. A tight pectoralis minor space (below the insertion of the pectoralis minor tendon into the coracoid process); hyper abduction of the arm closes the space.

Neurogenic Thoracic Outlet Syndrome

General Characteristics

1. The most frequent cause of TOS (hotly debated between neurologists, EMG specialists, and thoracic and specific groups of orthopedic surgeons)
2. High percentage of patients have an underlying anatomical variant:
   a. The four anatomical spaces of the thoracic outlet:
      i i. Sternocostovertebral space
      ii Scalene triangle (most frequently involved)
      iii Costoclavicular space

iv Pectoralis minor space

b. Congenital bands (12 types)
c. Cervical ribs
d. Long neck droopy shoulders
e. Tight thoracic inlet
f. Abnormal insertions of the anterior, middle or minimus scalene muscle

Clinical Manifestations

1. Abnormal posture of the affected extremity forward flexed and dropped shoulder as the position of comfort (weakness of the lower components of the trapezius muscle and the levator scapulae). There is often associated pathology of the ventral components of C2-C4.
1. Positive stretch maneuvers:
2. Roos' abduction stress maneuver is positive in approximately 60-70% of patients in one minute
3. Wright's maneuver is also frequently positive.
4. These maneuvers evoke heaviness and paresthesia in specific plexus sensory radiations within 1-2 minutes. Control patients can maintain these postures (surrender position of the arms) for at least three minutes
5. Positive Tinel's signs:
   a. Erb's point (supraclavicular plexus)
   b. Pectoralis minor space (lateral infraclavicular fossa)
   c. Compression of the neurovascular bundle (against the proximal humerus)
   d. At the cubital tunnel (ulnar nerve)
   e. At the Arcade of Frohse (dorsal radial sensory fibers). This Tinel's sign is invariably misdiagnosed as "tennis elbow".
   f. Pronator canal (median nerve)
   g. Occasionally the carpal tunnel and Guyon canal areas are mechanically sensitive.

Sensory loss in specific plexus distributions

1. Upper trunk:
   a. Trapezius ridge, deltoid and medial scapula border (C5-C6 sensory radiations)
   b. Pain or tenderness at the tip of the scapula is notalgia and is a C6 sensory nerve radiation, not T6 (most oftern).
2. Lower trunk:
   a. Medial arm and forearm distributions (brachial and antebrachial cutaneous nerve distributions)
   b. Radiation into the complete 4th finger (the ulnar nerve splits the fourth finger and supplies a small triangular area above the wrist). The lower trunk innervates the entire medial forearm and arm. The lower trunk

radiations are often misdiagnosed as ulnar nerve lesions.

c. Proximal lesions may be associated with a Horner's syndrome.

d. Lower trunk lesions are a common cause of chronic regional pain syndrome Type I and II that has severe somatosensory, motor, and autonomic features.

3. Lateral cord:
   a. Pain or paresthesia in the lateral forearm (lateral antebrachial cutaneous nerve) distribution
   b. Thumb, index, and radial side of the third finger have decreased sensation or paresthesias.
4. Medial cord:
   a. Medial forearm (territory of the medial antebrachial cutaneous nerve)
      i Rarely the brachial cutaneous nerve territory of the medial proximal upper arm is involved
   b. The ulnar side of the third finger and the complete 4th and 5th finger comprise the medial cord sensory topology in the hand
   c. There is frequent involvement of the intercostobrachial nerve concomitantly with medial cord injury; this causes pain in the anterior chest wall (T1-T3) and the lateral chest wall (anterior axillary line); paresthesia and pain may radiate under the breast to the middle of the epigastrium at the xiphoid process. These radiations are often misdiagnosed as visceral pain radiations
5. Posterior cord:
   a. Paresthesias of the triceps muscle and back of the arm
   b. Radiations to the dorsal forearm and base of the thumb and parts of the dorsal hand (posterior antebrachial radial cutaneous nerve)
6. Muscle weakness:
   a. Occurs in various components of the involved plexus; subscapularis, teres major, latissimus dorsi, deltoid, teres minor, triceps brachii, brachioradialis, extensor of the fingers and wrist, supinator and extensor and abductor muscles of thumb
7. Reflexes:
   a. Most often, they are normal.
   b. They may be increased if CRPS I or II has supervened which is more common with lower trunk lesions (sympathetic hyperactivity induces contraction of the intrafusal muscle fibers of the nuclear bag of the muscle spindle complex).

Neuropathology

1. Neurogenic thoracic outlet syndrome comprises approximately 90% of all patients suffering the syndrome.
   a. Most patients have suffered trauma with flexion-extension injuries of the

neck ("whiplash")

b. Repetitive movements commonly initiate the process.
c. Falls on the outstretched arms are common.
d. Most often, the process is neuropractic and recovers spontaneously. However, a small percentage of patients become chronic.
e. Secondary concomitant CRPS I and II may be caused by lower trunk trauma most often.

Specific Anatomic Causes of Neurogenic TOS

1. Cervical ribs:
   a. The incidence of cervical ribs in the population is estimated to be 0.3%.
   b. Women are affected two times more frequently than men
   c. Approximately 10% of patients with cervical ribs are symptomatic. Usually, symptoms are initiated by trauma.
   d. The Gruber classification of cervical ribs:
      i Type I:
         1. Protrudes slightly beyond the transverse process and attaches to the first rib by a tight fibrous band.
      ii Type II: 2.5 cm in length:
         1. Attaches to the first rib by a tight fibrous band.
         2. Rib and band lie within or on the medial border of the middle scalene muscle.
         3. This configuration narrows the scalene triangle.
      iii Type III:
         1. A complete rib with a fibrous connection to the first rib.
      iv Type IV:
         1. A complete rib with a cartilaginous joint at the first rib.
         2. The complete rib causes the neurovascular bundle to arch over the rib
         3. The neurovascular bundle is compressed when the shoulder girdle is depressed.

Ligaments and Fibrous Bands that Compress Cervical Spinal Nerves

1. Twelve different fibrous structures can compromise the thoracic outlet.
2. The most significant ligaments are:
   a. Transverse process of C7 to the first rib.
   b. Tip of the cervical rib that inserts on the first rib
   c. Ligaments that are within the body or on the anterior surface of the middle scalene muscle may affect C8-T1 spinal nerves of the lower trunk.
   d. Common anomalies:
      i Incomplete cervical rib on a long transverse process of C7 from which

a tight band inserts on the first rib.

Roos' Congenital Bands and Ligaments

1. Type I:
    a. Tip of an incomplete cervical rib ligament that inserts posteriorly to the scalene tubercle
2. Type II:
    a. The origin of the ligament is from the transverse process of C7 and inserts on the scalene tubercle
3. Type III:
    a. A ligament that originates and inserts on the first rib; the origin is posterior and the insertion is anterior.
4. Type IV:
    a. The ligament originates within the middle scalene (C2-C7)
    b. Courses on the anterior edge of the middle scalene.
    c. Inserts with the muscle on the first rib.
    d. The ligament is adjacent to C8, T1 spinal nerves
5. Type V:
    a. Scalenus minimus muscle is the Vth band.
    b. Origin is in the anterior scalene muscle (lower fibers)
    c. Courses behind the subclavian artery in front of the plexus to insert on the first rib.
6. Type VI:
    a. Scalenus minimus insertion into Sibson's' fascia over the cupola of the lung rather than the first rib.
7. Type VII:
    a. A fibrous cord that courses on the anterior surface of the anterior scalene muscle.
    b. Inserts on the costochondral junction of the sternum.
    c. The band lies behind the subclavian vein that it may compress.
8. Type VIII:
    a. Origin of the ligament is the middle scalene muscle.
    b. Courses under the subclavian artery and vein.
    c. Inserts on the costochondral junction
9. Type IX:
    a. A web of muscle and fascia that fills the posterior curve of the first rib.

The Rib-Band Syndrome of Gilliatt

General Characteristics

1. Primarily a lower trunk plexopathy.
2. Women are more often affected than men are.

Clinical Manifestations

1. Paresthesia of the 4th and 5th fingers, medial forearm to the medial humerus.
2. Atrophy of the thenar is greater than hypothenar muscles of the hand.

Neuropathology

1. A sharp fibrous band from the tip of an elongated C7 transverse process of a true cervical rib to the first rib.
2. A neuropraxic injury of the proximal lower trunk.

Neuroimaging

1. Plain x-ray:
    a. Prominent transverse process at C7
    b. Cervical rib
    c. The band cannot be appreciated by MRI
2. MRI micrography
3. Ultrasound

Laboratory Evaluation

1. 1. EMG:
    a. The median CMAP and medial antebrachial cutaneous SNAP amplitudes are reduced to a greater extent than the ulnar SNAP and CMAP.
        i Ulnar studies primarily assess C8 fibers

Brachial Plexus Injuries (Iatrogenic)

Brachial Plexus Surgery for Neurogenic Plexopathy

General Characteristics

1. No gender difference
2. Young and middle-aged patients are affected

Clinical Manifestations

1. Weakness of the intrinsic muscles of the hand noted immediately.
2. Pain may be the predominant symptom.
3. Lower trunk involvement is often associated with Type II complex regional pain syndrome.

Neuropathology

1. Most lesions occur during trans axillary first rib resection; less frequently with scalenectomy and neurolysis of the upper trunk in the supraclavicular fossa.
2. Direct surgical injury as traction (neuropraxis) plexus injury.
3. Phrenic nerve may be involved concomitantly (particularly if the procedure involves the middle scalene muscle).

4. Site of the lesion:
    a. Proximal lower trunk
    b. C8, T1 spinal nerves

Orthopedic Surgical Procedures that Injure the Plexus

General Characteristics

1. 1. Most common procedures are those for:
    a. Recurrent anterior shoulder dislocation
    b. Shoulder joint replacement
    c. Arthroscopy of the shoulder
    d. Surgical procedures that compromise the costoclavicular space
    e. Direct trauma from arteriography and cannulas
    f. Percutaneous cannulation of the subclavian and internal jugular vein
    g. Percutaneous brachial plexus block

Clinical Manifestations

1. Chronic recurrent anterior shoulder dislocation:
    a. Putti-Platt; Bristow procedures
    b. During surgery:
        i Direct trauma to the musculocutaneous nerve is the most frequent injury
        ii Median, ulnar, radial, and axillary nerves may be inured with clinically expected motor and sensory deficits
    c. Concomitant damage to the axillary artery and vein.
    d. Delayed onset of plexopathy following the modified Bristow procedure:
        i The bone screw that attaches the coronoid process to the glenoid rim works loose.
        ii Axillary artery may be pierced with pseudo aneurysm formation that compresses the infraclavicular plexus.

Shoulder Joint Replacement

1. Direct trauma to the axillary nerve and the supraclavicular plexus.

Arthroscopy of the Shoulder

1. Direct trauma to the infraclavicular nerves:
    a. Musculocutaneous
    b. Axillary
    c. Ulnar
    d. Radial

Neuropathology

1. Neuropraxis injuries of these nerves

Neuroimaging

1. Ultrasonography
2. MRI microneurography
3. EMG evaluation

Surgical procedures that compromise the costoclavicular space

1. Operations to correct Sprengel's deformity.
2. Midportion of the clavicle surgery (fracture repair or to obtain access to subclavian vessels); regeneration of the lateral clavicle with excess callus formation that compresses the upper trunk.

Direct Trauma from Arteriography and Cannulas

1. Trauma to the infraclavicular brachial plexus:
    a. Cords of the plexus are adjacent to the second segment of the axillary artery; the median nerve is on the surface of the artery
    b. Leakage of blood from the puncture site that causes direct compression of the terminal nerves: median > ulnar >radial
    c. Most often, there is a combination of median and ulnar nerve trauma.
    d. Pain, paresthesia, and arm weakness in characteristic patterns.
        i Onset of symptoms may be delayed for up to two weeks.
    e. Nerve lesions may occur from pressure (hematoma) in the medial brachial fascial compartment that:
        i Extends from the axilla to the elbow
        ii Formed by the medial intramuscular septum and the surface of the medial upper arm.
        iii Encloses the neurovascular bundle and fascial axillary sheath.
    f. Percutaneous cannulation of the subclavian and internal jugular vein:
        i Direct instrumentation induced trauma.
        ii Hematoma compression.
        iii Rarely axillary mononeuropathy
        iv Rarely upper trunk plexopathy
    g. Percutaneous brachial plexus block:
        i Injuries may be caused by:
            1. The block itself.
            2. Tourniquet-induced ischemia
            3. Post-operative casting
            4. The surgical procedure
        ii Axillary block approach causes more injuries than interscalene blocks
        iii Usual symptoms are paresthesia in the median and ulnar nerve distributions; usually slight weakness of the involved nerves.
        iv May have delayed onset (up to two days) following the procedure:
            1. Bupivacaine at 0.25% may demyelinate nerves.

Median Sternotomy

General Characteristics

1. Median sternotomies:
   a. Primarily open heart surgeries
   b. Thoracotomy
2. Brachial plexus injuries affect up to 5% of patients that undergo the procedure

Clinical Manifestations

1. Primarily affects the lower trunk
2. Sensory loss in the medial forearm and hand
3. Weakness of intrinsic hand muscles

Neuropathology

1. Neuropraxis injury of the lower trunk; usually recovers in months

Neuroimaging

1. Ultrasound evaluation of the plexus
2. MRI not effective in visualizing lesions that are neuropractic

Laboratory Evaluation

1. EMG:
   a. Usually, demonstrates a lower trunk lesion

Post Anesthesia Brachial Plexopathy

General Characteristics

1. Follows surgical procedures usually under general anesthesia
2. Abdominal operation (usually cholecystectomy or hysterectomy; now changing due to minimally invasive surgery)

Clinical Manifestations

1. Upper plexus more often involved than lower plexus; usually unilateral.
2. Weakness and paresthesia are the predominant signs and symptoms.
3. Rarely patients complain of pain
4. Rarely a Horner's syndrome
5. Recovery usually begins 2-3 weeks after onset and may require several months to be complete:
   a. Sensory loss recovers first followed in the lower plexus, then in the upper plexus and lastly motor function.

Neuropathology

1. A neuropractic injury
2. Positions associated with post-operative paralysis:
   a. Supine

b. Trendelenburg (steep and prolonged)
c. Abduction of one or both arms to 90 degrees or greater
d. Extension and external rotation
e. Rotation and lateral flexion of the head to the contralateral side
f. Lower shoulder and arm compressed
g. Flexed and prone position (back procedures)
h. Excessive abduction and arm flexion

Neuroimaging

1. 1. MRI/MRA:
    a. Microneurography to evaluate soft tissue and vascular components in the surgical field.
    b. Ultrasonography to evaluate terminal nerves

Postoperative Brachial Plexopathy (Thoracic Outlet Surgery)

General Characteristics

1. Surgery for neurogenic brachial plexopathy particularly performed without a clear anatomic target such as a cervical rib is fraught with complications

Clinical Manifestations

1. 1. First rib trans axillary resection:
    a. Weakness and wasting in a lower trunk distribution
    b. Paresthesias and burning pain in the 4th and 5th fingers and medial forearm.
    c. Less commonly:
        i Flail arm with numbness and pain of the entire upper extremity
        ii This pattern may evolve into a medial cord distribution of weakness.
2. Anterior scalenectomy and neurolysis:
    a. Pain across the trapezius ridge and down the medial scapular border.
    b. Minimal weakness of the rhomboids, supra and infraspinatus and biceps muscles
    c. Occasional paresthesia of the lateral deltoid and the lateral forearm
    d. Occasional weakness of the ipsilateral phrenic nerve

Neuropathology

1. Neuropractic, axonotmesis, and neurotmesis of components of the brachial plexus

Neuroimaging

1. MRI:
    a. To evaluate the surgical field for hematoma or bone defects (difficult to distinguish brachial plexus components with 1.5 Tesla magnet strength)
2. 2. Ultrasonography to evaluate terminal nerves

Laboratory Evaluation

1. EMG:
   a. After 14-21 days to evaluate the level and extent of the operative injury.

Gunshot Wounds/Laceration Injuries

General Characteristics

1. Gunshot wounds:
   a. 85% are in males
   b. the average age is 28 years

Clinical Manifestations

1. 80% of injuries affect the cords or terminal nerves
2. Majority of patients have plexus lesions in continuity
3. Laceration injuries:
   a. Knife injury or glass (fall through a glass window); propeller blades; chainsaw
   b. Clinical manifestations:
      i Associated damage to blood vessels of the neck, axilla, and upper lung
      ii 33% of injuries to the brachial plexus are in continuity
      iii Knife or glass injury tend to be focal

Neuropathology

1. Neuropractic (less often)
2. Usually neurotmesis injury

Neuroimaging

1. MRI/MRA
2. Ultrasonography

Laboratory Evaluation

1. EMG after 21 days demonstrates denervation in the injured components of the plexus

Backpack Palsy

General Characteristics

1. Noted in military personnel and civilians using improperly positioned heavy backpacks.
2. Males affected more often than females.
3. Related to backpack design and weight; multiple mechanical and time-dependent features.
4. Possible congenital structural or prior trauma as predisposing factors.
5. Hereditary neuropathy with susceptibility to pressure palsies

Clinical Manifestations

1. Preceded by transient episodes prior to the fully developed syndrome.
2. Muscle weakness of the shoulder, arm or forearm more than pain
3. Upper trunk > middle plexus innervated muscles are involved; the deltoid may be the most severely involved muscle.
4. Sensory loss and reflex changes are less apparent.

Neuropathology

1. Neuropraxic and axonometric injury

Neuroimaging

1. MRI:
   a. To rule out congenital defects and prior traumatic injury (excessive callus formation from a fractured clavicle)
2. Ultrasonography to evaluate the plexus and nerves

Laboratory Evaluation

1. EMG:
   a. To evaluate the location and severity of the injury

Shoulder Injuries with Concomitant Brachial Plexus Involvement

General Characteristics

1. Brachial plexus involvement is often overlooked in the context of shoulder pathology. Weakness is often ascribed to pain and joint pathology.
2. The usual injuries are:
   a. Humeral fracture or dislocation
   b. Scapular fracture
   c. Rotator cuff tear

Clinical Manifestations

1. Rotator cuff tear:
   a. Approximately 30% of these injuries are associated with brachial plexopathy.
   b. All components of the plexus may be injured.
   c. Posterior cord and middle trunk greater than upper trunk and lateral cord.
2. Humeral fractures and dislocation:
   a. Ischemic or a vascular compressive lesion
   b. Posterior cord and middle and lower trunk may have the greatest deficit
   c. Trunks and cords, as well as terminal nerves, may be involved with reductions of shoulder dislocations

Clavicular Fractures with Plexopathy

General Characteristics

1. Excess motion of the clavicle at the fracture site.
2. Exuberant callus formation
3. Tight figure of eight brace
4. Delayed onset (months to years)

Clinical Manifestations

1. Anterior division and upper trunk involvement with weakness of the innervated muscles
2. Upper arm pain exaggerated by arm elevation

Neuropathology

1. Primarily neuropractic and axonometric injury

Neuroimaging

1. MRI (local pathology)
2. Ultrasonography (terminal nerves) evaluation

Laboratory Evaluation

1. EMG:
    a. To evaluate location and extent of the injury

Burner/Stinger Syndrome

General Characteristics

1. Usual contact sports injury (shoulder trauma; face mask injury in football)

Clinical Manifestations

1. Severe pain and paresthesia in the arm without motor loss
2. Usual sensory radiation is from the neck to the fingers
3. Recovery within minutes

Neuropathology

1. Neuropractic stretch injury

Neuroimaging and Laboratory Evaluation

1. MRI and EMG:
    a. Not necessary unless symptoms persist; if symptoms are persistent then MRI and EMG are required

Arterial Vascular Thoracic Outlet Syndrome

General Characteristics

1. Extremely rare
2. May be seen in individuals that perform repetitive overhead/arm movements

(butchers, using saws; pitchers in baseball)

Clinical Manifestations

1. Adson's maneuver less often positive than in patients with true neurogenic thoracic outlet syndrome
2. Ischemia of the hands and fingers rather than specific neurogenic plexopathy is most common; some patients complain of heaviness and weakness of the arm in abduction; primarily upper trunk distribution
3. May have severe ischemic pain

Neuropathology

1. Bony abnormalities of the clavicle and first rib cause post stenosis dilatation then aneurysm formation of the subclavian or axillary artery.
2. Distal emboli from thrombi in the artery to the fingers

Neuroimaging

1. MRI:
   a. Evaluation of the local anatomy with particular reference to bony and congenital anomalies.
2. MRA:
   a. Evaluation of the arterial supply to the arm to rule out aneurysm of the subclavian or axillary arteries.

Laboratory Evaluation

1. EMG:
   a. Evaluation of the location and extent of any brachial plexus involvement

Effort Venous Thrombosis of the Upper Extremity (Paget-von Schroetter Disease)

General Characteristics

1. Thrombosis of the subclavian and axillary vein

Clinical Manifestations

1. Abrupt presentation
2. Upper extremity swelling cyanosis and livedo reticularis
3. Dilated venous collaterals over the chest and shoulder
4. Brachial plexus is not involved.

Neuropathology

1. Prolonged compression of the axillary vein on a hard surface (arm outside of the window and resting on the door of a car); compression of the subclavian vein between the clavicle and the first rib
2. May follow extreme exercise of the arm.
3. Bony, ligamentous and muscular anomalies

Neuroimaging

1. 1. MRA and MRV to evaluate the circulation to the arm

Immune Mediated Brachial Plexopathy

General Characteristics

1. Terminology:
   a. Acute brachial plexitis
   b. Neuralgic amyotrophy
   c. Parsonage-Turner Syndrome
2. Evidence suggesting an immune basis includes:
   a. May develop after an infection or vaccination
   b. Following bone marrow transplantation
   c. During treatment with immunomodulating agents:
      i Interferons
      ii Interleukin 2
      iii Tumor necrosis factor alpha blockers
   d. Antibodies against peripheral nerve myelin and soluble terminal complement complexes
   e. Response to steroids
   f. In association with some autoimmune diseases

Clinical Manifestations

1. Immune brachial plexus neuropathy usually presents with acute shoulder pain or forearm pain that is exacerbated by movement:
   a. The intense pain may last for days to weeks but usually evolves to a dull ache that may be persistent for several years.
2. Weakness is evident as pain dissipates and depends on the components of the plexus that is involved (trunks, divisions, cords or terminal nerves).
3. Patterns of weakness:
   a. The most common pattern of weakness involves muscles innervated by the upper trunk or multiple mononeuropathies that include:
      i Suprascapular nerves
      ii Long thoracic nerves
      iii Axillary nerves
   b. There may be concomitant involvement of the phrenic and interosseous nerves. These nerves may be involved in isolation
   c. Rarely cranial nerves IX, X, XI and XII can be involved
   d. Isolated spinal accessory involvement has been described

Neuropathology

1. Biopsy of immune brachial plexus neuropathy (IBPN) reveals:
   a. Perivascular perineural and endoneurial inflammatory infiltrates

2. Antigens have not been identified, but electrodiagnostic studies suggest they are axonal rather than epitopes of myelin.

Neuroimaging

1. MRI:
    a. May demonstrate increased T2 weighted signal intensity of the plexus that suggests inflammation with edema

Laboratory Evaluation

1. CSF:
    a. Approximately 10% of patients have increased spinal fluid protein with or without pleocytosis.
2. EMG:
    a. Electrodiagnostic studies depend on the component of the plexus that is involved.
    b. Nerve damage may be multifocal and is usually axonal
    c. The upper trunk is primarily involved:
        i Median and ulnar motor studies are positive in approximately 15% of patients; median and brachial SNAPs may be abnormal.
    d. 50% of patients demonstrate:
        i Decreased CMAP from the deltoid, biceps, and serratus anterior muscles
        ii Decreased SNAPs of the lateral, antebrachial, cutaneous and median sensory nerves
3. CSF:
    a. Slightly increased CSF protein with mild pleocytosis

Differential Diagnosis

1. Asymmetric form of chronic inflammatory demyelinating neuropathy
2. Multifocal acquired motor and sensory demyelinating neuropathy
3. Multifocal motor neuropathy

Hereditary Neurologic Amyotrophy

General Characteristics

1. AD; gene maps to chromosome 17q 25.3 (SEPT9)
    a. Encodes the septin-9 protein
2. A severe form of hereditary neuralgic amyotrophy without SEPT9 has been described
3. A novel locus on chromosome 21q21

Clinical Manifestations

1. A history of one or more sudden onset painful attacks that involve the neck, shoulder, or arm

2. Weakness in various affected components of the plexus
3. Associated features:
   a. Hypertelorism
   b. Occasional cleft palate:
      i Skin folds or creases on the neck or forearm
      ii Short stature
      iii Syndactyly

Neuropathology

1. Septins are involved in cytokinesis and cellular trafficking
2. Septin-9 protein localizes with other septins and with septin-intermediate filaments that interact with actin microfilaments and microtubules

Neuroimaging

1. MRI to rule out other causes of brachial plexopathy; STIR-MRI demonstrates hyperintense signals in the brachial plexus
2. Ultrasonography
3. Magnetic resonance neurography

Laboratory Evaluation

1. EMG:
   a. Similar to idiopathic brachial plexus neuropathy

Hereditary Neuropathy with Liability to Pressure Palsies

General Characteristics

1. PMP22 gene deletion; AD but gene de novo mutations occur; the gene is on chromosome 17p11.2.
2. The deletion of the 1.5 MB region is the same that is duplicated in CMT1a
3. Prevalence of 7.3/100,000 to 16/100,000 people

Clinical Manifestations

1. Age of onset is the second and third decade (but has been described to the 8th decade)
2. 60-70% of patients present with a single, focal acute neuropathy
3. Rare cranial nerve involvement that includes V, VII, XII, and components of X.
4. Brachial plexus involvement (12-27%):
   a. Possibly causative of backpack neuropathy
5. Painless recurrent plexopathy
6. Scapuloperoneal presentation (Davidenkov phenotype)
7. Muscle weakness and atrophy
8. Numbness in affected plexus distributions
9. Reduced or absent deep tendon reflexes (primarily ankle jerks)

10. Episodes may be preceded by minor compression of the affected nerve or the plexus
11. Rare vocal cord, phrenic nerve and root involvement

Neuropathology

1. Nerve biopsy demonstrates segmental demyelination with varying large-fiber loss.
2. Tomacula:
    a. Redundant or over folding layers of the myelin sheath of variable thickness are present
3. The 1.5 Mb deletion on chromosome 17p11.2 is found in approximately 85-90% of patients that are clinically affected
4. Mouse model demonstrates focal axonal constriction within tomacula.

Neuroimaging

1. MRI:
    a. CNS white matter lesions occur in isolated patients
2. Ultrasonography:
    a. Reveals hypertrophy at entrapment sites

Laboratory Evaluation

1. EMG:
    a. Increase in distal motor latencies especially of the median and peroneal nerves
    b. Focal motor slowing at entrapment sites
    c. NCV may be normal in some segments
    d. Sensory nerve conduction velocities may be decreased with decreased SNAP amplitudes
2. DNA testing for the deletion of the PMP22 gene

Neoplasms Affecting the Brachial Plexus

General Characteristics

1. Benign tumors:
    a. Neuronal sheath tumors:
        i 60-80% of brachial plexus tumors are neuronal sheath tumors
2. Includes:
    a. Schwannoma
    b. Neuroma
    c. Neurofibroma

Clinical Manifestations

1. Present as mass lesions in the supraclavicular fossa or axilla
2. Pain and paresthesia are early symptoms (distortion of nerve fibers without

conduction block, demyelination, or destruction of axons)

3. Later motor and sensory loss

Schwannoma

General Characteristics

1. Approximately 5% of benign and soft tissue neoplasms
2. Approximately 20% of tumors of the brachial plexus

Clinical Manifestations

1. Solitary
2. An adult tumor
3. Affects the upper plexus
4. Most often presents as a supraclavicular or axillary mass
5. May affect any organ and region including:
   a. Nasal septum
   b. Cervical sympathetic chain.
   c. Gingiva
   d. All cranial nerves; may be plexiform
   e. Base of the tongue
   f. Cecum and gastric mucosa
   g. Sublingual area
6. Affects the upper plexus most often
7. Sensory signs:
   a. Tender to palpation; radiating paresthesia is common
8. Later mild motor and sensory deficit referable to the involved dermatome and myotome of the nerve

Neuropathology

1. Benign and well encapsulated
2. Usually, affect the proximal components of the plexus
3. Degenerative changes and variable admixture of spindles (Antoni A), whorls, and hypocellular microcytic (Antoni B) areas with macrophages and collagen fibers; located near vessels and have a well formed collagenous capsule
4. Express S 100 protein and pericellular collagen type IV
5. Plexiform Schwannoma:
   a. A subtype that occurs in superficial cutaneous or subcutaneous locations.
   b. Intraneural pattern of growth
   c. Associated weakly with NF2 and Schwannomatosis (approximately 5% of patients); usually Antoini A pattern and is less encapsulated than classic Schwannomas

Neuroimaging

1. 1. MRI:

a. Homogeneously isointense on T1 weighted sequences and hyperintense on T2 images
b. Cystic degeneration may be noted in the usual Schwannoma

Laboratory Evaluation

1. EMG
2. Molecular genetics to evaluate for NFI

Neurofibroma

General Characteristics

3. Growth pattern is well-demarcated intraneural or diffuse infiltration of soft tissue at extraneural sites
4. Variants:
    a. Based on architectural growth and include localized, diffuse and plexiform subtypes:
        i Localized cutaneous neurofibroma is the most common:
            1. May involve a major nerve to cause a fusiform expansion of the nerve trunk (intraneural subtype)
            2. Diffuse neurofibromas cause a plaque-like enlargement (usually in the head and neck region)
        ii 10% of neurofibromas are seen with neurofibromatosis type I

Clinical Manifestations

1. Interdigitate more with nerve fibers within the nerve fascicle
2. In association with neurofibromatosis, they are often multiple and may affect a large portion of the brachial plexus.
3. Demonstrate motor and sensory deficits depending on which component of the plexus is affected
4. Neurofibromas associated with NFI:
    a. Occur both supra and infraclavicularly
    b. Are frequently multiple and plexiform
    c. Present at an earlier age than Schwannomas
    d. May extend intraspinally (dumbbell tumor) in the intradural extramedullary compartment
    e. Equal male and female incidence

Neuropathology

1. Neoplastic proliferation with Schwann cell differentiation:
    a. Wavy nuclear contours
    b. S-100 protein expression
2. Incorporate non-neoplastic peripheral nerve components that include axons, perineural cells, fibroblasts, mast cells, and lymphocytes

Neuroimaging

1. Plain films may demonstrate enlargement of an intra foraminal exit canal
2. MRI:
   a. Bag of worms appearance from diffuse involvement along a nerve segment
   b. Few flow voids within the lesion are seen in T2 weighted images
   c. Plexiform neurofibromas may present on imaging with an intermediate signal compared to muscle on T1 weighted images and with a hyperintense signal on T2 weighted sequences

Laboratory Evaluation

1. EMG

Perineurioma

General Characteristics

1. Advanced perineural differentiation
2. Two types of tumor have been described:
   a. Intraneural
   b. Soft tissue

Clinical Manifestations

1. A. Localized solitary expansion of peripheral nerve due to involvement of one or more nerve fascicles
2. Remain stable over time or progress slowly

Neuropathology

1. Perineurial cell proliferation that extends into the endoneurium that surrounds individual nerve fibers and capillaries that produce "pseudo-onion bulbs"
2. Soft tissue perineuromas lack an associated nerve
3. The most commonly utilized immunohistochemical marker is epithelial membrane antigen (EMA).

Neuroimaging and Laboratory Evaluation

1. Neuroimaging and electrodiagnostic features have not been described

Differential Diagnosis

1. Localized reactive Schwann cell proliferation (intraneural form)
2. Low-grade fibro myxoid sarcoma (soft tissue form)

Hybrid Benign Nerve Sheath Tumors

General Characteristics

1. Some arise in the setting of inherited syndromes the most common of which

is NFI.

Clinical Manifestations

1. A solitary painless nodule
2. Equal male to female incidence
3. Approximately 70% arise in the second to fifth decade
4. Wide distribution over the extremities and trunk.

Neuropathology

1. Usually well circumscribed; features of Schwannoma and soft tissue perineurioma
2. Encapsulated and composed of spindle cells.
3. EMA and S100 are histological markers

Neuroimaging and Laboratory Evaluation

1. Neuroimaging and electrodiagnostic features have not been well delineated.

Differential Diagnosis of Benign Non-Neural Sheath Plexus Tumors

1. Lipoma
2. Ganglioneuroma
3. Myoblastoma
4. Lymphangioma
5. Dermoid

Malignant Nerve Sheath Tumors that may involve the Brachial Plexus

General Characteristics

1. Approximately 15% of neural sheath tumors are malignant
2. They are primarily neurogenic sarcoma and fibrosarcoma
3. Malignant transformation of benign neural sheath tumors:
    a. Most common in von Recklinghausen's disease
    b. Late transformation (20-40 years) to sarcoma in patients who have been irradiated for breast cancer or Hodgkin disease

Metastatic Brachial Plexus Tumors

General Characteristics

1. Two-thirds originate from the lung or breast
2. Other metastatic lesions occur from:
    a. Larynx
    b. Pancreas
    c. Colon
    d. Bladder
    e. Testes

f. Thyroid
g. Esophagus
h. Lymphoma
i. Melanoma
j. Ewing's sarcoma

3. Metastatic tumors have often metastasized extensively prior to plexus involvement

Clinical Manifestations

1. Known malignant disease (rare for plexus involvement as a presentation).
2. A long latency from treatment of the primary tumor is not uncommon.
3. Pain in the arm and shoulder is often the first manifestation; weakness and sensory loss occur later
4. Associated extradural spread with cervical cord compression
5. Many breast cancer patients have received X-RT that involved the plexus prior to a metastatic disease presentation
6. Pancoast Syndrome:
   a. Direct spread from the apex of the lung (superior sulcus or thoracic inlet tumor)
   b. Usually, the syndrome is caused by a squamous cell carcinoma (rarely in the scar of a prior tuberculous infection) or an apical adenocarcinoma
   c. Pain in the shoulder, scapula or 4th and 5th finger that is often burning in quality
   d. Weakness wasting and sensory loss in the lower trunk distribution.
   e. Horner Syndrome
7. Primary lymphoma:
   a. Arising from the cervical or axillary lymph nodes may infiltrate the plexus.

Neuropathology

1. Metastatic lesions may grow along the components of the plexus.
2. Symptomatology may derive from expression of inflammatory cytokines as well as direct invasion of the tumor

Neuroimaging

1. Demonstrates thickening of plexus components; often contrast enhancement is noted
2. 18-FDG-SPECT:
   a. a. May demonstrate primary and other metastatic sites; useful in following the course of treatment
3. Ultrasonography

Laboratory Evaluation

1. Electrodiagnosis:
   a. Dependent upon the components of the plexus that is affected

Radiation-Induced Brachial Plexopathy

General Characteristics

1. Women irradiated for breast cancer is the most frequent cause followed by lung cancer and lymphoma X-RT treatment
2. Dosimetric considerations that induce lesions:
   a. Field size
   b. Amount of tissue irradiated
   c. Time period of the irradiation
   d. Number of fractions delivered
   e. Dose of each fraction
   f. Total dosage
3. Latent period of 0 to 34 years may occur after x-ray treatment

Clinical Manifestations

1. Paresthesias in the C5-C6 spinal nerve, lateral cord, and median nerve distributions
2. Pain may develop late and is usually of moderate severity.
3. Weakness of intrinsic hand muscles
4. All parts of the plexus may be involved, but the supraclavicular components of the plexus usually have greater involvement than the infraclavicular
5. Edema of the extremity may develop
6. Most patients have a progressive course although some patients plateau.
7. Rare clinical manifestations:
   a. Severe edema (possible compartment syndrome)
8. An acute onset ischemic process:
      i Injury to the subclavian artery
      ii Associated with painless weakness and sensory loss
      iii Segmental occlusion of the subclavian artery
   a. Reversible Plexopathy:
      i Develops 2-14 months after X-RT
      ii Hand and forearm paresthesia; shoulder pain; mild hand weakness.
      iii Chemotherapy after X-RT may be causative or associated.

Neuropathology

1. Extensive demyelination
2. Proliferative endarteritis of the vasa vasorum
3. Progressive fibrosis in the irradiated field

Neuroimaging

1. MRI with three Tesla magnet field strength which develops 3D isotropic sequences
2. Gadolinium enhancement is positive for tumor.

Laboratory Evaluation

1. EMG:
   a. a. Myokymic discharges in affected muscles

Differential points between X-RT damage and recurrent tumor

1. Tumor:
   a. Primarily the C8-T1 roots or the lower trunk is affected; rapidly progressive
   b. Severe burning pain and intrinsic hand muscle wasting
   c. Horner's Syndrome
   d. MRI:
      i May demonstrate thickening or mass in these plexus components
      ii Enhances with gadolinium
2. X-RT:
   a. Occurs primarily in the C5-C6 root or spinal nerve distribution
   b. Greater paresthesias than pain and weakness
   c. MRI:
      i Fibrosis of the plexus and surrounding tissue
      ii No enhancement with gadolinium
   d. EMG:
      i Myokymic discharges

Lumbosacral Plexus Lesions

Overview of Lumbosacral Plexopathy

Upper lumbar plexus lesions demonstrate various combinations of deficits in the iliohypogastric, ilioinguinal, genitofemoral, femoral and obturator nerve distributions. Weakness is seen in hip flexion, knee extension (concomitant inability to lock the leg on standing) and adduction of the thigh. Sensory loss is noted in the lower abdominal wall, inguinal, labial, and scrotal areas as well as the thigh and medial lower leg. An absent or a depressed knee reflex is noted.

Lower lumbar sacral plexus lesions cause deficits within the innervation territories of the gluteal, sciatic, tibial, and peroneal nerves. Weakness occurs in hip extension, and abduction, knee flexion, and all intrinsic foot musculature. Sensory loss occurs in the posterior thigh, anterior and posterior aspects of the lower leg below the knee and most of the foot. There are diminished or absent ankle reflexes. Gluteal and sciatic nerve weakness localizes a lesion to the sacral plexus.

Plexopathies are recognized when motor, sensory, and reflex deficits occur in multiple nerve and segmental distributions that affect one extremity.

Localization is often difficult due to the pathologies of the region, but usually in a broad sense can be divided into:

1. Lumbar plexopathy
2. Sacral plexopathy
3. Lumbosacral trunk lesions
4. Pan-plexopathy

In general, lumbar plexopathies evolve in a stepwise and dissociated manner.

In localization of lumbosacral plexopathies pathology of the cauda equina and conus medullaris has to be considered. Rarely, motor neuron disease may simulate plexopathy if deficits are without pain or sensory loss. Intraspinal lesions (lower spinal cord) tend to be bilateral with early bowel and bladder dysfunction rather than motor weakness. Cauda equina lesions are painful, and bladder dysfunction is seen early.

Differential points in the history or examination include:

1. Pain in the following territories define specific sensory roots and nerves:
   a. Hip (sclerotomal radiation of L5)
   b. Buttock (L5-S1 root); often have tenderness in the sciatic notch
   c. Proximal thigh laterally (L5); also may be caused by bursitis of the tensor fascia lata
   d. L1, L2, L3 roots innervate the dorsal thigh; this is also the sclerotomal distribution of the recurrent nerve of Spurling of L5. The usual problem is disc herniation that causes radiation to the dorsal thigh rather than its somatic dermatomal distribution.
   e. The medial thigh is innervated by the ilioinguinal nerve (L1, L2 roots)
   f. The groin is innervated by T12 and L1. It may also have a projected sclerotomal radiation from S1. Thus, S1 root irritation may radiate to the groin. This invariably is diagnosed as hip disease or an inguinal hernia.
   g. The straight leg raising test causes sciatic nerve pain (L5-S1 roots); the reverse SLR test stretches the femoral nerve (L2-L3 sensory roots are involved; often concomitant inguinal pain).
   h. In plexopathy, the Valsalva maneuver does not elicit pain as it frequently does with radiculopathy
   i. In peroneal nerve neuropathy with foot drop:
      i Inversion of the foot is normal
      ii Toe flexion and hip abduction are normal
      iii The ankle reflex is preserved
   j. Differential signs to distinguish lumbosacral trunk lesions from an L5 radiculopathy:
      i The lumbar trunk is formed primarily by the L5 spinal nerve with a

contribution from L4; peroneal sensation is normal which favors a trunk lesion.

- ii If the pattern of weakness is hip adductors, iliopsoas, and quadriceps a lumbar plexopathy rather than femoral or obturator nerve lesions is more likely

k. Simultaneous involvement of the lumbar and sacral roots is usual with external trauma; iatrogenic injury more often involves individual L5 plexus components.

Anatomical Relationship of the Lumbar and Sacral Plexus

1. The L1, L2, L3 ventral rami are the primary components of the lumbar plexus with contributions from T11 and T12.
   a. They traverse the posterior portion of the psoas muscle anterior to the vertebral transverse processes:
      i Femoral nerve (L2-L4 primary spinal nerves) also supplies sensation to the thigh and leg by:
         1. Medial and intermediate nerve of the thigh
         2. Saphenous nerve which provides sensation to the medial calf
2. Obturator nerve (L2-L4 spinal nerves):
   a. Innervates the adductor muscles of the thigh
   b. Provide cutaneous innervations to the medial thigh
3. Muscular branches that derive directly from the plexus:
   a. Iliopsoas (L1-L3 spinal nerves)
   b. Iliacus (L2-L3 spinal nerves)
4. Sensory nerves of the lumbar plexus:
   a. Iliohypogastric (L1 spinal root)
   b. Ilioinguinal nerve (L1 root) innervates:
      i Upper medial thigh
      ii Base of the penis and labia majora
   c. Genitofemoral nerve (L1-L2 root):
      i Innervates the upper anterior thigh
      ii Scrotum and labia majora
   d. d. Lateral cutaneous nerve of the thigh (L2-L3)
5. Lesions of the entire lumbosacral plexus:
   a. Are rare; most are incomplete
   b. Paralysis or paresis of the entire lower extremity with hypo or areflexia
   c. Sensory abnormalities that involve the entire lower extremity
6. Lesions of lumbar segments:
   a. Usually are incomplete
   b. Paresis and atrophy in the distribution of the femoral and obturator nerves:
      i Iliopsoas:

            1. Weakness of thigh flexion
        ii Quadriceps:
            1. Weakness of leg extension
        iii Sartorius:
            1. Weakness of thigh eversion
        iv Adductor muscles:
            1. Weakness of thigh adduction
    c. Sensory signs:
        i Sensory loss in the inguinal area and over the genitalia
            1. Iliohypogastric, ilioinguinal, and genitofemoral nerves are involved
        ii Lateral thigh:
            1. Lateral femoral cutaneous nerve
        iii Medial thigh:
            1. Obturator nerve
        iv Anterior thigh:
            1. Femoral nerve
        v Medial part of the lower leg:
            1. Saphenous nerve that is derived from the femoral nerve

Reflexes

1. Depressed or absent patellar reflex:
    a. Femoral nerve
2. Loss of cremasteric reflex:
    a. Genitofemoral nerve

Sacral Plexus

General Characteristics

1. S1-S3 ventral rami are the major roots:
    a. Contribution from L4-L5 and S4-S5 roots
2. The plexus overlies the lateral sacrum and the posterior lateral pelvic wall
3. Sciatic nerve (spinal nerves L4, L5, S1-S3):
    a. Innervates the hamstrings; all muscles below the knee
    b. All sensation below the knee except that supplied by the saphenous nerve (medial lower leg):
    c. At the sciatic notch it divides into the common peroneal and tibial nerves
4. Superior gluteal nerve (L4, L5 S1 spinal nerves):
    a. Innervates the gluteus medius and minimus muscles
5. Inferior gluteal nerve (L5, S1, S2 spinal nerves):
    a. Innervates the gluteus maximus muscles
6. Posterior femoral cutaneous nerve (S1, S2, S3):

a. Innervates the buttocks, perineum, posterior thigh
   i The cuneal branch innervates the posterior upper thigh and inferior buttock

Lesions of the Sacral Plexus

Complete Lesion

1. Motor signs:
   a. Paralysis or paresis of muscles innervated by the superior gluteal, inferior gluteal and the sciatic nerves
      i "Flail foot" from paralysis of both the dorsal and plantar foot musculature
   b. Weakness:
      i Knee flexion:
         1. Hamstrings
   c. Foot eversion:
         1. Peroneal
   d. Foot inversion (L4-S1 spinal roots):
      i Tibialis anterior and posterior tibial nerve
   e. Plantar flexion of the toes:
      i Medial plantar nerves (II – V digits)
      ii Tibial nerve innervates the flexor hallucis longus
   f. Extension of the toes:
      i i. Peroneal nerve innervates the extensor hallucis longus; L5-S1 roots
      ii ii. Deep fibular nerve (Extensor hallucis longus muscle – EHL)
   g. Abduction and internal rotation of the thigh:
      i i. Superior gluteal nerve
   h. Hip extension:
   i. Inferior gluteal nerve

Sensory Signs

1. Loss of sensation in the sciatic nerve distribution:
   a. Outer leg
   b. Dorsum, sole and inner aspect of the foot
2. Posterior thigh and popliteal fossa:
   a. Posterior femoral cutaneous nerve

Reflexes

1. Decreased Achilles reflex:
   a. Sciatic nerve
2. Depressed bulbocavernosus reflex

Sphincter Signs

1. Loss or dysfunction of bladder and bowel control:
    a. Pudendal nerve

Differential Diagnosis Features between Root and Lumbosacral Plexus Lesions

1. Positive mechanical signs favor a root lesion:
    a. Straight leg raising test (sciatic nerve and S1 root)
    b. Reverse SLR (places traction on the femoral nerve); the leg is extended with the patient lying on his stomach
    c. Valsalva maneuver that causes pain:
        i Root greater than plexus involvement
2. Warm, dry and red foot:
    a. Indicative of a plexus lesion
    b. Involvement of the retroperitoneal lumbar sympathetic nerves
3. Proximal > distal leg muscle weakness suggests a plexus lesion
4. Gluteus muscle innervations arise directly from the plexus
5. Iliopsoas muscle is not involved in a femoral nerve lesion because its innervation is directly from the plexus

Trauma of the Lumbosacral Plexus

General Characteristics

1. The lumbosacral plexus is often injured with trauma to the pelvic ring:
    a. Double fracture dislocation
    b. Traction injury from dislocation of the hip joint
2. Femoral nerve compression due to position:
    a. Occupies the gutter between the psoas and iliopsoas muscle above the inguinal ligament:
        i Surgical retraction (medially)
        ii Injured laterally by a hematoma between the iliacus fascia and the nerve
3. The lumbosacral cords are vulnerable to compression at the:
    a. Pelvis brim by the fetal head
    b. Obstetric forceps
4. Aneurysm of the common iliac or hypogastric arteries in the presacral areas
5. The femoral nerve is compressed by:
    a. Angulation under the inguinal ligament
    b. Prolonged flexion abduction of the thigh (dorsal lithotomy position under anesthesia)
6. Fixation points of the common peroneal nerve are at the sciatic notch and

fibular neck:
a. Vulnerable to traction injury

Clinical Manifestations

1. Fracture:
   a. Double vertical fracture dislocations of the pelvic bony ring:
      i 50% of patients suffer neurologic deficits
   b. The injury is usually ipsilateral to the iliac joint damage
   c. The lumbosacral plexus cord level is affected by consequent compromise of L5-S1 spinal nerve innervated muscles
2. Rupture, compression and traction injuries affect:
   a. Lumbosacral trunk:
      i Primarily L4 and L5 spinal nerves (L5 primarily)
      ii The spinal nerves are contiguous with the sacrum adjacent to the sacroiliac joint.
   b. Obturator and or superior gluteal nerves are often concomitantly injured
   c. L5-S3 anterior rami may be affected
   d. Concomitant vertebral body rupture
3. Intra-arterial injections:
   a. Injections into the buttock:
      i Ischemic injury due to vasoactive drugs that are injected into the inferior gluteal artery causing ischemia of the sciatic nerve
         1. Weakness, pain, and sensory loss in the sciatic nerve distribution occur minutes to a few hours after the injection
      ii Widespread lumbar plexus injury may occur due to retrograde extension of gluteal artery spasm to branches of the internal iliac artery
      iii Buttock skin may be painfully swollen, cyanotic and develop gangrene
      iv Painless lumbosacral plexopathy may follow cisplatin injection into the iliac artery
4. Obstetric and gynecologic procedures that damage the lumbosacral plexus:
   a. Risk factors:
      i Short women with large babies
      ii Prima gravida
   b. Postpartum weakness:
      i Lumbosacral trunk injury (primarily L5 spinal nerve) compression at the pelvic brim over the sacroiliac joint:
         1. Cephalic pelvic disproportion
         2. Protracted labor
         3. Mid pelvic forceps delivery
   c. Involvement of the quadriceps muscles:
      i Bilateral in 25% of patients

ii Concomitant with an obturator neuropathy

d. Causes of peripheral femoral neuropathy:
   i Lithotomy position under anesthesia during vaginal delivery (compression under the inguinal ligament)
   ii Separation of the symphysis pubis with direct compression of the nerve by the fetal head
   iii Epidural anesthesia:
   iv Paracervical block that affects the posterior femoral nerve (pain may be delayed by several days)
   v Lumbosacral plexus compressed at the pelvic brim by a uterine leiomyoma (accelerated growth during pregnancy)
   vi Intrapelvic Schwannoma

Catamenial Neuroendometriosis

General Characteristics

1. Usually the sciatic nerve is affected but all components of the lumbosacral plexus may be involved

Clinical Manifestations (sciatic)

1. Implantation of endometrial tissue either intra-abdominally or at the sciatic notch
2. Perimenstrual pain in the buttock or posterior thigh (sciatic involvement)
3. Weakness, sensory loss and reflex changes are dependent on the lumbosacral component or the terminal nerve that is affected

Neuropathology

1. Endometrial deposits in the sciatic notch may be associated with an out-pouching of a pocket of peritoneum
2. Endometrial perineural spread from the uterus to the sacral plexus along the pelvic autonomic nerves and then distally to the sciatic nerve or proximally to the lumbar plexus

Laboratory Evaluation

1. MRI:
   a. Delineates perineural spread and retrograde menstruation with peritoneal bleeding

Surgical Trauma of the Lumbosacral Plexus

1. Laterally placed retractor blades compress the femoral nerve between the iliac and psoas muscle during:
   a. Vaginal hysterectomy
   b. Modified lithotomy position (under anesthesia)
   c. Pelvic procedures (ovarian tumors and cysts)

2. Hip joint replacement:
    a. Approximately 0.7-1% of hip replacement surgeries are complicated by femoral, obturator or sciatic palsies
    b. Subclinical nerve damage occurs from:
        i Preoperative stretch injury due to hip dislocation
        ii Retroperitoneal hemorrhage
3. 3. Other surgical complications:
    a. Heat
    b. Toxicity from methyl methacrylate bone cement
    c. Direct trauma and that from retractor blades
    d. Postoperative aneurysm formation

Aneurysm of the Iliac or Hypogastric Artery (Vascular Injury during Lumbar Disc Surgery)

General Characteristics

1. Surgical repair has been associated with ischemic plexus lesions

Clinical Manifestations

1. Motor, sensory and reflex deficits are evident in multiple nerves or segmental distributions in the affected extremity
2. Rectal examination reveals a firm pulsatile mass
3. Hemorrhage from an aortic, iliac or a hypogastric aneurysm may compress the femoral nerve
4. Retroperitoneal hematoma occurs from abdominal aortic aneurysm leakage that may affect the lumbosacral plexus and femoral nerve

Neuropathology

1. Neuropractic and axonometric injury occurs with compression and traction injuries
2. Neuromeric injury is primary with high impact trauma and some surgical procedures

Neuroimaging

1. Ultrasonography of the plexus
2. MRI (conventional) to evaluate the plexus and soft tissue
3. CT to evaluate the bone at the site of injury

Neoplasms of the Lumbosacral Plexus

General Characteristics

1. Occur in less than 1% of patients with neoplasms
2. Direct extension from an intra-abdominal tumor occurs in 75% of patients while extra-abdominal sites are the source in approximately 25% of patients

3. The lower sacral plexus is involved in approximately 50% of patients followed by the upper plexus in 30% and panplexopathy in 18%
4. Bilateral plexopathy occurs in 25% of patients (usually of the upper extremities by breast cancer)
5. Involvement of the sacral sympathetic nerves occurs in approximately 10% of patients
6. Less commonly plexus invasion occurs from lymph nodes, metastases or bony structures

Clinical Manifestations

1. In approximately 15% of patients lumbosacral plexopathy is the initial presentation of an intra-abdominal tumor
2. The most frequent presentation in >90% of patients is with pain in the low back, buttock, hip or thigh:
    a. In 90% of patients the pain is unilateral in onset and is dull, constant aching and is rarely burning; cramping may occur in a radicular pattern
    b. Exacerbation may occur at night
    c. Patients find difficulty in achieving a comfortable position
    d. Position of comfort is with the legs and hips in flexion if the iliopsoas muscle is involved
    e. Pain is exacerbated by walking or sitting
    f. A warm and dry foot (often red) may be seen if the sympathetic chain is involved
    g. Pain may be present for approximately 3 months prior to the onset of other symptoms and signs
    h. Weakness and sensory loss due to involvement of different plexus components is seen in most patients; sensory loss occurs in between 50-75% of patients and is most severe in patients with concomitant weakness
    i. Progressive muscle weakness is diffuse and interferes with gait
    j. Incontinence and impotence occur in 10% of patients due to bilateral involvement
    k. Involvement of the lumbosacral trunk is associated with foot drop
    l. Sacral involvement causes weakness of foot flexion and hamstring muscle involvement
    m. Sensory deficits are most often unilateral
    n. The patellar reflex is depressed with an upper plexopathy and the ankle jerk is depressed with sacral involvement
    o. Peripheral edema occurs in 80% of patients with pan plexopathy, in 41% of patients with upper plexopathy and in 37% of patients with lower plexus involvement
    p. A rectal mass is found in 43% of patients with lower plexopathy and in 25% of patients with upper plexopathy and 15% with panplexopathy

q. Straight leg raising test occurs (is positive) in greater than 83% of patients with pan plexopathy
r. Pain may be increased with Valsalva maneuvers

Neuropathology

1. Intra-abdominal tumor extension to the lumbosacral plexus occurs in approximately 75% of affected patients:
    a. Tumor may invade directly
    b. May grow along the connective tissue, epineurium of nerve trunks or perineural spread
2. Most prevalent tumors are:
    a. Colorectal tumors (20%)
    b. Sarcomas (16%)
    c. Breast tumors (11%)
    d. Lymphoma (9%)
    e. Cervical tumors (9%)
    f. Other tumors including multiple myeloma account for 37% of intra-abdominal tumors
3. Metastatic lesions are from:
    a. Breast
    b. Lymphoma
    c. Sarcoma
    d. Lung
    e. Thyroid (rare)
    f. Melanoma
    g. Testicular
    h. Multiple myeloma
4. Primary pelvic plexus tumors are:
    a. Neurofibroma
    b. Schwannoma
    c. Sarcoma (degeneration of a benign Neurofibroma)
5. Benign tumors that affect the lumbosacral plexus
    a. Dermoid of the omentum
    b. Uterine leiomyoma

Laboratory Evaluation

1. Dependent on the type of underlying cancer and the extent of its involvement are increased
2. Sedimentation rate and C-reactive protein
3. Alkaline phosphatase
4. Protein electrophoresis
5. Prostate specific antigen

6. Uremia and hydronephrosis are associated with gynecologic malignancies

Neuroimaging

1. High resolution dedicated MR neurography
2. CT scan and conventional MRI are positive >80% of patients by the time of clinical presentation
3. Sacral bone involvement is often a sign of colorectal cancer

Radiation Therapy (X-RT) of the Lumbosacral Region

General Characteristics

1. Median time to the onset of symptoms is variable; the usual is five years; in some patient, symptoms may appear 20-30 years after treatment
2. There is no apparent relationship between the amount of X-RT and the latent period to symptoms
3. Signs rarely occur with less that 40gy rads

Clinical Manifestations

1. Bilateral or unilateral slowly progressive leg weakness
2. Starts distally usually in the L5-S1 roots; muscle wasting and absent reflexes
3. Numbness and paresthesia may be the presenting symptoms
4. Mild pain as a late symptom (approximately 50% of patients; aching, burning and lancinating in character)
5. May arrest after several years (usually five years)
6. Often associated bowel and bladder symptomatology treatment

Neuropathology

1. The usual cancers that are irradiated are:
    a. Lymphoma
    b. Testicular
    c. Ovarian
    d. Uterine
    e. Cervical
2. X-RT may induce:
    a. Malignant nerve sheath tumors
    b. Post-irradiation lower motor neuron syndrome
3. A dose above 1 Gy effects can be seen in:
    a. Schwann cells
    b. Fibroblasts
    c. Vascular and perineural cells
4. Injury may occur after:
    a. External beam photon therapy
    b. Intestinal or intracavitary radiation implants
    c. Combined photon and proton beam

5. The effect is dose dependent:
   a. Animal experiments demonstrate that the threshold dose is 20-25 Gy
   b. Accumulated doses below 40gy with conventional fractionation of 1.8-2.0 Gy are considered to have a low risk of injury to nervous tissue.
6. Late effects include proliferative endarteritis and fibrosis in the plexus and soft tissue; vascular permeability and venous exudation

Neuroimaging

1. MRI:
   a. Demonstrates thickening of the plexus with tumor and atrophy with X-RT; no enhancement with gadolinium with X-RT.
   b. Diffusivity measurements differentiate malignant lesions from irradiation injury
   c. High resolution MR neurography
2. Ultrasonography

Laboratory Evaluation

1. CSF:
   a. CSF protein may be slightly elevated
2. EMG:
   a. Myokymia may be demonstrated in approximately 60% of patients

Radiation vs. Tumor invasion of the Lumbosacral Plexus

Radiation Plexopathy

1. Insidious onset and progression:
   a. Sensory symptoms may begin at two months that may resolve after several months
   b. Presenting symptom and signs may be weakness
   c. Bilateral involvement
   d. Distal muscle weakness (L5-S1 roots)
   e. Atrophy and no enhancement on MRI; less diffusivity on DWI
   f. EMG may be normal or demonstrate myokymia and fasciculation

Tumor Invasion

1. Rapid onset and progressive course
2. Pain may be the initial symptom
3. Unilateral involvement
4. Proximal weakness (L1-L4 roots)
5. Enhancing mass on MRI (with gadolinium); destruction of bone

Post Irradiation Lower Motor Neuron Syndrome

General Characteristics

1. A heterogeneous group of syndromes has been described after irradiation of the distal spinal cord and cauda equine primarily as treatment for testicular cancer and lymphoma
2. The mean age at irradiation is 33 years of age (literature review)
3. The average irradiation dose is 5,225 cGy (range 3,000-14,600)
4. Latency between irradiation and symptom onset ranged from 3 months to 27 years
5. Also known as Post X-RT Cauda Equina Syndrome

Clinical Manifestations

1. Painless wasting and fasciculation of leg muscles
2. Most often a delayed onset from months to years after treatment
3. Mild sensory symptoms in some patients
4. A proportion of patients may develop sphincter involvement
5. Occasional periods of stability

Neuropathology

1. One autopsied patient that was uncomplicated by metastatic disease demonstrated:
   a. A radiation-induced vasculopathy of the proximal spinal roots
   b. Preservation of motor neuron cell bodies and the spinal cord architecture

Neuroimaging

1. Gadolinium enhancement on MRI of the cauda equine in approximately 50% of patients

Laboratory Evaluation

1. EMG:
   a. Patchy motor nerve root involvement
   b. Electrophysiological evaluation by magnetic stimulation:
      i Prolonged cauda equina conduction time that suggests focal demyelination of the nerve roots of the cauda equina

Medical Causes of Painful Lumbosacral Plexopathy

Diabetic Radiculoplexus Neuropathy

General Characteristics

1. Involves the nerve roots and the lumbosacral plexus most often in a setting of diabetic length-dependent neuropathy
2. Approximately 8% prevalence in type I and II diabetic patients

3. Rarely the presenting feature of diabetes
4. Often seen in Type II diabetic patients controlled by diet and oral hypoglycemic agents
5. Most common onset is the sixth to seventh decade
6. Rare to have concomitant nephropathy, retinopathy, or history of coma

Clinical Manifestations

1. Hip and anterior thigh pain are often the initial presenting symptoms
2. Leg weakness supervenes within a few days to weeks
3. Weakness predominates in a lumbar plexus distribution that affects:
   a. Hip flexion
   b. Adduction
   c. Knee extension
4. Approximately 2/3 of patients have weakness in the L5 myotome: 50% are weak in the S1 dermatome in addition to the proximal muscles innervated by L1-L4 roots. L5 and S1 innervated muscle weakness may occur without involvement of proximal muscle weakness
5. Sensory loss is common but often not noticed due to pain and weakness
6. A small percentage of patients have neuropathy of the lumbosacral trunk
7. Approximately 50% of patients have involvement of the autonomic nervous system that includes:
   a. Orthostatic hypotension
   b. Urinary dysfunction
   c. Impotence
   d. Constipation or nocturnal diarrhea
8. 75% of patients have concurrent length-dependent neuropathy
9. There may be gradual improvement of weakness over months, and the pain diminishes over weeks; proximal muscles are more likely to recover

Neuropathology

1. Microvasculitis:
   a. Epineural and perivascular inflammation
2. Multifocal fiber loss is demonstrated on nerve biopsy
3. The process is frequently bilateral

Laboratory Evaluation

1. The sed rate is elevated in 20% of patients
2. CSF:
   a. The protein may be elevated (120 % suggests root involvement)
3. EMG:
   a. EMG and nerve conduction velocities to evaluate the level and extent of the plexopathy as well as the often concurrent length dependent neuropathy

Neuroimaging

1. MRI:
   a. An early screen of the plexus to rule out other pathologies
   b. If malignant infiltration is suspected, CT may be added to imaging parameters as up to 40% of patients have epidural tumor extension with possible bone involvement

Painless Diabetic Radiculoplexus Neuropathy

General Characteristics

1. Motor polyradiculoneuropathies without pain occur in diabetes mellitus
2. Women and men are equally affected; the median age range is 62 years (age range between 36-78)
3. Patients had DM for a median duration of 5 ½ years (most with type 2 DM)
4. Diabetic complications of retinopathy and nephropathy occur in approximately 20% of patients
5. Weight loss is seen in approximately 80% of patients (> 10 pounds)

Clinical Manifestations

1. Symmetrical polyradicular pattern with greater distal than proximal involvement (in contrast to canonical diabetic lumbosacral radiculoplexus neuropathy (DLRPN))
2. Proximal segments are involved to the same degree as in DLRPN
3. The upper limb is involved in approximately 80% of patients: this involvement is more widespread and severe than with classical DLPRN

Neuropathology

1. Nerve biopsies:
   a. Ischemic injury and microvasculitis
   b. Focal or multifocal fiber loss
   c. Focal perineural degeneration or thickening
   d. Epineurial neovascularization
   e. Injury neuroma
   f. Perivascular and vascular inflammation of small arterioles, venules and capillaries

Laboratory Evaluation

1. A minority of patients have an elevated sed rate or laboratory results suggestive of an inflammatory process
2. CSF:
   a. Elevated protein with a normal cell count

3. EMG:
    a. Reduced or absent upper and lower limb sensory and compound muscle action potential amplitudes
    b. No temporal dispersion or conduction block
    c. Mild slowing of conduction velocities and prolongation of distal and F wave latencies
    d. Patchy and widespread involvement of lumbosacral myotomes by needle EMG

Idiopathic Lumbosacral Plexitis

General Characteristics

1. Phenotype is similar to that of diabetic radiculoplexus neuropathy
2. Lumbar plexus is more often affected than the sacral although pan plexopathies occur
3. Age of onset is 30 months to 81 years of age.
4. It is usually monophasic and mild but may be recurrent and have a progressive course
5. Bimodal incidence:
    a. Prior to age 20 years of age
    b. Between 40-60 years of age
6. Mild trauma, vaccination and viral illness have been reported to precede the illness in some patients
7. Children, in general, have a monophasic course; adults may have recurrences

Clinical Manifestations

1. Abrupt onset of unilateral pain in the anterior thigh (lumbar plexitis) and posterior thigh and buttock (sacral plexitis); some patients have a more prolonged onset with recurrent bouts of pain
2. Muscle weakness is observed within 5-10 days of onset of the pain; it may progress for days to weeks; the pain resolves as the weakness supervenes
3. Muscle weakness of L1-L4 roots is most common and is associated with a positive femoral reverse SLR nerve test and absent quadriceps reflex
4. Lower plexus involvement:
    a. Positive Tinel's sign at the sciatic notch and popliteal fossa
    b. Weakness of the anterior and posterior tibialis, everters of the ankle, foot flexors, and extensors
    c. Absent Achilles reflex
5. The process may be bilateral
6. Recovery is often prolonged (over months) and is often incomplete

Neuropathology

1. Impaired glucose tolerance has been reported in some patients

2. Nerve biopsy demonstrates demyelination and axon loss similar to diabetic patients
3. Probable microvasculitis; possibly immune-mediated

Neuroimaging

1. MRI:
   a. To rule out compressive or invasive lesions
   b. Gadolinium-enhanced lumbar and sacral roots, and trunks may be demonstrated

Laboratory Evaluation

1. EMG/NCV:
   a. To delineate the location and severity of the process
2. HbA1c (must be negative)
3. Sed rate elevated in some patients
4. CSF:
   a. Slight increase in protein has been demonstrated in some patients.

Differential Diagnosis of Medical Causes of Painful Lumbosacral Plexus Lesions

Vasculitis

General Characteristics

1. Usually a necrotizing vasculitis

Clinical Manifestations

1. Develops acutely
2. Painful; weakness with fixed sensory loss
3. Progresses in a step-wise manner
4. Constitutional symptoms are associated that include:
   a. Fatigue and weight loss
   b. Associated conditions:
      i Granulomas of the respiratory tract
      ii Retinitis
      iii Purpura
      iv CNS involvement
      v Eosinophilia
   c. Specific entities:
      i Diabetic microvasculitis
      ii SLE
      iii Periarteritis nodosa
      iv Sarcoid

v Steroid responsive lumbosacral plexopathy
vi Wegener's granulomatosis

Painful Infections Affecting the Lumbosacral Plexus

Abscess

1. Bacterial abscess whose origin is in the psoas or paraspinal musculature
2. Perirectal abscess:
   a. Immunocompromised patients
   b. Prior rectal surgery
   c. Fever in association with groin, abdominal or back pain
      i Usually sciatic nerve radiation
      ii L4-S2 motor/sensory deficits

Anogenital Herpes Simplex

1. General Characteristics:
   a. Less than 1% of women with primary anogenital infection develop plexopathy
   b. Most frequent incidence is in males with herpetic prostatitis
   c. HS type 2 greater than type 1
   d. The primary anogenital lesion may be on the cervix
   e. Rare plexopathy with recurrent attacks
2. Clinical features:
   a. Dermatomal leg weakness and sensory loss
   b. Paresthesias and sensory loss in the perineum, buttocks, and posterior thigh
   c. Urinary retention, constipation, and erectile dysfunction
   d. Reduced tone of the anal sphincter; sensory loss in sacral dermatomes; loss of the bulbocavernosus reflex
   e. May involve lower motor neurons of the sacrococcygeal plexus
   f. Mild meningeal irritation
   g. Symptoms and signs last 10 days to 3 weeks often with good recovery
3. Neuropathology:
   a. HS type 2 > than type 1
4. Laboratory evaluation:
   a. Diagnosis is confirmed by PCR
   b. CSF may demonstrate a lymphocytic pleocytosis

Cytomegalic Virus

1. Lumbosacral plexus noted in severely ill HIV patients
   a. $CD4^+$ count of <200 mm^3
2. Severe pain, paresthesia and weakness in a wide distribution of lower

extremity roots and the lumbosacral plexus

3. Associated retinitis

Herpes Zoster

1. L5-S1 roots most often affected

Tuberculosis

1. Cold abscess; involves the psoas and iliacus muscle; (T12-L4 roots)
2. Pyelonephritis:
3. Upper > lower plexus

Appendicitis

1. Upper roots of the lumbar plexus
2. Characteristic iliopsoas spasm
3. Hyperalgesia (mechanical of the lower abdomen)

Iliacus muscle abscess

1. Following laparoscopy
2. Upper plexus involvement

Lyme disease

1. L5 root most often affected

Brucellosis

1. L5 root is most often affected

Syphilis

1. Dorsal root entry zone; meninges are inflamed and involve the cervical roots
2. Pachymeningitis cervicalis
3. HIV-associated

Epidural Abscess

1. Surgery
2. Catheters (anesthesia for pain)
3. Osteomyelitis

IV Drug Abuse

1. Pyogenic organisms
2. Staph aureus is most common
3. Affects the disc space (end arterial supply)
    a. Severely painful (vibration of the bed causes pain)
    b. Very positive meningeal stretch signs
4. MRI:
    a. Involvement of both the anterior and posterior longitudinal ligaments
    b. Enhancement of the disc space, the nerve roots, and the paravertebral muscle
5. Contiguous spread of infection to nerve roots from osteomyelitis is the most common route of infections

EBV Infection

1. Upper lumbar plexus involvement most commonly affected

Retroperitoneal Hemorrhage

General Characteristics

1. The lumbar plexus may be compressed within the iliopsoas muscle
2. Femoral nerve in isolation may be compressed by an iliacus hematoma or hemorrhage (trauma or retractor)

Clinical Manifestations

1. Femoral nerve involvement
   a. The iliacus fascia is tighter than the psoas fascia; smaller hematomas produce femoral compression more frequently than diffuse lumbar plexopathy
2. Pain in the groin radiating to the anterior thigh and medial lower leg (primarily L3-L4 roots and the saphenous nerve)
3. Position of comfort is a flexed upper leg
4. Positive reverse straight leg raising test
5. Minimally painful Patrick's maneuver (internal/external rotation of the upper leg)
6. Weakness of the quadriceps; loss of sensation in the femoral nerve territory; loss of the quadriceps reflex
7. Grey-Turner's is sign in approximately 5-10 days over the costovertebral angle (purple blood breakdown products)
8. Clinical manifestations of psoas muscle hematoma:
   a. Severe groin and lower abdominal pain
   b. The upper leg is not usually flexed at the hip:
   c. Negative reverse SLR test (forced upper leg extension)
   d. Rarely hip flexion with external rotation of the leg is painful
   e. No palpable hematoma; rarely a groin mass in palpable
   f. Thigh adductor muscle weakness (obturator nerve)

Neuropathology

1. Iliacus and psoas hemorrhage; occur most often in anticoagulated patients
   a. May be associated with an abrupt drop in hemoglobin
   b. Rarely bilateral
   c. Heparin has a greater incidence than coumadin; the newer anticoagulants have not yet been reported.
   d. Often there is no preceding trauma
   e. Most often a neuropractic nerve injury

Neuroimaging

1. Loss of the psoas shadow on a routine abdominal flat plate

2. MRI demonstrates the hemorrhage

Differential Diagnosis of Hemorrhagic Plexus Lesions

1. Athletic injury; hyperextension and avulsion of the iliacus muscle from the ileum
2. Localized blunt trauma; pelvic fracture
3. Disseminated intravascular coagulation
4. Hemophilia and other clotting disorders
5. Leukemia
6. Aneurysmal rupture
7. Anticoagulation

Immune Mediated Causes of Painful Lumbosacral Plexopathy

1. AIDP (acute inflammatory demyelinating plexopathy) may involve the proximal plexus
2. CIDP (distal nerve involvement to a greater degree than proximal nerve roots)
3. Specific epitopes:
   a. GMI
   b. GalNAc-GTd
   c. Gd1b
   d. MAG
   e. SGPG
   f. Anti-sulfatide
4. Paraneoplastic Antibodies:
   a. Anti-Hu
   b. Anti-Yo
   c. Anti-MA
   d. Anti-TA
5. Post-vaccination
6. Post serum infusion with anti-venoms antibody preparations

Toxins/Anesthetics

1. Lidocaine/bupivacaine:
   a. 0.25% or greater concentration usually delivered by epidural catheter for severe neuropathic pain; demyelinating lesions of the roots
   b. Benzyl alcohol (adjuvant of anesthetics)
   c. Heroin (IV drug abuse); the adulterants may be talc or quinine to which there is an autoimmune response:
      i May have a delayed onset of symptoms and signs (1-2 days after

infusion)
- ii Diffuse lower extremity pain
- iii Minimal weakness or sensory loss
- iv Pain clears prior to recovery of motor function

Ischemic Lumbosacral Plexopathy

General Characteristics

1. There is a large arterial network with collaterals in the pelvis that usually permits ligation of an internal iliac artery with no adverse effects
2. The arterial network arises from anterior and posterior divisions of the internal iliac arteries which supply blood to the sciatic nerve and the gluteal musculature
3. The inferior gluteal artery supplies:
   a. A branch of the anterior division
1. The pelvic viscera
   a. The lower hip
   b. Back of the thigh
2. The posterior division:
   a. Gives origin to the superior gluteal artery that supplies:
      i The gluteal musculature
      ii The femoral nerve
      iii Sciatic nerve roots

Clinical Manifestations

1. Bilateral ischemic lumbosacral plexopathy from chronic aortoiliac occlusion:
   a. Presentation with progressive paraplegia
2. Gluteal muscle necrosis and lumbosacral plexopathy after renal transplantation:
   a. Diabetic patients may be at extreme risk
   b. Paraplegia has been reported following renal transplantation after ligation of the hypogastric artery
   c. Lumbosacral plexopathy has been reported after dual kidney transplantation and after pseudoaneurysm of the iliac artery in transplanted patients
   d. Mortality is extremely high in patients with gluteal necrosis
   e. Aortic aneurysms with hypogastric artery ligation during repair may be complicated by:
      i Gluteal necrosis and pain
      ii Rectal ischemia and pain
      iii Anal and bladder sphincter dysfunction

Neuropathology

1. Atherosclerotic aortoiliac occlusion

2. Severe diabetic vasculopathy of the internal iliac arteries
3. Following pelvic vessel embolization for post-partum hemorrhage
   a. May be associated with uterine necrosis

Laboratory Evaluation

1. Arteriography to evaluate the aorto0iliac circulation and to delineate aneurysm of these arteries
2. Recognition of gluteal necrosis:
   a. Occurs in approximately 3% of patients following internal iliac artery embolization performed in a traumatic situation
   b. Gluteal necrosis often misdiagnosed as a contusion or pressure ulcer; often extremely painful

Differential Diagnosis of Gadolinium Enhancement of the Lumbosacral Plexus

1. Carcinomatous meningitis
2. AIDP
3. CIDP
4. Arachnoiditis
5. Infections (CMV in particular)
6. Sarcoid
7. Leukemia/lymphoma
8. Tumor invasion

Differential Diagnosis of Unusual Lumbosacral Plexus Lesions

Acute Aortic Occlusion

1. Level of the lesion may be:
   a. Conus medullaris
   b. Cauda equina
   c. Proximal nerve trunks
   d. Lumbosacral plexus
2. Clinical manifestation:
   a. Acute lower extremity monoplegia

Neuromuscular Choristoma

General Characteristics

1. Rare congenital lesions
   a. Differentiated muscle intertwined with peripheral nerves and the lumbosacral plexus

Clinical Manifestations

1. Undergrowth of the affected limb
2. Primarily in the sciatic nerve:
   a. Progressive neuropathy
   b. Shortened atrophic limb
   c. Pes cavus
3. Undergrowth of bone with hip dysphasia

Neuropathology

1. Normal differential muscle within the affected nerve or plexus

Neuroimaging

1. Smoothly tapering fusiform enlargement of the sciatic nerve or brachial and or lumbar plexus components
2. T1 and T2 signal characteristics of muscle:
   a. Longitudinal bands of loss of T1 and T2 signal
3. Nerve fascicle thickening results in "coaxial cable" root presentation.
4. Bilateral lumbosacral plexopathy after mesenteric thrombosis
5. Lumbosacral plexopathy in the setting of pulmonary tuberculosis
6. Lumbosacral plexopathy from an internal iliac artery pseuroaneurysm

CHAPTER 3

PAINFUL NEUROPATHIES

Sodium Channelopathies

Nav1.7

General Characteristics

1. Painful neuropathies preferentially involve thinly myelinated A-delta and unmyelinated C-fibers
2. Voltage gated sodium channels generate and conduct action potentials in peripheral nociceptive pathways
3. Nav1.7 is encoded by the gene SCN9A that maps to chromosome 2q24.3
4. Inherited erythromelalgia and paroxysmal extreme pain disorder have been linked to a gain of function mutation of SCN9A
5. Heterozygous gain of function mutations in the SCN9A gene may also cause small fiber neuropathy

Clinical Manifestations of Hereditary Erythromelalgia

1. Episodic burning sensation of the hands and feet often associated with erythema and swelling
2. Often initiated in the first decade of life
3. Painful episodes can be precipitated by exercise, hot weather and viral illness
4. Attacks may be helped by cold
5. The pain is initially restricted to the surface of the affected body part but may also be perceived deeper within the tissue
6. Attacks at times can be aborted by cooling within the first 5 minutes

Neuropathology

1. Functional expression studies have demonstrated a variety of changes in channel function that include:
    a. The mutant channel being activated at more negative potentials
    b. Slower inactivation kinetics in peripheral sensory and sympathetic

neurons

c. Reduction of current thresholds in the DRG neurons that causes hyperexcitability and enhanced repetitive firing
d. Depolarizing shift in steady-steady activation that lowers the threshold for single action potentials and supports high frequency firing in DRG neurons.
e. Associated conditions with SCN9A mutations include:
   i Febrile seizures (familial, 3B)
   ii Hereditary sensory and autonomic neuropathy type IID (HSAN2D) (autosomal recessive)
   iii Congenital insensitivity to pain (autosomal recessive)
   iv Paroxysmal extreme pain disorder (autosomal dominant)
   v Small fiber neuropathy (autosomal dominant)
   vi Dravet syndrome (modifier) autosomal dominant

Laboratory Evaluation

1. Molecular genetic sequencing of the SCN9A mutation
2. Patch clamp studies

Paroxysmal Extreme Pain Disorder

General Characteristics

1. Paroxysmal Extreme Pain Disorder (PEPD) is caused by heterozygous mutation in the SCN9A gene that is autosomal dominant and maps to chromosome 2q24

Clinical Manifestations

1. Bouts of extreme pain usually within proximal regions of the body
2. Excruciating very brief pain of submandibular, ocular and rectal areas
3. Associated flushing of the surrounding skin
4. Autosomal dominant inheritance with incomplete penetrance of various pain components
5. Submandibular and ocular pain is described more consistently than rectal pain
6. Searing pain may be accompanied by bowel movements
7. Four types of painful episodes have been described:
   a. Birth crises:
      i Babies are born red and stiff
   b. Rectal crisis:
      i Triggered by defecation in infants and young children and emotional upset in older children and adults
   c. Ocular crisis:
      i Most often spontaneous severe ocular pain

   d. Mandibular crisis:
      i Triggered by eating and yawning
8. Accompanying autonomic manifestations include:
   a. Skin flushing
   b. Reflex asystolic syncopy
   c. Lacrimation
   d. Rhinorrhea
   e. Between episodes the physical examination is normal
   f. Rarely, pain may affect the entire body

Neuropathology

1. Functional analysis in vitro of 3 mutant Nav1.7 channels revealed:
   a. Reduction in fast inactivation that leads to a persistent sodium current

Laboratory Evaluation

1. Molecular genetic localization of the SCN9A mutation

SCN9A Mutations with Small Fiber Neuropathy

General Characteristics

1. A small fiber neuropathy is defined as a structural abnormality of small fibers (if painful A-delta 1-4 μ thinly myelinated and unmyelinated C-fibers) are involved
2. Characterized by degeneration of the distal terminations of their nerve endings
3. Gain of function mutations in voltage gated ion channels cause small fiber neuropathy in some instances. The fibers are hyperexcitable but are structurally intact
4. Somatosensory Aδ fibers and C-fibers that innervate the skin:
   a. Pass through the dermis to innervate cutaneous structures
   b. End as free endings in the epidermis (Aδ fibers become unmyelinated upon crossing the dermal-epidermal junction)
   c. Aδ fibers convey episodic well-localized fast pain and cold while C-fibers are slowly conducting and transmit:
      i Innocuous warm sensations
      ii Possibly some innocuous cold
      iii Burning pain
      iv Noxious input from high threshold mechanical, thermal and chemical stimuli
   d. Autonomic innervation:
      i Thinly myelinated fibers are a component of preganglionic innervation while C-fibers are a component of postganglionic fibers
      ii C-fibers innervate:

1. Sweat glands
2. Blood vessels
3. The heart

iii Mutations in nerve growth factor NGF or its high-affinity receptor NTRK1 cause degeneration of nociceptive and sympathetic neurons (HSAN type 5 and type 4 respectively)

e. Small fiber neuropathy (SFN) occurs with mutations in the SCN9A gene that encodes the Nav1.7 sodium channel

Clinical Manifestations

1. The typical sensory symptoms begin in the feet, progress proximally to involve the hands in a length dependent stocking-glove manner
2. Pain is most often the presenting symptom; it is usually spontaneous but may be evoked in some patients (mechanical hyperalgesia or allodynia)
3. The pain may be triggered by exercise or increased temperature (also occurs with Fabry's disease)
4. Motor function, coordination and deep tendon reflexes are normal as are the sensory modalities of light touch, vibration and proprioception
5. There is usually distal loss of pin-prick, thermal sensation and punctate hyperalgesia and dynamic allodynia are occasionally present

Neuropathology

1. Molecular genetic testing to delineate the SCN9A mutation

Laboratory Evaluation

1. Conventional nerve conduction studies are normal and are used to exclude an associated large fiber component of the neuropathy
2. In research laboratories lasers can be used to stimulate A-delta fibers to evoke cortical potentials
3. Microneurography has also been used (research settings) to record small fibers of peripheral nerve fascicles
4. Quantitative sensory testing :
   a. Delineates:
      i Detection thresholds
      ii Pain thresholds
      iii Stimulus response functions
   b. Is utilized for evaluation of A-beta, A-delta and C-fibers
5. Skin biopsy:
   a. A punch biopsy of 3 mm in diameter is a validated techniques for SFN in the usual circumstances (HIV, diabetes mellitus and amyloid)
   b. Morphometric analysis utilizing bright field immunohistochemistry or indirect immunofluorescence
   c. The biopsy is stained for the ubiquitin hydrolase PGD9.5

   d. Intra-epidermal nerve fiber density measurements are made and compared to international standards
   e. A decrease in intra-epidermal nerve fiber density with values below the fifth percentile relative to age and gender matched controls makes the diagnosis of SFN in those conditions with structural abnormalities
   f. In vivo corneal confocal microscopy is being assessed in the cornea which is innervated by C-fibers

Familial Episodic Pain Syndrome

General Characteristics

1. Described in a Columbian family

Clinical Manifestations

1. Episodes of upper body pain that begin in infancy
2. The pain is triggered by fasting or fatigue, cold temperature, illness and exertion

Neuropathology

1. The syndrome is autosomal dominant and is caused by mutations in the gene that encodes TRPA1 on chromosome 8
2. TRPA1 is a non-selective cation channel that is expressed in a sub-population of nociceptors that can be activated by extreme cold or endogenous ligands
3. The mutation is a substitution of a single amino acid in the S4-S5 region of TRPA1 that increases current flow through the activated channel

Laboratory Evaluation

1. Molecular genetic evaluation to delineate the mutation
2. QST
3. Skin biopsy

Pain Dysautonomia and Acromesomelia

General Characteristics

1. Described in a kindred with a novel Nav1.7 mutation

Clinical Manifestations

1. Erythema and burning pain in the hands since early childhood later spreading to the feet, cheeks and ears
2. Progressive muscle cramps
3. Autonomic features include:
   a. Hyperhidrosis
   b. Diarrhea or constipation
   c. Episodic dry eyes and mouth
   d. Hot flashes

e. Erectile dysfunction
4. Small hands and feet (acromesomelia); the brother and father were affected similarly

Neuropathology

1. Reduced intra-epidermal nerve fiber density
2. Missense mutation in the SCN9A gene (G856D; C2567G>A) in the proband, his father and brother
3. Functional analysis demonstrated:
   a. Hyperpolarization (-9.3 mV) channel activation
   b. Depolarizes (+6.2 mV) steady-state fast-inactivation
   c. Slows deactivation and enhances persistent current

Laboratory Evaluation

1. Molecular genetic evaluation to delineate the mutation
2. Skin biopsy

Congenital Insensitivity to Pain and Anhidrosis

General Characteristics

1. Congenital insensitivity to pain and anhidrosis is also known as hereditary sensory and autonomic neuropathy type IV (HSAN IV)
2. The condition is caused by a genetic loss-of-function of the NTRK1 gene on chromosome 1q23.1
3. The NTKR1 gene encodes the neurotrophic tyrosine kinase-1 receptor (TrKA)
4. Nerve growth factor function includes:
   a. Surveillance of nociceptive sensory neurons
   b. Sympathetic autonomic neuron maintenance
   c. A major component of homeostatic mechanisms and when deficient causes defects in development
   d. Bidirectional communication between the immune and central nervous system
   e. A component of osteoblast / osteo-progenitor differentiation and proliferation (important for fracture repair and consolidation) and normal bone metabolism

Clinical Manifestations

1. Insensitivity to pain
2. Anhidrosis
3. Cognitive deficiency
4. Less frequent findings:
   a. Impaired temperature sensation

b. Mandibular osteolysis
c. Dental caries
d. Premature tooth loss
e. Repetitive soft tissue and osseous infections (Staph aureus)
f. Self-mutilating behavior
g. Rare microcephaly
h. Urine and fecal incontinence
i. Growth retardation
j. Heterotopic ossification
k. Corneal ulcers
l. Painless fractures
m. Unexplained hyperthermic episodes
n. Repeated traumatic and thermal injuries; tips of the fingers and toes are typically involved

Neuropathology

1. There are three major mutations in the SCN9A gene that cause congenital insensitivity to pain:
   a. W897X located in the T-loop of domain 2
   b. 1767X located in the S2 segment of domain 2
   c. S459X located in the linker region between domains 1 and 2
2. The mutations result in a truncated non-functional protein

Laboratory Evaluation

1. Molecular genetic testing to delineate the mutation in SCN9A
2. Short-latency somatosensory evoked potentials:
   a. Marked prolongation of central conduction time
3. Microneurography:
   a. Delineates abnormal A-delta and C-fiber activity in the skin
4. A negative sympathetic skin response due to lack of sudomotor terminals in the skin
5. Pharmacologic tests of autonomic function are positive
6. Skin biopsy demonstrates:
   a. Hyperplastic epidermis with acanthosis and hyperkeratosis

Differential Diagnosis

1. Positive regulatory domain containing zinc finger protein 12 (PRDM 12)
   a. PRDM 12 proteins are epigenetic regulators that control neural specification and neurogenesis
   b. Mutations in the gene cause congenital insensitivity to pain
2. Hereditary sensory neuropathy (HSN I)
3. Hereditary sensory and autonomic neuropathy (HSN II)
4. Familial dysautonomia (Riley-Day syndrome) (HSN III)

5. Congenital indifference to pain (HSN V)
6. Lesch-Nyhan syndrome
7. Nav1.9 mutation (one variant)

Nav1.8 Small Fiber Neuropathy (SFN)

General Characteristics

1. Nav1.8 is encoded by SCN10A gene that maps to chromosome 3p22.2

Clinical Manifestations

1. Predominantly a painful sensory neuropathy
2. Infrequent signs and symptoms include:
   a. Dry eyes and dry mouth
   b. Orthostatic dizziness
   c. Palpitations
   d. Diarrhea and constipation
   e. Severe progressive gastroparesis (in one patient)
      i A novel heterozygous mutation in the SCN10A gene
   f. Brugada syndrome

Neuropathology

1. The Nav1.8 mutations:
   a. Accelerate recovery from inactivation
   b. Enhance response to slow depolarizations
   c. Enhance activation at the channel level
   d. Produce hyperexcitability of small dorsal root ganglion (DRG) neurons (nociceptors)

Laboratory Evaluation

1. Molecular genetic analysis to delineate the SCN10A mutation

Nav1.9 Small Fiber Neuropathy

General Characteristics

1. Nav1.7 and Nav1.8 channels are the main generators of the fast action potential in nociceptors
2. Nav1.9 channels modulate the threshold of nociceptor excitability through action on the resting membrane potential
3. Gain-of-function mutations in Nav1.9 may cause:
   a. Congenital insensitivity to pain
   b. Familial episodic pain
   c. Painful neuropathy

Clinical Manifestations

1. A family of mixed European ancestry:

a. Onset early in life
b. Rapid pain onset which lasts approximately 20-30 minutes
c. Triggers are gluten and low ambient temperature
d. Pain starts in the joints and then radiates to the arms and legs
e. Rarely pain is associated with neck and facial flushing
f. Pain episodes primarily occur in the afternoon
g. The quality of the pain is primarily burning
h. Clinical manifestations in Japanese families:
    i Infantile recurrent painful episodes; spontaneous relief around adolescence
    ii Autosomal dominant inheritance with mutation in the SCN11A gene that maps to chromosome 3p22
    iii Affected joints in order of frequency are knees, ankles, wrists and elbows
    iv The pain most often recurs on one side of the affected extremity
    v Rarely pain may be localized to the forearms, arm, palms, fingers, thigh and lower leg
    vi The painful episodes last for 15-30 minutes and recur several times per day; it is more frequent at night
    vii Night time crying and sleep disturbance were common in childhood
    viii The painful areas are cold and relief is obtained with warming
    ix The three major subtypes of clinical manifestations with Nav1.9 mutations:
        1. L811P mutation is associated with insensitivity to pain
        2. G699R, L1158P and 1381T are associated with small fiber neuropathy that occurs in the fifth or sixth decades and are associated with:
            a. Burning pain
            b. Skin discoloration
            c. Autonomic Dysregulation
        3. Familial episodic pain:
            a. This phenotype has been reported in two Chinese kindreds and a family of mixed European ancestry

Neuropathology

1. There are 12 amino acid substitutions of Nav1.9 that are associated with painful disorders
2. 7 mutations are associated with gain-of-function
3. Alterations in channel function include:
    a. Gating alterations despite no change in resting membrane potential or threshold; this mutation is in the S4 segment

Laboratory Evaluation

1. Molecular genetic testing to delineate mutations in the SCN11A gene in Japanese kindred

Metabolic Painful Peripheral Neuropathies

Diabetic Painful Neuropathy

General Characteristics

1. Diabetic peripheral neuropathy (DPN) can be generally separated into:
   a. Distal symmetric peripheral neuropathy (length dependent)
   b. Focal and multifocal neuropathies
      i Multiple mononeuropathy
      ii Lumbosacral, thoracic, and cervical radiculoplexus neuropathies
2. DPN occurs in patients with type 1 (T1DM) and type 2 diabetes mellitus (T2DM)
   a. Onset is insidious with a great number of patients remaining asymptomatic for a long period of time
3. DPN involves both large and small fibers in a length-dependent manner
4. Increased vibration and thermal thresholds occur early in the development of DPN
   a. DPN symptoms often develop earlier in the course of T1DM
   b. Large myelinated fibers may be more severely affected in Type I DPN whereas T2DM involves small nerve fibers
5. Type I and type 2 DM may respond differently to enhanced glucose control; more intense treatment of hyperglycemia in type 1 patients may lead to a lower incidence of neuropathy whereas it appears to have a minimal effect on type II patients
6. Hyperglycemia may be the primary driver of peripheral nerve injury in type I DM
7. Obesity, hypertension, low high density lipoprotein and hypertriglyceridemia may be risk factors for type II patients
8. Generalized risk factors for DPN include:
   a. Older age
   b. Long duration of diabetes
   c. Retinopathy
   d. Hypertension
   e. Dyslipidemia
   f. Hyperglycemic status
   g. Insulin treatment
   h. History of cerebrovascular disease
   i. Foot ulcers

Clinical Manifestations of Painful Diabetic Peripheral Neuropathy:

1. Acute painful diabetic neuropathy (APDN) is a distinctive polyneuropathy with two subtypes:
   a. Treatment-induced neuropathy (TIN)
   b. Diabetic neuropathic cachexia (DNC)
2. Acute painful diabetic neuropathy (APDN) manifestations include:
   a. Small-fiber involvement
   b. Occurrence after short-term good glycemic control
   c. Intense extremity pain
   d. Gradual recovery
3. Insulin-induced hypoglycemia may cause acute neuropathic pain
   a. Increased mechanical hypersensitivity
   b. Putatively the result of decreased glucose levels rather than insulin
4. Acute severe neuropathic pain in the extremities may occur during intensive treatment of patients with type 1 and type 2 diabetes
5. Asymmetric onset motor or sensory deficits (usually symmetrical) are frequently painful but are generally self-limited
6. Length dependent numbness and paresthesia more severe in the feet than the hands is most common. In general, the sensory signs are perceived above the knee before there is involvement in the upper extremities.
7. Less frequently there is lancinating and deep aching pain in the extremities in a length dependent pattern
8. Severe sensory loss is often associated with painless perforating foot ulcers accompanied by autonomic neuropathy
9. Patients with painless neuropathy are often areflexic, have all modality sensory impairment most prominent in the proprioceptive domain
10. A subgroup of patients have severe burning pain, only a slight diminution of proprioception and intact reflexes with concomitant autonomic neuropathy
11. Patients with impaired glucose tolerance may demonstrate burning foot syndrome

Neuropathology

1. The development of diabetic painful neuropathy is not understood but is generally considered to be a multifactorial process.
2. Putative mechanisms include:
   a. The polyol pathway:
      i Hyperglycemia is associated with increased concentration of intracellular glucose that saturates normal glycolytic pathways
      ii Glucose is shunted into the polyol pathway and is converted into sorbitol and fructose by aldose reductase and sorbitol dehydrogenases
      iii Increased concentrations of sorbitol and fructose cause:

1. Decreased nerve myoinositol
2. Decreased membrane Na^+ / K^+ - ATPase activity
3. Impaired axonal transport
4. Structural nerve changes

b. Advanced glycation products:
   i The non-enzymatic reaction of glucose with proteins, nucleotides and lipids causes advanced glycation end products (AGEs) that may interfere with neuronal metabolism and axonal transport

c. Oxidative stress:
   i Increased free radical production may occur with hyperglycemia that may damage blood vessels and cause nerve ischemia and facilitate AGE reactions

d. Activation of poly ADP ribosylation that facilitates the caspase 3 system and apoptosis

e. Activate genes that induce:
   i Cyclooxygenase-2 activation
      1. Cause endothelial dysfunction
      2. Decrease Na^+/K^+ -ATPase pump function

f. Impair C-peptide-related signaling pathways

g. Cause endoplasmic reticulum stress

h. Induces low grade inflammation

i. Neuronal death from hypoglycemia involves excitotoxicity and DNA damage

j. Mechanisms associated with pain in diabetic neuropathy:
   i In diabetic retinopathy, nephropathy and neuropathy there is upregulation of:
      1. Vascular endothelial growth factor (VEGF)
      2. Insulin growth factor (IGF)
      3. Mitogenic cytokines
      4. Inflammatory cytokines (TNF-α, IL-6, IL 8)

   ii Upregulation of these trophic factors and cytokines is associated with tight glycemic control and may be responsible for early acute pain

   iii There is experimental evidence for an increase in proinflammatory cytokines with hypoglycemia

Laboratory Evaluation

1. QST:
   a. Vibration thresholds detect mild or subclinical neuropathy
   b. Current perception threshold (CPT) to 2000 Hz stimulation correlates best with vibratory thresholds
2. Sudoscan detects electrochemical skin conductance:
   a. Proportional to the number of functioning sweat glands

3. Nerve conduction velocity (NCV):
   a. Slowed nerve conduction in nerve axons from segmental demyelination
   b. Quantifies spread of motor and sensory conduction, amplitude, distal latency and F wave latency
4. Skin biopsy:
   a. Assessment of intraepidermal nerve fiber density to detect small nerve fiber neuropathy
5. Corneal confocal microscopy:
   a. Assesses the corneal sub-basal plexes of nerve fibers that originate from the ophthalmic division of the Vth nerve:
      i Quantifies corneal nerve fiber length which is reproducible
      ii Sensitive to corneal nerve fiber damage in early stages of DPN

Vitamin B12 Deficiency

General Characteristics

1. Major causes of cobalamin (vitamin B12) deficiency are cobalamin malabsorption due to inability to release cobalamin from food or its binding proteins
2. Food-cobalamin malabsorption syndrome is caused by:
   a. Atrophic gastritis
   b. Related or unrelated to Helicobacter pylori infection
   c. Long-term ingestion of antacids and biguanides
   d. Mutations in genes encoding endocytic receptors involved in the ileal absorption and cellular uptake of cobalamin

Clinical Manifestations

1. There may be functional B12 deficiency in advanced malignancy:
   a. Elevated levels of B12-dependent metabolites, methyl malonic acid (MMA) and / or homocysteine in the face of normal B12 levels – possibly causing neuropathic pain putatively from oxidative stress
   b. Vitamin B12 deficiency may affect between 5-20% of older adults. Clinical manifestations in this population are primarily:
      i Cognitive impairment
      ii Dementia
      iii Depression
      iv Motor and sensory neuropathy
      v A combined sensation of numbness and deep aching pain in the legs is common. Active paresthesias occur in both upper and lower extremities
   c. Associated neurologic features include:
      i Optic neuropathy

   ii Slight ataxia
   iii Myelopathy
   iv Hyperactive reflexes in the face of atrophy and peripheral neuropathy are suggestive

Neuropathology

1. Vacuolar myelopathy particularly severe at cervical levels
2. Demyelinating peripheral neuropathy
3. Methyl cobalamin deficiency (the active form of vitamin B12) and is a coenzyme of methionine synthase that is required for DNA and protein methylation
4. Facilitates neurite outgrowth and inhibits neural apoptosis through the extracellular signal-regulated protein kinases 1 and 2 (ERK 1/2) and AkT signaling pathways

Laboratory Evaluation

1. Approximately 148 pmol/L (200 ng/L) is the usual set point for deficiency of vitamin B12
2. Serum B12 assays measure the sum of haptocorrin-bound and transcobalimin-bound (holotranscobalamin) B12; only holotranscobalamin is taken up by cells
3. Methionine synthase requires methylcobalamine for remethylation of methionine from homocysteine; homocysteine concentration of >20 μmol/L is suggestive of B12 deficiency in patients with normal folate concentrations
4. In B12 deficiency states increased methylmalonyl-CoA is hydrolyzed to methylmalonic acid. A serum concentration of >280 nmol/L is suggestive of B12 deficiency
5. EMG:
   a. A primarily demyelinative neuropathy
6. A low hemoglobin, RBC > 100μ and hypersegmented polymorphonuclear leukocytes; low platelets are characteristic

Neuroimaging

1. MRI:
   a. Methyl malonate increased concentration
      i Decreases total brain volume
   b. Homocysteine increased concentration
      i Increased white matter hyperintensities and cerebral infarcts

B6 Neuropathy

General Characteristics

1. Vitamin B6 in its active form, human pyridoxal kinase (hPL kinase) is a

cofactor for over 160 enzymatic reactions that are involved in:
   a. Neurotransmitter production
   b. Biosynthesis of D-aspartate, L-glutamate
   c. Glycine and GABA
   d. Serotonin
   e. Epinephrine and norepinephrine
   f. Histamine and dopamine
2. Pyridoxal (PL) is an inactive form of vitamin B6 and is converted to pyridoxal 5'-phosphate (PLP) by PL Kinase
3. Theophylline and Ginkotoxin (4'-0-methylpyridoxine), an analogue of vitamin B6 decrease PLP as does isoniazide
4. Risk factors for pyridoxine deficiency:
   a. Severe malnutrition
   b. Sickle cell disease
   c. Inflammatory conditions
   d. Rheumatoid arthritis
   e. Hepatitis and extrahepatic biliary obstruction
   f. Celiac disease
   g. Renal failure
   h. High alkaline phosphatase levels
5. Medical procedures:
   a. Hemodialysis
   b. Phototherapy for hyperbilirubinemia
6. Medications:
   a. Cycloserine
   b. Hydralazine
   c. D-penicillamine
   d. Isoniazid
   e. Pyrazinamide
7. Chronic alcoholism

Clinical Manifestations

1. Weakness and dizziness
2. Peripheral neuropathy:
   a. Early distal extremity numbness
   b. Bilateral distal limb burning paresthesias
   c. Late mild to moderate distal weakness
   d. Sensory ataxia
   e. Proprioception and vibration are more affected than pain and temperature
3. CNS manifestations:
   a. Depression and irritability
   b. Generalized seizures

4. Associated medical conditions:
    a. Cardiovascular:
        i Recurrent venous thromboembolism
        ii Possibly increased early myocardial infarction and stroke
        iii Accelerated atherosclerosis
    b. Glossitis and cheilosis
    c. Seborrheic dermatitis

Neuropathology

1. Large doses of pyridoxine cause peripheral neuropathy primarily of myelinated large fibers that arise from the DRG
2. Vacuolization, increased dense bodies, neurofilament aggregates and chromatolysis are noted in DRG neurons and myelinated fibers
3. Argyrophilic axonal neurodegenerative changes affect the dorsal columns
4. Putative mechanisms of increased pyridoxine toxicity include:
    a. Impairment of function of other B vitamins
    b. Competitive inhibition of pyridoxal phosphate
    c. Formation of reactive quinone methide
    d. Blockade of local chelation of magnesium
5. Deficiency of pyridoxine interferes with transamination, decarboxylation and synthetic pathways that involve carbohydrates, sphingolipids, sulfur containing amino acids, heme, and neurotransmitters; PLP is a cofactor for glutamic acid decarboxylase and thus its deficiency decreases GABA

Laboratory Evaluation

1. Levels of 4-pyridoxic acid are measured in the urine
2. PLP levels are dependent on albumin levels; low albumin levels can lead to a falsely low level
3. Erythrocyte aspartate aminotransferase (EAST) and the EAST activation coefficient (EAST-AC) are indicators of long term functional pyridoxine status

Vitamin B1 (Thiamine)

General Characteristics

1. Low levels of thiamine are usually encountered in a setting of malabsorption or inadequate oral intake
2. Risk factors for deficiency include:
    a. Alcoholism and associated malnutrition
    b. Renal dialysis
    c. Prolonged parenteral glucose (TPN)
    d. Bariatric surgery
    e. Long term diuretic therapy
    f. Hyperemesis gravidarum

   g. Cachectic cancer patients
3. Thiamine is a water-soluble vitamin absorbed in the jejunum
4. Thiamine combines with adenosine triphosphate (ATP) in the liver, kidneys and leucocytes which forms thiamine diphosphate its biologically active form
5. It is a coenzyme in carbohydrate metabolic pathways that include decarboxylation of pyruvic and alpha ketoacids as well as transketolations in the pentose monophosphate pathway

Clinical Manifestations

1. The mildest signs are muscle atrophy in the legs associated with tenderness on compression with loss or depression of ankle and knee reflexes; sensory loss early is in the legs with decreased touch and pain modalities
2. More advanced patients complain of weakness, paresthesias and pain that is insidiously progressive; a subgroup of patients have rapid progression of signs and symptoms that progress over days
3. Initial symptoms are in distal portions of the extremities and progress proximally with the feet more severely affected than the hands
4. In approximately 1/3 of patients the chief complaint is pain and paresthesia
5. Sensory complaints include:
   a. A dull constant ache of the feet and legs
   b. Sharp and lancinating extremity pain (similar to tabes dorsalis)
   c. Cramping and tightness in muscles of the feet and calves
   d. Band-like sensations around the legs
   e. Cold-like sensations of the feet
   f. Heat and burning sensation of the soles to a greater degree than the dorsum of the feet
   g. Patient's symptoms and signs fluctuate and at times are dominated by mechanical dynamic and static allodynia
   h. Most patients have greater distal than proximal weakness
   i. Severe deep muscle mechanical hyperalgesia is common which is most severe in the legs and feet
   j. Reflexes are depressed or absent at the knee and ankle while often preserved in the arms. In patients with severe pain and minimal weakness they may be slightly increased
   k. CNS manifestations:
      i Wernicke-Korsakoff syndrome:
         1. Wernicke's syndrome
            a. Ophthalmoplegia and nystagmus
            b. Ataxia
            c. Confusion
         2. Korsakoff's syndrome:
            a. Amnestic dementia

b. Confabulation

a. Associated medical conditions:

i Primarily severe cardiovascular signs and symptoms of heart failure

Neuropathology

1. Deficiency leads to decreased transketolase activity that increases pyruvic acid:
    a. It is not converted to acetyl-coA and does not enter the Krebs cycle for oxidative metabolism
    b. Pyruvic acid is metabolized anaerobically to lactic acid
2. Sural nerve biopsy:
    a. Primarily axonal degeneration with some fibers demonstrating segmental demyelination

Laboratory Evaluation

1. Increased blood pyruvate, alpha-ketoglutarate and lactate
2. Increased serum glycosylate
3. Urinary methyl glyoxal
4. Urinary thiamine and metabolites thiazole and pyrimidine

Neuroimaging

1. MRI: (Wernicke-Korsakoff):
    a. Hemorrhage and enlargement (acutely) of the mammillary bodies, dorsal medial thalamic nucleus and hypothalamus

Overview of Neurogenic Porphyria

General Characteristics

1. Porphyrins are precursors of heme that are synthesized in a multistep process. Enzymatic defects during the steps of heme synthesis cause distinct clinical syndromes that predominantly affect the skin or the liver and nervous system
2. The acute porphyrias that have periodic attacks of neurovisceral symptoms and neurologic deficits are:
    a. Doss porphyria (ALA dehydratase deficiency)
    b. Acute intermittent porphyria (AIP)
    c. Hereditary coproporphyria
    d. Variegate porphyria

Clinical Manifestations

1. Are dependent on the enzymatic defect and when it occurs in heme synthesis. Early defects in the synthetic cascades are associated with increased serum concentrations of aminolevulinic acid (ALA) and porphobilinogen (PBG). Enzymatic defects in the later part of heme synthesis cause photosensitivity due to porphyrin accumulation in the skin

Acute Intermittent Porphyria

General Characteristics

1. The liver is the major source of overproduction of heme pathway intermediates in the hepatic porphyrias of which AIP is the most common
2. AIP is caused by a heterozygous mutation in the gene encoding porphobilinogen deaminase (PBGD) that maps to chromosome 11q23.3. It is autosomal dominant

Clinical Manifestations

1. The initial and often the most prominent symptom is colicky abdominal pain that is most often generalized and is not associated with rigidity or rebound tenderness
2. Constipation and ileus are frequent concomitants of the pain
3. Attacks may last for days to weeks if not treated and are often associated with vomiting
4. Attacks may be precipitated by dieting, alcohol and estrogen as well as drugs that include:
   a. Phenobarbital
   b. Dilantin
   c. Sulfonamides
   d. Griseofulvin
   e. Succinimide anticonvulsants
5. The first attacks are rare prior to puberty and attacks are most dangerous during adolescence and early adulthood
6. Most often motor nerves are affected more than sensory but in some patients motor, sensory and autonomic nerves are affected concomitantly
7. Symptoms may begin in the feet and legs and ascend or less commonly there is asymmetric early involvement of the arms and hands and then spread to the trunk and legs
8. There may be proximal weakness of shoulder and pelvic girdle muscles with loss of knee jerks and preservation of ankle reflexes
9. There is rare facial paralysis, dysphagia and ocular muscle weakness
10. Sensory loss that may extend to the trunk is seen in approximately 50% of patients; may have pain in the chest and back
11. Acute neurovisceral pain may be associated with rapidly progressive quadriparesis resembling Guillain-Barré syndrome

12. CNS manifestations include:
    a. Confusion and delirium
    b. Visual field deficits
    c. Seizures
    d. Psychosis
13. Associated medical conditions:
    a. Tachycardia and hypertension occur in the acute stages (rarely hypotension)
    b. Fever and leukocytosis may occur during severe attacks
14. The neuropathy can rarely develop without other symptoms

Neuropathology

1. The mutation in PBGD is autosomal dominant with low penetrance. More than 300 PBGD gene mutations have been described all of which cause loss of enzymatic activity from the mutant allele
2. Acute attacks in AIP are precipitated by hormonal and environmental factors that induce hepatic 5-aminolevulinic synthase to produce the porphyrin precursors:
    a. ALA dehydratase
    b. Porphobilinogen
3. Demyelination of the cerebral cortex and cerebellum is seen in some patients
4. Chromatolysis in neurons of the spinal cord

Laboratory Evaluation

1. Patients during acute attacks have increases of 5-100 times the urine concentration of ALA and PBG
2. Hyponatremia is frequent; a patient has been studied who demonstrated median eminence of the hypothalamus and hypothalamic-hypophyseal tract lesions: patients may be hypomagnesemic
3. Molecular genetic testing to delineate the mutation in the PBGD gene
4. EMG / NCV
    a. The neuropathy may be predominately upper extremity, motor and proximal
    b. Predominately a motor axonal neuropathy

Neuroimaging

1. MRI:
    a. Multiple large, contrast-enhancing subcortical white matter lesions
    b. Diffusion-weighted MRI is normal
2. MR spectroscopy:
    a. Normal
3. The putative mechanism for the lesions is reversible vasogenic edema with transient disruption of the blood brain barrier

4. In many patients the white matter lesions are bioccipital and are partially or completely reversible

Doss Porphyria

General Characteristics

1. Also known as plumb porphyria is due to ALA dehydratase deficiency
2. The ALAD gene maps to chromosome 9q32 and encodes delta-amino levulinate dehydratase (porphobilinogen synthase)
3. It is a cytosolic enzyme that catalyzes the second step in the porphyrin and heme biosynthetic pathway
4. Clinical features are seen if there is greater than 90% deficiency of the enzyme
5. It is an autosomal recessive disorder

Clinical Manifestations

1. Colicky abdominal pain and vomiting
2. Primarily a motor neuropathy
3. In some patients the acute porphyria occurs during infusion of erythropoietin

Neuropathology

1. Putatively by stimulating heme synthesis, erythropoietin may unmask ALA dehydratase deficiency
2. Lead may unmask occult plumb-porphyria
3. Tyrosinemia type I may occur with the disorder

Laboratory Evaluation

1. There is markedly increased urinary ALA and coproporphyrin
2. Molecular genetic studies delineate the causative mutation
3. There is no urinary increase in PBG

Hereditary Coproporphyria (HCP)

General Characteristics

1. Hereditary coproporphyria (HCP) is caused by heterozygous mutation in the CPOX gene that maps to chromosome 3q11.2
2. Harderoporphyria is a subtype of HCP that is caused by a homozygous or compound heterozygous mutation in the CPOX gene
3. Inheritance is usually AD but AR patients have been reported

Clinical Manifestations

1. In general clinical features become manifest when there is ~50% enzyme activity (heterozygous mutation) or homozygous (<10% of activity) mutation
2. The neurovisceral manifestations are similar to those seen in AIP but are less severe

3. Neurologic defects are initiated by drugs, fasting, infections and the menstrual cycle
4. Approximately 50% of patients may be asymptomatic
5. Psychiatric symptoms occur
6. Peripheral neuropathy is primarily motor; sensory symptoms may include pain in the extremities
7. Cutaneous features occur in approximately 30% of patients and include:
    a. Vesiculobullous eruptions that involve the face, hands and sun-exposed skin areas
    b. Lesions may heal with scarring, increased pigmentation or hypertrichosis
8. Nausea, vomiting, diarrhea are frequent
9. Hypertension may occur during acute attacks
10. Generalized tonic-clonic seizures may occur

Neuropathology

1. HCP is caused by mutations in the CPOX gene that:
    a. Encodes the enzyme coproporphyrinogen oxidase. This enzyme is the sixth step in the heme biosynthetic pathway that converts coproporphyrinogen III to protoporphyrinogen IX

Laboratory Evaluation

1. Elevation of urinary ALA and PBG
2. ALA excretion exceeds that of PBG
3. Elevation of fecal coproporphyrin III alone without elevation of protoporphyrin IX distinguishes it from variegate porphyria (VP)
4. Fecal and urinary coproporphyrin III levels are increased 10-200 times normal levels
5. Molecular genetic delineation of the CPOX mutation

Neuroimaging

1. SPECT:
    a. Mild to moderate perfusion defects may be seen in the temporal lobes, frontal lobes and parietal lobes
2. MRI:
    a. In one of 7 patients white matter hypertensities (nonspecific) were detected

Variegate Porphyria

General Characteristics

1. Variegate porphyria is caused by heterozygous mutation in the PPOX gene that maps to chromosome 1q23.3 and encodes the enzyme protoporphyrinogen oxidase

2. Inheritance is autosomal dominant

Clinical Manifestations

1. The most prominent manifestation of variegate porphyria is an adult onset of cutaneous blistering skin lesions in sun-exposed areas
2. The lesions:
    a. The hands and face are prominently involved
    b. The lesions are subepidermal vesicles, bullae and erosions that crust and heal slowly
    c. Chronic skin characteristics are milia (small keratin filled cysts), scarring thickening and decreased pigmentation
    d. Facial hyperpigmentation and hypertrichosis may also occur
    e. Acute neurovisceral symptoms occur after puberty and include:
        i Highly variable attacks that may be similar from episode to episode; not all symptoms occur in a single attack and the acute symptoms may become chronic; attacks are common in women of child-bearing age
        ii Colicky abdominal pain with constipation
        iii Pain in the back, chest and extremities
        iv Seizures
        v Primarily a motor neuropathy that may progress to quadriparesis and respiratory failure
        vi Psychiatric symptoms
        vii Autonomic dysregulation (tachycardia and hypertension)
        viii The disease occurs in a worldwide distribution but is particularly prevalent in South Africa
        ix The homozygous variant of variegate porphyria is manifest by:
            1. Photosensitization in early childhood
            2. Skeletal hand abnormalities
            3. Less frequently: short stature, cognitive dysfunction and seizures

Neuropathology

1. The defect is a decreased activity of the enzyme protoporphyrinogen oxidase of approximately 50%
2. Predominant axonal neuropathy
3. Patchy demyelination in the CNS

Laboratory Evaluation

1. The diagnosis is secured by a combination of blood, urine and fecal tests
2. Biochemically active patients demonstrate:
    a. Increased PBG in a spot urine sample and/or increased plasma porphyrins (a distinctive fluorescence peak at 626-628 nm at neutral pH)

3. Increased fecal porphyrins with a predominance of both coproporphyrin III and protoporphyrin IX
4. Molecular genetic delineation of the mutation in the PPOX gene
5. CSF:
   a. Most often normal; rarely slightly increased protein
   b. EMG:
      i Denervation; some myopathic potentials
      ii CMAPs; small
      iii No demyelinative features
      iv Normal or small SNAPs

Fabry's Disease

General Characteristics

1. Fabry's disease is caused by mutations in the GLA gene that maps to Xq22.1
2. It encodes alpha-galactosidase A
3. Globotriaosylceramide (Gb3) and related glycosphingolipids accumulate in the plasma and tissue cellular lysosomes throughout the body. It is a progressive systemic disease affecting the kidneys, cerebral blood vessels and the heart. It may also manifests primarily as a small-fiber peripheral neuropathy.

Clinical Manifestations

1. Children and adolescents present with burning, symmetric pain in the palms of the hands and soles of the feet associated with extremity dysesthesias
2. Patients may suffer recurrent attacks of pain that are described as:
   a. Excruciating
   b. Lancinating and stabbing
   c. Begin distally in the extremities and spread proximally
   d. Episodes, ("pain crises") may occur daily
3. Attacks may be triggered by fever, stress, and physical activity putatively due to an inability to sweat. Rarer triggering events are exposure to cold, rapid humidity change and fatigue
4. A pain crisis may be associated with:
   a. Deep muscle aches
   b. Joint pain
   c. Unexplained fever
   d. Increased sedimentation rate
5. Neuropathic pain affects 60-80% of affected boys and 40-60% of girls (usually at a later age than boys)
6. Most adult males and approximately 60-90% of affected females have pain
7. During the course of the illness pain may diminish but rarely becomes more severe
8. Associated signs:

a. Angiokeratoma skin lesions:
   i Appear as clusters of individual punctate, dark red to blue-black angiectases in superficial skin layers; they are flat or slightly raised and do not blanch with pressure
   ii The greatest concentration of lesions is between the umbilicus and knees. Often they are in a "bathing suit distribution"; the oral mucosa, conjunctiva and other mucosae may be involved
   iii The number and size of the lesions increase with age
b. Ocular involvement:
   i A corneal opacity that is termed cornea verticillata (slit lamp) is seen in affected males and most heterozygous females
   ii Lenticular changes, or granular anterior capsular or subcapsular deposits and cataract are seen
   iii Aneurysmal dilatation and tortuosity of both conjunctival and retinal vessels is noted
c. Vascular disease:
   i Cardiac and cerebrovascular disease is present in most males by middle age
d. Renal involvement:
   i Progressive accumulation of glycosphingolipid in the kidney causes azotemia by the third to fifth decade
e. Males and females with the classic phenotype have involvement of gastrointestinal, pulmonary and lymphatic systems
f. Heterozygous females have a less severe course

Neuropathology

1. Deficiency of the lysosomal enzyme alpha-galactosidase A causes the systemic accumulation of globotriaosylceramide (Gb3) in the cellular lysosomes of vessels, nerves, tissues and bodily organs

Laboratory Evaluation

1. Small fiber dysfunction
2. Nerve biopsy:
   a. Length dependent neuropathy
   b. Reduction of thinly myelinated A-delta fibers (1-4 μ) and unmyelinated C-fibers (1 μ)
   c. Autonomic small fiber loss
3. Nerve conduction velocities:
   a. Motor and sensory NCV are normal early in the disease course
   b. Decreased CMAP amplitudes are seen more often than slow nerve conduction
4. Quantitative sensory testing:

   a. Reduction of small fiber modality function:
      i Raised cold and warm detection thresholds
5. Molecular genetic analysis of the GLA gene on Xq22.1 to delineate the mutation
6. Alpha galactosidase can be quantitated (and is decreased) in the plasma, urine and leucocytes
7. Cardiac evaluation:
   a. Left ventricular hypertrophy
   b. Concentric remodeling of the left ventricle
   c. Structural changes in the mitral valve (25% of male patients) and the aortic valve (10%) of male patients
8. Audiograms:
   a. Approximately 75% of male patients have high frequency sensorineural hearing loss
9. Renal disease:
   a. Manifest in more than 30% of male patients
10. Molecular genetic evaluation is the most reliable method of diagnosing female carriers as many carriers have normal α –Gal A enzyme activity

Chemotherapy Induced Peripheral Neuropathy (CIPN)

Overview

Chemotherapy-induced peripheral neuropathy affects approximately 30 to 40% of patients that undergo chemotherapy.

The major agents associated with CIPN are:

1. Thalidomide and its analogue lenalidomide
2. Epothilones (ixabepilone)
3. Vinca alkaloids (vincristine and vinblastine)
4. Taxanes (paclitaxel and docetaxel)
5. Proteasome inhibitors (bortezomib)
6. Platinum-based agents that include cisplatin, oxaliplatin, and carboplatin

The occurrence and degree of neuropathy with these agents is determined by the specific drug, the duration of treatment, the quantity administered and if the patient has a neuropathy prior to treatment. In general, the symptoms and signs are sensory but motor and autonomic nerves may be affected. CIPN may be initiated after the first dose and increases with treatment but plateaus by the end of therapy. However, platinum-based drugs demonstrate a "coasting effect" in which sensory modalities may continue for months after completion of treatment. The neuropathy in many patients is irreversible.

Mechanisms for pathogenesis of the neuropathy in CIPN include:

1. Activation of ion channels on pain dorsal root ganglia and spinal dorsal horn neurons that trigger secondary cascades leading to hyperexcitability
2. Opening of MPTP pores on mitochondria that induces intracellular calcium release
3. Activation of protein kinase C
4. Phosphorylation of TRPV receptors
5. Caspase / calpain activation
6. The generation of nitric oxide and free radicals that injures DNA and induces apoptosis of neurons and injures axons
7. Induces inflammatory processes in sensory pain projecting neurons (an inflammatory profile of cytokines and chemokines) that alters pain processing

Cisplatin

General Characteristics

1. Cisplatin (SP-4-2)-diamminedichloroplatinum(II) causes crosslinking of DNA that results in apoptosis
2. The usual cancers treated with cisplatin are:
   a. Sarcomas
   b. Some carcinomas
   c. Lymphomas
   d. Germ cell tumors
   e. Gynecological tumors
3. Cisplatins have a molecular affinity for peripheral nerves that are affected due to a less effective nerve-vascular barrier
4. It is a dose-dependent toxic neuropathy usually at a cumulative dose of 225-500 mg/m^2

Clinical Characteristics

1. The neurotoxic effects can manifest primarily as a sensory neuropathy or ganglionopathy primarily of large fibers
2. Patients develop paresthesias, hyperesthesias, decreased proprioception and vibration sensibility
3. Gait ataxia
4. Pseudoatheitoid movements of the extremities
5. Loss of muscle stretch reflexes in both upper and lower extremities
6. Lhermitte's sign (approximately 40% of patients)
7. Approximately 2% develop weakness
8. Onset of signs and symptoms may be delayed up to eight weeks after cessation of therapy; deficits may progress for up to 6 months following completion of therapy (coasting)
9. Patients may develop a paradoxical response to cold (perceived as heat)

10. Emerging reports of CNS toxicity with platinum-based chemotherapy include:
    a. Encephalopathy
    b. Seizures
    c. Transient blindness
    d. Aphasia
11. Ototoxicity:
    a. Hearing loss and tinnitus are frequently encountered

Neuropathology

1. Cisplatin causes covalence of DNA that produces intrastrand and interstrand cross-links; formation of these adducts inhibits transcription and replication and produces cell-cycle arrest
2. Inhibition of protein synthesis and axonal transport
3. Nerve biopsy (sural nerve):
    a. Large Aα and AB fiber loss > than A-delta (1-4μ) and unmyelinated (1μ) C-fibers
    b. Axonal degeneration with small clusters of regenerating fibers
    c. Secondary segmental demyelination

Laboratory Evaluation

1. QST Increased:
    a. Vibratory detection thresholds are decreased early
2. EMG:
    a. Low amplitude or unobtainable SNAPs
    b. Normal CMAPs and EMG

Oxaliplatin

General Characteristics

1. Oxaliplatin-based chemotherapy is the standard treatment for both adjuvant and metastatic colon cancer
2. Neurotoxic effects are a major cause of dose reduction and cessation of its administration

Clinical Manifestations

1. Acute neuropathy:
    a. Transient and develops either during or just after oxaliplatin infusion
    b. Rarely lasts more than 7 days
    c. It may be triggered by cold and manifests with:
        i Paresthesias and tingling
        ii Jaw spasm
        iii Limb stiffness

iv Muscle cramps

d. The incidence of acute neuropathy is 80-98%

2. Chronic neuropathy manifests with:
   a. Numbness or tingling of the hands and feet
   b. Develops in approximately 10-20% of patients after a cumulative dose of 750-850 mg/m2
   c. Signs and symptoms have been reported for 2-5 years after treatment

Neuropathology

1. The mechanism of oxaliplatin neuropathy is not known; putatively the acute form is related to chelation of calcium by oxalate, a metabolite of oxaliplatin that leads to sensory neuron hyperexcitability by failure of inhibition of calcium-dependent sodium channels
2. Oxaliplatin slows Na channel inactivation kinetics
3. Cell death of sensory neurons occurs in the DRG
4. Cold hyperalgesia in oxaliplatin has been posited to occur from:
   a. TRPA1 expression in small-diameter DRG neurons and by activation of p38 mitogen-activated kinase

Laboratory Evaluation

1. EMG:
   a. Low-amplitude or unobtainable SNAPs
   b. Normal CMAPs and needle EMG

Vincristine

General Characteristics

1. The neurotoxicity of the antitubulins is different in incidence, clinical manifestations and prognosis for each agent
2. Vincristine is the most neurotoxic and its severity is dose related commencing usually after administration of 4 mg/m^2
3. Vinblastine, vinflunine and vinorelbine are less toxic

Clinical Manifestations

1. Paresthesias and numbness that at times starts in the fingers prior to the toes
   a. Distal extremity weakness occurs in 25-35% of patients
   b. Autonomic involvement may cause constipation, urinary retention, impotence and orthostatic hypotension
   c. Rarely described are oculomotor palsies, facial and laryngeal weakness and hearing loss
   d. A subset of patients develops severe neuropathic extremity pain
   e. Symptoms and signs are usually prominent after a cumulative dose of 12mg although neuropathy can develop as early as two weeks after a

single 2 mg/m^2 dose

f. Approximately 30% of patients have a coasting effect for 1 month after termination of treatment
g. Symptoms and signs often remain for 3 months after treatment
h. Ankle reflexes may be lost prior to changes in sensory modalities

Neuropathology

1. Vincristine is a substrate of P-glycoprotein and is metabolized by the cytochrome P-450 (CYP) 3A5 and 3A4 isoforms; CYP3A5 clears 75% of the drug
2. CYP3A5 nonexpressor status is associated with peripheral neuropathy as its dysfunction leads to increased vincristine concentrations
3. Mutation in the centrosomal protein 72 gene that maps to chromosome 5p15.33 has been associated with vincristine neuropathy:
   a. The CEP72 gene:
      i Encodes a pericentriolar satellite protein that has a critical role in microtubule organization
      ii Impairs microtubule assembly by binding to tubulin
      iii Disrupts axonal transport
4. Nerve biopsy:
   a. Axonal degeneration of both myelinated and unmyelinated fibers
   b. Regenerating fiber clusters
   c. Some segmental demyelination

Laboratory Evaluation

1. Neurophysiology:
   a. Primarily an axonal sensorimotor peripheral neuropathy
   b. Motor and sensory nerve conduction studies demonstrate reduced amplitudes, normal or only slightly prolonged distal latencies and slowed conduction velocities
   c. Fibrillation and positive sharp waves may be demonstrated in distal muscles
2. QST:
   a. Decreased vibratory detection thresholds are decreased early

Vinorelbine

General Characteristics

1. Vinorelbine is a semisynthetic vinca alkaloid that is primarily used in the treatment of non-small-cell lung cancer. It is also used off label for metastatic breast cancer and rhabdomyosarcoma
2. It causes a dose-dependent peripheral neuropathy in 20-50% of patients

Clinical Manifestations

1. A progressive and often irreversible tingling numbness
2. A subset of patients have intense distal extremity neuropathic pain
3. Hypersensitivity to cold
4. Usually begins in the hands and feet with proximal progression
5. Autonomic symptomatology occurs but is not as severe as that which occurs with vincristine
6. A severe neuropathy only occurs in approximately 1% of patients
7. Motor weakness may occur after 3-6 months of treatment
8. Loss of ankle reflexes occurs after approximately 12 cycles

Neuropathology

1. Binds to tubulin which inhibits mitotic microtubule polymerization

Laboratory Evaluation

1. EMG/ NCV:
    a. Dose-dependent decrease of SNAP and CMAP amplitudes
    b. Normal distal latencies and conduction velocities

Taxanes (Paclitaxel, Docetaxel)

General Characteristics

1. Paclitaxel and docetaxel are used either alone or in combination with other agents in the treatment of breast, ovarian, lung and other cancers
2. Paclitaxel may be more neurotoxic than docetaxel

Clinical Manifestations

1. Sensory symptoms are most common and are dose dependent
2. A mild neuropathy develops in up to 85% of patients after 3 to 7 cycles of treatment with Taxol with administration of 135-200 mg/m^2
3. A severe neuropathy may occur in 2% of patients at this dosage
4. Doses between 250 and 350 mg/m^2 may cause symptoms after the first or second cycles at times within 24 hours of administration
5. Approximately 70% of patients develop a neuropathy after high dose regimes
6. Both paclitaxel and docetaxel cause:
    a. Paresthesias and dysesthetic pain in the feet and hands
    b. A predominant loss of vibration and proprioceptive modalities > pain and temperature (small fiber)
    c. Gait unsteadiness
    d. Sensory ataxia
    e. Weakness is usually minimal although motor neuropathy has been described; if weakness occurs it may be proximal

f. A severe neuropathy may develop if the patient has a preexisting neuropathy or has been treated with other neurotoxic agents (usually occurs with a cumulative dose >1500 mg/m2)
g. Taxane acute pain syndrome (TAPS) is characterized by:
    i Myalgias and arthralgias that start 1-3 days and last 5-7 days after taxane-based chemotherapy

Neuropathology

1. Taxanes may affect the neuronal cell body, the axon or both concomitantly
2. Taxol and taxotere increase tubulin polymerization that causes aggregation and an accumulation of abnormal bundles of microtubules in the DRG, axons and Schwann cells which putatively interfere with axonal transport
3. Nerve biopsy (sural nerve):
    a. Loss of large myelinated fibers
    b. Axonal degeneration with secondary demyelination and remyelination
    c. Electron microscopy:
    d. Tubular and membranous structures within axons
    e. Some small fiber involvement
    f. Small clusters of regenerating fibers

Laboratory Evaluation

1. Electrophysiology:
    a. Nerve conduction studies:
        i Reduced SNAP and CMAP amplitudes (correlate with dosage)
        ii Normal distal latencies and conduction velocities; rarely demyelinating features (slowed conduction velocities are demonstrated)
        iii Fibrillation potentials may occur in distal extremity muscles
2. QST
    a. Vibratory detection thresholds are more often impaired than thermal thresholds

Docetaxel (Taxotere)

General Characteristics

1. Primarily used for locally advanced or metastatic cancers:
    a. Breast cancer
    b. Head and neck cancer
    c. Gastric cancer
    d. Hormone-refractory prostate cancer
    e. Non-small cell lung cancer
2. Docetaxel may be twice as potent as paclitaxel but has comparable efficacy

Clinical Manifestations

1. Causes a dose-dependent primarily sensory neuropathy that is usually less severe than that which occurs with Taxol
2. Pain in the hands and feet
3. Lhermitte's sign may be present
4. Large fiber modalities of vibration are more affected than small fiber modalities
5. Reduced or absent ankle reflexes
6. Mild proximal and distal weakness occurs in 5-19% of patients
7. "Coasting" may occur for several months after treatment although many patients improve 1-2 months fallowing cessation of their protocols

Neuropathology

1. Binds to microtubules with high affinity which stabilizes them and prevents depolymerization / disassembly in the absence of GTP
2. Failure of disassembly causes a decrease in free tubulin needed for microtubule formation which causes inhibition of mitotic cell division between metaphase and anaphase
3. Microtubule accumulation intracellularly initiates apoptosis
4. Sensory nerve biopsy:
    a. Loss of large myelinated fibers
    b. Scattered fibers with axonal degeneration

Laboratory Evaluations

1. EMG/ NCV:
    a. Diminished amplitude of motor and sensory nerve amplitudes
    b. Mild slowing of conduction velocities

Epothilone

General Characteristics

1. Epothilones are microtubule stabilizing agents that are used in various types of refractory treatment-resistant cancer
2. Ixabelone is primarily used

Clinical Manifestations

1. Cumulative dose and possible preexisting neuropathy are risk factors
2. Primarily a sensory distal peripheral neuropathy similar to the taxanes

Neuropathology

1. Disruption of microtubules of the mitotic spindle
2. Interference with axon transport

Laboratory Evaluation

1. EMG/ NCV:

a. Axonal dose-dependent neuropathy

Suramin

General Characteristics

1. Suramin is a hexasulfonated naphthylurea
2. It is used either alone or in combination with other chemotherapeutic protocols for the treatment of hormone-resistant or metastatic prostate cancer

Clinical Manifestations

1. It causes a peripheral neuropathy in 25 to 90% of patients
2. Neurotoxicity is the dose-limiting side effect
3. A distal axonopathy is the more common neuropathy and is characterized by:
   a. Distal numbness and paresthesia
   b. Decreased light touch, pain and vibration sensibility
   c. Mild weakness of the distal extremities (toe extensors)
   d. Decreased ankle reflexes
   e. This form of neuropathy is reversible with cessation of treatment
4. Subacute sensorimotor demyelinating neuropathy:
   a. Is more severe than the axonal neuropathy and occurs in 10-20% of patients after 1-5 months of treatment
   b. It occurs when a peak plasma concentration of over 300 μg/L exposure to > 200 μg/L for 25 days per month or if a cumulative dose of 40,000 μg/L is attained
   c. Numbness and paresthesias of the distal extremities
   d. A symmetrical proximal > distal muscle weakness
   e. Decreased or absent reflexes in both upper and lower extremities
   f. The weakness can involve respiratory muscles and approximately 25% of patients require mechanical ventilation
   g. "Coasting" may occur for approximately 1 month following cessation of therapy
   h. Recovery occurs slowly and often there is residual weakness and numbness

Neuropathology

1. Suramin is pleiotropic and causes:
   a. Inhibition of apoptosis
   b. Suppression of proinflammatory cytokines
   c. Inactivates myofibroblasts
   d. Stimulates proliferation of renal epithelial cells
2. Action on nerves is not known. Suggested mechanisms include:
   a. Interference with neurotrophic factor interaction with their receptors

   b. Lysosomal dysfunction
   c. Possible immune-mediated demyelination
3. Sural nerve biopsy:
   a. Patients with subacute demyelinating polyradiculoneuropathy:
      i Loss of large and small myelinated fibers
      ii Secondary axonal degeneration
      iii Epi and endoneurial mononuclear inflammatory infiltrates
4. Accumulation of glycolipid lysosomal inclusions have been demonstrated in animal models

Laboratory Evaluation

1. Elevated CSF protein may be seen in the subacute demyelinating neuropathy
2. Patients with axonal neuropathy:
   a. EMG/ NCV:
      i Decreased amplitudes of SNAPs and CMAPs
      ii Minimal abnormalities of distal latencies and conduction velocities
3. Patients with the subacute sensorimotor polyradiculoneuropathy:
   a. EMG/ NCV:
      i Prolonged distal latencies and F-waves
      ii Slowed conduction velocities
      iii Temporal dispersion
      iv Conduction block
4. QST:
   a. Increased vibratory and cooling detection thresholds
5. Needle EMG:
   a. Decreased recruitment of MUAPs in proximal and distal muscles
   b. Occasional fibrillation potentials

Bortezamib (Velcade)

General Characteristics

1. Bortezomid is a polycyclic derivative of boronic acid that inhibits the mammalian 265 proteasome
2. Additional actions include:
   a. It suppresses secretion of bone marrow cytokines
   b. Increases oxidative stress

Clinical Manifestations

1. Neuropathy that is emergent or worsening of a preexisting neuropathy occurs in approximately 35% of patients in myeloma treatment trials
2. 1 to 1.3 mg/m2 appears to be the neurotoxic dose; the risk of neuropathy is dose dependent and approximately 50% of patients will be affected at a cumulative dose of 30 mg/m2

3. Sensory complaints are burning dysesthesia, paresthesias, and numbness in a length dependent manner
4. Autonomic dysfunction occurs that includes postural hypotension
5. Signs and symptoms usually improve in 3 to 4 months

Neuropathology

1. The boron atom in bortezomib binds the catalytic site of the 265 proteasome
2. Bortezomib causes a rapid change in the levels of intracellular peptides that may contribute to its biological effects
3. Increases oxidative stress
4. Suppresses bone marrow secretion of cytokines
5. One patient has been described with spongy degeneration of the DRGs

Laboratory Evaluation

1. NCS:
   a. Consistent with an axonal sensory neuropathy
2. QST:
   a. Early small fiber parameters are affected
   b. Increased temperature detection thresholds

Etoposide

General Characteristics (PV-16)

1. Belongs to the topoisomerase inhibitor class of drugs
2. It is used to treat:
   a. Kaposi's sarcoma
   b. Ewing's sarcoma
   c. Lung cancer
   d. Testicular cancer
   e. Lymphoma
   f. Non-lymphocytic leukemia
   g. Glioblastoma multiforma
3. It is also administered:
   a. In combination with bleomycin for testicular cancer
   b. As one of the conditioning agents prior to bone marrow or blood stem cell transplantation
   c. It is a semisynthetic derivative of podophyllotoxin

Clinical Manifestations

1. Causes a moderate-to-severe sensory axonal neuropathy or ganglionopathy in approximately 4 to 10% of patients
2. A subset of patients develop an autonomic neuropathy characterized by orthostatic hypotension and gastroparesis

Neuropathology

1. Etoposide forms a ternary complex with DNA and the topoisomerase 11 enzyme
    a. The complex prevents re-ligation of DNA strands and strand breaks
    b. Inhibits microtubule function

Laboratory Evaluation

1. NCS:
    a. Low amplitude SNAPs and CMAPs

Ifosfamide

General Characteristics

1. Ifosfamide is primarily used in the treatment of bone and soft tissue sarcomas in children and young adults
2. Ifosfamide is an alkylating agent (a cyclophosphamide analog)

Clinical Manifestations

1. The cumulative dose for toxicity is 14g/m^2
2. Peripheral neuropathy:
    a. Patients develop numbness and painful paresthesias that begin in the hands and feet approximately 10-14 days after cessation of treatment
    b. Rarely the neuropathy begins in the hands
    c. The neuropathy gradually resolves
    d. Encephalopathy:
        i Occurs in approximately 50% of patients
        i Putatively mediated by chloracetaldehyde (a break down product of ifosfamide)
        ii Patients may be just confused but others have developed delirium, status epilepticus and coma
        iii Methylene blue shortens the duration of the encephalopathy and may be prophylactic

Neuropathology

1. Ifosfamide is an alkylating agent that is a prodrug which requires activation by hepatic microsomal enzymes to ifosfamide mustard
2. It alkylates DNA which forms DNA-DNA cross-links that inhibit DNA synthesis

Laboratory Evaluation

1. NCS/EMG:
    a. Axonal neuropathy

Cytosine Arabinoside

General Characteristics

1. Is primarily used in the treatment of acute myeloid leukemia and non-Hodgkin lymphoma
2. Cytosine arabinoside is similar enough to human cytosine deoxyribose to be incorporated into human DNA which kills the cell
3. The drug alters the sugar component of nucleosides
4. Neuropathy may occur with cumulative doses that range from 60mg/m2 to 36 g/m^2

Clinical Manifestations

1. The neuropathy can begin within hours to weeks following treatment
2. A sensorimotor polyneuropathy occurs that resembles GBS after administration of high doses
3. Respiratory failure has been described with high dose therapy
4. A length-dependent sensory neuropathy occurs at low to intermediate doses

Neuropathology

1. Sural nerve biopsy:
   a. Demyelination or axonal degeneration
   b. Suggested mechanisms of action include:
      i Immune dysregulation
      ii Decreased protein synthesis that is necessary for myelin, axonal structure or transport
   c. High dose cytarabine has been associated with cerebral, cerebellar, spinal cord dysfunction and ocular pathology
   d. Cytosine arabinoside:
      i It is rapidly converted into cytosine arabinoside triphosphate which damages DNA in the S phase of the cell cycle (during DNA synthesis)
      ii Inhibits both DNA and RNA polymerases and nucleotide reductases

Laboratory Evaluation

1. Patients with GBS presentation:
   a. Demonstrate increased CSF protein
   b. EMG and NCS:
      i Demonstrate an acquired demyelinating sensorimotor polyneuropathy
      ii Primarily axonal neuropathy

Thalidomide

General Characteristics

1. Thalidomide is primarily used in the treatment of multiple myeloma, Waldenstrom's macroglobulinemia, acute myeloid leukemia

2. Lenalidomide (alpha-3-amino-phthalimido glutarimide) is an analogue of thalidomide with less toxicity

Clinical Manifestations

1. The peripheral neuropathy is frequently dose limiting
2. The usual cumulative dose that causes neuropathy is 7 grams; less than 10% of patients with a lesser dose are symptomatic
3. The usual symptoms are numbness, painful tingling and burning pain in the feet and hands (lenalidomide is similar but less toxic)
4. Muscle weakness occurs and is most prominent distally
5. Generalized hypo or areflexia
6. Large fiber modalities of sensation (12-20μ) for vibration and proprioception are more effected than small fiber modalities

Neuropathology

1. Sural nerve biopsy:
   a. Loss of large-diameter myelinated fibers; axonal degeneration
   b. Loss of DRG cells
   c. Thalidomide has pleiotropic effects:
      i Anti-angiogenic
      ii Anti-oxidative stress
      iii Inhibits TNF-α, IL-6, IL-10, and IL-12
      iv Modulates the production of IFN-γ
      v Decreases the production of IL-2, Il-4, and IL-5 by immune cells
      vi Decreases NF-KB and COX-2 activity
      vii Thalidomide binds cereblon which is a ubiquitin ligase substrate adapter protein and may be causative in its teratogenicity

Laboratory Evaluation

1. Nerve conduction studies:
   a. Reduced amplitudes or absence of SNAPs
   b. Usually preserved conduction velocities particularly of motor nerves

Late Neurologic Toxicity Associated with Peripheral Painful Neuropathy in Chemotherapy Induced Peripheral Neuropathy

Platinum Based Compounds

1. Symptoms and signs usually develop during treatment, but may progress ('coasting') for 2 to 6 months following its cessation:
   a. Approximately 20% of patients may be affected (based on a study of patients treated for testicular cancer 23 to 33 years following treatment)
   b. A similar study revealed that 28% of patients had an asymptomatic

neuropathy while 38% of patients were symptomatic after a median follow-up of 15 years

c. Other symptoms and signs include:
   - i Persisting taste and smell dysfunction
   - ii Oto and vestibular abnormalities
   - iii Raynaud's phenomenon
   - iv Mobility problems in older patients
   - v Persistent neuropathic pain

Oxaliplatin

1. Reversible in approximately 80% of patients; may completely resolve in 40% of patients at 6-8 months

5FU and Oxaliplatin

1. Frequently used in the treatment of gastrointestinal cancer
2. 92% of patients develop a sensory neuropathy which resolves in approximately 9 months
3. Dysesthesia and cold induced pain may be persistent

Platinum and Taxane Combinations

1. Approximately 15% persistent neuropathy at 6 months; at 48 months, 23% of patients have residual neuropathy

Vincristine

1. The neuropathy is often reversible after cessation of therapy. The median duration of paresthesia and weakness is 3 months
2. Cramps occur in the small muscles of the feet > hands

Taxane

1. Usually the neuropathy improves or resolves within 3-6 months after cessation of therapy

Thalidomide

1. The incidence of neuropathy varies from 25% to 83% and is dose dependent
2. Approximately 15% of patients interrupt therapy due to neurotoxicity
3. The neuropathy is often irreversible after a cumulative dose of 20 grams

Bortezomib

1. Signs and symptoms of neuropathy improve or resolve 3-4 months following treatment

Painful Toxic Neuropathies

Misonidazole

General Characteristics

1. Misonidazole is a nitroimidazole with both radiosensitizing and antineoplastic properties
2. Has been utilized as a radiotherapy sensitizer and for bladder cancer

Clinical Manifestations

1. The neuropathy usually starts after approximately 3 to 5 weeks of therapeutic drug administration to a total dose of > 18 grams
2. Patients get painful paresthesias primarily of the feet
3. Loss of both large and small fiber modalities
4. Distal muscle weakness occurs in a length dependent manner
5. Reflexes are preserved
6. The neuropathy occurs in approximately 40% of patients and 80% of patients have residual signs and symptoms three years after cessation of treatment

Neuropathology

1. Sural nerve biopsy:
   a. Decreased large myelinated fibers with axonal degeneration and swellings
   b. Segmental demyelination and remyelination
2. Electron microscopy
   a. Accumulation of neurofilaments with axon swelling
3. Misonidazole has high electron affinity, induces the formation of free radicals, and depletes radioprotective thiols that sensitize hypoxic cells to the cytotoxic effects of ionizing irradiation. The mechanism of action in producing neuropathy has not been established.

Laboratory Evaluation

1. Electrophysiology:
   a. Low amplitude or unobtainable SNAPs with slightly reduced CMAPs

Metronidazole

General Characteristics

1. A common antibacterial and antiprotozoal agent that has wide global usage
2. It is a synthetic 5-nitro-imidazole

Clinical Manifestations

1. Painful extremity paresthesias
2. Loss of both small and large fiber sensory modalities
3. Rarely distal weakness in a length dependent manner
4. Metallic taste
5. Central neurological characteristics:
   a. Seizures
   b. Diffuse encephalopathy

   c. Acute and chronic cerebellar toxicity

Neuropathology

1. Sural nerve biopsy:
   a. Axonal degeneration
2. It inhibits nucleic acid synthesis by disrupting DNA of mitochondrial cells

Laboratory Evaluation

1. Electrophysiology
   a. Low-amplitude or unobtainable SNAPs with normal CMAPs

Amiodarone

General Characteristics

1. Amiodarone is a class III antiarrhythmic drug used for both ventricular and atrial arrhythmias; it is also indicated for recurrent ventricular fibrillation or hemodynamically-unstable ventricular tachycardia

Clinical Manifestations

1. Patients develop a neuromyopathy similar to that induced by chloroquine
2. Patients develop distal extremity sensory loss manifest by tingling and burning pain
3. Severe proximal and distal muscle weakness may develop which is worse in the legs than the arms
4. Two to three years of use is required for the induction of the neuromyopathy
5. Reduced sensation to all modalities
6. Decreased or absent muscle stretch reflexes
7. Associated medical conditions include:
   a. Tremor
   b. Thyroid dysfunction
   c. Pulmonary fibrosis
   d. Parotid gland hypertrophy
   e. Corneal micro deposits
   f. Light-sensitive blue-gray skin discoloration

Neuropathology

1. Sural nerve biopsy:
   a. Segmental demyelination and axonal degeneration
2. Electron microscopy:
   a. Lamellar or dense inclusions in Schwann cells, pericytes and endothelial cells
3. Muscle biopsy:
   a. Electron microscopy:
      i Autophagic vacuoles with myeloid and dense inclusions

    ii Neurogenic atrophy in distal muscles
4. In immortalized adult rat Schwann cells amiodarone caused:
    a. Accumulation of phospholipids and neutral lipids
    b. Upregulation of the expression of gangliosides
    c. Increased oxidative stress
    d. Impaired lysosomal degradation in Schwann cells

Laboratory Evaluation

1. Electrophysiology (EMG/ NCV):
    a. Low-amplitude or unobtainable SNAP
    b. Normal or reduced CMAP amplitudes
    c. Irritable and myopathic MUAPs in proximal muscles of patients with myopathy
    d. Needle EMG demonstrates distal denervation with fibrillations, positive sharp waves and occasional myotonic discharges
    e. Sensory NCS:
        i Moderately slow conduction velocities and prolonged distal latencies

Disulfiram

General Characteristics

1. Disulfiram is characteristically used as a second-line agent for treating chronic alcoholism
2. Alcohol is metabolized by alcohol dehydrogenase to acetaldehyde, which is then metabolized by aldehyde dehydrogenase to acetic acid and excreted
3. Disulfiram inhibits aldehyde dehydrogenase which increases the serum concentration of acetaldehyde to cause symptoms of a "hangover"

Clinical Manifestations

1. The onset of disulfiram neuropathy is over weeks rather than over months which is characteristic of alcohol
2. Muscle tenderness
3. Hyperhidrosis of distal limbs
4. A subset of patients have painful lower extremity burning paresthesias
5. Numbness and pain in the soles of the feet that then progresses in a length-dependent pattern
6. Weakness of lower extremity distal musculature
7. Depressed ankle jerks
8. Loss of both large and small fiber sensory modalities below the knees

Neuropathology

1. Sural nerve biopsy:
    a. Loss of large-diameter myelinated fibers is predominate and although

there may be significant concomitant loss of small-diameter fibers
   b. Axonal degeneration
   c. Segmental demyelination
   d. Electron microscopy:
      i Axonal swelling due to the accumulation of neurofilament debris
2. Possible effects from carbon disulfide that is a metabolite of disulfiram metabolism in the liver
3. Degeneration of DRG

Laboratory Evaluation

1. Electrophysiology (EMG/ NCV):
   a. Low amplitude or unobtainable SNAPs with normal or reduced CMAP amplitudes
   b. Needle EMG:
      i Positive sharp waves and fibrillation potentials in distal muscles
      ii Decreased recruitment of neurogenic MUAPs

Thallium

General Characteristics

1. Thallium is a highly reactive heavy metal that exists in monovalent and trivalent forms
2. It is odorless and tasteless; in the past was widely used as a rodenticide
3. It is primarily used in the electronic industry, pharmaceutical industry and glass manufacturing
4. Exposure can occur by the respiratory route, skin absorption or oral intake

Clinical Manifestations

1. Neurologic signs and symptoms usually start within 2-5 days; rarely patients may be symptomatic neurologically < 24 hours post exposure
2. Pain and paresthesias of the hands and lower extremities especially the soles of the feet
3. Painful length-dependent sensory symptoms
4. Distal muscle weakness more severe in the legs than arms
5. Less frequently:
   a. Ataxia
   b. Tremor
   c. Athetosis
   d. Cranial nerve palsies
   e. Headache
   f. Seizures
   g. Insomnia
   h. Coma

i. Autonomic dysfunction
j. Neuropsychiatric manifestations
k. Associated medical conditions:
    i Gastrointestinal symptoms occur within the first 3-4 hours that include abdominal pain, nausea, vomiting, diarrhea or constipation
    ii Ocular dysfunction includes abnormal color vision, diplopia and decreased visual acuity from optic neuropathy
    iii The first cutaneous signs are scaling of the palms and soles with an acneiform or pustular rash of the face
    iv During 2-3 weeks, following exposure there is diffuse alopecia. The scalp, temporal parts of the eye brows, eyelashes and limbs
    v Mees lines occur in the nail plate (transverse white lines)
    vi Tachycardia, hypertension and pleuritic chest pain occur

Neuropathology

1. Axonal degeneration
2. Chromatolytic changes in anterior horn cells
3. Experimental studies demonstrate large intra-axonal vacuoles at the nodes of Ranvier

Laboratory Evaluation

1. Thallium can be recovered in the hair, nails, feces, saliva, and urine. A 24 hour thallium concentration evaluation by atomic absorption spectrometry is standard and should be <5 meq/L
2. EMG/ NCV:
    a. Low-amplitude or unobtainable SNAPs with normal or decreased CMAP amplitudes

Arsenic

General Characteristics

1. Arsenicals are still used in some agricultural pesticides
2. Chronic toxicity from ingestion or inhalation may be occupational or environmental (wells from water sheds near old mines)
3. Acute toxicity occurs with accidental ingestion, suicide attempts and intentional poisoning
4. Arsenic may be in Chinese herbal balls and Korean herbal medications
5. Arsenic is used to treat and preserve lumber, in wallpaper, to strengthen lead and in the glassmaking industry

Clinical Manifestations

1. Acute intoxication:
    a. A burning sensation in the mouth and throat

   b. Severe abdominal pain, cramping, diarrhea and vomiting
   c. Breath and stool smells like garlic
   d. Vertigo is followed by delirium, convulsions and coma
   e. Circulatory collapse followed by hepatic and renal failure
   f. Severe acute axonal neuropathy has followed treatment with arsenic trioxide for acute promyelocytic leukemia
2. Subacute arsenic toxicity:
   a. Abdominal pain
   b. A length dependent primarily sensory neuropathy characterized by burning pain and paresthesia
   c. Generalized muscle weakness
   d. Autonomic dysregulation
   e. A Guillain-Barré syndrome presentation

Neuropathology

1. Enzyme systems with sulfhydryl groups are particularly vulnerable to arsenicals
2. Pyruvate dehydrogenase may be inhibited by conversion of the cofactor lipoic acid, which contains a dithiol group, to lipoate arsenate. This reaction inhibits the conversion of pyruvate to acetyl CoA which inhibits the Krebs cycle
3. Sural nerve biopsy:
   a. Primarily axonal degeneration

Laboratory Evaluation

1. Patients with long-term exposure develop a microcytic, hypochromic anemia; eosinophilia and neutropenia may be concomitant
2. A 24 hour urine collection for total arsenic is diagnostic; it is also stored in hair and fingernails; the usual dose of arsenic excreted in the urine of symptomatic patients is 100-400 mcg/ 24 hours
3. EMG/ NCV:
   a. Low amplitude or unobtainable SNAPs with normal or reduced CMAPs
   b. Demyelinating features
   c. Prolonged distal latencies
   d. Slow conduction velocities

Nitrofurantoin

General Characteristics

1. Nitrofurantoin is an antibiotic primarily utilized for urinary tract infections

Clinical Manifestations

1. Patients most often develop sensory complaints of numbness and painful

paresthesias
2. Motor weakness may be severe and lead to quadriparesis
3. Elderly patients and those with poor renal function are at greatest risk
4. There is decreased sensation to all modalities in a length-dependent manner
5. Distal muscle weakness
6. Loss or decreased muscle stretch reflexes

Neuropathology

1. Axonal degeneration
2. Degeneration of DRG and anterior horn cells
3. Skin biopsy (1 patient):
    a. Clustered terminal nerve swellings without nerve terminal degeneration

Laboratory Evaluation

1. EMG/ NCV:
    a. Low amplitude or unobtainable SNAPs
    b. Normal or reduced CMAP amplitude
    c. Normal conduction velocities in the patient with small fiber presentation

Isoniazid

General Characteristics

1. Isonicotinylhydrazide (INH) is an antibiotic used as a first-line drug for the treatment and prevention of latent and active tubercular infections
2. It is utilized for typical and atypical mycobacterium (M. kansasii and M. xenopi)
3. INH blocks the formation of mycolic acids that are required for synthesis of the mycobacterial cell wall

Clinical Manifestations

1. Approximately 20% of patients taking >6 mg/kg/d develop a peripheral neuropathy
2. The standard dose of 3-5 mg/kg/d causes neuropathy in approximately 2% of patients
3. Elderly, malnourished patients and "slow acetylators" are at risk for peripheral neuropathy
4. The neuropathy usually develops after 6 months of therapy but has been described within weeks in patients taking high doses
5. Patients present with numbness and tingling of their hands and feet
6. During continued therapy, painful dysesthesia may appear in a length-dependent manner along with distal weakness
7. Examination reveals loss of all sensory modalities, distal muscle weakness and atrophy

8. Rare sensory ataxia
9. Generalized reduction or loss of muscle stretch reflexes

Neuropathology

1. Sural nerve biopsy:
   a. Loss of both myelinated and unmyelinated nerve fibers
   b. Axonal degeneration
2. Degeneration of the dorsal columns
3. INH causes pyridoxine deficiency by inhibiting pyridoxal phosphatase

Laboratory Evaluation

1. EMG/ NCV:
   a. Electrophysiology
      i Decreased or unobtainable SNAPs with less severe involvement of CMAPs

Nucleoside Neuropathies

General Characteristics

1. Zalcitabine (dideoxycytibine; ddC)
2. Didanosine (dideoxyinosine; ddI)
3. Stavudine (d4T)
4. Lamivudine (3Tc)
5. Antiviral nucleoside reverse transcriptase inhibitors
6. The above agents are all used in the treatment of HIV patients

Zalcitabine (ddC)

General Characteristics

1. At doses greater than 0.18mg/kg/d ddC causes neuropathy
2. DdC is a nucleoside analog reverse transcriptase; it is less potent than some other reverse transcriptase inhibitors (RTIs)
3. It is an analog of pyrimidine, is phosphorylated in T cells and other HIV target cells to its active triphosphate form ddCTP. This metabolite is a substrate for HIV reverse transcriptase and is incorporated into viral DNA. This terminates chain elongation due to lack of the hydroxyl group. Its activity is limited to retroviruses

Clinical Manifestations

1. On doses of 0.03 mg/kg/d approximately 1/3 of patients develop a peripheral neuropathy within 1 week to 1 year (mean of 16 weeks) from onset of therapy
2. Patients develop a length dependent extremity hyperpathia
3. Small fiber modality decrease of pinprick and temperature sensation are more affected than large fiber vibration and position sense

4. Mild weakness of intrinsic foot and ankle musculature occurs
5. Decreased muscle stretch reflexes at the ankle
6. The "coasting affect" may be seen 2-3 weeks following cessation of therapy

Neuropathology

1. Nucleoside reverse transcription inhibitors:
   a. Have varying affinities for human mitochondrial DNA polymerase γ (POLG) which is the primary enzyme for mitochondrial replication
   b. Loss of mitochondrial replication causes:
      i Impaired oxidative phosphorylation
      ii Increased production of free radicals
      iii Oxidative stress
      iv Specific NRTIs are more neurotoxic than others
         1. ddC is more toxic than ddI or d4T and the combination of ddI/ d4T
         2. The differences in neurotoxicity may be related to their affinities for specific thymidine kinase isoforms

Laboratory Evaluation

1. EMG/ NCV:
   a. Reduced or absent SNAPs

Painful Infectious Neuropathies

Lyme Disease

General Characteristics

1. Lyme disease is due to infection with Borrelia burgdorferi that is transmitted by the deer tick Ixodes dammini
2. It requires 12 to 24 hours of tick attachment to infect the human host
3. The three stages of Lyme disease are:
   a. Early infection characterized by localized erythema migrans
   b. Disseminated infection associated with systemic symptoms that include:
      i Fever and chills
      ii Localized adenopathy
      iii Fatigue
      iv Myalgia and headache
      v Neck and back pain
      vi Pericarditis and heart block
      vii Inflammatory changes of large and small joints
      viii Erythema migrans in other parts of the body
   c. Neurologic complications develop during second and third stages of the infection

Clinical Manifestations

1. Facial palsy may be bilateral
2. The neuropathy may be asymmetric
3. Approximately 50% of patients develop numbness, paresthesias, cramps and weakness distally in the extremities
4. Greater loss of vibration and proprioception than small fiber modalities
5. Muscle stretch reflexes are depressed
6. In addition to peripheral neuropathy (length dependent) patients may have:
    a. Mononeuropathies
    b. Mononeuropathy multiplex
    c. Painful radiculopathy
    d. Plexopathies
7. Associated neurologic manifestations include:
    a. Encephalitis / meningitis
    b. Myelitis
    c. Cranial neuropathies (VIIth nerve palsy most commonly)
    d. An inflammatory myopathy
    e. Acrodermatitis chromica atrophicans, a bluish discoloration of the skin, along with continued joint destruction may be seen late in the disease course

Neuropathology

1. Sural nerve biopsy:
    a. Perivascular infiltrates of plasma cells and lymphocytes around small endoneurial, perineurial and epineurial small blood vessels
    b. Experimental studies in Rhesus DRG explants exposed to live B burgdorferi organisms reveal:
        i CCL2 and IL-6 in sensory neurons, satellite glial cells and Schwann cells
        i IL-8 in satellite glial cells and Schwann cells
        ii Neuronal apoptosis
        iii B. Burgdorferi is internalized through the endo-lysosomal pathway that activates intracellular pathogen recognition receptors

Laboratory Evaluation

1. Immunofluorescent or enzyme-linked immunosorbent assays may be an initial screen
2. Western blot assays are utilized to confirm a positive enzyme-linked immunosorbent assay
3. CSF evaluation in patients with polyradiculitis, cranial nerve and central nervous system manifestation demonstrates:
    a. Lymphocytic pleocytosis

   b. Mild to moderately increased protein
4. EMG/ NCV:
   a. Dependent on the specific peripheral nerve involvement
      i A primary axonopathy in peripheral nerves
      ii Mononeuropathy or mononeuropathy multiplex
         1. Reduced CMAPs and SNAPs
         2. Absent H-reflexes
      iii Facial palsy:
         1. Decreased facial nerve CMAPs
         2. Abnormal blink reflexes
      iv Electrophysiological characteristics are often asymmetric
      v Needle EMG:
         1. Increased insertional and spontaneous activity
         2. Positive sharp waves and fibrillation potentials
         3. Decreased recruitment of MUAPs that have neurogenic characteristics

Human Immunodeficiency Virus

General Characteristics

1. Approximately 20% of patients that are affected by HIV develop a painful neuropathy from the infection itself or other associated viral infections such as CMV
2. A significant number of patients develop neuropathy from the neurotoxic effects of nucleoside analogs:
   a. Spontaneous pain that may be lancinating
   b. Associated autonomic neuropathy
   c. Mechanical allodynia

Clinical Manifestations

1. Distal Symmetric Polyneuropathy:
   a. DSP is the most common painful neuropathy associated with HIV infection and AIDs
   b. Numbness and painful paresthesias affect the distal legs and arms
   c. There is reduced sensibility to all modalities
   d. Mild distal extremity weakness is seen early in the infection; proximal leg and distal arm weakness is a feature of late disease
   e. Muscle stretch reflexes are decreased in the ankles but retained at the knees and in the upper extremities

Neuropathology

1. Sural nerve biopsy:
   a. Loss of both myelinated and unmyelinated axons

b. Loss of neurons in the DRG and secondary degeneration of the posterior columns
c. Perivascular inflammation composed of macrophages, T lymphocytes and increased expression of proinflammatory cytokines
d. Skin biopsy:
    i Decreased density of small myelinated (A-delta fibers) epidermal fibers is demonstrated

Clinical Manifestations Associated with CMV Infections

1. CMV Infection:
    a. An acute progressive lumbosacral polyradiculoneuropathy may be seen in severely ill AIDs patients
    b. CD4+ count is often less than 50 cells/mm3
    c. Patients present with severe radicular pain in the lower extremities
    d. Asymmetric leg weakness
    e. Loss of perineal sensation associated with bowel and bladder incontinence
    f. Less frequently the arms and cranial nerves may be affected
    g. Decreased or absent muscle stretch reflexes occur in the lower extremities
    h. Babinski sign may be demonstrated if there is an associated CMV transverse myelitis
    i. CMV associated retinitis may be associated

Neuropathology Associated with CMV Infections

1. Ventral and dorsal root inflammation is evident most severely in the lumbosacral areas
2. Less frequently there is involvement of cranial nerve roots as they exit the brainstem with associated myelitis
3. CMV inclusions are seen in endothelial cells and macrophages in nerve roots
4. Neurons may be damaged by CMV directly or by ischemia from a secondary vasculitis

Laboratory Evaluation Associated with CMV Infections

1. CSF:
    a. A neutrophilic pleocytosis that is associated with a low glucose and high protein
    b. Positive CMV cultures can be obtained from the CSF, blood and urine
2. Electrodiagnostic studies:
    a. NCS:
        i Asymmetric decreased amplitudes of SNAPs and CMAPs
        ii EMG (needle):
            1. Active denervation in the muscles innervated by the affected roots

Differential Diagnosis of Acute Cauda Equina Syndrome in the HIV Positive Patient

1. Infectious causes include:
    a. CMV
    b. Herpes simplex virus (1 and 2)
    c. Varicella zoster virus
    d. Mycobacterium tuberculosis

HIV Mononeuritis Multiplex

1. Multiple mononeuropathies are seen in patients with HIV infection associated with AIDS.
    a. Patients present with paresthesias and pain, numbness, weakness and loss of reflexes in the territory of the affected nerve

Neuropathology

1. Axonal neuropathy that may be caused by a necrotizing vasculitis or perivascular inflammation
2. Putative deposition of HIV antigen-antibody complexes on blood vessel walls
3. Associated hepatitis B and C infection or CMV involvement

Laboratory Evaluation

1. CSF:
    a. Mononuclear pleocytosis
    b. Elevated protein
2. EMG/ NCV:
    a. NCS and EMG evaluation is compatible with vasculitis

Herpes Varicella Zoster

General Characteristics

1. Herpes varicella zoster (HVZ) causes peripheral neuropathy from
2. Reactivation of latent virus or a primary infection. Severe disseminated zoster occurs in immunosuppressed patients while dermal zoster is associated with reactivation in later life
3. The reactivation rate is approximately 33% in seropositive individuals over age 50

Clinical Manifestations

1. Approximately 2/3 of infections in adults are manifested as dermal zoster
2. Severe pain and paresthesias develop in a dermatomal distribution:
    a. Thoracic dermatomes are affected in 50% of patients
    b. Trigeminal distributions in 18%
    c. Cervical dermatomes in 14% of patients
3. 25% of patients develop postherpetic neuralgia

4. The rash develops approximately 1-2 weeks following dermatomal pain. It is vesicular and appears in the affected dermatome
5. Weakness in the affected roots occurs in 5-30% of patients which develops within 2 weeks of the skin eruption but can vary from hours to a month
6. Segmental zoster paresis occurs:
    a. Involvement of thoracic dermatomes may cause abdominal hernias
    b. Unilateral phrenic nerve involvement with diaphragmatic paralysis has been described
7. CNS involvement:
    a. Encephalitis (particularly with V1 involvement)
    b. Meningitis
    c. Transverse myelitis
    d. MCA and carotid artery stroke
8. Neurological complications occasionally occur without a rash
9. Postherpetic neuralgia:
    a. Pain in affected dermatome for more than 3 months after the skin lesions have healed
    b. Pain is seen in 9 to 15% of patients after one month and in approximately 2 to 5% of patients at one year
    c. The pain may be spontaneous and burning, stimulus evoked or lancinating

Neuropathology

1. Evaluation of spinal nerves:
    a. Axonal degeneration with secondary demyelination
    b. Destruction of DRG neurons
    c. Secondary degeneration of the posterior columns
2. Following primary infection, a latent infection is established in neurons of the DRG:
    a. Latent viral DNA is in an "end-less' state such that the ends of the virus genome are joined to form structures consistent with unit length episomes and concatemers from which viral gene transcription is restricted
    b. Upon reactivation the virus travels down the sensory nerves to involve both motor and cutaneous innervations

Laboratory Evaluation

1. CSF:
    a. Elevated protein with or without pleocytosis
    b. Polymerase chain reaction to confirm the diagnosis
    c. Electrodiagnostic studies:
        i NCS
            1. Decreased or absent SNAPs in affected nerves

2. Normal or decreased CMAP amplitudes
ii Needle EMG:
1. Positive sharp waves and fibrillation potentials
2. Neurogenic like MUAPs recruitment in affected muscles

Herpes Simplex

General Characteristics

1. HSV-1 infection most commonly causes oral mucosal infection and facial skin lesions
2. HSV-2 causes genital mucosal ulceration; HSV-2 patients may not develop clinical disease but shed virus from the genital tract intermittently
3. HSV becomes latent in sensory ganglia following infection that is permanent

Clinical Manifestations

1. Both HSV1 and HSV-2 may cause meningitis
2. HSV-1 has been described in a patient with:
   a. Atypical lumbosacral pain
   b. Weakness of motor roots L4-S1
3. HSV-2 infection may cause:
   a. Weakness in L4-S2-S4 dermatomes
   b. Paresis of the urinary and anal sphincters
   c. Paresthesia and pain in the buttocks and lower extremities
   d. Patients may develop peripheral signs and symptoms after herpetic meningitis and encephalitis have cleared
   e. Shooting lancinating pain may occur prior to blister formation with genital HSV-2 infection (in genital areas)
   f. The first episode of infection may be the most severe and can be associated with fever, muscle pain, swollen lymph nodes
   g. Associated neurologic conditions:
      i Herpes keratitis
      ii Herpes encephalitis
      iii Severe neurologic complications occur in immunosuppressed patients

Neuropathology

1. Herpes is contracted through direct contact with an active lesion or body fluid
2. Virus gains entry into neurons by entry receptors that include nectin, HVEM and 3-0 sulfated heparin sulfate
3. Herpetic CNS lesions:
   a. Intense hemorrhagic necrosis of the inferior and medial temporal lobes
   b. Lesions may also occur in the cingulate gyri and insular cortex
   c. Acute stage demonstrates intranuclear eosinophilic inclusions in neurons

and glial cells

Laboratory Evaluation

1. CSF:
   a. A lymphocytic pleocytosis of 10-200 cells/mm3
   b. RBCs may be seen as is xanthochromia in some patients
   c. Rare hypoglycorrhachia with sugars below 40mg/dL
   d. Moderate increase of protein
2. PCR is positive in the serum and the CSF

Neuroimaging

1. MRI
   a. Classic medial and inferior temporal lobe hemorrhagic lesions

Syphilis

General Characteristics

1. Syphilis has reemerged worldwide in the late 1990s
2. Patients with concurrent HIV may comprise from 1/3 to 2/3 of new patients in some populations
3. Syphilis may increase viral loads in HIV patients with concomitant decrease of CD4 cell counts
4. Patients with HIV have an increased risk of developing neurologic complications

Clinical Manifestations

1. The treponeme most often invades the CNS within 3 to 18 months after infection
2. The initial occurrence that causes neurosyphilis is meningitis which occurs in approximately 25% of all patients
3. Clinical syndromes include:
   a. Syphilitic meningitis
   b. Meningovascular syphilis
   c. General paresis
   d. Tabes dorsalis
   e. Optic atrophy
   f. Meningomyelitis
4. There is usually a combination of two or more syndromes with one predominant

Tabes dorsalis

1. Tabes dorsalis usually develops 15 to 20 years after the initial infection
2. The major symptoms are lightening pains, ataxia and urinary incontinence
3. Neurologic examination reveals:

a. Impaired or absent vibratory and position sense in the lower extremities
b. Positive Romberg sign
c. Absent knee and ankle muscle stretch reflexes
d. Sensory ataxia
e. Minimal or no motor weakness
f. Lightening pains:
    i Occur in more than 90% of patients
    ii They are sharp and lancinating, more frequent in the legs but can occur from the face to the feet
    iii Rarely they are persistent in one location
    iv Associated paresthesias include that of coldness, numbness and tingling
    v The lancinating pain and paresthesias are intermittent and may last for hours or days
    vi There is loss of thermal, pain and tactile modalities in affected areas
    vii Often associated neurological complications include:
        1. An insensitive and hypotonic bladder that causes overflow incontinence
        2. Impotence
        3. Constipation and megacolon
        4. A staggering stamping gait
        5. Trophic foot ulcers and Charcot joints are characteristic; Charcot joints occur in approximately 10% of tabetic patients and affect the hip and knee joints most frequently
    viii Rarely seen is gastric crisis:
        1. The patient suddenly experiences epigastric pain that spreads around the body or up over the chest
        2. Patients may sense a feeling of thoracic constriction that is associated with nausea and vomiting; symptoms may last for days; attacks end abruptly
        3. Patients have residual soreness of the epigastric skin
        4. Other paroxysmal pain attacks that occur with tabes dorsalis include:
            a. Intestinal crisis with colicky abdominal pain and diarrhea
            b. Laryngeal pain
            c. Laryngeal pain with associated:
                i. Gulping movements
                ii. Dyspnea
            d. Rectal pain with associated:
                i. Tenesmus
            e. Bladder crisis with dysuria

Neuropathology

1. Atrophy of the posterior roots most prominently of the lumbosacral roots
2. Degeneration of the dorsal columns
3. Loss of neurons in the DRG
4. Normal peripheral nerves
5. The major mechanism appears to be inflammation along the posterior roots

Laboratory Evaluation

1. The CSF:
   a. Mild pleocytosis (lymphocytic)
   b. Minimal to moderate protein elevation with positive IgG oligoclonal bands
   c. Normal glucose
   d. In long standing patients, the spinal fluid can be normal
2. The standard serum evaluations:
   a. VDRL
   b. FTA-ABS
   c. Rapid plasma reagin (RPR)
   d. Treponema pallidum particle agglutination assay (TPPA)
3. 47-PCR and polA-PCR for CSF analysis

CHAPTER 4

PAINFUL VASCULITIC NEUROPATHIES

Overview

Vasculitides are immune mediated diseases that affect blood vessels and become symptomatic due to end-organ ischemia.

They are usually classified according to:

1. The size of the blood vessel involved (small, medium or large)
2. Whether it is primary or secondary
3. Or if it is isolated to the peripheral nervous system.

General clinical peripheral presentations include:

1. A mononeuropathy
2. Multiple mononeuropathies
3. Distal symmetric polyneuropathy (often asymmetric by EMG evaluation).

In patients with mononeuropathy, additional specific nerves become involved over time that causes a pattern of asymmetric peripheral nerve dysfunction. If there is a pattern of overlapping mononeuropathies, specific nerves are involved bilaterally to varying degrees that leads to a generalized, asymmetric process. If the process is insidious with a gradual progression, patients may appear to have a symmetric polyneuropathy. Approximately 60% of patients present with a mononeuritis multiplex pattern and 40% with a distal symmetric polyneuropathy. Patients with mononeuropathies most often complain of burning pain in the affected nerve's distribution. Neurologic examination reveals weakness and sensory involvement. Less frequently the presentation may be pure sensory. Muscle stretch reflexes are variably affected.

Laboratory evaluation usually demonstrates an inflammatory profile with an elevated sedimentation rate and C-reactive protein. Some of the vasculitides are associated with specific antibodies as exemplified by anti-neutrophil cytoplasmic antibodies (ANCA), antinuclear antibodies (ANAs) or cryoglobulins and rheumatoid factor.

Leukocytosis and a moderate anemia are often concomitants. The affected nerves are enlarged and hypoechoic by ultrasound. Electrodiagnostic studies most often reveal absent or reduced motor and sensory amplitudes. The examination is most often asymmetric. Distal latencies may be normal or slightly prolonged. Conduction velocities are normal or only minimally slowed. Rarely, pseudoconduction block can be seen in affected nerves. Needle EMG shows asymmetric denervation.

Sensory nerve biopsy reveals asymmetric nerve fiber loss between and within individual nerve fascicles with primarily axonal degeneration. Immunostaining may reveal IgM or IgG, complement and membrane attack complexes on or within blood vessels. Mononuclear cells, epineurial, perineurial and endoneurial vessels may be positive for the receptor for advanced glycosylation end products, nuclear factor kappa B. Interleukin 6 may be demonstrated along with CD4(+), CD8(+) and CD68(+) cells that invade the nerves. Blood vessels in muscle often demonstrate transmural inflammatory cell infiltration and necrosis. Matrix metalloproteinases, primarily MMP-9 are upregulated.

Painful Primary Systemic Vasculitis Diseases that Affect Large and Medium-sized Blood Vessels

Giant Cell Arteritis

General Characteristics

1. Temporal arteritis and Takayasu arteritis are the two large artery arthritides.
2. Peripheral neuropathy is only seen with temporal arteritis

Clinical Manifestations

1. Giant cell arteritis (GCA) affects medium and large caliber blood vessels that include the aortic arch, the internal and external carotid arteries and less frequently the vertebral arteries
2. Other cranial arteries than the temporal arteries can be involved in GCA which include:
   a. Branches of the external carotid artery the most important of which are the posterior ciliary arteries that affect the optic nerve
   b. Primary and secondary branches of the aorta
   c. Lower extremity arteries (rare)
   d. Mesenteric arteries (rare)
3. Typical clinical manifestations with temporal artery involvement:
   a. Preceding symptoms of fatigue, weight loss, and in some patients a generalized muscle and joint ache
   b. Headache (often burning) associated with scalp tenderness
   c. Jaw and tongue claudication (rarely ischemic tongue and nasal septum ischemic lesions)
   d. Sudden loss of vision from ischemic optic neuropathy

e. Peripheral nerve manifestations:
    i Occur in approximately 15% of patients and include:
        1. Mononeuritis multiplex
        2. Radiculopathy
        3. Brachial and lumbosacral plexopathy
        4. Generalized sensorimotor peripheral neuropathy
f. Peripheral tenderness of the temporal artery with nodularity (a cord) is apparent in less than 50% of patients

Neuropathology

1. GCA demonstrates an inflammatory infiltration of the arterial wall by lymphocytes, macrophages and giant cells
2. Only approximately 50% of patients have multinucleated giant cells
3. The inflammation is characteristically at the transition from the adventitia to the muscularis or less frequently to the adventitia and rarely the vasa vasorum
4. The internal elastic lamina is fragmented and the lumen is distorted; inflammation is most often segmental

Laboratory Evaluation

1. The ESR and CRP are elevated in 77 to 86% in the former (mean values approximately 90 mm/hr) and 95-98% in the latter (90 mg/dl).
2. Less than 5% of GCA have no increased serological inflammatory markers
3. Normochromic normocytic anemia, leukocytosis and or thrombocytosis are seen
4. Increased acute-phase proteins
5. Antiferritin autoantibodies are seen in approximately 90% of patients but also occur in other inflammatory and rheumatic diseases

Neuroimaging techniques

1. Color-coded duplex sonography:
    a. Inflammatory changes can be detected in the temporal arteries, extracranial vessels, the occipital and subclavian arteries
2. Edema of the vascular wall is seen as hypoechoic wall thickening ("halo" sign) often associated with stenosis and occlusions
3. Duplex sonography evaluates arterial flow that is accelerated in stenotic areas. The sensitivity of the technique is 85% and its specificity exceeds 90%. Reversal of flow through the temporal artery is a contraindication to temporal artery biopsy
4. The "halo" sign may disappear after 2-3 weeks of steroid therapy
5. High-resolution magnetic resonance imaging (MRI):
    a. The scanners utilized are 1.5T to 3T:
        i Swollen wall segments from inflammation can be differentiated from

unaffected vessels which may guide biopsy sites

b. MRA angiography to evaluate the aorta, supra-aortic arteries, visceral and extremity arteries if clinically indicated

c. ^{18}FDG-PET scan demonstrates GCA in arteries that are larger than 4mm in diameter

Polymyalgia Rheumatic (PMR)

General Characteristics

1. Approximately 15% of patients with PMR develop giant cell arteritis and 40-50% of patients with GCA have concomitant PMR
2. In the USA the incidence of PMR is 52.5 patients / 100,000 persons more than 50 years: the prevalence is approximately 0.5-0.7%
3. Caucasian patients are affected to a greater extent than other ethnicities, women are more affected than men and the disorder is rare in African-American individuals

Clinical Manifestations

1. Diagnostic criteria include:
   a. Age of onset 50 years or older
   b. Pain persisting for more than 1 month that involves at least two of the following areas: neck, shoulders and pelvic girdle
   c. Absence of other disorders that may cause similar symptoms
   d. Morning stiffness that lasts more than 1hr
   e. Rapid response to prednisone (<20mg)

Neuropathology

1. PMR is associated with the HLA-DR4 haplotype
2. IL-1 and TNFα gene polymorphisms are weakly associated with GCA and PMR
3. Absence of significant involvement of blood vessels
4. Synovitis, bursitis and tenosynovitis of the shoulder, hip, knee, wrist and metacarpal phalangeal joints may be seen
5. Putative recognition of an unknown antigen by dendritic cells or macrophages
6. There is systemic activation of both T and B cells; patients have an elevated IL-6 during exacerbations

Laboratory Evaluation

1. Muscle biopsy and EMG are normal
2. The ESR is mildly elevated in 7-20% of patients; it is usually greater than 40mm/hr and rarely may exceed 100 mm/hr
3. The CRP is often elevated and parallels the ESR

4. Normocytic normochromic anemia is common as is an elevated platelet count
5. Antinuclear antibodies, complement, rheumatoid factor and anti-CCP are usually normal; IL-6 is elevated during exacerbations and follows disease activity; serum B-cell activating factor (BAFF) is also associated with disease activity
6. MRI:
   a. Evaluation of the shoulder demonstrates subacromial, subdeltoid bursitis and glenohumeral joint synovitis; inflammation of the tendon sheaths in the hands has been described
7. ^{18}FDG PET has demonstrated inflammation of the subclavian arteries as well as uptake in the shoulders, hips and spinous processes of the cervical and lumbar vertebrae

Polyarteritis Nodosa (PAN)

General Characteristics

1. PAN is the most common necrotizing vasculitis; its incidence ranges from 2 to 9 patients per million population

Clinical Manifestations

1. Mononeuropathy is the most common pattern of peripheral nerve involvement
2. The sciatic nerve itself or its peroneal or tibial branches are the most commonly involved
3. Cranial neuropathy or CNS vascular disease occurs in <2% of patients
4. Myalgias and arthralgias occur in 30-70% of patients
5. Constitutional symptoms of fatigue, weight loss and fever are common
6. Associated organ involvement includes:
   a. Liver, kidney, gastrointestinal tract and skin
   b. The lungs are usually spared
   c. Abdominal pain, gastrointestinal bleeding and retroperitoneal hemorrhage occur
   d. Skin lesions include:
      i Petechia and livedo reticularis
      ii Subcutaneous nodules
      iii Distal gangrene

Neuropathology

1. Medium sized arteries are the most frequently involved although small arteries can be affected
2. Approximately 1/3 of patients have hepatitis B antigens; it is also seen concomitantly with hepatitis C and HIV

3. Nerve biopsy:
   a. Supplying vessels demonstrate CD8+ T cell, macrophage and PML invasion associated with fibrinoid necrosis of the vessel wall
   b. IgM, IgG, complement and membrane attack complexes are seen in the vessel walls
   c. Thrombosis and ischemic damage of the vasa nervorum is seen
4. The pain in vasculitic neuropathy may be associated with an increased expression of nerve growth factor (NGF)
5. The ulnar nerve is most frequently involved in the upper extremity
6. Approximately 75% of PAN patients have a neuropathy

Laboratory Evaluation

1. Electrodiagnosis:
   a. A multifocal axonal neuropathy with decreased compound muscle action potentials (CMAP) amplitudes
   b. Needle EMG:
      i A neurogenic pattern with spontaneous muscle fiber activity, polyphasic and high-amplitude MUAPs
2. Elevated sed rate
3. Other medium-sized vessel vasculitides include Kawasaki disease and thromboangiitis obliterans. They are not associated with peripheral neuropathy.

Small Vessel Vasculitis

Chung-Strauss Syndrome (CSS)

General Characteristics

1. CSS is a vasculitis that affects small blood vessels and manifests with symptoms that are similar to PAN
2. It has an incidence of approximately 1/3 of PAN
3. In contradistinction to PAN the respiratory system is frequently involved but neurological symptomatology is equal
4. Patients usually have had a long preceding period of asthma and rhinitis which then evolve into an intermittent phase of primarily pulmonary eosinophilic infiltrates
5. Vasculitic manifestations involve the skin, gastrointestinal tract, sinuses, joints and peripheral nerves

Clinical Manifestations

1. Involvement of the peripheral nervous system occurs in approximately 75-80% of patients
2. The neuropathy is primarily that of mononeuropathy multiplex but can be a pure sensory or axonal sensorimotor neuropathy

3. Patients often present with late onset asthma (>35 years of age)
4. Systemic vasculitis occurs approximately 3 years after the onset of asthma
5. 16-49% of patients develop a necrotizing glomerulonephritis in contradistinction to PAN which is on an ischemic basis
6. Patients have been described that were administered leukotriene antagonists

Neuropathology

1. Sural nerve biopsy:
    a. Necrotizing vasculitis with CD8+ cytotoxic T lymphocytes, CD4+ cells and slight eosinophilic infiltrates
    b. Less frequently both intravascular and extravascular granulomas are demonstrated around affected blood vessels
    c. Granulomatous vasculitis effects small and medium-sized arteries, arterioles, capillaries and venules

Laboratory Evaluation

1. Serum reveals eosinophilia, leukocytosis, elevated ESR and C-reactive protein, rheumatoid factor and IgG and IgM
1. 40-70% of patients have pANCA or myeloperoxidase antibodies
2. Approximately 50% of patients have positive pulmonary infiltrates on chest x-ray
3. EMG:
    a. A multifocal axonal neuropathy
    b. Mononeuropathy

Wegener's Granulomatosis (Granulomatosis with Polyangiitis)

General Characteristics

1. Wegener's granulomatosis has been recently renamed granulomatosis with polyangiitis
2. It is an autoimmune disease associated with granulomatous inflammation and anti-neutrophil cytoplasmic (ANCA) associated small vessel vasculitis

Clinical Manifestations

1. The prevalence of granulomatosis with polyangiitis is 5 patients per 100,000 of the population with its greater incidence being in northern Europe
2. GPA is seen in all ethnicities but its highest prevalence is in Caucasians
3. GPA granulomatosis is a necrotizing vasculitis that involves the upper and lower respiratory tract and causes glomerulonephritis
4. The early symptoms are nasal discharge, chronic cough, hemoptysis that evolves to dyspnea
5. Approximately 20-50% of patients develop neurological complications and include:

   a. Mononeuropathy multiplex
   b. Cranial neuropathies
   c. Distal symmetric polyneuropathy
6. CNS manifestations:
   a. Stroke
   b. Pachymeningitis
   c. Seizures
   d. Reversible posterior leukoencephalopathy
7. Neuropathy occurs more frequently
8. The peak incidence occurs between 64-75 years of age
9. The most common cranial nerves affected are the II, VIth and VIIth nerves:
   a. Cranial nerve involvement is seen in 5-10% of patients
   b. Caused by extension of the nasal or paranasal granulomas rather than by vasculitis

Neuropathology

1. GPA is a necrotizing vasculitis of arterioles, capillaries and venules
2. Clinical and experimental evidence has shown that myeloperoxidase (MPO), proteinase 3 (PR3) and lysosomal-associated membrane protein 2 (LAMP2) are major antigenic targets for ANCA in neutrophils
3. Tumor necrosis factor (TNF)-alpha and interleukin (IL)-1 induce the translocation of proteinase 3 to the endothelial surface that causes the adherence of neutrophils to endothelial cells. This induces degranulation of the neutrophils which damages the endothelial surface of small blood vessels

Laboratory Evaluation

1. The serum contains ANCA antibodies directed against proteinase-3 that has a specificity of 98% and a sensitivity of 95%
2. The absence of peripheral eosinophilia is a distinguishing point that differentiates the disorder from Chung-Strauss syndrome
3. Electrodiagnostic studies:
   a. Multiple mononeuropathies
   b. Symmetrical polyneuropathy

Microscopic Polyangiitis (MPA)

General Characteristics

1. Microscopic polyangiitis (MPA) is a necrotizing vasculitis primarily affecting the lung and kidney capillaries
2. Neuropathy occurs in 10-50% of patients

Clinical Manifestations

1. Mononeuritis multiplex is the most common peripheral manifestation

2. Similar to PAN and CSS; age at onset: 50 years
3. Skin purpura and abdominal pain

Neuropathology

1. There is severe involvement of pulmonary capillaries that leads to alveolar hemorrhage and interstitial fibrosis
2. MPA is a necrotizing arteritis that involves small vessels (capillaries, venules, and arterioles). Rarely medium sized arteries are involved
3. There is scant immune deposition in vessels and granulomatous inflammation is absent
4. ANCA in MPA is directed against myeloperoxidase and rarely against proteinase 3; it is an antineutrophil cytoplasmic antibody associated vasculitis
5. The kidneys may be affected with a pauci-immune necrotizing and crescentic glomerulonephritis

Laboratory Evaluation

1. Most often associated with p-ANCA and less commonly c-ANCA
2. Lung and kidney involvement
3. Electrodiagnosis:
    a. Most frequently a mononeuritis multiplex

Behcet's Disease

General Characteristics

1. Behcet's disease involves small and medium sized blood vessels
2. There is a relationship between HLA-B51; there is also a strong association with leukocyte antigen-B

Clinical Manifestations

1. Recurrent oral and genital painful ulcers; rarely sharply punched out skin ulcers are seen
2. There are inflammatory lesions of the eye, arthritis (often large joints), gastrointestinal lesions and thrombophlebitis of the hepatic venous and lower extremity systems
3. Neurologic complications:
    a. CNS:
        i Headache
        ii Meningoencephalitis
        iii Stroke
        iv Cerebral venous thrombosis
        v Arterial aneurysms
        vi Myelitis (rare)
        vii Psychosis

   b. Peripheral neuropathy is rare

Neuropathology

1. A vasculitic disorder of small to medium sized blood vessels
2. Studies suggest a T-helper type 1 (TH1) predominant response to as of yet unknown stimulus
3. Increased CD4 and CD8 lymphocytes are found in the peripheral blood in association with IL-2 and interferon-γ (gamma)

Laboratory Evaluation

1. HLA-B5 may be an associated genetic factor
2. Hypercoagulable state
3. Lower extremity Doppler ultrasonography:
   a. Symmetric venous involvement of all deep and superficial veins of the lower extremities

Secondary Systemic Vasculitides

Connective Tissue Diseases

Systemic Lupus Erythematosus

1. Approximately 20% of SLE patients develop a neuropathy during the course of their illness

Clinical Manifestations

1. Distal-symmetric
2. Mononeuritis multiplex
3. Approximately 70 to 80% are axonal and 20% are demyelinating
4. One third of patients develop autonomic involvement

Systemic Sclerosis

1. Approximately 30% of systemic sclerosis patients develop a neuropathy

Clinical Manifestations

1. Most often a predominant sensory neuropathy
2. Small fiber neuropathy
3. Autonomic neuropathy of the gastrointestinal tract
4. The "numb chin" syndrome (mental nerve involvement)
5. Carpal and tarsal tunnel syndrome

Sjogren's Syndrome

1. Incidence of neuropathy in both primary and secondary Sjogren's syndrome varies widely (2 to 64%)

Clinical Manifestations

1. Symmetrical and asymmetric neuropathies
2. Small fiber neuropathy
3. Trigeminal nerve involvement
4. Autonomic neuropathy

Rheumatoid Arthritis

1. Neuropathy is demonstrated in 15 to 50% of rheumatoid arthritis patients
2. Distal symmetric sensorimotor neuropathy
3. Associated carpal and tarsal tunnel compression is associated as is drug-induced neuropathy

Paraneoplastic Vasculitic Neuropathy

1. The most common malignancies associated with paraneoplastic neuropathies are:
   a. Small cell lung cancer
   b. Gynecological cancer
   c. Lymphoma
2. Less frequent malignancies are:
   a. Carcinoma of the kidneys
   b. Myelodysplastic syndromes
   c. Leukemias
   d. Bile duct
   e. Prostate
   f. Stomach
3. Lymphoma causes:
   a. Mononeuritis multiplex
   b. Generalized sensorimotor neuropathy
   c. Direct nerve infiltration

Clinical Manifestations

1. Pure sensory neuronopathy:
   a. Often burning quality
2. All forms of peripheral neuropathy have been described
3. High CSF protein and high sedimentation rate may be suggestive of paraneoplastic vasculitic neuropathy
4. Anti-Hu antibody may be seen in paraneoplastic vasculitic neuropathy from an underlying small cell lung cancer

Infection Associated Vasculitic Neuropathy

Hepatitis C Cryoglobulinemia

1. Cryoglobulins are immunoglobulins that precipitate at temperatures <37°C
2. The cryoglobulins are often asymptomatic or can induce a small-vessel

immune-complex-mediated vasculitis

3. Although most patients with hepatitis C infection develop cryoglobulinemia only 15% demonstrate vasculitis
4. Approximately 30-70% of patients develop:
   a. Small fiber neuropathy (painful)
   b. Mononeuritis multiplex
   c. Sensorimotor neuropathy (often asymmetric)
   d. Associations include:
      i Purpura of the skin (particularly severe in the distal extremities)
      ii Arthralgias
      iii Renal involvement
5. Other infections associated with vasculitic neuropathy include:
   a. AIDs
   b. Cytomegalovirus
   c. Epstein Barr virus
   d. Herpes varicella zoster

Rarer Secondary Systemic Vasculitides

1. Sarcoidosis:
   a. Mononeuritis multiplex
   b. CIDP
   c. VIIth nerve involvement
2. Inflammatory bowel disease:
   a. Incidence of 0.7% of vasculitic neuropathy; most associated neuropathies are nonvasculitic

Drug-Induced Hypersensitivity Vasculitis

1. Hypersensitivity vasculitis is most often secondary to drug reactions:
   a. Naproxen:
      i Rarely induces a leukoclastic vasculitis with neuropathy
   b. Minocycline:
      i Induces a vasculitic neuropathy
   c. Other drugs inducing a vasculitic neuropathy are:
      i Penicillin
      ii Cocaine
      iii Heroine
      iv Phenytoin
   d. Vasculitis may involve the CNS
   e. Petechiae are common
   f. Pathogenesis may be a complement mediated leukoclastic reaction

Nonsystemic Vasculitis of the Peripheral Nervous System

1. Vasculitic neuropathy can occur without systemic involvement (NSVN)

Clinical Manifestations

1. NSVN is seen in 60% of vasculitic neuropathies primarily in adult patients
2. The neuropathy is insidious and progressive in 1/3 of patients
3. Patients develop mononeuritis multiplex or a generalized slightly asymmetric generalized sensorimotor neuropathy

Neuropathology

1. Small and medium sized vessels are affected
2. Nerve biopsy:
   a. Axonal neuropathy
3. Intramural infiltration of epineurium and perineurium with T cells
4. Increased MMPs 2 and 9 that are secreted from T and stromal cells that:
   a. Destroy the subendothelial basement membrane
   b. Disrupt the nerve-blood barrier
   c. Allow inflammatory cell infiltration of the peripheral nerves

Laboratory Evaluation

1. Elevated sedimentation rate; positive ANA titers in some patients
2. Electrodiagnosis:
   a. EMG:
      i Mononeuritis multiplex
      ii Sight asymmetric sensorimotor neuropathy

Diabetic Lumbosacral Radiculoplexus Neuropathy (DLRPN)

1. The disorder is not associated with the severity of the diabetes and may affect patients in good glycemic control

Clinical Manifestations

1. Most patients have painful lower limb nerve roots, lumbosacral plexus and peripheral nerves
2. The disorder may develop acutely or insidiously
3. An upper limb variant has been described

Neuropathology

1. Nerve ischemia due to a microvasculitis

Vasculitis and Neuropathy from Essential Mixed Cryoglobulinemia

General Characteristics

1. Cryoglobulins:
   a. Are circulating immune complexes that consist of immunoglobulins
   b. They are temperature dependent and precipitate with a drop in

temperature and redissolve upon warming

2. The incidence of essential mixed cryoglobulinemia is high in areas where there is low HCV infection prevalence
3. Cryoglobulin classification:
   a. Type I:
      i Cryoglobulins are monoclonal immunoglobins, primarily IgM_{K}, that are directed against polyclonal IgG immunoglobulins
      ii They are most often detected in patients with lymphoid malignancies exemplified by multiple myeloma
   b. Type II cryoglobulins:
      i They are a mixture of monoclonal IgM and polyclonal immunoglobulins that are directed against polyclonal IgG antigens
   c. Type III cryoglobulins:
      i Are composed of a mixture of polyclonal IgM, IgG and IgA that are directed against polyclonal IgG
   d. Mixed cryoglobulinemia:
      i Consist of type II and III cryoglobulins
      ii Encountered in connective tissue diseases and with infection by hepatitis B and C
      iii Essential mixed cryoglobulinemia is:
         1. When mixed cryoglobulinemia occurs in the absence of an underlying disorder other than viral hepatitis
         2. The majority of patients with essential mixed cryoglobulinemia have associated hepatitis C antigenemia

Clinical Manifestation

1. A peripheral neuropathy is encountered in 25-90% of patients with cryoglobulinemia of any type
2. The neuropathy of essential mixed cryoglobulinemia is manifest by:
   a. Pain in a distal extremity distribution
   b. A symmetric sensory or sensorimotor polyneuropathy
   c. Mononeuropathy multiplex
   d. Pure small fiber neuropathy (rare)

Neuropathology

1. The mechanism suggested for the neuropathy is a virus triggered immune-mediated attack on nerves rather than direct nerve invasion as HCV replication in nerves has not been demonstrated
2. Putative mechanisms for the neuropathy include:
   a. Ischemia from hyperviscosity
   b. Vasculitis related to immune complex deposition in epineurial blood vessels

Laboratory Evaluation

1. Electrodiagnosis:
   a. NCS are similar to those of PAN
   b. One patient has demonstrated conduction block on motor NCS

Widespread Painful Disorders

Complex Regional Pain Syndrome Type II (CRPS II)

General Characteristics

1. Most patients that develop CRPS have suffered either an injury to terminal twigs (peripheral fibers) of C and Aδ nociceptive afferents (type I CRPS) in soft tissue, or have a frank nerve injury (type II CRPS), bone fracture, or have undergone a surgical procedure. Cluster analysis reveals that the signs and symptoms of the syndrome may be separated into distinct factors
2. CRPS affects more females than males (relative risk 2:1-4:1)
3. Average age of onset 37-60 years
4. Type I (small fiber axonal injury) is far more common than type II (injury to a major nerve)

Clinical Manifestations

1. Continued regional pain:
   a. Disproportionate to the inciting event
   b. Most often burning in quality associated with a deep ache
   c. Episodes of lancinating pain
2. Sensory signs and symptoms:
   a. Mechanical hyperalgesia
   b. Mechanical static and dynamic allodynia
   c. Thermal hyperalgesia
      i Cold lowers pain thresholds more than warm
   d. Pain spread from the initial area of injury most often distally to proximally
      i Rarely pain may be initially proximal to the area of injury
      ii Frequently over time the pain may be generalized to envelop the entire body
   e. After sensations:
      i Pain continues after the stimulus is withdrawn. It is not stimulus bound
   f. Mirror pain:
      i The pain is experienced in a similar distribution contralaterally to the injury
   g. Vasomotor motor dysfunction:

- i Temperature asymmetry
- ii Skin color changes:
  1. Livedo reticularis
- iii Sweating asymmetry

h. Sudomotor dysfunction and edema:
- i Swelling due to fluid in the body's tissue
- ii Hyper or hypohidrosis
- iii Sweating asymmetry

i. Motor and trophic alterations:
- i Decreased range of motion
- ii Motor dysfunction:
  1. Weakness
  2. Dystonia
  3. Myoclonus
  4. Rapid tremor
- iii Dystrophic changes:

j. Hair:
- i Early in the course of illness, there is hypertrichosis; the hair is thicker and more curly than normal. Over time patients lose hair in affected areas

k. Nails:
- i Become ridged and brittle

l. Skin is frequently erythematous, thickened and demonstrates livedo reticularis

m. Bones are demineralized and fracture easily

The clinical diagnosis requires at least one symptom in each of the factors and one sign in at least two of the factors. CRPS I and CRPS II manifest similar symptoms and signs. Multiple studies have demonstrated that the spread of CRPS is a common phenomenon with time in refractory patients. Mirror spread and contiguous extremity spread are the most common patterns. Rapid new contiguous spread has also been described. A study of the natural history of CRPS demonstrated that 92% of 656 patients reported the spread of pain in some pattern over the course of their illness. CRPS spreads and may encompass the entire body surface in a significant portion of long standing refractory patients.

Neuropathology

1. Peripheral afferent and efferent and central involvement that causes neurogenic inflammation (secretion of substance P and calcitonin gene related peptide) from injured nerve terminals
2. Activation of the immune system that causes an exaggerated inflammatory response
3. Maladaptive plasticity in both the central and peripheral nervous systems

4. Central sensitization is likely to play a role in contiguous spread, ipsilateral involvement and the generalized spread of CRPSII. It is manifested by:
    a. Spontaneous pain at the site of injury and beyond its spatial extent
    b. Mechanical pain hypersensitivity (AB fiber dynamic mechano-allodynia) and punctate and pressure hyperalgesia
    c. Temporal summation ("windup")
5. Mechanisms include:
    a. Enhanced membrane excitability, increased synaptic efficacy of pain projections and disinhibition of PTNs (pain transmission neurons). Increases of previously subthreshold synaptic afferent input to nociceptors above and below the affected segments (carried by Lissauer's tract in the spinal cord) discharges PTNS and increases their receptive field size. PTNs also receive small amplitude low threshold mechano-afferent (AB input) and nociceptive inputs outside of their receptive fields that become functional during central sensitization that further decreases receptive field threshold, increases receptive field size, and amplifies temporal summation.
    b. It has been recently demonstrated that generalized whole body allodynia and hyperalgesia can be produced by a migraine attack. Functional magnetic resonance imaging in migraine patients with generalized mechanical allodynia demonstrated acute thalamic activation to dynamic mechano-allodynia and heat stimuli. The authors postulated that central sensitization of thalamic neurons with total body receptive fields occurs or that there is pain-facilitation from "on" cells of the rostral medullary nucleus that project to the thalamus or descend to the spinal cord and induce hyperexcitability of PTNs at all spinal levels
6. Pain facilitation by central sensitization may also occur from neuro-immune interactions that cause:
    a. Activation of microglial cells and support their role in the initiation of neuropathic pain and that of astrocytes in its maintenance
    b. Nerve injury:
        i Has been implicated in the disruption of the blood-spinal cord barrier that:
            1. Results in an influx of inflammatory mediators
            2. The segmental spinal recruitment of T-cells and monocytes. The chemokines CCL2 and CCL20 are pivotal in this process
    c. There is support for the mechanism that neuro autoantibodies initiate a spreading inflammatory response throughout the neuroaxis. Radiolabelled PK11195, a biomarker of microglial activation, has demonstrated activation at the first dorsal horn synapse and in a minority of patients, trans synaptic activation in the thalamus
    d. An autopsied patient with long standing generalized CRPS demonstrated

significant posterior horn cell loss and activation of both microglia and astrocytes, most prominently at the index level (L5) but extending throughout the spinal cord.

e. A possible mechanism for both symptom spread and neuronal loss is activated glial secretion of pro-inflammatory cytokines, nitric oxide, excitatory amino acids, prostaglandins and adenosine triphosphate

f. Reorganization of the somatosensory cortex occurs after peripheral nerve injury; demonstrated by functional MRI:

   i The pain matrix which encompasses discriminative, affective, motivational and inhibitory components is modulated in CRPSII that may have a major effect on both the development and maintenance of widespread pain

g. Increased levels of proinflammatory cytokines that include TNF-α, interleukin 1-B, IL-2 and Il-6 and decreased levels of anti-inflammatory cytokines IL-4 and IL-10 have been identified in the plasma and cerebrospinal fluid and within affected extremities of CRPS II patients

Laboratory Evaluation

1. Quantitative sensory testing
2. EMG and NCS to evaluate the peripheral nerve injury
3. Triple phase bone scan
4. Plain radiographs:
   a. Generalized osteopenia, bone lakes and periarticular osteopenia

Fibromyalgia

General Characteristics

1. Fibromyalgia is a disorder of widespread pain and tenderness that has been continuous for at least 3 months
2. The pain is on both sides of the body, above and below the waist and includes the axial spine
3. The 2010 ACR criteria require:
   a. Fatigue
   b. Sleep disorder
   c. Cognitive dysfunction
4. The physician assessment:
   a. Physicians to evaluate patients by questions to determine scores on a widespread pain index (WPI) and a symptom severity (SS) scale
      i The WPI is a 0-19 scale that assesses pain in 19 different body regions that include:
         1. Shoulder girdle
         2. Hip

3. Jaw
4. Upper arm
5. Upper leg
6. Lower arm and lower leg
7. Upper and lower back
8. Chest
9. Neck
10. Abdomen

ii The pain is evaluated over the past week

iii The SS scale quantifies symptom severity in a 0-12 scale for:

1. Cognitive dysfunction
2. Fatigue
3. Unrefreshed sleep

Clinical Manifestations

1. Painful tender points as detailed by the manual tender point survey (MTPS) method
2. Other than the tender points outlined in the MTPS the physical examination is negative
3. The tender points are evaluated over the:
   a. Cervical spine
   b. Trapezius ridge
   c. Arcade of Frohse
   d. Medial scapular border
   e. LS vertebra
   f. Mid to lower back
   g. Medial knee
   h. Anterior chest

Neuropathology

1. Structural brain changes in patients with fibromyalgia have demonstrated:
   a. Moderate evidence that central sensitization is correlated with gray matter volume loss in the anterior cingulate and prefrontal cortex
   b. Global gray matter volume is unchanged
2. Functional MRI has demonstrated that brain activity is response to a nociceptive stimulus:
   a. Is similar in pattern to activation of the pain matrix but has greater activation than normal controls
   b. Some evidence for decreased functional connectivity in the descending pain-modulating system in FM patients
   c. Functional MRI evidence that the default mode network to insula

connectivity is associated with spontaneous pain in fibromyalgia patients

d. Altered fMRI activity in FMS has also been demonstrated:
   i Between the DMN and the anterior mid cingulate cortex, the right parahippocampal gyrus, left superior parietal lobule and the left inferior temporal gyrus
   ii Reduced functional connectivity between the DMN and the right parahippocampal gyrus has been demonstrated by correlation analysis to be associated with longer duration of disease
e. The translocator protein is upregulated during glial activation in chronic pain patients and is:
   i The rate-limiting step in neurosteroid synthesis
   ii Modulates synaptic transmission
   iii Related serotonergic mechanisms determine if pro- or anti- nociceptive neurosteroids are synthesized
   iv Fibromyalgia patients with the high TSPO (translocator protein) affinity binding genotype:
      1. Have higher pain intensity and more severe fibromyalgia as compared to patients with mixed / low affinity binders
      2. The effects are modulated by interaction with the serotonin transporter gene
f. A subset of patients with fibromyalgia have a large fiber demyelinating neuropathy similar to chronic inflammatory demyelinating polyneuropathy (CIDP)
g. There is mounting evidence to support a contribution of small fiber neuropathy to a subgroup of patients with FMS

Laboratory Evaluation

1. There is no consistent or characteristic abnormality on laboratory testing for fibromyalgia
2. Diagnostic evaluation is to rule out diseases with similar manifestations or to diagnose concomitant disorders
3. Skin biopsy to evaluate epidermal nerve fiber density

Small Fiber Neuropathy (SFN) as a Cause of Widespread Somatic Pain

General Characteristics

1. Definition:
   a. A small fiber neuropathy is a structural abnormality of small nerve fibers that is characterized pathologically by degeneration of the distal small fiber nerve endings
   b. Small fibers are unmyelinated C-fibers (1μ) and Aδ fibers (1-4μ) that

traverse the dermis to innervate cutaneous structures. Both types of fibers terminate as free endings in the skin

c. Aδ fibers carry epicritic fast pain, well localized and lancinating in quality as well as cold sensation
d. C-fibers transmit innocuous warm and possibly innocuous cold sensibility as well as nociception from high threshold mechanical, thermal and chemical stimuli
e. There is active interplay between fiber types on pain transmission neurons that also result in specific sensations as exemplified by the thermal grill illusion
f. Small fibers are a major component of the autonomic nervous system:
   i Thinly myelinated fibers are preganglionic
   ii C-fibers contribute to postganglionic fibers that innervate sweat glands, blood vessels and the heart
g. Nerve growth factor interacts with and is trophic for these small fiber neurons
h. Mutations in both NGF or its high-affinity receptor NTRK1 cause:
   i Degeneration of nociceptors and sympathetic neurons
   ii The cause of autonomic neuropathy type V (nociceptors) and type IV (sympathetic neurons)
i. Incidence and prevalence of SFN has not been established

Clinical Manifestations

1. Symptoms are variable both in severity and progression in patients with SFN
2. Symptoms usually start in the feet and progress proximally in a length-dependent manner. When the neuropathy crosses the knees patients note hand involvement. The pattern is that of stocking and glove sensory abnormality
3. Pain may be the presenting symptom. It is characterized by:
   a. Spontaneous (stimulus independent) but can be evoked by mechanical stimuli
   b. It is most often described as burning or prickling and in some patients has a pruritic element
   c. Pain attacks triggered by exercise or temperature suggest:
      i Nav1.7 mutations
      ii Fabry's disease
4. SFN may present with a patchy loss of sensation that involves the face or trunk which suggests an autoimmune cause
5. Autonomic dysfunction manifests with:
   a. Constipation and diarrhea
   b. Impotence
   c. Postural hypotension:
      i If severe, amyloid neuropathy may be causative

6. Trophic changes:
   a. Dry, cracked, erythematous and shiny skin (particularly prominent in CRPSI)
7. Motor function is normal
8. Reflexes are normal but in a subset of patients may be slightly hyperactive
9. Cerebellar and sensory coordinative function is normal
10. Large fiber sensory modalities of vibration, proprioception and light touch are normal
11. A distal loss of pin-prick or thermal sensation (easily tested with a cold tuning fork) are diminished. A subset of patients has punctate mechanical hyperalgesia and dynamic mechanical allodynia (pain evoked from lightly brushing the skin)
12. Resting tachycardia with a postural drop in blood pressure suggests autonomic fiber involvement
13. Diagnostic criteria for SFN in diabetes mellitus include:
   a. Possible - length-dependent symptoms and / or clinical signs (hypoesthesia in small fiber modalities)
   b. Probable – length dependent symptoms, clinical signs of small fiber damage and normal nerve conduction studies
   c. Definite – length dependent symptoms, clinical signs of small fiber damage, normal nerve conduction studies, and altered intra-epidermal nerve fiber density at the ankle and / or abnormal quantitative sensory testing of thermal thresholds at the foot

Neuropathology

1. Skin biopsy:
   a. A skin punch biopsy 3 mm in diameter is usually obtained 10 cm proximal to the lateral malleolus; alternatively, the biopsy site is the proximal thigh 20 cm below the iliac spine. In combination with the distal biopsy site may help in the differential between a neuropathy and neuronopathy
   b. Morphometric analysis:
      i Bright field immunochemistry or indirect immunofluorescence are the techniques utilized for routine diagnostics (bright field immunohistochemistry is most commonly utilized)
      ii The biopsy is stained for the PGP9.5 antigen a ubiquitin hydrolase that is found in all nerve fibers
      iii Intra-epidermal nerve fiber density measurements quantify the number of nerve fibers that cross the dermal-epidermal junction per millimeter of epidermal surface
      iv Values below the fifth quartile compared to age and gender matched controls are diagnostic of a SFN
      v Qualitative assessments of small nerve fibers include:

1. Axonal swelling, a marker of predegenerative change
2. Weaker PGP9.5 staining

vi In vivo corneal confocal microscopy can measure Aδ and C-fibers that originate in the ophthalmic division of the Vth nerve; corneal nerve bundle density inversely correlates with the severity of neuropathy

Laboratory Evaluation

1. The specific biomarkers of the disorders that cause SFN
2. Quantitative sensory testing
   a. Detection thresholds, pain thresholds (for mechanical and thermal stimuli) and stimulus-response functions (exemplified by "wind up") are evaluated
   b. Thermal detection and pain thresholds are most important for SFN
3. Electrodiagnostic evaluation:
   a. NCS primarily assess large myelinated fibers (AB fibers 12-22μ) and are unable to measure small fibers
   b. Conventional NCS are utilized in SFN workup to rule out a large fiber component (would suggest an autoimmune etiology)
   c. Laser evoked potentials:
      i Lasers can stimulate Aδ –fibers and their evoked cortical potentials allow evaluation of the somatosensory pathways from Aδ-fiber terminals in the skin to cortical terminations (SI, SII, insular cortex among others)
   d. Microneurography:
      i Recording microelectrodes are inserted into nerve fascicles that allow multiple small fiber recording. The function of small fibers can be directly determined but at the moment this is a research tool
   e. Autonomic nervous system testing:
      i The Ewing protocol for cardiovascular reflex testing
      ii Sympathetic skin response
      iii Quantitative sweat testing

Painful Channelopathies

General Characteristics

1. In these rare inherited conditions small fibers are dysfunctional but structurally intact
2. Inherited erythromelalgia (IE):
   a. IE is caused by mutations of the SCN9A gene that maps to chromosome 2q24.3 and is AD
   b. The gene encodes the Nav1.7 sodium channel

Clinical Manifestations

1. Episodes of symmetrical burning pain of the feet or legs associated with erythema
2. There is usually a family history but sporadic patients are seen
3. The usual onset is in the first two decades of life: late onset patients, in the sixth decade have been described with minimal ion channel dysfunction
4. The attacks may be triggered by a mildly warm stimulus or exercise and may be ameliorated by cooling (some patients place their affected extremities in ice-water)

Neuropathology

1. There have been 20 gain of function mutations in the Nav1.7 channel that cause IE
2. The mutations lower pain projection neuron firing thresholds which allows the channel to be activated by smaller depolarizations
3. Slow deactivation kinetics which keep the channel open longer once it is activated
4. Dorsal root ganglia pain projecting neurons are hyperactive

Laboratory Evaluation

1. Molecular genetic testing to delineate the specific SCN9A mutation

Paroxysmal Extreme Pain Disorder (PEPD)

General Characteristics

1. The mutation is in the SCN9A gene that encodes Nav1.7 that maps to chromosome 2q24.3

Clinical Manifestations

1. These patients suffer paroxysmal attacks of pain in the lower body, often the rectum
2. Pain may be experienced in the eyes, jaw and is often associated with flushing of the affected site
3. Attacks may be precipitated by defecation, crying or yawning or occur spontaneously

Neuropathology

1. The SCN9A mutations that are seen in PEPD impair inactivation of the Nav1.7 channel that causes an enhanced persistent current

Laboratory Evaluation

1. Molecular genetic analysis to delineate the SCN9A gene mutation that leads to the mutated Nav1.7 channel

Familial Episodic Pain Syndrome

General Characteristics

1. Recently described in one Columbian family

Clinical Manifestations

1. Severe upper body pain that begins in infancy
2. Upper body pain that is triggered by fasting or fatigue, illness, cold or exercise

Neuropathology

1. It is an autosomal dominant mutation in the TRPA1 gene that maps to chromosome 8q21.11
2. Encodes a non-selective cation channel that is expressed in a sub-population of nociceptors that can be activated by endogenous ligands or extreme cold
3. The biophysical kinetics of the TRPA1 channel are altered which increases current flow when the channel is activated
4. The mutation causes a single substitution in the S4-S5 region of the receptor which increases chemical sensitivity of TRPA1 but does not change its voltage sensitivity
5. This R852A mutation causes:
    a. Increased basal channel activity
    b. A loss of Ca (2+) - induced potentiation
    c. Accelerated Ca (2+) - dependent inactivation
    d. Putatively, the inter-subunit salt bridges between adjacent S4-S5 regions stabilize the conformations associated with the chemical and voltage gating of the channel

Laboratory Evaluation

1. Molecular genetic analysis to delineate the mutation of the TRPa1 gene

Infantile Pain Episodes Associated with Nav1.9 Mutations in Familial Episodic Pain Syndrome in Japanese Families

General Characteristics

1. The mutation in Nav1.9 was discovered by exome analysis with 12 affected and nine unaffected members in 2 families
2. Two missense mutations were identified in the SCN11A gene that maps to chromosome 3p22
3. Nav1.9:
    a. Is a tetrodotoxin (TTx) – resistant channel that is expressed in nociceptors
    b. It has hyperpolarized voltage-dependent activation that is close to the resting membrane potential
    c. It inactivates slowly which leads to a persistent current
    d. Mutations in Nav 1.9 have caused both gain of function and loss of function channel kinetics that cause painful and painless peripheral

neuropathy and autonomic symptoms

Clinical Manifestations (novel 1.9 variants, R222H and R2225) in Japanese families

1. A childhood onset; a subset of patients have onset of pain in infancy
2. In some patients, painful episodes decrease in adolescence
3. There are 3 subtypes of clinical manifestations with SCN11A missense mutations:
   a. Loss of pain (L811P)
   b. Painful small fiber neuropathy
      i G699R, L1158P and 1381T variants
      ii Cause painful small fiber symptomatology
      iii Late onset – the fifth or sixth decade
      iv Associated with:
         1. Skin discoloration
         2. Burning pain
         3. Autonomic dysfunction manifested by:
            a. Dry eyes
            b. Diarrhea
            c. Urinary alterations
            d. Palpitations
            e. Orthostatic dizziness
6. Familial episodic pain:
   a. Early infantile onset of episodic pain
   b. Gradual amelioration in adolescence
   c. Pain is primarily in the lower extremities
   d. Induced by cold and barometric pressure changes
   e. Relief of pain with anti-inflammatory medication and by warming the affected extremities

Neuropathology

1. In Japanese patients, all subjects had mutations at the arginine amino acid in position 222
2. Experimental evidence suggests that the mutation may impair axonal channel components that are important for AP firing, channel localization and distribution

Laboratory Evaluation

1. Molecular genetic analysis of the SCN11A gene to delineate the mutation

Primary Small Fiber Neuropathy

Genetic Causes

1. Nav 1.7 mutations
2. Nav 1.8 mutations
3. Nav 1.9 mutations

Familial Amyloid Polyneuropathy (FAP)

General Characteristics

1. Is caused by mutations in the TTR gene that maps to chromosome 18q12.1
2. Greater than 100 missense mutations in the TTR gene have been delineated worldwide (not all are amyloidogenic). The variants are primarily seen in single individuals or within a few families
3. TTR-FAP has a prevalence of 1 in 100,000 individuals in the USA and Europe; it is endemic in northern Portugal, Sweden, Cyprus, Majorca and Japan
4. It is heterogeneous as regards to signs and symptoms among individuals and between geographic locations

Clinical Manifestations (TTR met 30 type)

1. The most common form of familial amyloid polyneuropathy
2. Most often symmetric, distal neuropathy that begins in the lower extremities, progresses to the arms and then to the proximal extremities and trunk
3. Upper extremity involvement is predominant in the TTR184s and TTR L58H variants
4. Patients may complain of pain and small fiber symptomatology
5. Autonomic dysfunction is manifested as impotence and urinary dysfunction
6. Late onset progressive transthyretin-related amyloid neuropathy
7. All late-onset TTR-mutant patients manifest:
    a. Distal weakness
    b. Sensory loss to all modalities
    c. Loss of deep tendon reflexes
    d. Sensorimotor hand involvement
    e. Sensory-ataxic gait (92% of patients)
    f. TTR may manifest with congestive heart failure and postural hypotension

Neuropathology

1. TTR is a transport protein for thyroxine in plasma and retinol (Vitamin A)
2. TTR circulates as a tetramer of four identical subunits; it is synthesized by the liver and the choroid plexus
3. TTR mutations:
    a. Accelerate TTR amyloid formation
    b. Most mutations are associated with cardiac and/or nerve involvement
    c. Variably involved are:
        i The gastrointestinal tract

    ii Vitreous
    iii Lungs
    iv Carpal tunnel ligaments
  d. The described single point mutations cause destabilization of the quaternary structure into B-plated sheet predominant insoluble and inactive forms
  e. Tetramer dissociation is a required and rate-limiting process in the formation of amyloid fibrils
  f. Amyloidogenic mutations:
    i Destabilize the quaternary and tertiary TTR structure
    ii Induce conformational changes that lead to dissociation of the tetramers that then reassemble into partially unfolded species that form amyloid fibrils that deposit into the peripheral nerves and heart

Laboratory Evaluation

1. Skin biopsy
2. QST
3. Molecular genetic analysis to delineate the mutation in the TTR gene

Fabry's Disease

General Characteristics

1. Fabry's disease is an X-linked lysosomal storage disease due to a lack of alpha-galactosidase A
2. Its incidence is 1 patient in 40,000 males
3. Heterozygous females may be asymptomatic or due to lyonization or random X-inactivation may be severely affected

Clinical Manifestations

1. A large proportion of patients present with burning or lancinating pain in their distal extremities
2. Angiokeratomas:
   a. Reddish or purple maculopapular lesions are found:
      i In the bathing suit distribution (scrotum, inguinal and perineum)
      ii The umbilicus
3. Angiectasias:
   a. Small red lesions may occur in the nail beds, conjunctiva and oral mucosa
4. Associated medical complications:
   a. Small vessel cerebrovascular disease with stroke
   b. 0.0167% of all causes of end stage renal disease
   c. Hypertension
   d. Atherosclerosis with myocardial infarction
   e. Patients succumb by the fifth decade

Neuropathology

1. Sural nerve biopsy:
   a. Decreased small myelinated (1-4μ) and unmyelinated C-fibers (1-μ)
2. Glycolipid granules in DRG cells of the peripheral and sympathetic nervous system
3. Skin biopsy:
   a. Decreased epidermal nerve fiber density
4. The disease is caused by mutation of Xq21-22 that leads to decreased α-galactosidase and the consequent accumulation of ceramide trihexoside in peripheral nerves and vascular endothelial cells of organs

Laboratory Evaluation

1. A-galactosidase deficiency can be demonstrated in leukocytes and cultured fibroblasts
2. Molecular genetic analysis to delineate the mutation
3. NCS:
   a. Decreased amplitudes of motor and sensory nerves
4. QST:
   a. Increased temperature detection thresholds

Tangier Disease (TGD)

General Characteristics

1. Tangier disease is caused by homozygous or compound heterozygous mutation in the ABCA1gene that maps to chromosome 9q81; it is autosomal recessive
2. Families have been described from Chesapeake Bay, Missouri and Kentucky

Clinical Manifestations

1. Major presentations include:
   a. An asymmetric mononeuropathy multiplex
   b. A slowly progressive symmetric polyneuropathy affecting the legs > arms. Remitting and relapsing in some patients.
   c. A pseudosyringomyelia presentation with dissociation between loss of pain and temperature with maintenance of large fiber modalities of vibration and position sense in the arms
2. Large, yellow-orange tonsils
3. Enlarged liver, spleen and lymph nodes

Neuropathology

1. Tangier disease patients have elevated plasma triglyceride concentrations and almost absent HDL that result from mutations in the ATP binding cassette transporter A1(ABCA1)

2. The ABCA1 transporter:
   a. Facilitates the efflux of cellular phospholipid and free cholesterol to aggregate with apolipoprotein A-1 (apoA-1) to form HDL particles
3. Plasma deficiency or absence of HDL, apolipoprotein A-1 (apoA-1, the major HDL apolipoprotein) causes the accumulation of cholesteryl esters in many body tissues
4. Nerve biopsy:
   a. Axonal degeneration with both de- and re-myelination
   b. Electron microscopy:
      i Abnormal accumulation of cholesteryl esters in Schwann cells including those associated with thinly or unmyelinated nerve fibers
5. Skin biopsy:
   a. Decreased intradermal small fiber density

Laboratory Evaluation

1. Plasma HDL concentration of less than 5mg/dl
2. Low total plasma cholesterol (below 150mg/dl)
3. Normal or high plasma triglycerides
4. Electrodiagnosis:
   a. Motor and sensory NCS are normal or have moderate decreased amplitudes, prolonged distal latencies and slow conduction velocities

Other Causes of Small Fiber Painful Neuropathy

Idiopathic

1. Idiopathic small fiber neuropathy:
   a. In approximately 50% of patients with SFN no specific etiology can be determined
2. Sulfoglucuronosyl paragloboside epitopes
3. TTR met 30
4. Sulfatide epitopes
5. GALOP epitopes
6. Familial amyloid neuropathy

Burning Mouth Syndrome

General Characteristics

1. Burning mouth syndrome is also named stomatodynia, glossodynia
2. Definition:
   a. Any form of burning or stinging sensation in the mouth in association with a normal mucosa in the absence of local or systemic disease

Clinical Manifestations

1. The intra-oral burning or dysesthetic sensation recurs daily for more than 2h

/ day for more than 3 months
2. Most often encountered in perimenopausal or menopausal aged women
3. There is a female / male ratio of 7:1
4. The anterior 2/3 of the tongue is most commonly affected
5. Taste alterations and dryness are associated

Neuropathology

1. Putatively a neuropathic condition; possible small fiber neuropathy

Laboratory Evaluation

1. Neurotransmitter positron tomography has demonstrated hypofunction of the dopaminergic system of the basal ganglia:
   a. Spatial and temporal brain responses to noxious heat thermal stimuli are different in burning mouth syndrome as compared to controls

Ehlers Danlos Syndrome

General Characteristics

1. Ehlers-Danlos syndrome may be caused by mutation in:
   a. The alpha-1 (V) gene COL5A1 that maps to chromosome 9q34
   b. Alpha-2 (V) gene COL5A2 that maps to chromosome 2q31
   c. Alpha-1(1) gene COL1A1 gene on chromosome 17q
2. There are 6 major EDS variants the most common of which are:
   a. Hypermobility (hEDS)
   b. Chronic (cEDS)
   c. Vascular (vEDS)
3. There is a recently described overlap between hEDS and the joint hypermobility syndrome (JHS)

Clinical Manifestations

1. Pain is common in the various EDS types particularly in JHS/hEDs and manifests with:
   a. Recurrent / migratory onset of arthralgias in childhood
   b. An evolution by slow progression to a widespread chronic pain syndrome in adults and elderly patients
2. Patients experience:
   a. Burning pain (hands and feet)
   b. Dysesthesia
   c. Paresthesias
   d. Mechanical allodynia
   e. Cramps
   f. Diffuse myalgias
3. Most EDS patients have moderate to severe autonomic dysfunction

Neuropathology

1. Skin biopsy:
   a. A decrease of IENFD as compared with age and sex-matched controls

Laboratory Evaluation

1. Sural SNAP and conduction velocities are normal

Idiopathic Small Fiber Neuropathy (Possible Glucose Intolerance)

General Characteristics

1. Approximately 50% of small fiber neuropathies are idiopathic (no specific underlying etiology can be determined)
2. Approximately 50% of idiopathic SFN have abnormal 2-hour glucose tolerance tests or an abnormal fasting glucose which may be seen despite a normal glycosylated hemoglobin
3. Risk factors for the development of SFN:
   a. All of the features between prediabetes and metabolic syndrome:
      i Hyperlipidemia
      ii Hypertension
      iii Obesity
      iv Insulin resistance

Clinical Manifestations

1. Symptoms vary widely that often start as vague unpleasant sensations in the feet
2. Cold like pain, tingling and a pins and needle sensation that evolves into burning pain
3. The pain may be persistent but varies in intensity throughout the day
4. Lancinating electric shock-like pain, that lasts for seconds, may be superimposed on persistent pain
5. Symptoms may increase at night and during periods of inactivity
6. Mechanical hyperesthesia and dynamic and static allodynia may affect the lower extremities
7. Autonomic dysregulation may manifest as:
   a. Dry eyes and dry mouth
   b. Postural lightheadedness, presyncope and syncope
   c. Hypo or hyperhidrosis
   d. Erectile dysfunction
   e. Urinary frequency, nocturia and difficulty voiding
   f. Gastrointestinal manifestations:
      i Nausea and vomiting
      ii Constipation or diarrhea

        iii Early satiety
8. Motor and coordinative function is usually normal
9. Large fiber modalities of sensation that include proprioception, vibration and light touch are intact
10. Affected extremities have decreased thermal sensitivity and "pin-prick" sensitivity; a subset have mechanical hyperalgesia and allodynia
11. Some patients demonstrate dystrophic skin changes

Neuropathology

1. No specific etiology can be determined
2. Skin biopsy:
    a. Decreased intraepidermal small nerve terminal fibers (A-delta and C-fibers); lowest quartile
    b. Terminal axonal swelling and often abnormalities of sweat glands

Laboratory Evaluation

1. QST:
    a. Heat or heat-pain detection thresholds may be the most specific for SFN
2. Contact heat evoked potentials (CHEPs):
    a. Provides rapid cycles of heat that produce evoked cortical potentials that are linearly correlated between CHEP amplitude and cutaneous nerve fiber density
3. Quantitative Sudomotor Axon Reflex Testing (QSART):
    a. A measure of postganglionic sympathetic cholinergic function
    b. QSART is abnormal in approximately 75% of patients with SFN and sudomotor dysfunction can precede neuropathic signs and symptoms
    c. Other tests for autonomic sweat testing include:
        i Sweat imprint
        ii Thermoregulatory sweat testing
        iii Quantitative direct and indirect sudomotor tests

Primary Causes of Small Fiber Neuropathy

Idiopathic

1. Idiopathic SFN
2. Burning mouth syndrome
3. Fibromyalgia
4. Significant number of patients with glucose intolerance

Channelopathies

1. Nav 1.7 mutations:
    a. Inherited erythromelalgia
    b. Paroxysmal extreme pain disorder

2. Nav 1.8:
    a. Severe pain
    b. Brugada syndrome
3. Nav 1.9:
    a. Familial episodic pain syndrome
    b. Infantile pain episodes

Genetic Causes of Small Fiber Neuropathy

1. Fabry's disease
2. Tangier's disease
3. Ehlers-Danlos
4. TTR met 30
5. Sulfoglucuronosyl paragloboside (SGPG)
6. Sulfatide
7. GALOP

Secondary Causes of SFN

1. Impaired glucose tolerance
2. Diabetes mellitus
3. Rapid glycemic control "insulin neuritis"
4. Vitamin B12 deficiency
5. Dyslipidemia
6. Hypothyroidism
7. Chronic kidney disease
8. Hepatitis

Infections

1. HIV
2. Hepatitis C
3. Influenza
4. Erythromelalgia-related poxviruses
5. Idiopathic autonomic neuropathy (often preceded by upper respiratory or gastrointestinal infections)
6. Epstein-Barr virus-associated acute autonomic neuropathy
7. Chagas disease (chronic phase)
8. Mycoplasma infection

Toxins / Drugs

1. Anti-retrovirals:
    a. CART therapy
2. Antibiotics:
    a. Metronidazole
    b. Nitrofurantoin

   c. Linezolid
3. Chemotherapeutic agents:
   a. Bortezomib
   b. Bortezomib-thalidomide (used in the treatment of multiple myeloma)
4. Other Causes:
   a. Flecainide
   b. Statins
   c. Alcohol
   d. Vitamin B6 toxicity

Immune Mediated

1. Guillain-Barre syndrome (a component of the immune attack)
2. Chronic inflammatory demyelinating polyneuropathy (a component of the neuropathy)
3. Celiac disease
4. Sarcoid
5. Sjogren's syndrome
6. Systemic lupus erythematosus
7. Peripheral Nerve Vasculitis:
   a. Primary Vasculitides:
      i Periarteritis nodosa
      ii Chung-Strauss syndrome
      iii Granulomatosis with polyangiitis
      iv IgG4-related disease
      v Microscopic polyangiitis
   b. Secondary Systemic Vasculitides:
      i Systemic lupus erythematosus
      ii Systemic sclerosis
      iii Sjogren's syndrome
      iv Rheumatoid arthritis
      v Paraneoplastic vasculitic neuropathy
      vi Hepatitis C cryoglobulinemia
      vii Vasculitis without any systemic involvement (NSVN)
      viii Inflammatory bowel disease
      ix Paraneoplastic neuropathies
      x Amyloid
      xi Monoclonal gammopathy
      xii Mixed cryoglobulinemia

Other Causes of SFN

1. Critical illness
2. Complex regional pain syndrome type I (CRPS I)

CHAPTER 5

PAIN SENSITIVE CRANIAL STRUCTURES

Overview

The major pain sensitive structures of the head are:

1. The skin, subcutaneous tissues, muscles, extracranial arteries and external periosteum of the skull;
2. Eye, ear, nasal cavities and paranasal sinuses;
3. Intracranial venous sinus system;
4. The dura within the cranial fossae and primarily the proximal anterior, middle and intracranial segment of the carotid arteries;
5. Cervical nerves 1-3 and the cranial nerves as they traverse the dura

The pia-arachnoid, brain parenchyma, ependyma, and choroid plexus are insensitive to pain.

An understanding of pain radiations is critical for differential diagnosis of craniofacial pain. Middle meningeal artery pathology radiates retro-orbitally and to the temporal region. Pain that originates from the intracranial carotid, proximal middle and anterior cerebral arteries radiates to the eye and orbito-temporal areas. The first and second divisions of the trigeminal nerve transmit pain from the forehead, orbit, anterior and medial skull fossae and the upper surface of the tentorium. Sphenopalatine branches of the facial nerve subserve the nasoorbital areas. The ninth and tenth cranial nerves and the first three cervical nerves subserve the posterior fossa and the undersurface of the tentorium. Cranial nerves IX and X transmit pain to the soft palate and fauces of the tonsils. Cervical nerve one has no external pain radiation and innervates the odontoid process. Cervical nerves C2-C4 form the lesser occipital, pre and postauricular nerves and the third occipital nerve that innervate the posterior cranium and the external ear. Pressure on the tentorium may radiate pain into the inner ear. C2 irritation may be felt above the eyebrow. Diaphragma sellae distortion may be perceived as infrabrow pain. The tentorium delineates the trigeminal from the cervical-vagal-glossopharyngeal innervation territories. The trigeminal nerve carries sympathetic fibers from the first three cervical ganglia and parasympathetic fibers from the sphenopalatine and otic ganglia.

General rules of pain referral:

1. Supratentorial pathology refers pain to the anterior 2/3 of the head in the distribution of V1 and V2 of the trigeminal nerve
2. Infratentorial pathology refers pain to the vertex, brow, and neck primarily by the C2 root.

There is convergence of trigeminal and cervical afferents on dorsal horn pain projecting neurons at the C2 segmental level which is the anatomical basis for pain from the neck and occipital areas to project to the forehead (extremely common with C2 involvement in elderly patients with cervical spondylosis and during cough with Chiari malformations). The seventh nerve refers pain to the mastoid region, nine and 10 cranial nerves to the soft palate, fauces of the tonsils and eardrum (X) and larynx. The vertebral artery may refer pain to the lateral eyebrow. Dental and temporomandibular pain is carried by V2 and V3 (alveolar and buccal nerves). Cervical carotid arterial pain may also refer rarely to the eyebrow. Angina characteristically may radiate to the jaw and rarely to the cranial vertex.

Mechanisms of Cranial Pain

Intracranial lesions cause pain by distorting blood vessels and the dura at the base of the brain that may occur before there is increased intracranial pressure. Patients with increased intracranial pressure have bioccipital and bifrontal headache.

The Trigeminal Innervation of Blood Vessels

The proximal portions of large intracerebral blood vessels, nervous sinuses and the pial vessels are innervated by unmyelinated C-fibers. The unmyelinated C-fibers' origin is the ophthalmic division (V1) of the trigeminal nerve and the upper cervical roots (posterior fossa structures). These C-fibers co-release the vasoactive neuropeptides substance P and calcitonin gene related peptide in addition to glutamate when the trigeminal ganglia are stimulated. Some form of sensitization of these thinly myelinated and unmyelinated blood vessels occurs during migraine and other forms of vasodilatory headache.

Specific headaches are thought to occur from dilatation of intracranial and extracranial blood vessels that may also have sensitized nociceptive C and A-delta fibers in their walls. These include seizures, alcohol intoxication, nitrate ingestion, and monosodium glutamate (MSG). Compression of the carotid or superficial temporal artery may partially relieve this form of headache by decreasing arterial pulsation. Rapid arterial pressure increases that occur with pheochromocytoma, malignant hypertension, Valsalva maneuvers (intercourse) and with monoamine oxidase inhibitors may also be caused by arterial dilatation.

Vasodilation of Vessels Innervated by the Sensitized Trigeminal System

Inflammation of the extracranial temporal and occipital arteries (from giant cell arteritis) frequently causes burning persistent scalp pain early in its course and then becomes diffuse (activation of C-fibers for burning pain). Ischemic vascular disease in and of itself does not cause pain. Dissection of the carotid artery projects pain to the ipsilateral face, eye, brow, and forehead. Dissection of a vertebral artery projects pain postauricularly, to the upper neck and rarely to the outer 1/3 of the ipsilateral eyebrow. Basilar artery thrombosis causes a pain radiation to the basi-occiput and rarely to the forehead. Posterior communicating or distal internal carotid artery pain causes retroorbital pain.

Paranasal sinus pain or blockage accrues from infection of the maxillary or frontal sinuses. There is usually mechanical hyperalgesia over the sinuses. The ethmoid sinus causes pain deep in the midline behind the root of the nose. The sphenoid sinus may project pain to the vertex of the cranium (controversial lower face pain). The putative mechanism for these pains is activation of nociceptors in the sinus walls. The pain of frontal and ethmoidal sinusitis is at its maximum upon awakening and lessens with upright posture. The reverse is true for maxillary and sphenoid sinusitis. These symptoms are dependent on intrasinus pressure (activation of sensitized ASIC receptors; these are upregulated in nociceptive afferents when hydrogen ion is generated by the infection).

Ocular induced headaches are primarily localized to the orbit, forehead, temple, or the eye itself. In general, it follows a prolonged use requiring adduction and is steady and aching. It is usually caused by astigmatism, hypermetropia, and rarely myopia. Refractive error may also cause headache. Diplopia and eye patching are associated with frontal headache. Acute angle glaucoma causes raised intraocular pressure and steady, aching eye pain that radiates to the forehead. It is accompanied by an erythematous conjunctiva and may be precipitated by anything that dilates the pupil.

Meningeal irritation from blood or infection is most often acute (in the case of subarachnoid hemorrhage) and may be insidious with fungal or tuberculous infection. SAH causes severe generalized headaches that reach maximum intensity almost immediately and is associated with nausea, vomiting, and neck stiffness. A major component of meningeal irritation is pro-inflammatory cytokines released from immune cells, prostaglandins (PGE2), kinins, serotonin, and blood components. Sensitized blood vessel and meningeal nociceptors may also be activated by increased intracranial pressure. Sudden severe headaches ("thunderclap") are also caused by posterior reversible encephalopathy syndrome, eclampsia, migraine, dissection of major arteries but most importantly subarachnoid hemorrhage from any source.

Low CSF pressure headaches are most frequently caused by lumbar puncture. They may occur spontaneously from leakage of CSF from perineural cysts or dural tears. They are associated with a steady occipital nuchal and frontal headache that occurs with erect posture and are relieved rapidly with recumbency. The headache may be exacerbated by jugular vein pressure. It is often associated with mild nausea and is purported to be caused by traction of dural structures by caudal brain displacement.

Postural headaches, particularly those with recumbency occur with subdural hematoma (may also be exacerbated by the upright posture) and with posterior fossa mass lesions. The headache of idiopathic intracranial hypertension (pseudotumor cerebri) may also be worse in the morning.

Tension Headache

General Characteristics

1. Tension type headache is classified as:
   a. Infrequent episodic
      i Fewer than one headache per month
   b. Frequent episodic TTH
      i Two to 14 headaches per month
   c. Chronic TTH
      i 15 or more headache days a month
   d. Tension headache has been estimated to affect more than 4% of the population and is more prevalent in women

Clinical Manifestations

1. The onset is usually in middle age rather than childhood or adolescence
2. It is typically bilaterally located in occipital nuchal, temporal or frontal areas
3. The pain is usually dull, aching or tightness and pressure from a band surrounding the cranium; in some instances, they may have a throbbing quality.
4. There are no migraine type auras and the headaches usually do not interfere with activities of daily living
5. The onset is often gradual and once established may be very long-lasting; from 30 minutes to 7 days
6. They are more variable in duration, more quality specific and less severe than migraine
7. Migraine and traumatic headaches may be complicated by tension headache.

Neuropathology

1. Pressure pain thresholds over the temporalis, masseter and frontalis muscles are lower in TTH than age-matched controls
2. Increased presence and tenderness of myofascial trigger points may sensitize central pain projecting neurons

Neuroimaging

1. MRI to delineate a structural cause of headache
2. Sedimentation rate to rule out giant cell arteritis

Brain Tumor Headache

General Characteristics

1. Headache occurs in approximately 1/3 to 50% of patients with brain tumors.

It is rare to be the initial symptom that brings the patient for an examination

Clinical Manifestations

1. There are no specific features that delineate brain tumor headaches
2. In general, it is felt as deep seated, usually steady (rarely throbbing), and may be described as aching.
3. Physical activity may be provoking and rest may be a relieving factor
4. Nocturnal awakening due to pain is unusual and is caused by cluster headache, hypnic headaches or caffeine withdrawal
5. Projectile vomiting without nausea may occur in late stages in adults or in posterior fossa tumors that irritate the vomit center in the floor of the IVth ventricle. It is more common in children with posterior fossa tumors
6. If the headache is unilateral it is on the same side as the tumor
7. Bifrontal and bioccipital headache after a period of unilateral headache suggests hydrocephalus
8. Colloid cysts of the IIIrd ventricle or those that obstruct the foramina of Monroe as well as giant subependymal astrocytomas at this site frequently are associated with headache
9. Paroxysmal headaches have been described with both intra and peri-ventricular brain tumors. Their characteristics are:
   a. Severity
   b. Reach maximum intensity in a few seconds
   c. Last for minutes to an hour and then rapidly subside
10. Brain tumors with greatly elevated intracranial pressure cause:
    a. Vomiting
    b. Transient obscuration of vision (suprachiasmatic cistern pressure that renders the chiasm ischemic)
    c. Leg weakness with "drop attacks"
    d. Loss of consciousness
    e. These paroxysmal attacks have been described with colloid cysts of the IIIrd ventricle, craniopharyngiomas, pinealomas and cerebellar tumors

Neuropathology

1. Headaches of brain tumors are caused by displacement of major cerebral blood vessels or hydrocephalus from blockage of CSF flow at different levels. Unilateral ventricular enlargement from a choroid plexus papilloma may cause headache on the ipsilesional side

Laboratory Evaluation

1. Sed rate to rule out inflammatory conditions

Neuroimaging

1. MRI:

   a. To delineate the mass lesion and consequent cerebral edema
   b. To rule out multiple intraparenchymal lesions
   c. To rule out brain tumor mimics that include subdural hematoma and abscess as well as hemorrhage or unusual pathologies associated with mass lesions
2. Electroencephalogram:
   a. To evaluate seizure potential

Post-Traumatic Headache

General Characteristics

1. Impact-related mild traumatic brain injury is primarily caused by contact sports, motor vehicle accidents, falls and assaults
2. It is estimated that approximately 1.6-3.8 million mild TBI occur each year in the USA

Clinical Manifestations

1. Longitudinal studies demonstrate an incidence of 71% of headache after moderate (mTBI) or severe TBI and a cumulative incidence of 91% after mild mTBI; prevalence remains at 44% over one year with moderate TBI and 54% after mTBI
2. A prior history of headache is associated with a higher risk of PTH
3. Five symptom clusters are identified in patients with mTBI:
   a. Post-traumatic headache / migraine
   b. Nausea
   c. Emotional / affective
   d. Fatigue / malaise
   e. Dizziness / mild cognitive impairment
4. The most common headache phenotypes utilizing ICHD-3 criteria with mTBI are:
   a. Migraine / probable migraine in 50% of patients with headache
   b. Tension type headache

Neuropathology

1. Concussion is associated with diffuse axonal injury that may not be detectable with conventional MRI
2. In mTBI:
   a. Biomechanical forces cause linear and rotational acceleration-deceleration of the brain that creates diffuse shear strains on parenchymal tissue
   b. Axonal injury in mTBI develops over days to weeks after the injury
   c. Present theories support a post-traumatic metabolic cascade that involves glutamate release, ion fluxes and free radicals that cause mitochondrial dysfunction and calcium sequestration

   d. Energy crisis with lack of ATP leads to cytoskeletal damage as excess intracellular calcium damages myelin and oligodendrocytes
   e. Impaired axonal transport may cause secondary axonal disconnection and Wallerian degeneration
   f. Global and regional decreased blood flow also occur with concussion and with cerebral hypoperfusion there is oxidative stress
   g. Histopathology:
      i Axonal bulbs, irregular tortuous axonal varicosities and small globoids of degraded myelin sheath are described
      ii Mechanical strains that are diffuse along the length of an axon cause an elongated pattern of axonal swelling

Laboratory Evaluation

1. Relationship between the apolipoprotein E gene and headache following concussion
   a. Patients with the APOe4 allele may be more likely to sustain a post-concussion headache
   b. Headache may be more severe after the concussion'

Neuroimaging

1. Myelin water imaging:
   a. Evaluates changes in myelin water fraction derived from the T2 decay signal
   b. After 2 weeks post-injury (concussion) decreased myelin water fraction in:
      i The splenium of the corpus callosum
      ii Posterior thalamic radiations
      iii Superior corona radiata
      iv Superior longitudinal fasciculus
      v Posterior limb of the internal capsule
      vi Myelin water fraction recovers to pre-injury values by 2 months post-injury

Laboratory Evaluation

1. Relationship between the apolipoprotein E gene and headache following concussion:
   a. Patients with the APOe4 allele may be more likely to sustain a post-concussion headache
   b. Headache may be more severe after the concussion

Subdural Hematoma (SDH)

General Characteristics

1. Definition:
   a. A subdural hematoma is loculation of blood below the inner layer of the dura but external to the brain parenchyma
   b. Acute SDH are less than 72 hours old. The subacute phase is thought to begin 3 to 7 days following acute injury
   c. Chronic SDH develop over weeks

Clinical Manifestations

1. Lucid intervals (following concussions) occur in approximately 40% of patients with acute SDH
2. Acute subdural hematomas are more likely than chronic ones to be associated with primary brain injury
3. More than 50% of comatose patients with acute SDH suffer parenchymal contusions
4. Headache of chronic subdural hematoma:
   a. Deep seated and dull
   b. Steady and is unilateral (the scalp may be tender to mechanical stimuli)
   c. May be associated with lethargy, confusion and fluctuating hemiparesis
   d. In acute SDH:
      i Positional exacerbation of pain after recumbency or leaning the head to one side
      ii The headache increases in frequency and severity over weeks
   e. Tentorial hematomas may cause pain in the eye

Neuropathology

1. Acute SDHs are caused by high-impact trauma to the skull with consequent acceleration-deceleration brain tissue movement relative to fixed blood vessel and dural structures
2. The usual ruptured vessels are those that connect the cortical surface to a dural sinus, the bridging veins
3. Bridging veins are stretched with brain parenchymal atrophy; less frequently, a cortical vein or small artery may be torn by direct trauma. One study has demonstrated that ruptured cortical arteries are located around the Sylvian fissure.
4. Associated with the head trauma are:
   a. Parenchymal hematomas
   b. Contusions
   c. Subarachnoid hemorrhage
   d. Diffuse axonal injury
5. Low pressure venous bleeding from ruptured cortical veins dissects the arachnoid from the dura and then layers out over the convexity
6. In the subacute phase the clotted blood liquefies (a hematocrit-like effect)

7. The chronic phase demonstrates that cellular elements disintegrate leaving serous fluid in the subdural space which rarely calcifies
8. The rate of acceleration-deceleration of the head determines bridging vein failure
9. Risk factors for chronic SDH include:
    a. Chronic alcoholism
    b. Seizures
    c. Coagulopathy
    d. Arachnoid cysts
    e. Anticoagulant therapy
    f. Hypertension
    g. Arteriosclerosis
    h. Thrombocytopenia
    i. Diabetes mellitus

Laboratory Evaluation

1. Initial blood tests:
    a. Complete blood count
    b. Coagulation profile
    c. Metabolic panel:
        i Serum sodium is of particular importance as hyponatremia is seen in 5-12% of patients with head injury and exacerbates cerebral edema and lowers seizure threshold

Neuroimaging

1. CT scan:
    a. Images can be obtained within 5 minutes
    b. Highly sensitive to acute blood
2. MRI:
    a. Sensitive to the size of the hematoma and to soft tissue pathology

Mimics of Subdural Hematoma

1. Metastasis
2. Lymphoma
3. Sarcoma
4. Infections
5. Autoimmune disorders

Headache of Temporal Arteritis (GCA)

General Characteristics

1. A very important headache in older patients; almost all patients are older than 65 years of age
2. Giant cell arteritis primarily involves the major branches of the aorta with

typical involvement of the extra-cranial branches of the carotid artery

Clinical Manifestations

1. Constitutional symptoms are present in a significant number of patients that consist of a low-grade fever, weight loss and associated mild anemia
2. The headache:
    a. Insidious throbbing or non-throbbing headache with superimposed lancinating pain
    b. Rarely the headache has an explosive onset
    c. The pain is usually unilateral, less frequently bilateral and often localized to the affected arteries
    d. Approximately 50% of patients have aching in the proximal limb girdle muscles that is associated with polymyalgia rheumatica
    e. The headache pain is persistent throughout the day and is often exacerbated at night
    f. If untreated, the headache may last for months
    g. Associated symptoms include:
        i Jaw claudication
        ii A burning scalp
        iii Episodes of amaurosis fugax:
            1. Transient monocular blindness or looking through a haze with loss of visual acuity
            2. Rare ophthalmoplegia
    h. Ischemic nodules in the scalp, a perforated nasal septum and tongue lesions that resemble squamous cell carcinoma have been described
    i. The superficial temporal and other scalp arteries may be thickened and tender

Neuropathology

1. Temporal artery biopsy demonstrates:
    a. An intense granulomatous or "giant cell" arteritis
2. Recent experimental work supports the role of cytokine pathways that include:
    a. Pro-inflammatory interleukins
    b. IL-6-IL-17 axis
    c. IL-12 interferon-gamma-axis

Laboratory Evaluation

1. The sedimentation rate is usually >50mm/h and often >75mm/h
2. The C-reactive protein is more sensitive than the sedimentation rate and is particularly helpful if the sed rate is only mildly elevated
3. A subgroup of patients have leukocytosis
4. Ultrasonography:

   a. May demonstrate a halo and irregularly thickened vessel walls
5. Temporal artery biopsy is the gold standard for diagnosis; occasionally extracranial external arteriography is utilized for selection of the biopsy site

Headache of Idiopathic Intracranial Hypertension (IIH)

General Characteristics

1. Definition – IIH is characterized by increased intracranial pressure without radiological and laboratory evidence of intracranial pathology except for an empty sellae, optic nerve sheaths distended with cerebrospinal fluid and smooth-walled non-flow-related venous sinus stenosis or compression
2. The most commonly affected patients are obese women of child-bearing age but it is described in patients of any age or sex
3. The incidence of IIH varies from 0.03 to 2.36/100,000/year of the total population

Clinical Manifestations

1. Headache is the most common symptom and is present in 80-90% of patients
2. Headache characteristics:
   a. Typically frontal or retro-orbital pressure-like or less frequently throbbing
   b. May be associated with nausea, vomiting and transient visual obscurations
   c. Some patients note exacerbation with recumbency
   d. There is no relationship between the severity or frequency of the headache and the intracranial pressure
   e. Approximately 40% of IIH patients have a migraine headache history
   f. Headache may resemble a tension-type pattern
3. Visual deficits:
   a. Transient visual obscurations
      i Loss or graying out of vision (looking through "gauze") for less than 30 seconds (usually a few seconds) is seen in 68% of patients and is due to ischemia of the optic chiasm from pressure on the suprachiasmatic cistern); other mechanisms proposed are ischemia of the optic nerve head and herniation of the parahippocampal gyrus into the tentorial notch
      ii Tunnel vision
      iii Decreased visual acuity
      iv Papilledema
      v Pulsatile tinnitus is reported in 52% of patients; rarely low-frequency hearing loss and vertigo are reported
      vi Diplopia from VIth nerve palsy

Neuropathology

1. The cause of IIH is being evaluated. The link between obstructive segments in the distal transverse sinus and increased arterial inflow is a possible mechanism
2. It is seen in association with:
   a. Metabolic disorders
   b. Drugs and their withdrawal
   c. Disruption of venous outflow from the brain
   d. Systemic diseases

Laboratory Evaluation

1. Complete blood count
2. Pro-coagulant profile
3. Serum iron and iron-binding capacity
4. Antinuclear antigen
5. Lyme screen
6. Lumbar puncture:
   a. CSF is under pressure but otherwise negative; rarely the protein is low

Neuroimaging

1. MRI:
   a. Imaging of the head and orbit with contrast and magnetic resonance venography (MRV)
   b. MRI features:
      i Empty sellae
      ii Narrowing of the trigeminal cave
      iii Enlargement of the foramen ovale; less frequent enlargement of the jugular foramen and hypoglossal canal
      iv Slit ventricles
      v Stenosis of the transverse sinus
      vi Enlarged optic nerve sheaths
      vii Flattening of the posterior globe

Low CSF Pressure Headache

General Characteristics

1. Spontaneous intracranial hypotension most often occurs from cerebrospinal leaks at the spinal level and rarely from the skull base
2. The leaks cause loss of CSF volume that may be associated with subdural fluid collections

Clinical Manifestations

1. The headaches' most distinguishing feature is exacerbation with the upright

posture and relief with recumbency
2. If untreated the headache may last for days or weeks
3. The headache may be at the brow the back of the skull and radiates to the upper back of the neck and thoracic spine and shoulders
4. The headache is often associated with nausea, neck stiffness and vomiting
5. Tinnitus, vertigo and VIth nerve palsy are not uncommon
6. Self-audible bruit

Neuropathology

1. The syndrome is posited to be caused by downward displacement of the upper brainstem and posterior fossa with the upright posture; the VI nerve may be trapped under the petroclinoid ligament
2. The CSF pressure may be extremely low (60mm H2O) or not measurable
3. Rupture of a perineurial spinal nerve sleeve may be causitive
4. Connective tissue diseases that include Marfan's syndrome, Ehlers-Danlos syndrome and autosomal dominant polycystic kidney disease may be associated

Laboratory Evaluation

1. CSF:
   a. A subgroup of patients may demonstrate a mild lymphocytic pleocytosis; slight to moderate elevated protein and normal glucose concentration

Neuroimaging

1. MRI:
   a. Subdural fluid collections, pachymeningeal enhancement, engorgement of venous structures, pituitary hyperemia and sagging of the brain
   b. Radioisotope cisternography and CT myelography are utilized to delineate the site of CSF leakage

Cough Headache

General Characteristics

1. A headache that is precipitated by coughing or straining in the absence of intracranial disorder lasting up to 30 minutes

Clinical Manifestations

1. Cough headache is usually bilateral but can be unilateral
2. Most often is localized to the fronto-temporal areas of the cranium
3. Usually affects individuals over 40 years of age
4. Usually lasts for 1 second to 30 minutes but longer duration headaches have been described (a few patients with headaches lasting 2 hours)
5. Cough headache can be triggered by other Valsalva maneuvers but not by exercise

6. Nausea, vomiting photo- and phonophobia are distinctly rare
7. The pain may have a bursting quality
8. May be so severe as to simulate headache of subarachnoid hemorrhage

Symptomatic Cough Headache

General Characteristics

1. Underlying etiologies are present in approximately 40% of patients with cough headache and are primarily caused by Chiari type I malformation

Clinical Manifestations

1. Patients with an underlying etiology for cough headache:
    a. Have more associated symptoms that depend on the etiology
    b. Have additional headache triggers
    c. More severe pain
    d. More diverse headache durations
2. Etiologies of symptomatic cough headache include:
    a. Chiari I malformation
    b. Posterior fossa lesions (vascular malformations)
    c. Low cerebrospinal pressure
    d. Obstructive hydrocephalus
    e. Arachnoid cysts (posterior fossa)
    f. Dermoid tumor (posterior fossa)
    g. Meningioma (posterior fossa)
    h. Os odontoideum
3. Headache characteristics of cough headache from an underlying etiology:
    a. Occipital or suboccipital location
    b. Explosive, lancinating, pressure or mixed in quality
    c. Duration is typically seconds or more than 1 minute
    d. Triggers include postural movements, laughing and defecation
    e. A proportion of patients have:
        i Dizziness, unsteadiness, facial and upper extremity numbness, vertigo and syncope
        ii Unusual triggers for symptomatic cough headache:
            1. Carotid artery disease
            2. Non-ruptured cerebral aneurysm

Neuropathology (Primary Cough Headache)

1. Increased intracranial pressure caused by coughing due to increased intra-thoracic and intra-abdominal pressure that causes increased central venous pressure that leads to ICP in primary cough headache
2. Putative mechanisms for primary cough headache include:
    a. Transverse or jugular vein stenosis that leads to increased venous cerebral

pressure

b. Hypersensitive pressure receptors on venous vessel walls
c. CSF hypervolemia
d. Crowded posterior fossa

3. Increased intracranial pressure is posited to be the mechanism for symptomatic cough headache:
   a. Chiari I malformation:
      i Descent of the cerebellar tonsils below the foramen magnum
      ii A craniospinal pressure dissociation with greater pressure in the ventricles than the lumbar subarachnoid space such that coughing would displace the tonsils further into the foramen magnum

Laboratory Evaluation

1. MRI:
   a. To delineate structural lesions of the posterior fossa or craniovertebral junction

Other Headache Disorders Triggered or Aggravated by Coughing Include

1. Idiopathic increased intracranial pressure
2. Post-ictal headache
3. High-altitude headache
4. Migraine
5. Tension-type headache
6. Cluster headache

Exertional Headache

General Characteristics

1. Athletes and runners as well as weight lifters are primarily involved

Clinical Manifestations (Weight-Lifters Headache)

1. May occur as a single event or repeatedly over months
2. Each episode may last for hours or days
3. The pain begins immediately or within minutes of heavy lifting
4. Indomethacin is generally effective in treatment of exertional headache

Neuropathology

1. Need to rule out subarachnoid hemorrhage
2. Increased ICP

Laboratory Evaluation

1. CT to evaluate for blood
2. MRI to delineate any structural lesion

3. LP to rule out subarachnoid hemorrhage if there is neck stiffness

Sexual Headache

General Characteristics

1. Sexual activity may cause a tension-type headache or a severe sudden headache with orgasm

Clinical Manifestations (Orgasmic Headache)

1. The headache occurs with orgasm and may last for minutes to hours
2. The headache may occur several times and then abate

Neuropathology

1. Need to rule out hypertensive and aneurysmal bleeds, vascular malformation with bleeding and carotid artery dissection
2. Probable cause is increased intracranial pressure
3. Indomethacin is often effective therapy

Laboratory Evaluation

1. Lumbar puncture to rule out SAH on the first occasion
2. CT
3. MRI

Thunderclap Headache

General Characteristics

1. Definition:
   a. Thunderclap headache is an acute and severe headache that has its maximum intensity at onset; it can be primary or secondary

Clinical Manifestations

1. Primary thunderclap headache is diagnosed when no underlying cause can be found
2. The headache is severe, may be diffuse or frontal and reaches maximum intensity immediately
3. It may be accompanied by nausea and vomiting and infrequently by hypertension

Neuropathology

1. Most thunderclap headaches are benign
2. Secondary forms include:
   a. Migraine
   b. Aneurysmal SAH
   c. Perimesencephalic hemorrhage

   d. Arteriovenous malformation
   e. Dural arteriovenous fistula
   f. Reversible vasoconstriction syndrome
   g. Conditions that may present with or without thunderclap headache include:
      i Pituitary apoplexy
      ii Cervical artery dissection
      iii Cerebral venous thrombosis
      iv Posterior reversible leukoencephalopathy
      v Cocaine and / or adrenergic agents
3. Non-vascular causes of TCH include:
   a. Colloid cyst of the IIIrd ventricle
   b. Spontaneous intracranial hypotension

Laboratory Evaluation

1. CT to evaluate for blood
2. MRI to delineate a structural lesion
3. Judicious use of LP if there is any neck stiffness or neurologic sign

Headaches from Secreting Endocrine Tumors

General Characteristics

1. This type of headache most often occurs with tumors that either secrete vaso-active substances or cause accelerated hypertension

Clinical Manifestations

1. The headache is intense and throbbing
2. It is associated with flushing of the hands and face and on occasion with numbness and paresthesias of the fingers
3. Episodes occur upon awakening

Neuropathology

1. The endocrine tumors in which this type of headache has been reported are:
   a. Mastocytosis:
      i Tissue is infiltrated by mast cells that secrete histamine, heparin and serotonin
   b. Carcinoid tumors
   c. Serotonin secreting tumors
   d. Pancreatic islet tumors
   e. Pheochromocytoma

Laboratory Evaluation

1. Serum analysis to delineate the secreted endocrine or neurotransmitter

Neuroimaging

1. MRI:
    a. To rule out a structural lesion
    b. MRA to evaluate for vasospasm

Migraine Headache

Overview

At present, both clinical and experimental evidence supports the hypothesis that the pathophysiology of migraine headache involves:

1. Inherited alteration of brain excitability
2. Intracranial arterial dilatation
3. Recurrent activation and sensitization of the trigeminovascular system
4. Structural and functional alterations in a subset of patients

Altered brain excitability has been derived from the study of sensory auras, ictal, and interictal hyper-responsiveness to visual, auditory, and olfactory stimuli in conjunction with decreased descending inhibition of pain by the conditioned pain system. There is activation and sensitization of the trigeminovascular system that is demonstrated by pain in specific radiations of the Vth nerve and central sensitization of the pain matrix that causes progressive cephalic and whole body dynamic and static mechanoallodynia during a migraine attack. Structural changes include subcortical white matter hyperintensities (consistent with small vessel vascular disease) and thickening of cortical areas involved in sensory processing. Cortical spreading depression has been proffered as the mechanism for migraine aura.

Migraine

General Characteristics

1. Migraine is frequently divided as to patients with aura and those without aura. The first has been termed classic migraine and the latter common migraine
2. The ratio of classic to common migraine is 1:5

Clinical Manifestations

1. Both types may have preceding changes in mood, appetite and fatigue

Migraine with Aura

1. The auras effect vision, motor and sensory function that are followed in a few minutes to hours by a hemicranial headache
2. Approximately 1/3 of patients suffer bilateral headache that is frequently associated with nausea, vomiting, photophobia and phonophobia
3. The headache usually lasts for hours or a day or two
4. Migraine without aura has an insidious onset over minutes to an hour of a

hemicranial or generalized headache that may or may not be associated with nausea and vomiting

5. Both types have sensitivity to light, sounds and smells
6. Head movement exacerbates the headache in both types
7. A distinguishing feature of the headache is its throbbing quality. Most often one side of the head is affected more often than the other but the headache shifts sides in some attacks
8. In 60 to 80% of patients an inherited pattern is discerned although it is not as evident with common migraine
9. Onset is in adolescence to middle aged adults; children are involved; it is more common in women
10. The headache is often premenstrual in younger women; in approximately 15% of women they may be solely premenstrual (catamenial)
11. In 75-80% of pregnant patients, migraine decreases or ceases during the last two trimesters; rarely migraine may start in the first trimester
12. Migraine may exacerbate in post-menopausal women and has a variable response to estrogen
13. In many migraineurs, birth control pills are associated with both an increased frequency and severity of headaches
14. Triggers for migraine include specific foods, alcohol, a low barometric pressure, glare (particularly from computer screens), cervical nerve root irritation, caffeine withdrawal and strong sensory stimuli
15. Frequently has its onset with awakening but may occur at any time during the day
16. In the preceding day, patients may note a change of mood which may be either euphoria or depression without an obvious trigger
17. Hunger, drowsiness and yawning may be precedents
18. The onset of the aura may be abrupt if visual:
    a. Unformed flashes of light, rarely multicolored (photopsia) that are followed by an enlarging blind spot with a shimmering edge that advances across the visual field at approximately 3mm/s
    b. Fortification spectra (zig-zag lines)
    c. Blurred vision with decreased visual acuity
    d. Patients may be left with a scotomata often homonymous that supports a visual cortical origin
    e. There are rare retinal changes or alterations in optic nerve vessels
19. Other focal neurologic phenomena include:
    a. Numbness and tingling of the face, lips and hand (cheiro-oral pattern)
    b. Cognitive dysfunction
    c. Mild aphasia or dysarthria
    d. Slight weakness of an extremity

e. Patients may have one or a few neurologic deficits which in general have the same pattern with each attack
f. The neurologic deficits last for approximately 30 minutes; characteristically weakness or numbness spreads from one part of the body to another slowly (minutes) in contradistinction to an embolus in which all areas are affected simultaneously or with a seizure in which the spread occurs over seconds
g. After the aura, patients experience a dull headache which occurs and evolves in intensity and becomes pulsatile, most often on the side of the affected cerebral hemisphere
h. Patients are relieved with rest in a recumbent posture in a dark room. Most are nauseated but rarely vomit
i. Between attacks patients with migraine are normal although many patients have motion sickness
j. Auras may occur without headaches and rarely precede or accompany the headache
k. Persistent migraine aura:
    i Persistent migraine aura without infarction lasts longer than 1 week. It consists of:
        1. Persistent primary visual disturbance (PPVD)
        2. Typical aura
l. Recently recognized auras include:
    i Brainstem localizing symptoms
    ii Lateralizing weakness
    iii Monocular visual loss

Hemiplegic Migraine

General Characteristics

1. Two forms are primary:
    a. Familial hemiplegic migraine
    b. Sporadic hemiplegic migraine
    c. The two forms are phenotypically similar
    d. Familial hemiplegic migraine-1 (FHM1) is caused by heterozygous mutation in the CACNA1A gene that maps to chromosome 19p13.13 and is autosomal dominant
    e. FHM2 is caused by mutation in the ATP1A2 gene and FHM3 is caused by SCN1A gene; a fourth gene for FHM has been mapped to chromosome 1q31
    f. Approximately 50% of patients have a defined locus, the most common of which is the CACNA1A gene that encodes the P/Q calcium channel α

subunit; the ATP1A2 gene encodes the Na+/K+ -adenosine triphosphatase channel and the SCNA1 gene encodes the α-subunit of the sodium channel

Clinical Manifestations (FHM-1)

1. Recurrent headaches associated with hemiparesis or hemiplegia
2. May be associated with hemisensory numbness and tingling
3. Less frequently associated with speech disturbance
4. The neurologic deficit may precede or be associated with the deficit; the hemiparesis persist for days or weeks or resolves prior to the headache
5. Other migraine symptoms may occur during the episode
6. Disturbances of consciousness and rarely coma has been described
7. The neurologic deficit usually clears in minutes to hours
8. Less frequent neurologic deficits:
    a. Cerebellar ataxia
    b. Retinal degeneration
    c. Nystagmus
9. Age of onset varies from 5 to 30 years of age

Neuropathology

1. Experimental evidence in a transgenic mouse model:
    a. Demonstrates increased Cav 1.2 in cultured granule cells
    b. Increased susceptibility to cortical spreading depression
2. Ischemic stroke

Laboratory Evaluation

1. Molecular genetic analysis to delineate the mutation
2. Spectroscopy:
    a. FHM1 patients demonstrate:
        i Decreased N-acetyl aspartate (NAA)
        ii Increased myoinositol
        iii Decreased glutamate in the cerebellum

Neuroimaging

1. MRI:
    a. In patients with cerebellar signs:
        i Less gray matter and less white matter with more CSF in the cerebellum

Alternating Hemiplegia of Childhood

General Characteristics

1. Alternating hemiplegia of childhood-1 (AHC1) is caused by heterozygous mutation in the ATP1A2gene that is autosomal dominant and maps to

chromosome 1q23.2

2. It overlaps with familial hemiplegic migraine and GLUT1 deficiency

Clinical Manifestations

1. The onset is before 18 months of age
2. It is chronically progressive
3. Is associated with headache and vomiting
4. Loss of consciousness
5. Autonomic dysfunction
6. Cognitive dysfunction
7. Paroxysmal ocular palsy
8. Choreoathetosis
9. The expanding spectrum of phenotypes with ATP1A3 mutations include:
    a. Alternating hemiplegia of childhood
    b. Rapid-onset dystonia Parkinsonism and CAPOS
10. Triggering episodes are environmental stress, water exposure, physical activity and possibly specific foods
11. Episodic manifestations cease with sleep and may return shortly after awakening

Neuropathology

1. The α1 isoform for the NA $^{(+)}$/K$^{(+)}$ ATPase is ubiquitously expressed in the adult CNS whereas α2 isoform is expressed in neurons
2. The α1 and α3 isoforms of the Na^{+}/K^{+} ATPases restore neuronal membrane potential after depolarization and maintain neuronal excitability
3. The α3 isoform, putatively is important in the re-uptake of neurotransmitters

Laboratory Evaluation

1. Molecular genetic analysis to delineate the mutation in the ATPase gene
2. SPECT:
    a. Has demonstrated progressive decrease in cerebral perfusion during attacks

Differential Diagnoses

1. Moyamoya disease
2. MELAS
3. Mutations in CACN1A, ATP1A2 and SCNA1 genes

Migraine with Brainstem Aura (Basilar Artery Migraine)

General Characteristics

1. Most often seen in young women and adolescent girls but is increasingly recognized in all age groups in both males and females with 3:1 ratio of female

to males

2. Members of one family have been described with a mutation in the ATP1A2 gene

Clinical Manifestations

1. Patients have:
   a. Dysarthria
   b. Vertigo
   c. Tinnitus
   d. Hypacusis
   e. Diplopia
   f. Ataxia
   g. Decreased level of consciousness
   h. No motor weakness
2. At least one aura symptom that spreads gradually over 5 minutes or more and / or two or more symptoms occur in succession:
   a. Each individual aura symptom lasts 5 to 60 minutes
   b. At least one aura symptom is unilateral
   c. The aura is accompanied or followed within 60 minutes by headache

Neuropathology

1. The headache and signs and symptoms originate from the brainstem and are neuronal in origin
2. If there is motor weakness the disorder is familial hemiplegic or sporadic hemiplegic migraine

Neuroimaging

1. MRI / MRA:
   a. To rule out vascular or other structural lesions

Laboratory Evaluation

1. EEG:
   a. To delineate a possible seizure disorder

Retinal Migraine

General Characteristics

1. Retinal migraine is a monocular visual alteration that causes scintillations, scotomas or blindness
2. Typical migraine with aura involves the cerebral cortex and is associated with binocular visual phenomena
3. Retinal migraine affects approximately 1 out of every 200 patients who suffer migraines
4. Approximately 30% of patients have a past history of nonretinal migraine

with or without aura. 25% have a relative with retinal migraine

Clinical Manifestations

1. A fully reversible monocular positive and / or negative scintillating scotomata or blindness
2. Monocular visual field defect that occurs during an attack
3. Migraine headache without aura that begins during the visual symptoms or follows them within 60 minutes
4. Normal ophthalmological examination between attacks
5. Patients have been described who have visual symptoms without headaches and have permanent visual scotomas (rare)
6. Negative symptoms:
    a. Black, grey, white or shaded areas that vary in size that can appear abruptly or gradually progress inwardly from the peripheral visual field
    b. Positive symptoms:
        i Flashing lights or scintillating scotomata
    c. Symptoms are always monocular and typically last 5-20 minutes; they may occur several times per day

Neuropathology

1. Direct ophthalmoscopic evaluation during episodes have demonstrated retinal artery attenuation; rarely retinal hemorrhages have been described
2. Retinal nerve fiber analysis:
    a. Mean retinal nerve fiber layer (RNFL) thickness for nasal and nasal inferior quadrants were seen to be significantly thinner than controls in patients with migraine
    b. Mean choroid thickness at the fovea was also thinner in migraineurs but the macular thickness was equal to control subjects
3. A putative mechanism for retinal migraine is deficient retinal and choroidal blood flow due to activation of the trigeminovascular system and consequent release of vasoactive neuropeptides onto the arterioles that supply the retina and choroid

Laboratory Evaluation

1. CBC, sedimentation rate
2. Coagulation panel
3. EKG
4. Doppler ultrasonography of the carotid
5. Transthoracic echocardiogram

Recurrent Painful Ophthalmoplegic Neuropathy (RPON) (Ophthalmoplegic Migraine)

General Characteristics

1. Most patients have a history of migraine and the headache during the episode has features of migraine

Clinical Manifestations

1. Migrainous-type headache that accompanies or is followed by weakness of cranial nerve III, IV or VI
2. There is often a latent period of up to few days from the onset of the headache to the onset of the ophthalmoplegia
3. A transient third-nerve palsy with ptosis with or without pupillary involvement is usual. Much less frequently, the VIth nerve is involved. It is very rare in adults
4. The ocular paresis may outlast the headache for days or weeks
5. After multiple attacks there may be slight mydriasis and oculomotor paresis

Neuropathology

1. Not ascertained

Laboratory Evaluation

1. LP:
    a. To rule out lymphoma, leukemia or other infiltrating pathologies
2. Detailed medical evaluation to rule out the usual causes of IIIrd nerve palsy

Neuroimaging

1. MRI / MRA:
    a. Has demonstrated gadolinium enhancement of the cisternal component of the affected nerve
    b. MRA:
        i To rule out a posterior communicating artery aneurysm

Differential diagnosis of painful ophthalmoplegia

1. Tolosa-Hunt syndrome
2. Sphenoid sinus mucocele
3. Cavernous sinus thrombosis
4. Sellar and parasellar tumors
5. Sinus infections

Migraine and Stroke

General Characteristics

1. Meta-analyses have consistently demonstrated an association between migraine and stroke. It is particularly well delineated for ischemic stroke and for migraine with aura
2. Neuroimaging studies utilizing MRI have demonstrated:

a. Migraineurs have an increased incidence of subclinical brain infarction in the posterior circulation
b. There is an increased incidence of white matter hyperintensities (putatively arteriolar ischemia) in female patients
3. A controversial relationship exists between patients with migraine and PFO
4. There is also controversy surrounding the relationship of migraine with cervical artery dissection

Clinical Manifestations

1. Case-control studies have shown that ischemic stroke risk parallels an increase in frequency of migraine attacks; possibly patients with greater than 13 attacks / year have a 10-fold higher risk of stroke (patients were 20-44 years of age)
2. Women's Health study (5,130 women with migraine):
   a. Had a higher risk ratio for stroke if they suffered 1 attack with aura / week
3. Migrainous infarction:
   a. Occurs in a patient with migrainous aura which is typical of previous attacks with one or more aura symptoms that lasts for >60 minutes
   b. Neuroimaging demonstrates the ischemic infarction in the appropriate area
   c. Possible prevalence of migrainous infarction is between 0.5 and 1.5% of all ischemic strokes; possibly 10 to 14% of ischemic stroke in young patients in the posterior circulation. Young women with migraine with aura are primarily affected
4. A cross-sectional Dutch study of adults aged 30-60 revealed:
   a. High white matter lesions occur in women with migraine which increase with attack frequency but are equal in patients with or without aura
   b. Longitudinal studies have demonstrated that migraine sufferers are not at increased risk of cognitive impairment from their white matter lesion load
5. Silent-infarct-like lesions:
   a. Are more common in migraine patients than controls; the association is greater in patients with migraine and aura than patients without aura
   b. Approximately 90% of the infratentorial infarct-like lesions were in a vascular border zone location in the cerebellum
6. Migraine and hemorrhagic stroke:
   a. There is an association of women that have migraine with aura and hemorrhagic stroke at four patients per 10,000 females
7. Migraine and cryptogenic TIA and stroke:
   a. In a population-based study, cryptogenic TIA and ischemic stroke have an association with previous migraine. The association is strongest in the patients >65 years of age

   b. The risk of ischemic stroke increases with migraine attack frequency, migraine with aura and in young women
   c. Most ischemic events that occur in patients with migraine happen many years after their first attack which suggest shared risk factors on a genetic basis shared with both conditions
8. Migraine and patent foramen ovale (PFO):
   a. Patent foramen ovale has been documented in 40-60% of patients with migraine and aura and only 25% of the normal population
   b. Possibly a 2.5 increased risk of stroke in patients with PFO and migraine
   c. Patients with a PFO have a fivefold higher risk of having migraine

Migraine and Stroke from a Common Cause

1. Several vascular disorders are associated with a high risk of both migraine (usually with aura) and stroke:
   a. Arteriovenous malformations:
      i The side of the aura is contralateral and the headache is ipsilesional to the AVM
      ii Migraine with aura may be associated with Sturge-Weber syndrome (leptomeningeal angiomatosis)
2. Syndromes associated with migraine include:
   a. CADASIL
   b. MELAS
   c. HERNS (cerebroretinal vasculopathy, and hereditary endotheliopathy with retinopathy, nephropathy and stroke)
3. General vascular conditions that may occur with migraine with aura and ischemic stroke include:
   a. PFO and mitral valve prolapse
   b. Essential thrombocythemia, thrombocytopenia, leukemia
   c. SLE and antiphospholipid syndrome
4. Monogenic Migraine:
   a. The mutations in three well-described genes in familial hemiplegic migraine at the present are the only monogenic cause of migraine. They include:
      i FHM 1:
         1. Caused by mutation in the CACN1A gene that maps to chromosome 19p13
         2. Encodes the pore forming α1 subunit of the cav2.1 channel (P/Q type)
      ii FHM 2:
         1. Caused by mutations in the ATP1A2 gene that maps to chromosome 1q23
         2. Encodes the α2 subunit of sodium-potassium pump ATPases

   iii FHM 3:
      1. Caused by mutation of the SCN1A gene that maps to chromosome 2q24
      2. Encodes the α1 subunit of the neuronal voltage-gated sodium channel $Na_v1.1$
- b. A putative mechanism for the association of these mutations with migraine is that they increase the glutamate and potassium concentration in the synaptic cleft that may increase cortical spreading depression (CSD). There is solid support for CSD engaging the trigeminovascular system that has been shown to be a major component of migraine pathogenesis

Migraine Susceptibility Genes and Cerebral Ischemia

1. Genetic variants putatively associated with migraine include:
   a. Neurotransmitter pathway genes:
      i Dopamine D2 receptor (DRD2)
      ii Human serotonin transporter (HSERT)
      iii Catechol-o-methyltransferase (COMT) and dopamine b-hydroxylase (DBH)
   b. Genes involved in vascular physiology:
      i 5, 10-methylenetetrahydrofolate reductase (MTHFR)
      ii Angiotensin1-converting enzyme (ACE)
      iii Endothelin type A (ETA) receptor
   c. Genes involved in hormone physiology:
      i Estrogen receptor 1(ESR1)
      ii Progesterone receptor (PGR)
      iii Androgen receptor (AR)

The C6771 polymorphism of the MTHFR gene may be a link between migraine and ischemic stroke due to its effect on homocysteine levels. Low dietary folate in patients with migraine and this MTHFR polymorphism have higher homocysteine levels which has been implicated in endothelial dysfunction

Neuropathology

1. Possible mechanisms for ischemic stroke in patients with migraine:
   a. Hemodynamic factors:
      i Cortical spreading depression induces an early increase in cerebral blood flow that is followed by oligemia that causes an increase in vascular resistance. This is manifested by arterial constriction particularly in the posterior circulation
      ii The reduced blood flow may be due to increased vascular resistance rather than active vasoconstriction; neutrally mediated vasodilatation may cause low flow in major intracranial vessels during migraine

auras

2. Inflammation:
    a. Cortical spreading depression causes vasodilatation of extraparenchymal vessels that induces the release of vasoactive peptides (CGRP and substance P), activates pro-inflammatory cytokines and upregulates adhesion molecules and nitric oxide synthase all of which are prothrombotic
    b. Vasospasm was previously thought to be the mechanism for migraine aura from the release of vasoactive agents such as serotonin or endothelin. There is documented evidence that this mechanism may be involved in rare instances of migrainous infarction
3. Coagulation cascades:
    a. During a migraine attack there may be activation of thrombotic factors:
        i Platelets and mast cells may release platelet activating factor which induces platelet aggregation
        ii PAF is a component in the release of von Willebrand factor and the activation of the platelet II B/IIIa receptor that is essential for binding fibrinogen
        iii The activation of these coagulation factors occur during migraine attacks
4. Endothelial Dysfunction:
    a. Endothelial dysfunction is manifested by:
        i A reduction of the bioavailability of vasodilators (nitric oxide)
        ii An increase of endothelial derived contracting molecules which impairs blood vessel reactivity in both conducting vessels and the microcirculation
        iii Decreased endothelial activation which is characterized by a procoagulant, proinflammatory and proliferative state
        iv A major component of endothelial dysfunction is oxidative stress the markers of which are higher in migraineurs both during attacks and in the interictal period
        v Reduced endothelial repair capacity in migraineurs has been demonstrated by:
            1. Decreased levels of endothelial progenitor cells (measured by flow cytometry) predominantly in patients with aura
            2. Decreased migratory capacity of endothelial cells
            3. Increased markers of senescence

Neuroimaging

1. MRI:
    a. Most common lesions are white matter hyperintensities in the deep or periventricular white matter on T2-weighted or Fluid Attenuated Inversion Recovery (FLAIR) sequences

b. The WMH are typically multiple, small and punctate
c. Perfusion weighted MRI deficits in migraineurs' aura are not limited to a single vascular territory, may be bilateral in approximately 20-25% of patients and have a posterior circulation predominance
d. Strokes with migraine have predominance in the posterior circulation
e. Hypoperfusion in a watershed distribution may be seen in the cerebellar vasculature

Migraine with CSF Pleocytosis

General Characteristics

1. A syndrome of transient headache and neurological deficits with CSF lymphocytosis
2. Is a diagnosis of exclusion

Clinical Manifestations

1. Transient neurologic deficits that last hours
2. Migraine-like headaches
3. Rare fever without stiff neck
4. Transient deficits are primarily sensorimotor and aphasia
5. Small percentage of patients have visual symptomatology
6. Some patients have had a history of prior migraine and others a viral-like illness during the preceding 3 weeks

Neuropathology

1. Possibly aseptic meningitis with an associated migraine headache
2. Possible human herpes virus type 7 (HH-7) infection

Laboratory Evaluation

1. CSF:
   a. The CSF may have between 10 to several hundred lymphocytes
   b. The protein is mildly to moderately elevated

Neuroimaging

1. MRI:
   a. Normal

Menstrual (Catamenial Migraine) Migraine

General Characteristics

1. Definition
   a. Attacks of migraine that occur regularly in at least 2 of 3 consecutive menstrual cycles and occur exclusively on day 1 to 2 of menstruation but may range 2 days before to 3 days after with the first day of menstruation as day one

2. The two subtypes are:
    a. Pure menstrual migraine
    b. Menstrually related migraine

Clinical Manifestations

1. Pure menstrual migraine there are no aura and no migraine other than that which occurs with the menstrual cycle
2. Menstrually related migraine occurs in 2 of 3 consecutive menstrual cycles primarily on days 1 and 2 of menstruation but may also occur outside of the menstrual cycle

Neuropathology

1. "Estrogen withdrawal" migraine-triggering hypothesis posits the cause of the headache is lack of estrogen in the late luteal phase
2. Recent studies of estrogen levels in patients with migraine demonstrate:
    a. There is no significant difference in estrogen peak levels or mean daily levels of estrogen between migraineurs and controls
    b. There is a significant difference in the rate of estrogen decline in the late luteal phase
    c. There is no difference in the rate of decline in the periovulatory phase
    d. In patients with migraine, the rate of estrogen decline cannot distinguish cycles with and without an acute headache

Neuroimaging

1. MRI or CT to exclude any structural lesion otherwise normal

Status Migrainosus

General Characteristics

1. Status migrainosus is a debilitating migraine attack that lasts for longer than 72 hours

Clinical Manifestations

1. Migraine attacks may increase in frequency for several months often up to 3 to 4 / week:
    a. The scalp may become tender on the side of the headache
    b. The pain is initially unilateral and later generalizes
    c. The pain may be throbbing but has an associated ache
    d. There is a history of migraine
    e. The headache is debilitating

Neuropathology

1. Rarely this form of headache is initiated by head trauma or viral infection
2. The headache may be perpetuated by medication rebound

Laboratory Evaluation

1. Rule out narcotic or other medication overuse

Neuroimaging

1. MRI:
    a. To rule out a structural lesion

Vestibular Migraine

General Characteristics

1. Vestibular migraine is the most common cause of episodic vertigo in both adults and children
2. The diagnosis depends on the patient's history as there are no clinically useful biomarkers
3. Vestibular migraine has a lifetime prevalence of approximately 1% and a 1-year prevalence of 0.9% in the general population
4. It occurs 1.5 to 5 times more often in women than men
5. Migraine-related syndromes are the most common cause of vertigo and dizziness in children

Clinical Manifestations

1. Vertigo in patients with migraine may manifest as:
    a. Spontaneous vertigo in 21 to 83% of patients
    b. Positional vertigo and dizziness in 17 to 65% of patients
    c. Head motion intolerance in 31 to 77% of patients
2. Vertigo may be induced by moving visual objects
3. Additional symptoms:
    a. Unsteadiness
    b. Balance problems
4. Attack duration may vary from seconds to days; diagnostic criteria for vestibular migraine require a 5 min minimum duration
5. Vertigo can precede or occur during or after the headache
6. A small group of patients have isolated vertigo attacks that alternate with migraine
7. Approximately 40% of patients have tinnitus, hearing disturbances and aural pressure
8. Neurological examination between episodes is usually normal
9. Canal paresis and bilateral vestibular failure occur in 8 to 22% and 11% respectively
10. During attacks patients may demonstrate:
    a. Central vestibular ocular motor abnormalities
    b. Gaze induced nystagmus
    c. Deficiencies of saccadic pursuit

    d. Central positional nystagmus
11. Interictal ocular motor deficits increase over time
12. During acute attacks:
    a. Central vestibular dysfunction occurs in 50% of patients and peripheral dysfunction in 15%
    b. Hearing is not affected and the site of pathology may not be determined in 35% of patients

Neuropathology

1. Interactions of vestibular and pain pathways at several levels i.e. from the inner ear to the thalamus and cortex
2. fMRI study:
    a. Increased activation of the temporo-parietal-insular areas and bilateral thalami during an attack (2 patients):
        i Possible activation of the vestibulo-thalamo-cortical pathways
    b. fMRI of vestibulo migraine patients during cold caloric stimulation
        i Increased thalamic activation
3. FDG-PET study:
    a. An increase of metabolic activity was demonstrated bilaterally in the ventral-anterior thalamus during an attack
4. Voxel-based morphometric MRI study demonstrated:
    a. Reduction of gray matter volume in the superior, inferior and middle temporal gyri
    b. Decreased tissue mid-cingulate, dorsolateral, prefrontal, insula, parietal and occipital cortices

Laboratory Evaluation

1. Posturography, vestibular evoked myogenic potentials (VEMPs) and evaluation of the subjective visual vertical (SVV) have been inconsistent
2. Inner ear MRI study:
    a. Utilizing gadolinium contrast transtympanically demonstrated cochlear and vestibular endolymphatic hydrops in 4/19 vestibular migraine patients

Differential Diagnosis of Vestibular Migraine

1. Meniere's disease
2. Benign paroxysmal positional vertigo (BPPV) in those patients with positional vertigo attacks
3. Anxiety associated migraine with vestibular disorders MARD (migraine anxiety-related dizziness)

Cluster Headache

General Characteristics

1. Cluster headache (CH) is the most common of the autonomic cephalalgias
2. It has a prevalence of 0.1% in the general population and is more frequent in males with a ratio of 2.5 to 7.1:1
3. The lifetime incidence of CH is 124 patients / 100,000 of the population

Clinical Manifestations

1. CH is most frequently seen in adult men between 20 to 50 years of age
2. It is severe unilateral pain typically retro-orbital and fronto-temporal that is associated with:
    a. Conjunctival injection
    b. Tearing
    c. Eyelid edema
    d. Miosis
    e. Ptosis
    f. Nasal congestion
    g. Rhinorrhea
    h. Facial hyperhidrosis
3. The pain around the eye is felt as deep, extremely intense and is non-throbbing. It may radiate to the forehead, temple, cheek, and less frequently to the ear, occiput, and neck.
4. It occurs typically at night between 1 to 2 hours after sleep onset or several times during the night on several or more consecutive days
5. Less often the headache occurs during the day (up to eight times / day) or during the early evening. There is no aura or vomiting.
6. The headache may occur with the same periodicity each night for periods of weeks; it may cease and not recur for months or rarely for years. In a few patients it may become chronic
7. The autonomic symptoms last for approximately 45 minutes (range of 15 to 180 minutes)
8. There is frequent slight ptosis that may become permanent
9. During an attack the temporal artery on the homolateral side and the scalp may demonstrate mechanical hyperalgesia
10. Few patients can lay quietly during an attack. Most hold their head, sit in a chair or pace. The headache may cease abruptly or back away gradually
11. Usually the same orbit is involved during a particular cluster or in future attacks

Neuropathology

1. The pain of CH is generally thought to occur from activation of the trigeminovascular system:
    a. The activation occurs both in the brainstem and in cranio-facial

sympathetic neurons that cause the autonomic signs and symptoms

b. It is posited that retrograde activation of trigeminal fibers releases vasoactive neuropeptides, the most important of which is calcitonin gene related peptide (CGRP) that innervate cranial blood vessels. Upon release, CGRP induces intracranial vasodilatation and can cause sterile neurogenic inflammation that consists of edema and protein leakage into the dura. Nociceptive activation from this sterile inflammation are transmitted from the trigeminal ganglion to the trigeminal cervical complex (TCC) and projected to the thalamus and cortex. Substance P, another vasoactive neuropeptide, may also be involved in this process. Both oxygen and sumatriptans lower CGRP levels.
c. Activation of the superior salivatory nucleus may cause the cranial autonomic signs and symptoms of CH:
    i Its parasympathetic outflow is transmitted primarily via the sphenopalatine ganglion
    ii It causes the tearing, conjunctival injection, nasal congestion, and rhinorrhea seen during attacks. These effects are due to the release of acetylcholine and vasoactive intestinal peptide (VIP). During CH attacks CGRP and VIP levels are increased which supports the hypothesis that the trigeminal-parasympathetic reflex is a component of CH pathology.
    iii It is posited that the Vth nerve concomitantly activates the trigeminovascular pain system and the superior salivatory nucleus. At present, it is not known what causes the initial activation of the trigeminovascular system or the trigeminal-parasympathetic reflex.

2. There is evidence that CH has a primary central origin initiated from the hypothalamus:
    a. Support for a hypothalamic role is:
        i The circadian periodicity of attacks and that the clusters most often occur during the spring and fall.
        ii There are direct connections from the locus coeruleus and the dorsal raphe nuclei to the hypothalamus and alteration of these monoaminergic nuclei may be a component of hypothalamic regulation
        iii Direct connections from the posterior hypothalamus to the pain TCC (trigeminal) complex have also been demonstrated
        iv Several hypothalamic nuclei are important for pain perception
        v Central sensitization of pain projecting neurons and the pain matrix may play a role in CH
        vi Stimulation of the posterior hypothalamus is effective in controlling CH in some patients
        vii During attacks, the pain matrix demonstrates increased blood flow.

b. These areas are:
   i Anterior cingulate gyrus
   ii Prefrontal cortex
   iii Thalamus
   iv Periaqueductal grey
   v Basal ganglia
   vi Insula
   vii Cerebellum
c. Imaging studies have also demonstrated alterations in the diffuse nociceptive inhibitory complex (DNIC) system in patients with CH

Laboratory Evaluation

1. Cluster headache is a clinical diagnosis; there are no biomarkers

Trigeminal Autonomic Cephalalgias

Overview

Trigeminal autonomic cephalalgias (TAC) are classified as a group due to a common pathophysiology based on activation of the trigeminovascular system, the trigemino parasympathetic reflex, and dysregulation of circadian rhythm. The clinical pain syndromes are in the trigeminal distribution and all have autonomic activation. Clinical features among the syndromes overlap but treatment responses are relatively specific which helps in the diagnosis. TACs may be an expression of an underlying pathologic process.

Paroxysmal Hemicrania

General Characteristics

1. The prevalence of paroxysmal hemicranias is approximately 2-20 per 100,000 of the population
2. There is no male or female predominance

Clinical Manifestations

1. The mean age at onset is between 31-41 years of age; it has been reported in children and in adults up to 81 years of age
2. Approximately 20% of paroxysmal hemicranias are episodic
3. The patient suffers severe orbital or periorbital pain that is unilateral and rarely may become bilateral
4. Pain may also be felt in temporal, periauricular, maxillary and infrequently in occipital areas
5. Pain radiates commonly to the shoulder, neck and arm
6. Severe pain may radiate across the midline
7. Most attacks do not change sides
8. Attacks usually last from 2-20 minutes but have been described for as long

as an hour

9. The onset of pain is abrupt and reaches maximum intensity in less than 5 minutes; its quality is throbbing, lancinating or boring
10. It is associated with some of the ipsilateral autonomic phenomena that include:
    a. Conjunctival erythema and injection with lacrimation
    b. Nasal congestion and rhinorrhea
    c. Eyelid edema
    d. Forehead and facial hyperhidrosis
    e. Miosis and slight ptosis
11. More than 5 attacks per day; a usual frequency may be between 8to 30 episodes over a 24 hour period:
    a. One to 5 attacks per 24 hours have been reported
    b. Approximately 30% of patients report REM-related nocturnal attacks that awaken patients
12. An absolute response to indomethacin therapy
13. Autonomic phenomena may be seen bilaterally but are worse on the symptomatic side
14. Secondary paroxysmal hemicrania has been described with:
    a. Malignant and benign tumors
    b. Systemic disease

Neuropathology

1. Activation of the trigeminovascular system has been posited to cause the pain
2. Activation of the trigeminoparasympathetic reflex initiates the autonomic phenomena

Neuroimaging

1. MRI:
    a. Imaging of the head to rule out secondary causes of paroxysmal hemicrania
    b. Medical evaluation to evaluate for underlying systemic disease

Short-lasting, Unilateral, Neuralgiform Headache Attacks with Conjunctival Injection and Tearing (SUNCT)

General Characteristics

1. The syndrome in many ways is similar to trigeminal neuralgia and some believe it to be a variant

Clinical Manifestations

1. A unilateral ocular and periocular pain, that is less severe than trigeminal neuralgia and may also involve the temporal, auricular and occipital areas
2. The quality of the pain is lancinating, pulsating and infrequently stabbing or

burning
3. It rarely spreads across the midline or changes sides
4. The pain typically lasts from 5 to 240 seconds (mean of 1 minute)
5. Longer-lasting attacks of 250, 600 seconds and to 2-3 hours have been described
6. Rarely SUNCT status pain can last for 1-3 days (occurring most of each day)
7. Low-grade background pain may be a concomitant of the intermittent exacerbations
8. The patterns of attacks are:
    a. Single clonic attacks
    b. Groups of stabs that occur with a series of attacks
    c. "Sawtooth" pattern with stabbing pains that last for minutes
9. The frequency of attacks is from 3 to 200 daily which varies widely both to season and diurnally:
    a. The average is 28/day
    b. Attacks are bimodal occurring in the morning and late afternoon
    c. <2% of attacks occur at night
10. Mechanical stimuli in trigeminal areas can trigger pain. There is a short latency from the stimulus to pain onset
11. Neck movement, out of the trigeminal territory may also trigger pain; alcohol does not exacerbate pain
12. After a painful episode there is no refractory period which differentiates SUNCT from trigeminal neuralgia
13. Ipsilateral conjunctival injection and lacrimation are concurrent with the onset of pain
14. Nasal congestion and rhinorrhea may be similar but hyperhidrosis is less frequent and may be subclinical

Neuropathology

1. Activation of the trigeminovascular system has been posited to cause the pain
2. Activation of the trigeminoparasympathetic reflex initiates the autonomic phenomena
3. Secondary SUNCT has been reported with:
    a. Pontine and brainstem infarction
    b. Cerebellopontine arteriovenous malformations
    c. Cerebellopontine astrocytomas, tumors and cysts
    d. Brainstem cavernous hemangioma
    e. Tumor of the cavernous sinus
    f. Extraorbital cystic mass
    g. Vertebral artery dissection
    h. Neurofibromatosis
    i. Eye trauma

   j. In association with HIV and osteogenesis imperfect
   k. 5% of pituitary tumor patients may have SUNCT

Laboratory Evaluation

1. MRI / CT to rule out secondary causes of SUNCT

Short-lasting Unilateral Neuralgiform Headache Attacks with Cranial Autonomic Features (SUNA)

General Characteristics

1. Similar to SUNCT
2. SUNCT / SUNA may be as common as paroxysmal hemicranias

Clinical Manifestations

1. SUNA may be differentiated from SUNCT by:
   a. SUNA may be associated with any autonomic sign
   b. Attack duration may be up to 10 minutes

Neuropathology

1. Activation of the trigeminovascular system causes the pain and activation of the trigeminoparasympathetic system; the autonomic phenomena
2. Secondary causes of SUNA are similar to those of SUNCT and include vascular disease, tumors, and malformations of the brainstem and posterior fossa

Laboratory Evaluation

1. MRI / CT to rule out secondary causes

Hemicrania Continua

General Characteristics

1. The female to male ratio is 2.8:1

Clinical Manifestations

1. The headache is unilateral and lasts > than 3 months
2. Pain is localized frontally and in temporal regions as well as periorbitally
3. Rarely the pain can alternate sides. A few bilateral patients have been reported
4. The pain occurs daily and is continuous
5. Pain characteristics:
   a. The pain is of moderate severity with a VAS of 4.7
   b. 74% of patients report fluctuations in pain severity
   c. 40% of patients have disabling exacerbations with severe pain (VAS 9.3) which may last for 30 minutes for 10 hours and up to 2-5 days
   d. During the exacerbations hemicrania continua is very similar to severe migraine

e. Some pain is described as jabs and jolts
f. Approximately 20% of patients describe a foreign body feeling in the eye that may precede or accompany the headache
g. Patients describe throbbing as the severity of the headache increases
h. During exacerbations patients get:
    i Conjunctival injection with lacrimation
    ii Nasal congestion and rhinorrhea
    iii Miosis and ptosis
i. The remitting form of hemicranias continua is characterized by:
    i Headache that lasts for a few days that is followed by a remission from 2-15 days
    ii This pattern is present in approximately 50% of patients; the other 50% have continuous pain from the onset of the headache
    iii Approximately 1/3 of remitting patients evolve to the chronic form in a mean of 7.8 years
j. Nocturnal attacks are seen in approximately 50% of patients
k. Triggers that exacerbate the pain are:
    i Menses
    ii Postural changes
    iii Strong smells
    iv Stress
    v Alcohol (some patients)
l. Autonomic signs are minimal except during exacerbations that suggest that autonomic activation is dependent on pain severity. The most common autonomic phenomena are photophobia, nausea, conjunctival injection, phonophobia, and tearing.
m. Hemicrania continua may be associated with aura
n. Approximately 15-18% of patients report nasal stuffiness or rhinorrhea
o. There is no significant age difference between those with a remitting onset (mean of 32 years) and those with a continuous onset (34 years)

Neuropathology

1. The pattern of activation links the pathophysiology of hemicrania continua to both cluster headache and migraine
2. Secondary hemicrania continua:
    a. Medication abuse
    b. Mesenchymal tumor of the sphenoid bone
    c. Mild to moderate head trauma

Neuroimaging

1. fMRI:
    a. Activation of the posterior hypothalamus and the dorsal rostral pons

2. MRI /CT of the head to rule out secondary causes of HC otherwise normal

Differential Diagnosis of TAC

1. Orofacial pain:
    a. Pain referral patterns with TACs may involve intraoral and non-trigeminal distributions:
        i Cluster headache and paroxysmal hemicrania may simulate dental pain
2. Regional tumors:
    a. May occur in 0.8-5% of facial pain patients
3. Trigeminal neuralgia:
    a. Lacrimation may be associated with involvement of any division
    b. SUNCT / SUNA and cluster may be misdiagnosed
    c. SUNCT:
        i Does not respond to sodium channel blockers
        ii Multiple and obvious autonomic signs
        iii Has no refractory period
        iv Cluster-tic syndrome:
            1. The combination of cluster headache and trigeminal neuralgia:
                a. Neck movements may be a trigger in approximately 40% of patients
                b. A form of cluster-tic syndrome has very short attacks that are difficult to distinguish between SUNCT and paroxysmal hemicranias
            2. CPH-tic syndrome and mixed attacks are difficult to discriminate from SUNCT

Major Differential Points that Distinguish TACs

1. Attack duration and frequency:
    a. Unilateral headache with ipsilateral autonomic signs of less than 2 minutes is most likely SUNCT:
        i Trigeminal neuralgia with associated autonomic signs is also possible. It would be favored if there is a refractory period
        ii SUNA attacks are longer, lasting in general for minutes (overlap with short paroxysmal hemicranias)
    b. Headaches that last for more than 4 hours accompanied by autonomic symptomatology are usually migraine or one of its variants. The diagnosis is more secure if the upper third of the head is involved:
        i Rarely cluster headache may last for up to 48 hours
        ii There are similarities between long lasting cluster headache and migraine
        iii The pain of cluster headache is more severe than migraine and

resembles that of trigeminal neuralgia or SUNCT

iv Migraine attacks may occur in clusters and have a cyclical pattern

v Circadian pattern or cluster attacks may occur with hemicrania continua and paroxysmal hemicrania. The majority of patients with paroxysmal hemicrania have a chronic rather than episodic pattern that distinguishes them from the usual episodic circadian cluster headache

Coronal Linear Headache

General Characteristics

1. Linear headache is a new form of headache or a variant of migraine

Clinical Manifestations

1. Paroxysmal or chronic fixed headache or head pain
2. Restricted in a linear trajectory that connects the occiput or occipitocervical area to the ipsilateral nasion or forehead
3. A subgroup of patients have associated nausea, vomiting and dizziness
4. Most attacks are spontaneous but triggers include noise, stress, lack of sleep or rest after physical exertion
5. Paroxysms of pain may last for hours to days in the majority of patients; some patient attacks are only of a few minute duration
6. The pain is of moderate intensity and is described as pulsating or pressure-like
7. The frequency of attacks varies from one attack / day to 5 or 6 attacks per year; there are long term remissions in some patients
8. In twenty patients that have been described, the age at onset ranges from 20-73 years of age
9. There is a female predominance of 1:5:1
10. The width of the painful area is between 5 and 10 mm; the linear trajectory is parallel to the sagittal plane of the head

Neuropathology

1. The pathogenesis is unknown but a migraine mechanism has been posited:
    a. A linear area of meningeal nociceptors parallel to the superior sagittal sinus is activated by cortical spreading depression (CSD) that activates the trigeminovascular pathway as occurs with migraine

Laboratory Evaluation

1. MRI of the head and cervical spine to rule out an alternate diagnosis

Epicrania Fugax

General Characteristics

1. Epicrania fugax is a recently described primary headache

Clinical Manifestations

1. Paroxysmal, short lasting, 1-10 seconds, of moderate pain
2. Is initiated in a specific area of the posterior scalp and rapidly radiates anteriorly in a linear trajectory to the forehead, eye or nose
3. The quality of the pain is moving, stabbing, electric-like or lancinating
4. The pattern of movement may be zig-zag which may cross the midline
5. At the cessation of the attack, patients may have ipsilateral autonomic signs that include lacrimation, conjunctival injection or rhinorrhea
6. Patients are usually symptom free between attacks
7. The mean age of onset is 49 years (range 34-75 years)

Neuropathology

1. The pathophysiology is not known
2. Probable activation of the trigeminovascular system that causes the pain and the trigeminoparasympathetic reflex that causes the autonomic phenomena

Laboratory Evaluation

1. MRI of the head and cervical spine to rule out structural lesions

Cervicogenic Headache

General Characteristics

1. The incidence and prevalence of cervicogenic headache is not clear. It has been estimated that approximately 4% of the population may at some point suffer cervicogenic headache
2. It may comprise 0.4-15% of the headache population and possibly 15-20% of all chronic and recurrent headaches
3. Possibly women are affected more frequently than men

Clinical Manifestations

1. Unilateral head pain primarily in the parietal and frontal areas that is initiated occipitally; a particular radiation to the brow
2. Provoked by unphysiologic neck positions; limitation of motion of the neck to all planes but particularly to extension
3. Primarily C5, C6, C7 upper arm radiations; no radiation into the hand; atrophy of the deltoid cap and biceps; frequently associated inverted radial reflex
4. Diffuse arm pain primarily C5-C7 distribution
5. Pain is initiated in the occipital area and radiates anteriorly
6. The pain is most often a dull ache

Neuropathology

1. Facet joints, cervical muscles, intervertebral discs, nerve roots, the vertebral arteries and uncovertebral joints have all been associated with cervical headaches

2. The greater, lesser and third occipital nerves cause the headache as does cervical plexus injury from whiplash or surgical procedures
3. Cervicogenic related structures are supplied by the upper cervical nerve roots that relay sensory information into the spinal tract of the trigeminal nucleus that is the anatomical basis for pain radiations to frontal and orbital areas. Recent evidence from anesthetic blocks support an association of cervical headache pain from mid-cervical segments
4. The pain may be triggered by cortical spreading depression activation of meningeal nociceptors that initiates the trigeminovascular pain pathways similar to what has been described with lesser and greater occipital nerve neuralgia

Laboratory Evaluation

1. Cervical spine MRI to delineate specific pathology
2. Diagnostic nerve blocks

Hypnic Headache

General Characteristics

1. Hypnic headache is a rare primary headache disorder with exclusively sleep related headache attacks

Clinical Manifestations

1. The headache occurs only during sleep which awakens the patient
2. It occurs more frequently than 15 times / month
3. It persists for longer than 15 minutes after the patient awakens
4. Starts after age 50
5. The pain is mild to moderate but is severe in approximately 20% of patients
6. The pain is bilateral in 2/3 of patients
7. Attacks are typically 15 to 180 minutes although longer episodes have been described
8. There are no autonomic symptoms and no more than one symptom of nausea, photophobia or phonophobia
9. Spontaneous remissions can occur
10. Most patients show motor activity during attacks

Neuropathology

1. Abnormality of the circadian rhythm; posterior hypothalamic dysregulation of the circadian rhythm possibly similar to that described in cluster headache

Neuroimaging:

1. MRI of the head to rule out any structural lesions

Differential Points in Regard to Sleep-related Headache

1. Headaches that are intrinsically related to sleep include:

   a. Migraine with and without aura
   b. Cluster headache
   c. Hypnic headache
   d. Paroxysmal hemicrania
2. Headaches that cause a sleep disorder:
   a. Chronic migraine
   b. Chronic tension headache
   c. Medication overuse headache
3. Headaches that are a symptom of a sleep disorder:
   a. Obstructive sleep apnea
4. Headaches from a systemic condition:
   a. Anemia
   b. Hypoxemia
5. Chronobiological dysfunction:
   a. Involvement of the hypothalamus
   b. Cluster headache (circadian and circannual rhythmicity)
   c. Hypnic headache (an alarm clock pattern)
6. Possible relation of headache to REM sleep:
   a. Cluster headache
   b. Hypnic headache
   c. Paroxysmal hemicrania
7. Headaches associated with obstructive sleep apnea:
   a. Cluster headache
   b. Hypnic headache
   c. Sleep apnea headache
8. Headaches associated with insomnia:
   a. Chronic migraine
   b. Medication overuse
   c. Psychiatric comorbidity
   d. Chronic tension-type

Cranio-Facial Pain

Trigeminal Neuralgia (TN)

General Characteristics

1. A new classification proposes 3 diagnostic categories:
   a. Classic TN that is caused by morphologic changes in the trigeminal nerve root from vascular compression
   b. Secondary TN due to a neurologic disease
   c. Idiopathic when the etiology cannot be identified

Clinical Manifestations

1. Onset is usually middle age or later in life
2. There is the sudden onset of severe stabbing pain in the mandibular and maxillary division of the Vth nerve and much less frequently the first division
3. The pain is usually only of seconds duration or rarely a minute and is often accompanied by a wince or "tic"
4. The patient has trigger areas that initiate the pain which are usually around the mouth (lips, gums, cheeks)
5. The paroxysms occur both during the day and night and if untreated may last for weeks to months
6. In general there is no motor or sensory loss in the affected Vth nerve distribution
7. A subgroup of patients have a continuous low level discomfort, itch or sensitivity in affected areas
8. Usually spatial and temporal summation of a mechanical stimulus in a trigger zone is necessary to trigger pain
9. After a paroxysm there is a 2-3 minute refractory period
10. The pain cannot extend to the cervical nerve territory that includes the posterior 1/3 of the scalp, the back of the ear or the angle of the jaw
11. The territory of the mandibular division of the Vth nerve extends to the temple so that patients may experience pain in the lip and the cranium
12. If two trigeminal divisions are involved they are contiguous which occurs most frequently with the mandibular and maxillary divisions
13. First division involvement may be caused by specific neuropathology
14. TN may remit for weeks to years in a significant proportion of patients
15. TN is overwhelmingly unilateral. Bilateral TN is usually caused by multiple sclerosis (possibly 10% of MS associated TN)
16. The sensory quality of pain in TN may change over time
17. Stimulus evoked pain:
    a. Innocuous mechanical stimuli in a branch territory of the Vth nerve
    b. The stimulus may be a primary touch or a whiff of air. Maneuvers that are more complex usually are a combination of tactile stimuli and facial movement. The evoked pain may not be felt at the site of the stimulation and may radiate
    c. In general, the trigger zones are small and may even be punctate and are usually in the central portion of the face that includes the nasolabial fold, nose and the mouth
18. A sensory deficit is most often associated with underlying pathology
19. TN with continuous pain:
    a. A subgroup of TN patients has pain between attacks. Its characteristics are:

i It is continuous
ii Is not associated with any other cause for facial pain
iii It is described as dull, burning or tingling
iv It localizes in the same distribution as the paroxysmal pain, fluctuates in intensity, has periods of remission and exacerbation similar to that of paroxysmal pain
v Continuous pain occurs in idiopathic, classical or secondary TN

Neuropathology

1. In classic TN, there is dislocation or atrophy of the trigeminal nerve root at its entry zone into the brainstem. Flattening and atrophy of the nerve root are signs of clinically relevant compression
2. Secondary TN is caused by pathologic processes that affect the nerve
   a. Cerebellopontine angle tumors or MS cause TN in 15% of patients
   b. Tumors are usually benign and include acoustic or trigeminal schwannoma, meningioma, or epidermoids that usually affect the root at the nerve entry zone to the pons. Its mechanism of action is putatively focal demyelination with ephaptic conduction. Malignant tumors infiltrate the nerve, cause axonal degeneration and have a different clinical profile
3. TN occurs in 2-5% of patients with MS and MS occurs in 2-14% of patients with TN. Demyelinating plaques in the pons have been demonstrated
4. Less frequent pathologies that cause TN include:
   a. Aneurysm or dolichoectasia of the basilar artery
   b. Brain arteriovenous malformations
5. As noted, approximately 80-90% of primary TGN are caused by vascular compression of the TG nerve at the root entry zone by the superior cerebellar or anterior inferior cerebellar arteries

Neuroimaging

1. Morphologic changes of the nerve and the root entry zone rather than mere contact of the artery with the nerve increase diagnostic specificity dramatically
2. 3D reconstruction with MRI delineates the anatomy of the trigeminal nerve and its entry zone:
   a. 3DT2 weighted MRI, driven equilibrium or constructive interference in steady state delineates the external and cavernous portion of the nerve
   b. 3D time of flight magnetic resonance angiography delineates arteries while 3D T1-weighted MRI with contrast or phase-contrast MRI delineates veins
3. The anatomical changes in the nerve itself can be discerned with diffusion tensor imaging (DTI) and fiber tractography

Glossopharyngeal Neuralgia

General Characteristics

1. Glossopharyngeal neuralgia is rare with an incidence of 0.2 to 0.7 per 100,000 individuals/year
2. It is classified as classical or symptomatic
3. It has many clinical similarities to trigeminal neuralgia

Clinical Manifestations

1. Paroxysmal attacks of pain that usually last for a fraction of a second to rarely up to 2 minutes
2. The pain characteristics include:
    a. Localization to the posterior tongue, tonsillar fossa, pharynx, beneath the angle of the jaw and the ear (auricular branch of the vagus nerve)
    b. The pain is sharp, lancinating and severe
    c. Triggers most commonly are swallowing, chewing, speaking, coughing, fear of eating and yawning
    d. Attacks are stereotyped in each patient
    e. There is no clinically definable neurologic deficit
    f. Rarely, there is varied distribution of the pain with overlap amongst the trigeminal, vagal and facial nerves:
        i Unusual manifestations include:
            1. Cardiac arrhythmias associated with pain episodes
            2. Fear to eat
            3. Syncope
    g. The pain often occurs in clusters, is lancinating and most often is initiated in the throat and radiates to the ear (rarely vice versa). Alternatively, pain may radiate from the pharynx, tonsil and posterior tongue base to the eustachian tube and inner ear or mandibular angle
    h. The pain may recur after a brief period of remission. There may be residual pain in the affected distributions
    i. Attacks usually occur during the day and may occur for weeks or months if untreated:
        i Unusual triggers include:
            1. Sudden head movement
            2. Swallowing cold liquids
            3. Raising the arm on the side of the pain
            4. Lateral movement of the jaw
            5. Touching the external auditory canal, the side of the neck and the pretragus of the painful side
        ii Unusual manifestations:
            1. Tinnitus

2. Vomiting
3. Vertigo
4. Swelling sensation
5. Involuntary movements

j. Vagoglossopharyngeal neuralgia:
   i Is due to the complex anatomy between the nervus intermedius, vagus and glossopharyngeal nerves
   ii It may manifest as cardiac asystole, convulsions or syncope
k. Cardiovascular phenomena occur during the paroxysms of pain or immediately following its cessation
l. There is a subset of patients that have the cardiac manifestations without the neuralgia

Neuropathology

1. Neurovascular nerve compression at the root entry zone is the major pathology of many patients with idiopathic glossopharyngeal neuralgia. The usual arteries that compress the nerve are:
   a. Posterior inferior cerebellar artery
   b. Vertebral artery
   c. The vertebral artery plus the anterior inferior cerebellar artery
2. Secondary pathologies that cause glossopharyngeal neuralgia are:
   a. Cerebellar pontine angle mass lesions (benign tumors and cysts)
   b. Oropharyngeal tumors
   c. Arachnoiditis
   d. Stylohyoid ligament ossification
   e. Multiple sclerosis
   f. Vascular malformations

Laboratory Evaluation

1. Complete blood count, erythrocyte sedimentation rate, anti-nuclear antibody to rule out underlying systemic disease

Neuroimaging

1. MRI, MRA and 3-dimensional computed tomography angiography (3D-CTA) to rule out vascular compression
2. High resolution MRI and image processing with 3D constructive interference in steady state (CISS) to evaluate neurovascular compression
3. Radiological findings suggestive of glossopharyngeal neuralgia from vascular compression:
   a. High origin of PICA
   b. PICA making an upward loop

   c. PICA causing and compressing the supraolivary cistern
4. MRI of the neck is required to rule out tumors of the hypopharynx, larynx or piriform sinus
5. A cervical radiograph will identify an elongated stylohyoid bone (Eagle's syndrome)

Herpes Zoster

General Characteristics

1. Herpes zoster (HZ) is caused by the reactivation of varicella – zoster virus (VZV) that has established latency in sensory ganglia after initial infection (chicken pox)
2. It will affect approximately 1 in 3 people in the USA during their lifetime. There are approximately 1 million HZ patients annually in the United States
3. Major risk factors are older age and diminished VZV-specific cell-mediated immunity
4. Other risk factors for HZ are:
   a. Family history; the association is highest with first-degree or multiple relatives
   b. Prior HZ episodes
   c. Sleep disturbance
   d. Stress
5. HZ is not associated with trauma, smoking, tonsillectomy, diet, exposure to pesticides or herbicides

Clinical Manifestations

1. Neuralgia associated with a vesicular eruption that affects cranial and peripheral nerves (DRG).
2. HZ auricularis:
   a. Vesicular eruption of the external auditory meatus and pinna and less frequently the palate and occipital area
   b. It may be associated with or without loss of hearing, tinnitus and vertigo
   c. Facial paralysis
   d. These signs are accompanied by severe neuropathic pain
3. The more common involvement is that of the Gasserian ganglion which usually affects the first division of V (herpes zoster ophthalmicus):
   a. The rash usually occurs 4-5 days after the onset of pain. Rarely there is no skin rash
4. Elderly patients are more likely to develop chronic and intractable pain
5. The pain of post herpetic neuralgia:
   a. Most often is burning with super-imposed waves of lancinating pain
   b. The dermatomes or cranial nerve territory that is affected may

demonstrate:
  i Mechanical hyperalgesia and dynamic mechanical allodynia
  ii Increased threshold to pin-prick and thermal sensitivity

Neuropathology

1. The pathologic changes in HZ infections are usually limited to the dorsal root ganglion (DRG) or a sensory nerve or the nerve root close to the affected ganglion
2. In trigeminal ganglia infection, the component of the ganglia that supplies VI is most severely affected:
    a. The ganglia is swollen and congested and in severe cases the adjacent spinal cord is affected
    b. There is intense primarily lymphocytic infiltration of the affected ganglion; necrosis in the walls of small blood vessels
    c. Degenerative changes in sensory neurons

Laboratory Evaluation

1. Direct fluorescent antibody testing of vesicular fluid
2. PCR testing of vesicular fluid or a corneal lesion

Trochlear Headache

General Characteristics

1. The trochlear nerve innervates the superior oblique muscle that depresses and adducts the eye
2. The muscle tendon is located in the trochlea, a cartilaginous structure in the superomedial orbit. Inflammation of the trochlea can occur either idiopathically or from primary autoimmune connective tissue disease
3. Primary trochlear headache has been described

Clinical Manifestations (Primary Trochlear Headache)

1. The headache is not associated with inflammation
2. 80% of patients are female of a mean age of 46 years (range of 18 to 77 years)
3. The headache is continuous, dull of moderate-to-severe intensity located periorbitally (medial eyebrow, orbit or forehead)
4. May be associated with photophobia and diplopia
5. The pain is aggravated by eye movement or reading; paradoxically the pain is exacerbated by looking up although the action of the superior oblique muscle is to depress and adduct the eye

Neuropathology

1. Approximately 50% of patients with trochleitis, that demonstrated clinically apparent trochlear edema, had Behcet's syndrome, granulomatosis polyangiitis (formally Wegener's syndrome), lymphoma or Tolosa-Hunt syndrome

Laboratory Evaluation

1. Evaluation for systemic autoimmune or neoplastic causes

Neuroimaging

1. MRI:
   a. Negative orbital study in patients with primary trochlear headache
   b. Trochlear tendon swelling and edema with secondary causes

Occipital Neuralgia

General Characteristics

1. Occipital neuralgia is recurring paroxysmal attacks of pain in the distribution of the greater occipital nerve (GON), lesser occipital nerve (LON) or third occipital nerve
2. There are connections of the C2 dorsal root component of the occipital nerve with cranial nerves VIII, IX, and X which enlarges the spectrum of symptoms from irritation of these nerves
3. The greater occipital nerve is most commonly involved, followed by the LON and rarely the third occipital nerve
4. The GON and LON are involved concomitantly in 9% of patients
5. The anatomy of the GON:
   a. The GON takes origin from the dorsal ramus of C2 (medial branch) ascends superiorly between the inferior oblique capitis and the semispinalis capitis muscles. It continues rostrolaterally deep to the trapezius muscle. It pierces the trapezius aponeurosis inferior to the nuchal ridge, becomes subcutaneous, and is located medially to the occipital artery. It provides sensory innervation from the external occipital protuberance to the vertex of the cranium
   b. The lesser occipital nerve arises from branches of C2 and C3 of the cervical plexus and extends superiorly along the posterior border of the sternocleidomastoid muscle. Its innervation territory is the lateral scalp and posterior to the ear.
   c. The third occipital nerve is a branch of C3, emerges inferiorly to supply sensation to the upper neck and lower portion of the occipital scalp

Clinical Manifestations

1. Most often the pain is unilateral and most severe in the occipital region
2. Pain quality is lancinating and stabbing often initiated from the neck and radiating to the posterior cranium; less frequent radiations are to parietal and temporal scalp and rarely to the fronto-orbital region
3. Due to dorsal root connections of C2 with cranial nerves VIII, IX and X; patients may have:
   a. Tinnitus, dizziness and nausea

4. Palpation and percussion of the GON:
    a. 2cm lateral and 2cm inferior to the external occipital protuberance
    b. Tenderness and a positive Tinel's sign may be elicited along the course of the nerve
    c. The LON is lateral to the GON and is most easily percussed along the superior nuchal ridge one-third lateral to the external occipital protuberance and medial to the mastoid

Neuropathology

1. Most injuries of the nerves are neuropractic
2. The usual injuries are concussions, whiplash that occur with motor vehicle accidents, contact sports and falls
3. Secondary pathologies that cause occipital neuralgias are:
    a. Compression of the cervical roots from cervical spondylosis
    b. Malignant infiltration
    c. Giant cell arteritis
    d. Bony callus formation after vertebral fractures
    e. Atlantoaxial lateral mass osteoarthritis
    f. Hypertrophic cervical pachymeningitis
    g. Cervical cord tumor
    h. C1-C2 arthrosis syndrome
    i. Chiari malformation
    j. Fracture of the atlas
    k. Pachymeningitis cervicalis associated with syphilis
    l. Third nerve occipital neuralgia:
        i Degenerative or traumatic arthropathy that involves the C2 and C3 apophyseal joints that impinges on a branch of the C3 dorsal ramus

Neuroimaging

1. Cervical spine radiographs with particular attention to the open mouth view
2. CT scan of the craniocervical junction (high cervical trauma)
3. MRI scan to delineate any spinal cord or soft tissue pathology

Carotidynia and Pain from Extracranial Arterial Dissection

Carotidynia

General Characteristics

1. Cervicofacial pain that can be elicited by pressure over the common carotid artery

Clinical Manifestations

1. Compression of the common carotid artery at or near its bifurcation causes a dull pain that is referred to the ipsilateral face, ear, jaw, orally and into the neck
2. Variant carotidynia (described by Roseman)
   a. Occurs in young adults
   b. Recurrent and self-limited pain and tenderness at the carotid bifurcation that may last for up to two weeks
   c. Exacerbating factors include head movement, chewing and swallowing
3. Carotidynia with migraine headaches:
   a. May be seen at any stage of adult life
   b. Attacks last for minutes to hours and are associated with a throbbing headache similar to migraine without aura
4. Carotid or vertebral artery dissection:
   a. In general, pain is localized to the area of injury in the anterior neck or face (carotid) or the posterior neck and lateral eyebrow (vertebral artery)
   b. Some dissections present with "thunderclap headaches" rather than neck pain; many patients have a throbbing headache over days that has been described bilaterally
   c. Carotid dissection is often associated with neck pain, pain over the eye and a partial Horner's syndrome

Neuropathology

1. Causes of carotidynia include:
   a. Giant cell arteritis
   b. Takayasu's arteritis
   c. Migraine and cluster headache
   d. Displacement of the carotid artery by tumor
   e. Dissecting aneurysm
   f. Fibromuscular dysplasia
   g. Atherosclerosis
   h. Intraluminal hemorrhage
   i. Aneurysm
2. Idiopathic carotidynia:
   a. Posited to be caused by edema or inflammation of tissues surrounding the carotid bifurcation

Laboratory Evaluation

1. A thorough medical evaluation to rule out an autoimmune or inflammatory condition

Neuroimaging

1. MRI (cervical):
   a. Enhancing tissue surrounding the symptomatic carotid artery at the level

of the distal common carotid and carotid bifurcation

b. The enhancing rim of tissue (5 patients) measured 6-8 mm; the length of the enhancing segment varied between 1.5-3.5 cm which included the distal common carotid and portions of the carotid bulb
c. Enhancing tissue was consistent with the fascia of the carotid sheath
d. The caliber of the carotid vessel is normal and demonstrates normal flow voids.

Temporomandibular Joint Disorder

General Characteristics

1. It is estimated that 10 million people in the USA have temporomandibular joint disorder and that a significant portion of individuals in the general population will develop it (~25%) at some point during life
2. The female to male ratio is 4:1
3. Rarely occurs in children

Clinical Manifestations

1. The highest incidence occurs in adults aged 20 to 40
2. The pain generally occurs unilaterally in the muscles of mastication
3. The pain radiates to the ear and jaw and is exacerbated with chewing
4. The jaw may lock with mouth opening
5. If there is displacement of the articular disc patients may have ear clicking or popping
6. Rarely patients complain of unilateral headache without concomitant jaw pain
7. Rarely patients may have back and shoulder pain
8. Bruxism during sleep and teeth clenching during the day
9. There may be progressive pain during the day
10. There is limitation of jaw opening. The normal aperture from lower to upper anterior teeth is 40mm
11. Masseter and internal pterygoid muscle spasm
12. Rarely ipsilateral facial swelling
13. Clicking and popping in the TMJ with jaw movement
14. Tenderness of the TMJ by palpation in the external auditory meatus while the patient opens the mouth
15. Crepitus in the joint
16. Deviation of the jaw to the affected side

Neuropathology

1. Macro and microfacial trauma
2. Malocclusion due to loss of molars or ill-fitting dentures
3. Arthritic changes

4. Repetitive trauma associated with age and tooth loss
5. TMJ disc displacement is associated with mandibular asymmetry
6. Most craniofacial dysmorphisms are not associated with temporomandibular dysfunction; a large study has demonstrated that temporomandibular disorders are not associated with vertical craniofacial morphology

Laboratory Evaluation

1. Complete blood count, calcium, phosphate and alkaline phosphatase (bone disease), uric acid (gout), creatine phosphokinase (muscle disease), sedimentation rate (temporal arteritis) and rheumatoid factor (rheumatoid arthritis)

Neuroimaging

1. MRI:
   a. There is a significant correlation between disc length, condyle morphology and disc displacement
   b. A series of 794 patients with clinical TMJ demonstrated by MRI (T1 and T2 weighted sequences):
      i 62% had physiological disc position
      ii 35% have anterior displacement
      iii 3% a posterior disc position

Persistent Idiopathic Facial Pain (PIFP)

General Characteristics

1. PIFP is the new terminology for atypical facial pain
2. Definition:
   a. A persistent facial pain that does not have the characteristics of the cranial neuralgias and is not attributed to another disorder
3. Atypical odontagia may be a sub-type of atypical facial pain (AFP) in which the pain is confined to the teeth or gums:
   a. Definition:
      i It is a pain with no demonstrable cause which is perceived to be coming from a tooth or multiple teeth and is not relieved by standard treatments to alleviate dental pain
4. PIFP or atypical facial pain has been classified as a component of the symptom complex of chronic facial pain that also includes:
   a. Burning mouth syndrome
   b. Temporomandibular joint dysfunction (TMD)
   c. Atypical odontalgia
5. Recent research supports the hypothesis that PIFP is a neuropathic pain

Clinical Manifestations

1. The pain is frequently poorly localized. It occurs more often in the maxilla

than the mandible. Both may be affected.

2. The pain is not perceived in the distribution of the trigeminal nerve and is usually unilateral
3. The pain may be located in the socket of an extracted tooth or to an area of a previous surgical procedure
4. The pain may spread to other sites, if the teeth are involved a quadrant of the mouth may be affected
5. The onset is often attributable by the patient to a dental procedure. The pain is continuous for months to years with intermittent exacerbations. It gradually increases with time.
6. The pain is variously described as deep, pressure-like, crushing or burning
7. The pain does not respect the midline or a dermatomal distribution. It may radiate to the temple, neck or occiput
8. The pain is associated with depression and anxiety as well as with other chronic pain syndromes. Xerostomia and dysgusia may be prominent
9. The pain is persistent throughout the day; less frequently it is intermittent
10. There are no precipitating or relieving factors and no "trigger zones"; facial movements do not exacerbate the pain and non-steroidal analgesics are not effective
11. The pain is moderate to severe; usually does not disturb sleep

Neuropathology

1. Putative central sensitization of trigeminal nociceptive neurons in the brainstem
2. Central sensitization has been demonstrated after pulpectomy or transection of dental nerves as well as from inflammation of peripheral tissue
3. Neuralgia-inducing cavitational osteonecrosis (controversial term and entity) refers to degeneration of the bone marrow in the maxilla or mandible on an ischemic basis. Most often, it is painless, but in some patients causes neuropathic pain. Degenerative extracellular cystic spaces are seen in the bone marrow

Laboratory Evaluation

1. Radiographs, cone beam CT, and MRI to exclude other pathology that includes arteriovenous malformation, tumor, temporomandibular joint disorder or MS

Intraoral non-Dental Pain

1. Atypical odontalgia
2. Post-traumatic trigeminal neuropathy
3. Burning mouth syndrome

Extraoral Pain with or without Intraoral Pain

1. Temporomandibular disorders
2. Trigeminal neuralgia
3. Glossopharyngeal neuralgia
4. Persistent idiopathic facial pain
5. Giant cell arteritis
6. Migraine / neurovascular orofacial pain

Sinusitis

General Characteristics

1. Sinusitis is very common and thought to effect 10 to 30% of the USA and European population per year
2. Women are more frequently affected than men
3. Chronic sinusitis affects approximately 12% of the population
4. Sinusitis is inflammation of the mucous membrane of the paranasal sinuses and is classified according to anatomic site:
    a. Maxillary
    b. Ethmoidal
    c. Frontal
    d. Sphenoidal
5. Pathogenic organism (viral, bacterial or fungal)
6. Associated factors:
    a. Nasal polyposis
    b. Immunosuppression
    c. Anatomic variants
7. Acute rhinosinusitis:
    a. An infection that may be present for four weeks
8. Recurrent acute rhinosinusitis:
    a. Four or more separate episodes of acute sinusitis within one year
9. Subacute rhinosinusitis:
    a. An infection that persists for four to 12 weeks; posited to be a transition between acute and chronic infection
10. Chronic rhinosinusitis:
    a. Signs and symptoms that persist for more than 12 weeks

Clinical Manifestations

1. Headache or facial pain over the affected sinuses is seen in both acute and chronic sinusitis
2. The quality of the pain is constant, dull or aching
3. The pain is typically localized to the involved sinus:
    a. Maxillary sinus:
        i The pain is experienced most often in the cheek or as a generalized

headache, or toothache

b. Frontal sinus:
    i The pain is experienced in the brow, forehead and above the eyes
c. Ethmoidal sinus:
    i Pain is between or behind the eyes, the medial canthi, and may be associated with generalized headache
d. Sphenoidal sinus:
    i Pain or pressure behind the eyes; frequently radiates to the vertex of the skull, the mastoid process or occipitally
    ii Pain is exacerbated with bending over or with recumbency
    iii Pain may start unilaterally and then progress bilaterally
    iv Tilting the head forward and a Valsalva maneuver exacerbate the pain which are differential points from toothache
    v Less frequent symptoms and signs of sinus infections:
        1. Infection of the orbit (most often from ethmoid sinusitis)
        2. Osteomyelitis of the forehead and facial bones (Pott's puffy tumor)
        3. Middle ear symptoms:
            a. Due to congestion of the nasal passages
            b. Pressure in the head or vibrating feeling in the head
        4. Halitosis

Neuropathology

Basic Mechanisms of Sinus Pathology

1. Obstruction of sinus drainage
    a. Obstruction of sinus ostia prevents normal mucous drainage. Causes of ostial obstruction include:
        i Trauma
        ii Rhinitis
        iii Inflammatory systemic disorders
        iv Immune deficiency
        v Disorders of mucociliary clearance:
            1. Cystic fibrosis
            2. Respiratory allergies
            3. Primary ciliary dyskinesia (Kartagener syndrome)
        vi Patients with immunodeficiency:
            1. Agammaglobulinemia
            2. Decreased IgG and IgA
        vii Mechanical obstruction of ostia:
            1. Nasal polyps
            2. Foreign body

3. Deviated septa
4. Anatomical variants that narrow the osteomeatal complex

viii A combination of anaerobic and aerobic bacteria is associated with chronic sinusitis. Common organisms include:
1. Staphylococcus aureus
2. Coagulase-negative staphylococci
3. Gram negative enteric organisms
4. Chronic rhinosinusitis is a multifactorial inflammatory disorder rather than a persistent bacterial infection

ix It has been posited that biofilm bacterial infections may be a cause of antibiotic-refractory chronic sinusitis:
1. A biofilm is a complex aggregate of extracellular matrix and inter-dependent microorganisms from multiple species. Bacteria in microfilms have much greater resistance to antibiotics than free-living bacteria

x Major associated complications of sinusitis:
1. Often involve the frontal, sphenoidal and ethmoidal sinuses include:
    a. Brain abscess from invasion of bacteria through affected bones and blood vessels
    b. Meningitis
    c. Orbital infections from continguous spread from the ethmoid sinus by anterior and posterior ethmoidal veins thrombophlebitis. The infection spreads to the lateral or orbital side of the ethmoid labyrinth
    d. Central nervous-system spread to involve the cavernous sinus
2. Maxillary sinusitis from an odontogenic origin is well described

Laboratory Evaluation

1. In context, nasal cytology to delineate:
    a. Allergic rhinitis
    b. Eosinophilia
    c. Nasal polyposis
    d. Aspirin sensitivity
2. Recurrent infection:
    a. Immunoglobulin evaluation

Neuroimaging

1. CT with frontal and coronal planes
2. MRI with contrast is the method of choice for intraorbital or intracranial complications

Silent Sinus Syndrome (SSS)

General Characteristics

1. A syndrome that is usually painless and demonstrates unilateral enophthalmos and hypoglobus

Clinical Manifestations

1. Enophthalmos is universally present
2. Upper lid retraction, lid lag and restriction of gaze
3. Normal visual acuity but some patients develop diplopia
4. Males and females are affected equally and the disease presents in the third to the fifth decade
5. Facial asymmetry
6. Progressive changes over weeks to months
7. Rarely patients have headaches and nondermatomal facial pain

Neuropathology

1. There is support for the hypothesis that SSS may be a variant of chronic maxillary atelectasis
2. Obstruction of outflow theory:
   a. An acquired obstruction of the maxillary infundibulum causes hypoventilation of the sinus with accumulation of secretions. The reabsorption of secretions causes a negative pressure in the maxillary antrum
   b. Infundibular obstruction may be caused by aberrant nasal anatomy such as lateral deviation of the middle turbinate
   c. Other causes of occlusion are mucous plugging, mucocoele and nasal polyps. Surgery may damage the osteomeatal complex

Laboratory Evaluation

1. CT evaluation:
   a. Occlusion of the maxillary infundibulum due to lateral retraction of the uncinate process with apposition against the inferiomedial aspect of the orbital wall
   b. The orbital floor is inferiorly displaced and there is increased concavity of the medial and lateral maxillary wall toward the antrum
   c. There is a loss of antral volume

Complex Regional Pain Syndrome

General Characteristics

1. Complex regional pain syndrome is a neuropathic pain syndrome that is divided into type I in which no specific large nerve is injured and type II in

which a specific nerve injury can be identified

2. Type I CRPS is most common and there is supporting evidence for it as a small fiber neuropathy
3. CRPS characteristically follows injury to an extremity or a surgical procedure

Clinical Manifestations

1. Following soft tissue or nerve injury patients develop:
    a. Pain in the injured part out of a nerve root or dermatomal distribution that characteristically:
        i Is spontaneous and more severe than the injury would suggest
        ii Demonstrates mechanical and thermal hyperalgesia, allodynia and when evoked is not stimulus bound
        iii Progressively spreads in most patients
        iv Autonomic dysregulation characterized by either an increase or decrease of blood flow (usually the former in acute injury) and hyper or hypohidrosis
        v Neurogenic edema of the affected part
        vi A movement disorder that includes:
            1. Difficulty initiating and sustaining movement
            2. Weakness
            3. Myoclonic jerks
            4. Tremor
            5. Spasm
            6. Increased reflexes
            7. Dystonia
        vii Trophic changes in which nails and hair grow too rapidly and then thin and may fall out (hair); loss of muscle and subcutaneous tissue
        viii If the face is involved there is erythema, neurogenic edema, severe pain with mechanical and thermal hyperalgesia and allodynia:
            1. Myokymia of the orbicularis oculi
            2. No dystrophy of subcutaneous tissue but frequent poor dentition with loss of teeth
            3. Red and hot ears
        ix The upper extremity is frequently involved with the face

Neuropathology

1. The cervical plexus and usually the upper components of the brachial plexus have undergone a neuropractic injury from a motor vehicle accident, fall or surgical procedure (damage to the supra orbital nerve from plastic surgery)
2. The process is thought to occur from a continued peripheral nerve drive on pain projecting neurons of the dorsal root ganglion that causes sensitization of both peripheral and central pain projecting neurons throughout the pain

matrix. The process is one of maladaptive neuroplasticity

3. The warmth and neurogenic edema is secondary to release of substance P and calcitonin gene related peptide (vasoactive neuropeptides) that dilate and increase permeability of peripheral blood vessels

Laboratory Evaluation

1. EMG:
   a. To evaluate large nerve dysfunction and to delineate any possible relieving factors
2. Skin biopsy:
   a. Demonstrates small fiber loss and abnormalities of sweat glands
3. QST:
   a. Demonstrates mechanical and thermal decreased perception thresholds in some patients
   b. Decreased thresholds for cold and heat pain
   c. Increased temporal summation ("wind up")
4. Autonomic testing:
   a. Abnormal quantitative sweat test

Neuroimaging

1. MRI of the cervical spine and the brachial plexus to rule out underlying pathology

Neck-Tongue Syndrome

General Characteristics

1. A rare syndrome that involves the neck and the tongue when suddenly turning the head

Clinical Manifestations

1. Sudden rotation of the neck and head causes lancinating pain of the upper neck or occiput
2. This pain is immediately followed by transient ipsilateral numbness of the tongue. Rarely there is numbness in the back of the palate
3. Symptoms are usually seconds to 1 minute

Neuropathology

1. Abnormal subluxation of one lateral atlanto-axial joint with compression of the C2 ventral ramus against the articular process
2. The posterior cervical plexus joins the first 3 cervical roots. The pain in the occiput suggests stimulation of the second and third cervical roots
3. The C2 root is compressed between the atlas and axis during excessive rotation of the neck
4. The lingual nerve forms a communication with the hypoglossal nerve as they

course over the hyoglossus muscle below the tongue. The hypoglossal nerve is connected by a loop between the first and second cervical roots

5. Thus there are anatomical connections from the lingual nerve via the hypoglossal nerve to the second cervical root that may explain tongue numbness when the C2 root is compressed

Laboratory Evaluation

1. CT of the cervical spine and craniocervical junction to evaluate the origin of the C2-C3 cervical roots and the atlanto-axial anatomy

Dry Eye Disease (DED)

General Characteristics

1. DED is also known as keratoconjunctivitis sicca, affects the ocular surface due to alterations in the quality or quantity of the tear film
2. The multiple etiologies cause an unstable tear film
3. A classification divides the syndrome into:
   a. Aqueous-deficient dry eye
   b. Evaporation dry eye
   c. Aqueous deficient dry eye is classified as:
      i Sjogren's syndrome
      ii Non-Sjogren's syndrome

Clinical Manifestations

1. Ocular discomfort
2. A feeling of dryness in the eye
3. Photophobia
4. Blurred and fluctuating vision
5. Often associated dry mouth

Neuropathology

1. Sjogren's syndrome with an autoimmune attack of the salivary and lacrimal glands
2. In normal individuals, the precorneal tear film covers the exposed ocular surface that continuously evaporates. Tears are replenished by the lacrimal glands which moisten the nonkeratinized epithelium of the cornea
3. During interblink intervals, there is a rapid drop of eye surface temperature due to tear evaporation. There is a concomitant increase of osmolality of the tear film.
4. Thinning and disruption of the precorneal tear film causes mechanical stress of the cells and nerve fibers of the superficial epithelial corneal layers which releases inflammatory mediators

5. These physical changes increase excitability of corneal cold trigeminal neurons due to an increase in sodium currents and a decrease of potassium currents
6. Corneal polymodal receptors demonstrate increased sodium currents
7. Experimental evidence shows that cold thermoreceptors contribute to the detection and signaling of ocular surface wetness. Under dry eye conditions, they develop injury-evoked neuropathic discharge that may underlie the ocular discomfort of DED patients

Laboratory Evaluation

1. The biomarkers for primary Sjogren's disease are anti-SS-A(Ro) or SS-B(La) antibodies
2. Elevated antinuclear antibodies (ANA) or increased rheumatoid factor are found in other autoimmune diseases that are a component of secondary SS
3. Novel autoantibodies for early SS are to:
   a. Salivary protein 1 (SP-1)
   b. Parotid secretory protein 1 (PSP-1)
   c. Carbonic anhydrase VI (CA-6)

Neck Pain

Overview

The primarily neuropathic causes of neck pain have been covered in the discussion of cervical and pharyngeal plexus disorders, congenital anatomical variants of the cranial cervical junction, disc disease, spondylosis, facet and spondylolisthesis, and spinal cord pain.

This discussion is of neck pain caused by myofascial syndromes, retropharyngeal disorders and tendinitis of neck muscles that are associated with pain.

Cervical Myofascial Pain

General Characteristics

1. Myofascial pain is caused by muscles and their surrounding fascia
2. The muscles primarily involved in cervical myofascial pain are the:
   a. Trapezius
   b. Levator scapulae
   c. Rhomboids
   d. Supraspinatus
   e. Infraspinatus
3. Cervical myofascial pain most often occurs in a setting of overuse or trauma
4. Myofascial pain is common in the general population and maybe 21% of patients seen in orthopedic clinics. It is more common among women and occurs more frequently with increasing age until midlife when its incidence

gradually declines

Clinical Manifestations

1. This is a clinical diagnosis with no generally accepted biomarkers
2. Many patients present with a history of trauma and persistent muscle pain. Others have an insidious onset associated with repetitive upper extremity movement, poor posture and stress
3. Poor posture includes dropped and forward flexed shoulders with protracted scapulae
4. Trigger points are found in the trapezius, supraspinatus, infraspinatus, rhomboids and levator scapulae muscles
5. A palpable taut band is noted in the affected skeletal muscle or its surrounding fascia. A local twitch response can be induced with palpation
6. Range of cervical spine movement is usually restricted with pain elicited in positions that stretch the affected muscle
7. Strength of the upper extremity is normal. Radiating pain into the hand and fingers supports an associated brachial plexus involvement
8. Sensation is normal

Neuropathology

1. Myofascial pain is associated with trigger points in the affected skeletal muscle
2. A trigger point is a hyperirritable area that is in a palpable taut band of muscle fibers. Palpation of trigger points elicits local pain and referred pain
3. Trigger points may have associated autonomic phenomena

Neuroimaging

1. MRI to rule out any structural cervical spine lesions

Laboratory Evaluation

1. EMG evaluation of trigger points has been found to be contradictory and controversial

Retropharyngeal Tendinitis

General Characteristics

1. Acute calcific tendinitis of the longus colli muscle is an aseptic inflammatory process that is located in the prevertebral space
2. The longus colli muscle is located in the prevertebral space and is composed of upper oblique, vertical, and lower oblique fibers. The upper oblique fibers take origin from the anterior tubercles of the transverse processes of the C3-C5 vertebrae and insert on the anterior tubercle of the atlas
3. Vertical fibers arise from the bodies of the upper thoracic and lower cervical vertebrae and insert on the bodies of the upper cervical vertebrae

4. Oblique fibers arise from the anterior areas of T1-T3 and insert on the anterior tubercles of the transverse processes of the C5-C6 vertebrae

Clinical Manifestations

1. Acute neck pain and stiffness
2. Odynophagia
3. Less frequent signs and symptoms include:
   a. Dysphagia
   b. Sore throat
   c. Limited range of cervical motion
   d. Pharyngeal edema
   e. Erythema of the nasopharynx
   f. Neck spasm

Neuropathology

1. It has been proposed that the natural history of retropharyngeal calcinosis consists of 5 phases:
   a. Precalcific
   b. Formative
   c. Resting
   d. Resorptive
   e. Postcalcific
2. Endochondral ossification has been proposed which is similar to that which occurs in the Achilles tendon. This model proposes that fibrocartilaginous metaplasia is the initiating event
3. Erroneous differentiation of tendon-derived stem cells into chondrocytes or osteoblasts may be causative
4. Calcium hydroxyapatite crystal deposition occurs; rupture of these crystals causes an aseptic foreign-body type inflammatory response that leads to formation of fluid in the retropharyngeal space surrounding the longus colli muscle

Laboratory Evaluation

1. Mild elevation of the sedimentation rate with low-grade leukocytosis

Neuroimaging

1. CT scan detects both the prevertebral edema and calcium hydroxyapatite crystals that are deposited in the longus colli tendon. CT is considered more sensitive in distinguishing retropharyngeal tendinitis from abscess
2. MRI demonstrates the prevertebral edema and is less sensitive for depicting the calcific deposits

Differential Diagnosis

1. Meningitis (stiff neck and painful range of motion)

2. Retropharyngeal abscess
3. Neoplasm
4. Cervical disc
5. Fracture dislocation
6. Spondylolisthesis

Ossification of the Posterior Longitudinal Ligament (OPLL)

General Characteristics

1. The ossification of the ligament is most often at cervical levels C2-C4
2. The ratio of males to females is 2:1
3. In Japanese patients, the prevalence of OPLL is 1.8-4%. The prevalence in North America is much lower, possibly 0.12%
4. The genetics is most often sporadic but there have been some familial patients in Caucasian and European populations

Clinical Manifestations

1. The majority of patients are asymptomatic. The posterior longitudinal ligament extends from the occiput to the sacrum and is located posterior to the vertebral bodies and dorsal to the intervertebral discs
2. Ossification and hypertrophy of the ligament presents with a progressive neurologic deficit, pain or acute neurologic symptoms
3. In a large Japanese study, 17% of patients that were followed for 18 years developed myelopathy
4. Cervical myelopathy with neck pain and progressive weakness, sphincter involvement and hyperreflexia comprise its natural history. Radiculopathy may be prominent

Neuropathology

1. Ossification of the posterior longitudinal ligament is a multifactorial and polygenic disease
2. RSPO2 (encoding R-spondin 2) has been identified by genome-wide association studies as a susceptibility gene which is a secreted agonist of canonical Wnt/β-catenin signaling. The most significant SNP in the GWAS locus maps to chromosome 8q23.1 which is located in the chondrocyte promotor region of the RSPO2 gene
3. Ossification and hypertrophy of the ligament decreases the cervical spine diameter, compresses the spinal cord which causes an ischemic myelopathy
4. The cord parenchyma is also damaged by repeated trauma to the ventral spinal cord by the hypertrophied and ossified ligament

Neuroimaging

1. CT:

a. Delineates early OPLL that demonstrates multiple small areas of bone within an enlarged ligament that over time coalesce to form a large bony plaque within the ligament ventral to the spinal cord.
b. A "single-layer sign" signifies dense ossification within the ligament that extends to the periphery
c. A "double-layer sign" in which there is ossification of the ligament behind the vertebral body as well as in the posterior longitudinal ligament
d. The dura may be penetrated by the bony mass in the ligament to cause a CSF leak

2. MRI:
   a. Early OPLL is seen dorsal to the interspaces; over time there are areas of new bone formation demonstrated by increased signal on T1-weighted sequences in the ligament. There is no enhancement with gadolinium.

Superior Laryngeal Neuralgia

General Characteristics

1. The superior laryngeal nerve is a branch of the vagus nerve. Its origin is from the middle of the nodose ganglion
2. The cricothyroid muscles are innervated by the superior laryngeal nerve while all other intrinsic laryngeal muscles are innervated by the recurrent laryngeal nerve
3. The nerve descends lateral to the pharynx, behind the internal carotid artery and divides into the external laryngeal and internal laryngeal nerves

Clinical Manifestations

1. The superior laryngeal nerve is the closest nerve contiguous to the bifurcation of the carotid artery
2. Paroxysms of pain along the anterior cervical triangle
3. Radiations may extend to the ipsilateral ear and eye
4. The pain may last for minutes to hours
5. Triggering factors are:
   a. Swallowing
   b. Straining the voice
   c. Head turning
6. A common trigger point is on the lateral aspect of the throat overlying the thyrohyoid membrane. Other trigger points include:
   a. At the foramen of the internal branch of the superior laryngeal nerve
   b. In the pyriform sinus where the superior laryngeal nerve is superficial

Neuropathology

1. May occur from upper respiratory infection such as influenza
2. Laryngitis

3. Trauma, particularly carotid endarterectomy as the nerve lies in close proximity to the carotid bifurcation
4. Prior tonsillectomy
5. Lateral pharyngeal diverticulum
6. Compression by the superior thyroid artery and / or vein

Laboratory Evaluation

1. EMG to evaluate the function of the laryngeal musculature

Neuroimaging

1. MRI:
   a. To rule out pathology of the larynx and perilaryngeal structures

Eagle Syndrome

General Characteristics

1. The disorder is caused by an elongated or misshaped styloid process and / or calcification of the stylohyoid ligament. The incidence of Eagle's syndrome is approximately 0.16% of the population

Clinical Manifestations

1. Lancinating pain that radiates to the jaw, back of the throat, base of the tongue, face, ear or neck
2. Dysphagia
3. A foreign object sensation in the throat
4. Triggers for pain include:
   a. Chewing
   b. Swallowing
   c. Turning the head
   d. Touching the back of the throat
5. Tinnitus
6. The elongated styloid process can at times be palpated behind the tonsillar fossa
7. Vascular Eagle syndrome:
   a. The elongated styloid process may compress the internal carotid artery below the skull:
      i Rarely may cause TIA or stroke

Neuropathology

1. The styloid may be elongated, >30 millimeters in length, in approximately 4% of the population (~4% of these patients are symptomatic)
2. Styloid / C1 transverse process juxtaposition may be a cause. In these patients, the distance between the styloid process and the transverse process of C1 ranged from 0.05-0.46 cm; the length of the process ranged from 2.4 – 8.5

cm.

3. Calcification of the stylohyoid ligament

Neuroimaging

1. CT:
   a. The normal length of the styloid in an adult is approximately 2.5cm; an elongated process is generally > 3cm in length
   b. Lateral deviation of the process may be symptomatic

Cricoid Cartilage Syndrome

General Characteristics

1. The cricoid cartilage is inferior to the thyroid cartilage in the neck at the C6 vertebral level to which it is connected by the median cricothyroid ligament medially and postero-laterally by the cricothyroid joints.
2. The cricoid is attached to the first tracheal ring by the cricotracheal ligament
3. It is a component of the attachment of the cricothyroid muscle, posterior cricoarytenoid muscle and lateral cricoarytenoid muscles

Clinical Manifestation

1. Anterior cervical or throat pain

Neuropathology

1. Calcification with age
2. Composed of hyaline cartilage

Neuroimaging

1. MRI:
   a. To rule out any pathology or structural lesion

Hyoid Syndrome

General Characteristics

1. The hyoid bone is the only bone in the human body with no direct contact with any other bone
2. It forms a moveable base for the tongue; it is U shaped and is located between the root of the tongue, mandible and thyroid cartilage
3. Its muscle associations include:
   a. Mylohyoid (mandible)
   b. Hypoglossus (tongue)
   c. Stylohyoid (skull)
   d. Thyrohyoid (thyroid cartilage)
   e. Sternohyoid (sternum)
   f. Omohyoid (the medial border of the scapular notch

Clinical Manifestations

1. Pain on swallowing in the region of the hyoid (anterior cervical pain)
2. Common radiations are to the ear, face, lower jaw and pharynx
3. Less common radiations:
   a. Zygomatic arch
   b. Temporomandibular joint
   c. Mandibular molar teeth
   d. Very rarely the sternum
4. Palpation and pressure on the greater cornu of the hyoid bone causes local pain and specific pain radiations

Neuropathology

1. Trauma to the greater cornu of the hyoid bone
2. In a subset of patients, tenosynovitis of the intermediate tendon of the digastric muscle
3. The bone may be involved by chondrosarcoma which presents as a slow-growing painless mass in the neck
4. Osteonecrosis of the hyoid bone after radiation therapy for carcinoma of the head or neck

Neuroimaging

1. MRI:
   a. To delineate pathology or structural lesions
   b. To rule out a recurrent neoplasm

Ernest Syndrome

General Characteristics

1. Ernest syndrome is insertion tendinosis of the stylomandibular ligament at its insertion into the mandible
2. The function of the ligament is to limit the maximum opening and protrusion of the mandible
3. The ligament is derived from the first branchial arch and is posited to be innervated by a branch of the third division of the trigeminal nerve

Clinical Manifestations

1. Throat pain
2. Pain around the TMJ
3. Ear fullness and pain
4. Anterior temporal pain and headache
5. Pain in the body of the mandible
6. Eye pain
7. Odontalgia

Neuropathology

1. Degenerative changes at the insertion zone in the muscle or ligament; Sharpey's fibers are affected usually after repetitive movement or trauma

Neuroimaging

1. MRI to rule out any other pathology

Superior Pharyngeal Constrictor Syndrome

General Characteristics

1. A myofascial disorder of the superior pharyngeal constrictor muscle
2. The muscle is large, is quadrilateral and has 4 origins:
   a. The inferior medial plate and pterygoid hamulus of the sphenoid bone
   b. The pterygomandibular raphe
   c. The medial surface of the mandible
   d. The lateral surface of the body of the tongue
3. The insertion is into the median raphe of the posterior pharyngeal wall
4. The muscle is innervated by the pharyngeal plexus which is formed by branches of the glossopharyngeal and vagus nerves

Clinical Manifestations

1. Pain in the throat
2. Radiation to the TMJ area
3. Swallowing triggers pain
4. Otalgia
5. Radiation to the temple
6. Dysfunction of the swallowing reflex
7. Pain on mechanical pressure of the posterior and lateral areas of the pharyngeal wall posterior to the pterygoid hamulus

Neuropathology

1. Putatively biomechanical stress of the muscle when the mouth is widely opened
2. May be injured during intubation for general anesthesia
3. Injured during the Halstead technique for injecting the alveolar nerve

Neuroimaging

1. MRI to delineate any other cervical pathology
2. Flexible laryngoscopy

Superior Thyroid Cornu Syndrome

General Characteristics

1. Ossification of a superior thyroid cornu

Clinical Manifestations

1. Throat pain
2. Dysphagia
3. Odynophagia
4. Foreign body sensation in the throat
5. Symptoms may develop years after trauma

Neuropathology

1. Displacement of the superior cornu following neck trauma or congenitally
2. The displacement is usually medial and anterior to its normal position which produces a protruding mass impinging upon the lumen of the pharynx; a similar effect occurs if the superior thyroid cornu is elongated by ossification
3. Strangulation, external compression and endotracheal intubation may cause repositioning of the superior cornu towards the lumen of the larynx
4. Congenital defects are due to maldevelopment of the fourth branchial arch
5. Ossification of thyroid cartilage begins at 20-23 years of age at its inferior margin

Laboratory Evaluation

1. Flexible endoscopy
2. CT scanning with 3D reconstruction

Lateral Thyrohyoid Ligament Syndrome

General Characteristics

1. The lateral thyrohyoid ligament forms the posterior border of the thyrohyoid membrane and passes between the tip of the superior cornu of the thyroid cartilage and greater cornu of the hyoid bone
2. The recurrent laryngeal nerve lies laterally

Clinical Manifestations

1. Chronic unilateral neck pain associated with painful swallowing (some patients)
2. 1/3 of patients have a foreign body sensation in the throat
3. Severe pain on palpation either at the superior lateral thyroid cartilage or in the ligament that extends to the hyoid bone

Neuropathology

1. Initiating factors that have been reported are trumpet playing, severe cough, excessive voice use and strenuous physical activity
2. Inflammation of the ligament that is frequently responsive to steroids

Laboratory Evaluation

1. Flexible laryngoscopy

Neuroimaging:

1. MRI to rule out other pathology

Thyroid Cartilage and Mastoid Process Syndromes

General Characteristics

1. The thyroid cartilage is composed of two plates or lamina that connect anteriorly at an angle of 90 to 120 degrees
2. The cartilage is a component of voice production by facilitating vibration of the vocal cords
3. It forms attachments for laryngeal muscles and protects the vocal folds
4. The cricothyroid joint joins the cricoid and thyroid cartilage and changes the tension (assists in this action) and pressure on the vocal cords which helps to adjust the pitch of the voice

Clinical Manifestations

1. Tenderness to mechanical stimuli over the thyroid cartilage and the area of insertion of the sternocleidomastoid muscle on the mastoid process

Neuropathology

1. Fracture of the cartilage
2. Increased tension or stress on the muscles that surround the cartilage
3. Putative inflammation of the cartilage

Laboratory Evaluation

1. Flexible laryngoscopy

Neuroimaging

1. MRI to rule out other pathologies

Rare Syndromes Causing Pain in the Throat

1. Eagle syndrome
2. Ernest syndrome
3. Hyoid bone syndrome
4. Thyroid cartilage and mastoid process syndrome
5. Cricoid cartilage syndrome
6. Superior laryngeal nerve neuralgia
7. Neck tongue syndrome
8. Retropharyngeal tendinitis
9. Posterior longitudinal ligament calcification syndrome
10. Superior cornu of the thyroid cartilage syndrome
11. Superior pharyngeal constrictor syndrome

CHAPTER 6

SOMATIC CHEST WALL PAIN

Overview

1. Chest wall pain may be caused by:
    a. Musculoskeletal disorders
    b. Direct injury to the roots and nerves that supply the sensory innervation of the thorax
    c. Referral from a visceral source
    d. Central nervous system disorders that disrupt somatosensory input or its processing

Musculoskeletal Chest Wall Pain

General Characteristics

1. The prevalence of musculoskeletal chest wall pain is unknown but has been estimated to affect 10% of patients that present with chest pain
2. Anatomy:
    a. The ribs articulate posteriorly with the vertebral bodies and their transverse processes at the costovertebral and costotransverse joints which are diarthroidal synovial joints
    b. The second to 10th ribs articulate with two hemifacets with two adjacent vertebra separated by an intervertebral disc
    c. The joint is divided by an intra-articular ligament and attaches the head of the rib to the intervertebral disc
    d. The first, eleventh and twelfth ribs articulate by a single facet with its own vertebral body
    e. Ribs are attached to the costal cartilages by costochondral articulations that are synchondroses
    f. The first to seventh ribs are vertebrosternal in that their costal cartilages

join the sternum at the chondrosternal joints

g. The cartilages of the 8th, 9th and 10th ribs articulate with the cartilage above them and are vertebrochondral ribs; the 11th and 12th ribs are free at the cartilaginous ends.
h. The costal cartilage of the first rib attaches to the manubrium by a synchondrosis. The remaining six pairs of chondrosternal articulations are synovial lined and contain an intra-articular ligament
i. There may be synovial membrane interchondral articulations between the fifth to ninth costal cartilages. These joints may degenerate with age.
j. The medial end of the clavicle articulates with the manubrium by its costal cartilage to form the sternoclavicular joint. The joint is divided into two synovial membrane-lined cavities by an intra articular fibrocartilaginous disc
k. The manubriosternal joint attaches the manubrium with the body of the sternum. It is a synchondrosis and is composed of a fibrocartilaginous disc. In approximately 1/3 of adults, there is resorption of the central component of the disc that then forms a synovial membrane lined joint. Ossification of the disc and synostosis of the joint occurs in 10% of adults.
l. The xiphisternal joint (at the most ventral aspect of the sternum) is a synchondrosis between the body of the sternum and the xiphoid cartilage that may ossify over time.

Clinical Manifestations of Musculoskeletal Chest Wall Pain

1. The onset is usually insidious. Precipitating features may be repetitive movements, minor trauma or unusual physical exertion
2. The pain is usually localized to the affected site and may be a deep ache or lancinating; it may radiate widely
3. Exacerbating factors are positional changes such as turning of the chest, deep breathing or movement of the shoulder girdle
4. Local chest wall tenderness (mechanical hyperalgesia)
5. Duplication of pain by specific movements or by chest wall palpation
6. A small number of tender areas that are asymmetric and grouped in a single area support a referred pain
7. Widespread pain tender points that are symmetrical and are associated with diffuse aching, stiffness and sleep disruption support a diagnosis of fibromyalgia

Local Chest Wall Pain - Tietze's Syndrome and Costochondritis

General Considerations

1. Tietze's syndrome as originally described in 1921 is characterized by painful

nonsuppurative swelling of the cartilaginous articulations of the anterior chest wall

2. Costochondritis causes pain and swelling of the costochondral articulations
3. There is no ethnic or geographic predispositions but clustering of patients has been reported

Clinical Manifestations (Tietze's syndrome)

1. Pain in the anterior chest wall is the primary symptom
2. The pain varies in intensity and is usually localized to the involved synchondrosis
3. The disorder has a predilection for the second and third costochondral junctions. Less frequently, the chondrosternal, manubrial, sternal sternoclavicular and xiphisternal articulations are involved
4. In more than 70% of patients, the lesions are unilateral and single. If the lesions are multiple they usually affect contiguous articulations on the same side
5. Some patients have a history of excessive coughing during the course of a prior upper respiratory infection
6. Exacerbating factors are coughing, deep breathing and lying prone
7. The affected cartilage is mechanically tender and swollen but not warm or erythematous. There are no constitutional symptoms.
8. The disorder is self-limited but has remissions and exacerbations
9. Pain may stop spontaneously within weeks or months but the cartilaginous swelling may persist
10. More common in patients <40 years of age

Neuropathology

1. There are few pathological studies. Some specimens have demonstrated degenerated costal cartilage with minor inflammatory changes in the perichondrium with primary Tietze's syndrome.
2. Secondary Tietze's syndrome includes:
    a. Infectious involvement of the costochondral joints
    b. Chest wall tumors
    c. Osteomyelitis of the sternum and ribs as a complication of median sternotomy
    d. Fungal costochondritis with Candida, Aspergillus, Blastomyces and Actinomyces are the major fungal organisms

Laboratory Evaluation

1. Appropriate studies to delineate rheumatic or autoimmune involvement of cartilage (rheumatoid arthritis, relapsing polychondritis)
2. Sedimentation rate, C-reactive protein if infection or autoimmune disorders are suspected

Neuroimaging

1. MRI:
   a. Is superior to CT for detecting cartilaginous damage and bone marrow edema
   b. The MRI pattern of primary Tietze's Syndrome includes:
      i Thickened and enlarged cartilage at the affected joints
      ii Focal or widespread increased signal intensities are demonstrated in both T2-weighted and STIR or FAT SAT sequences
      iii Bone marrow edema in the subchondral bone is noted in approximately 50% of patients
      iv Gadolinium enhancement occurs in the areas of thickened cartilage, subchondral bone marrow, joint capsule and ligaments

Costochondritis

General Characteristics

1. Costochondritis and costosternal syndrome are used interchangeably
2. It is a not uncommon disorder and may occur as a primary disease or in combination with median sternotomy or trauma

Clinical Manifestations

1. Pain occurs at the costochondral or chondrosternal articulations with swelling which is a differential point from Tietze's Syndrome
2. In 90% of patients, multiple lesions are seen. The second to fifth costal cartilages are most frequently affected
3. The major physical finding is diffuse tenderness to mechanical stimuli over the involved costal cartilages:
   a. Pain may be provoked by the "crowing rooster" sign in which the cervical spine is extended and traction is placed on the posteriorly extended arms or traction is applied to an adducted arm with the head rotated to the ipsilateral side
   b. The disorder is self-limited but there are recurrences during its course
   c. More common in patients > 40 years of age

Neuropathology

1. The etiology of costochondritis has not been defined
2. It has been associated with minor trauma
3. Less frequently, it has been seen in intravenous drug users from bacterial and fungus infections
4. In the course of thoracic surgery in patients who have had a median sternotomy incision
5. Costochondritis has also been described with vitamin D deficiency

Laboratory Evaluation

1. Medical evaluation to delineate causes of atypical chest pain

Neuroimaging

1. MRI to evaluate cartilage and subchondral bone

Rib Trauma

General Characteristics

1. Rib fractures are the most common injury from blunt chest trauma and account for > 50% of thoracic injuries from non-penetrating trauma
2. Approximately 10% of patients admitted to hospital after blunt chest trauma have one or more rib fractures
3. Rib fractures in the elderly are common from falls: in adults, motor vehicle accidents is the most frequent mechanism and in youths, sport injury and violence are frequently causative

Clinical Manifestations

1. Point tenderness and local swelling at the site of trauma
2. Pain is exacerbated by deep breathing and various movements
3. In elderly patients each additional rib fracture increases the odds of dying by 19% and of developing pneumonia by 27%
4. First rib fractures have an association with spinal and vascular injuries. They are the rarest of all rib fractures
5. Fracture of the lower ribs are associated with abdominal organ injury
6. Left lower rib fractures may injure the spleen; right lower rib fractures are associated with liver injury
7. Fracture of ribs 11 and 12 are associated with renal injury

Neuropathology

1. Stress fractures of the ribs and long bones are associated with:
   a. Rheumatoid arthritis
   b. Osteoporosis
   c. Osteomalacia
   d. Paget's disease of bone
2. Patients with long standing deforming rheumatoid arthritis with affected shoulders may have rib erosions that involve the outer areas of the second to sixth ribs that are usually painless
3. Carcinoma of the lung, breast, thyroid, kidney, and prostate are the most common tumors that metastasize to the ribs. They present with painful swelling or as a pathologic fracture
4. Primary neoplasms of the ribs are rare and include:
   a. Ostechondroma

   b. Multiple exostoses
   c. Chondrosarcoma
   d. Multiple myeloma
   e. Eosinophilic granuloma
5. Rarely the ribs may be involved by bacterial, syphilitic, tuberculous or fungal infections

Laboratory Evaluation

1. Radiographs demonstrate approximately ½ to 2/3 of fractures
2. After several weeks, a callus that forms with healing may be demonstrated
3. Bone scanning and MRI with contrast are extensively utilized if metastases or tumors are sought

The Slipping Rib Syndrome

General Characteristics

1. The syndrome is caused by hypermobility of the interchondral fibrous attachments of the anterior attachments of ribs 8 to 10. This allows the costal cartilage tips to subluxate and impinge upon the intercostal nerves.

Clinical Manifestations

1. Some patients have a history of trauma to the chest on the affected side
2. The onset is insidious usually over several months
3. The pain is unilateral, intermittent in the anterior ends of the lower costal cartilages (the tenth is most often involved)
4. Lancinating pain may occur in the anterior costal margin and the abdominal wall
5. Specific movements may elicit a painful click over the tip of the involved costal cartilage
6. The pain may be duplicated by the "hooking" maneuver in which the fingers are placed under the anterior costal margin and then the rib cage is pulled anteriorly. The maneuver may produce a palpable click as the ribs slip over one another
7. The syndrome can occur at any age but most often is seen in middle-aged patients. Men and women are affected equally.

Neuropathology

1. Traumatic rupture of the fibro-cartilaginous band that connects ribs 8 to 10
2. The involved cartilage is tender and hyper mobile
3. A rib tip subluxates upward to override the rib above and impinges upon the intercostal nerve

Laboratory Evaluation

1. This is a clinical diagnosis

Neuroimaging

1. Radiographs and MRI to rule out other pathologies
2. Bone scan to evaluate for costochondritis

Differential diagnosis

1. Rib fracture
2. Tietze's Syndrome
3. Bone metastases
4. Muscle tears
5. Pleuritic disease

Pain from the Sternum and its Articulations

Sternoclavicular Hyperostosis (SCCH)

General Characteristics

1. Sternoclavicular hyperostosis is a chronic inflammatory disorder that presents with erythema, swelling and pain in the sternoclavicular joint

Clinical Manifestations

1. Erythema, swelling and pain in the sternoclavicular joint
2. Approximately 50% of patients have acne or pustular lesions the best described of which is palmoplantar pustulosis (PPP)
3. Extrasternal articular disease is seen in approximately 25% of patients
4. The age of onset is between 24-79 years: it is usually a disorder of middle life
5. The usual presentation is pain and palpable tenderness in the sternoclavicular region that may radiate to the upper chest wall
6. The process is usually bilateral but unilateral involvement occurs
7. The process is chronic and follows a relapsing remitting course
8. Pain may radiate to the shoulder, neck, or anterior upper chest wall in association with the swelling and tenderness of the sternoclavicular joint
9. Motion of the ipsilateral shoulder is restricted due to medial clavicle involvement
10. Exacerbating factors are shrugging or retracting the ipsilateral shoulder; if severe, the shoulder girdle becomes fixed in a "squared shoulder" position
11. Extrasternal articular manifestations include:
    a. The axial skeleton is involved in 50% of patients
    b. Symptomatic peripheral arthritis occurs in approximately 20% of patients and primarily affects large joints. The knee and ankle are most frequently involved. Less frequently involved are the wrist and interphalangeal joints
12. SCCH is classically associated with pustulotic skin changes that include:
    a. Palmar and plantar pustulosis (PPP)
    b. Pustular psoriasis

   c. Acne conglobata
   d. Acne fulminans
   e. Hidradenitis suppurativa
   f. Psoriasis vulgaris
13. In 70% of patients, the interval between the onset of skeletal symptomatology and skin disease is 2 years although patients may present with PPP before or after
14. The disease follows a relapsing remitting course. Associated disorders that have been reported are subclavian vein occlusion and thoracic outlet syndrome

Neuropathology

1. The anatomy of the sternoclavicular joint is complex:
   a. It is a synovial lined articulation that is composed of the inferior medial head of the clavicle, the upper outer portion of the sternum and the cartilage of the first rib
   b. The joint is divided into two compartments that are separated by an intra-articular disc
   c. The articular capsule that surrounds the joint is reinforced by ligaments
   d. SCCH starts as a nonspecific inflammation of the ligaments (sternoclavicular) and surrounding soft tissue
   e. Perichondritis is early and then evolves to an erosive arthritis; endosteal and periosteal bone formation occurs along with the growth of fibrous tissue
   f. The chronic inflammation causes a progressive hyperostosis which over time causes soft tissue ossification and fusion of the sternoclavicular joints
   g. Concomitantly with disease of the sternoclavicular joint, enthesopathic and hyperostotic changes may involve the shafts of long bones, the sacroiliac joints and large peripheral joints
   h. Histologically SCCH is similar to the inflammatory response seen in chronic osteomyelitis or Paget's disease. It is an ossifying periostitis associated with general hyperostosis

Laboratory Evaluation

1. Normal serum alkaline phosphatase and urinary hydroxyproline distinguish the process from Paget's disease

Neuroimaging

1. Radiographs:
   a. Ossification that progresses to hyperostosis of the clavicles, sternum and anterior upper ribs
   b. Early in the process the joint spaces in the sternoclavicular region are preserved but develop erosive changes over time

c. Usually the first to fourth rib are involved; the seventh rib may be involved but ossification beyond the eighth rib has been described.
d. Erosive changes and exuberant bone formation can occur along the anterior aspects of the vertebral bodies. The radiographic changes may be sclerotic rather than proliferative or destructive. Any area of the cervical, thoracic or lumbar spine can be involved
e. Inflammatory enthesopathy (the attachment of a ligament or tendon to a bone) of the costoclavicular ligament and the small hyperostotic foci of at least 5 mm diameter of the sternal end of the first pair of ribs are early diagnostic signs
f. Scintigraphy may demonstrate uptake early in the course of the disorder prior to positive radiographs. Increased uptake is seen in the sternoclavicular joint, the costal cartilage of the first and second ribs and the manubrium

Condensing Osteitis of the Clavicle

General Characteristics

1. A painful expansion and sclerosis of the medial end of the clavicle

Clinical Manifestations

1. This is a disorder of young and middle aged women
2. There may be a history of stress of the joint from heavy lifting
3. There is unilateral or bilateral painful expansion and sclerosis of the medial end of the clavicle without sternal hyperostosis or sternoclavicular synostosis
4. There is pain on abduction of the arm which may radiate to the ipsilateral shoulder or to the subscapular region

Neuropathology

1. Histologic examination reveals an ossifying periostitis with increased thickness of cancellous bone

Neuroimaging

1. Radiographs reveal preservation of the joint space and lack of manubrial involvement which differentiates it from osteoarthritis
2. MRI:
   a. T2-weighted sequences in areas of clavicular sclerosis demonstrate varying signal intensity that ranges from low intermediate to high signal intensity putatively related to the degree of bone marrow edema
   b. Contrast-enhanced T1-weighted sequences demonstrate intra-osseous and periosseous enhancement

Manubriosternal Joint

General Characteristics

1. Manubriosternal arthritis is a rare cause of upper sternal pain

Clinical Manifestations

1. The pain is localized to the joint or radiates along the upper ribs to the shoulder simulating angina
2. Localized tenderness and swelling of the joint
3. Affects young males performing heavy manual labor

Neuropathology

1. The manubriosternal joint is a cartilaginous joint (symphysis) in which a thick layer of hyaline cartilage covers the articular surfaces with an intervening fibrocartilage disc
2. Cavitation in the disc is common which occurs in 30% of patients
3. The joint is most commonly involved in rheumatoid arthritis, gout, ankylosing spondylitis and psoriatic arthritis
4. Rarely the joint can be affected by infection (tuberculosis) or osteoarthritis

Laboratory Evaluation

1. Appropriate studies to rule out ischemic heart or lung disease and inflammatory arthritides

Neuroimaging

1. Lateral radiographs of the chest may demonstrate erosive joint changes
2. CT scan of the chest
   a. May demonstrate cyst formation in the joint

Xiphoid Cartilage and Xiphisternal Joint

General Characteristics

1. The xiphoid process is a small cartilaginous extension of the lower sternum. It is at the level of the 9th thoracic vertebra and the T6 dermatome. At age 15 to 29, the xiphoid fuses to the body of the sternum with a fibrous joint. The joint ossifies around 40 years of age

Clinical Manifestations

1. The chief complaint is usually low substernal or epigastric pain
2. The pain may radiate to the precordium or abdomen
3. The xiphoid cartilage is tender and pressure reduplicates the pain and its radiation
4. The process may run a self-limited course
5. Pain in the joint may be elicited by lifting or bending

Neuropathology

1. Direct damage to the cartilage and joint from blunt chest trauma

2. Some consider it to be Tietze's syndrome of the xiphisternal joint

Laboratory Evaluation

1. Appropriate studies to rule out thoracic or abdominal pathologies

Neuroimaging

1. Radiograph of the joint

Traumatic Muscle Pain

General Characteristics

1. Intercostal and accessory thoracic muscle pain is usually traumatic or from unaccustomed or excessive muscle activity

Clinical Manifestations

1. The onset may be sudden or gradual with localized pain and mechanical sensitivity of the affected muscle
2. Pain is exacerbated by maneuvers that stretch the involved muscles

Neuropathology

1. Trigger points that are areas of local mechanical hyperalgesia in muscle but also can be demonstrated in ligaments, tendons and the periosteum
2. If a trigger point is mechanically stimulated, a taut band within the muscle contracts; they may be associated with a local muscle twitch response

Laboratory Evaluation

1. Radiograph to rule out other pathology

Precordial Catch Syndrome

General Characteristics

1. A rare benign self-limited disorder most often of children and adolescents

Clinical Manifestations

1. Occurs primarily in young healthy persons
2. Sharp pains are felt in the anterior chest wall ("catches" or "stitches")
3. The pain is often at the left parasternal area or near the cardiac apex
4. Pain may occur with a forward flexed posture
5. The pain lasts for 30 seconds to 3 minutes
6. The pain may be exacerbated by deep inspiration and is relieved by a change of posture or shallow breathing
7. There is no local tenderness

Neuropathology

1. Putative irritation of the parietal pleura

Neuroimaging

1. Chest radiograph to rule out pathology

Epidemic Myalgia (Bornholm Disease)

General Characteristics

1. An acute viral illness that causes severe pain in the chest wall and the epigastrium

Clinical Manifestations

1. The disorder affects the intercostal and upper abdominal wall muscles
2. Usually there is a prodrome of 1-10 days of viral illness. After that, the patient experiences severe lancinating pain in the lateral chest wall usually the size of a palm (in adults). The upper epigastrium is primarily affected in children
3. The pain is exacerbated by breathing, coughing and other chest movement
4. Paroxysms of severe lancinating pain occur between symptom free intervals
5. Involved muscles are tender
6. Patients have fever, headache and pharyngitis concomitantly and approximately 10% have pleurisy
7. The illness usually lasts for 3 to 7 days but relapses can occur. The disorder is self-limited

Neuropathology

1. The usual viruses causing epidemic myalgia are:
   a. Group B coxsackie virus
   b. In sporadic cases coxsackie type A and echoviruses are more frequent. Human parechovirus type 3 has recently been described

Laboratory Evaluation

1. Isolation of the virus from the throat or feces early in the course of the illness
2. Demonstration of a rising titer of type-specific neutralizing antibodies

Disorders of the Posterior Chest Wall

1. Pain and local tenderness in the posterior chest wall may be caused by:
   a. Trauma
   b. Metabolic bone disease
   c. Infections
   d. Juvenile kyphosis (Scheuermann's disease)
   e. Thoracic disc disease
   f. Costovertebral arthritis
   g. Diffuse idiopathic skeletal hyperostosis
   h. Ankylosing spondylitis

Thoracic Disc Disease

General Characteristics

1. Symptomatic thoracic disc disease is rare but may be accompanied by serious spinal cord compression due to the small diameter of the spinal canal at this level
2. Precipitating factors are heavy lifting, trauma and infection (IV drug abuse)

Clinical Manifestations

1. Occurrence is most common at the mid to lower thoracic levels and in men in the fifth decade
2. In some patients there may be preceding back pain for weeks or months due to disc annulus degeneration
3. Thoracic disc pain may radiate anteriorly and mimic cardiac pain although in this instance it is usually lancinating and in an intercostal nerve distribution
4. Posterolateral disc herniations cause compression of nerve roots with associated unilateral chest wall pain while posterior herniations cause myelopathy

Neuropathology

1. Annulus fibrosis degeneration and tears with disc pulp protrusion
2. An inflammatory response from the extruded nucleus pulposis with local leukocytosis, cytokine and chemokine expression from immune cells

Neuroimaging

1. MRI

Differential diagnosis

1. Early ankylosing spondylitis
2. Costovertebral joint syndrome
3. Metastases

Costovertebral Arthritis

General Characteristics

1. Costovertebral and costotransverse arthritis may be seen with osteoarthritis, ankylosing spondylitis and rarely with other inflammatory arthritides

Clinical Manifestations

1. The pain is usually at the first, eleventh and 12th costovertebral joints as they have the most mobility
2. The pain is exacerbated by deep inspiration, coughing or chest compression
3. The pain is characteristically a dull ache

Neuropathology

1. The usual underlying disorders are osteoarthritis, ankylosing spondylitis and psoriatic arthritis

Laboratory Evaluation

1. MRI:
   a. A positive spinal MRI for inflammation is the presence of anterior / posterior spondylitis in >3 sites
   b. Fatty deposition at several vertebral corners are an early sign of axial ankylosing spondylitis
   c. Radiographs:
      i Joint space narrowing, subchondral bony sclerosis and marginal osteophytes
   d. Osteophytes and disc herniations in spinal radiculopathy can be differentiated by susceptibility-weighted MRI

Diffuse Skeletal Hyperostosis (DISH)

General Characteristics

1. Diffuse idiopathic skeletal hyperostosis is a non-inflammatory degenerative disease that causes ossification of spinal ligaments and decreased spinal mobility
2. Possibly present in 19% of men and 4% of women that are older than 50 years of age

Clinical Manifestations

1. This is a disorder primarily of middle aged and elderly men
2. Pain and stiffness of the thoracolumbar spine
3. In general the pain is mild, dull and nonradiating; it is exacerbated by inactivity and cold
4. There is a slight increase in dorsal kyphosis, a minimal decrease in thoracic range of motion and chest expansion; there is occasional local tenderness

Neuropathology

1. An increase of vertebral fractures on a hyperostotic fused spine
2. DISH is associated with an increased risk of metabolic syndrome (odds ratio of 3.88)
3. Serum levels of the natural osteogenesis inhibitor Dickkopf-1 (DKK-1) are low
4. The diagnosis requires at least two or three contiguous intervertebral bridges without severe disc changes (seen in degenerative spine disease) or ankylosis of the sacroiliac or facet joints (in contrast to spondyloarthritis)
5. Partial or complete bone bridges that consist of cortical woven bone that are accompanied by morphological changes in the adjoining part of the intervertebral disc

Laboratory Evaluation

1. Low levels of the natural osteogenesis inhibitor Dickkopf-1 (DKK1) encoded from the HGNC gene that maps to chromosome 10q21.1

Neuroimaging

1. Radiographs:
   a. Undulating anterior ossification of 2-4 or more contiguous thoracic vertebrae with space between the deposited bone and the underlying vertebral bodies with relative preservation of the intervertebral disc height. It is distinguished from ankylosing spondylitis by the absence of sacroiliitis, true syndesmophytes and apophyseal joint ankylosis

Ankylosing Spondylitis

General Characteristics

1. Spondyloarthritis (SpA) is a group of disorders that includes:
   a. Ankylosing spondylitis (AS)
   b. Psoriatic arthritis (PsA)
   c. Inflammatory bowel disease-associated arthritis
   d. Reactive arthritis
   e. Undifferentiated SpA
2. All of these disorders primarily affect the axial skeleton, erosions, and new bone formation in the sacroiliac joints and in the spine.
3. Other associated clinical manifestations are:
   a. Asymmetrical oligoarthritis
   b. Enthesitis
   c. Dactylitis
   d. Extraskeletal manifestations that include:
      i Psoriasis
      ii Uveitis
      iii Chronic inflammatory bowel disease
4. Axial spondyloarthritis SpA is a subset of patients without radiographic sacroiliitis and may represent an earlier stage of anklyosing spondylitis. The criteria for AxSpA include:
   a. Evidence of sacroiliitis by MRI
   b. Chronic back pain
   c. HLA-B27 positivity
   d. Nonarticular symptoms
5. Susceptibility to ankylosing spondylitis is conferred by variations in the HLA-B27 gene allele that maps to chromosome 6p21.3:
   a. Functions in antigen presentation
6. Other associated genes include:

a. 2q12.1 locus
    i Modulator of inflammation
b. IL-1 gene that maps to chromosome 22q13.2
    i Metabolism of xenobiotics
c. CYP2D6 gene that maps to chromosome 5q15
    i An endoplasmic reticulum aminopeptidase
d. IL23 receptor gene that maps to chromosome 1p31.1

Clinical Manifestations of Ankylosing Spondylitis

1. Insidious onset of thoracic and low back pain
2. Onset of signs and symptoms prior to age 40
3. Symptoms are worse in the morning or with inactivity
4. Improvement of symptoms with exercise
5. Inflammatory back pain is the most common symptom and presenting manifestation of 75% of patients; it often is dull and diffusely localized to the sacroiliac and buttock areas
6. The onset is insidious over months to years with at least three months of symptomatology prior to presentation. Most patients suffer chronic disease with intermittent exacerbations
7. The pain begins unilaterally and intermittently in the sacroiliac area, progresses and becomes bilateral and more proximal
8. Morning stiffness is common and usually lasts for 30 minutes. It may awaken the patient in the early morning
9. Nocturnal back pain during the second half of the night
10. Alternating buttock pain
11. Peripheral musculoskeletal involvement is seen in 30-50% of patients
12. Peripheral enthesitis (inflammation at the site of insertion of ligaments and tendons on bone) occurs at:
    a. Achilles tendon insertion
    b. The plantar fascia on the calcaneus or the metatarsal heads
    c. Base of the fifth metatarsal head
    d. Tibial tuberosity
    e. Superior and inferior poles of the patella
    f. Iliac crest

Neuropathology

1. The initial involvement is in the S1 joint which is followed by involvement of discovertebral, apophyseal, costovertebral and costotransverse joints
2. The early lesion is subchondral granulation tissue that erodes the joint and is gradually replaced by fibrocartilage and then ossifies
3. The initial process occurs at the junction of the vertebra and the annulus fibrosus of the intervertebral discs. The outer fibers of the disc undergo

ossification that forms syndesmophytes

4. Extraarticular involvement includes:
    a. Acute anterior uveitis
    b. Aortitis
    c. Cardiac arrhythmias (generally a late manifestation)
    d. Restrictive lung disease

Laboratory Evaluation

1. Molecular genetic evaluation to delineate gene mutations particularly allelic variations of HLA-B27

Neuroimaging

1. Radiographs:
    a. Early signs of enthesitis (site of tendon or ligamentous bone attachments) include squaring off of the vertebral bodies due to erosions of their superior and inferior margins which erases the normal concave contour of their anterior surface
    b. Inflammatory lesions of enthuses cause sclerosis of the superior and inferior margins of the vertebral bodies
2. CT and MRI Imaging
    a. Reveal early sacroiliitis, erosions and enthesitis that may not be evident on radiographs

Fibromyalgia

General Characteristics

1. Frequently utilized diagnostic criteria for fibromyalgia include:
    a. Diffuse widespread musculoskeletal pain and stiffness that may affect the back, neck and shoulders
    b. The pain is modulated by weather (particularly a drop of barometric pressure), activity and fatigue
    c. Localized tenderness at specific sites
    d. Disturbed sleep with fatigue, aching and stiffness upon awakening
    e. Associated tension headache, irritable bowel syndrome
    f. Normal laboratory and radiographic studies; newer information supports a small fiber neuropathy as causative in a subgroup of patients

Clinical Manifestations

1. The chest wall is a common localization for pain (often in the distribution of the intercostobrachial nerve)
2. The disorder is predominant in the third or fourth decades and affects women in a ratio of 5:1
3. The most common symptoms are pain, aching and stiffness throughout the

body but including the chest wall and periscapular areas

4. Tender points and pain are often elicited in the foraminal exit areas of the cervical roots (C2-C4), the supraclavicular fossa (upper trunk of the brachial plexus), the infraclavicular fossa (primarily the lower trunk of the brachial plexus), and the neurovascular bundle that contains the entire plexus (activated when compressed against the upper humerus). Pain one inch from the medial scapular border (an upper trunk radiation of the brachial plexus) is common
5. It may be associated with some features of neurogenic edema (erythema and swelling) as noted in type I CRPS.
6. Exacerbating factors are:
    a. Cold
    b. Air conditioning
    c. Poor sleep
    d. Fatigue
    e. Stress
    f. Inactivity
    g. Increased exercise
7. The pain fluctuates from day to day and in some patients by the hour

Neuropathology

1. Trigger points and taut muscle bands within affected muscles are the hallmarks of the disorder

Laboratory Evaluation

1. No signs of inflammation. The sedimentation rate and C-reactive protein are negative
2. There is mounting evidence for a small fiber neuropathy as causative in a subgroup of patients

Neuroimaging

1. Neuroimaging with MRI is to rule out other pathologies

Clinical Summary of Isolated Musculoskeletal Chest Wall Pain

1. Costochondritis:
    a. Costochondral or costosternal junction tenderness
    b. Affects the second to fifth ribs
    c. No swelling
2. Lower rib pain syndrome:
    a. Pain over the 10th to 12th rib or the upper abdomen
    b. A tender area over the costal margin that reproduces the pain when palpated

3. Sternalis syndrome:
   a. Localized tenderness of the body of the sternum or the sternalis muscle
   b. Mechanical pressure may cause bilateral pain radiations
4. Thoracic costovertebral joint dysfunction:
   a. Pain 3-4 cm from the midline that is localized
   b. Referred pain from the posterior midline to the lateral and anterior chest wall
5. Fibromyalgia:
   a. Widespread musculoskeletal (a subgroup with neuropathic) pain and tenderness
   b. Many tender points are cervical and brachial plexus areas
   c. Fatigue, anxiety and sleep disturbance

Rheumatic Autoimmune Causes

1. Rheumatoid arthritis:
   a. Swelling and tenderness primarily of multiple small joints although large synovial joints are affected
   b. Thoracic costovertebral joints and costoclavicular joints may be affected
   c. Positive rheumatoid factor, anticitrullinated protein antibody and abnormal C-reactive protein and sedimentation rate are documented
2. Axial Spondyloarthropathy:
   a. Back pain of insidious onset and of at least 3 months duration
   b. Onset < than 45 years of age
   c. Imaging studies that demonstrate sacroiliitis by MRI, radiographs (one other feature of SpA)
   d. HLA-B27 and 2 other features of SpA
3. Psoriatic Arthritis:
   a. Inflammatory articular disease of joints, the spine or entheseal areas with three out of five of the following:
      i Current psoriasis, a past history or a family history of psoriasis
      ii Psoriatic nail changes
      iii Negative for rheumatoid factor
      iv History of dactylitis (inflammation of an entire finger or toe)
      v X-ray evidence of juxta-articular new bone formation in the hands or feet

Non-rheumatic Causes of Musculoskeletal Chest Wall Pain

1. Osteoporotic fracture:
   a. Acute back pain
   b. Insidious loss of height and or kyphosis with thoracic fractures
   c. Acute localized pain over the fracture site
   d. Often underlying risk factors

2. Neoplasms with pathologic fractures or bone pain:
   a. Severe boring pain often most severe at night
   b. Mechanically sensitive areas of metastases or pathologic fracture
   c. Radiographic evidence of posterior element involvement (facet) or vertebral body involvement)
   d. Not very responsive to opioids. If responsive to NSAIDs possible osteoid osteoma

CHAPTER 7

REFERRED PAIN

Overview

Referred pain is the perception of pain at a site that is different from the origin of the painful stimulus. Its origin is in visceral organs and it is projected to different areas of the body surface and somatic tissues. The origin of the referred pain is presently thought to depend on the organization of neural circuits that process somatic and visceral pain. In general, it is thought that there is somatovisceral integration at peripheral, spinal and supraspinal levels. A number of recent studies have demonstrated unit responses of dorsal horn neurons to both visceral and somatic afferents. Spinal lamina I neurons have been demonstrated as an essential early element in the processing of nociceptive input. They receive afferences from the skin, joints, muscles and the viscera that project to the brain-stem, thalamus and other components of the pain matrix. It has been demonstrated that both A-delta (thinly myelinated 1-4μ) and C-fibers (unmyelinated) from multiple dorsal roots can synapse directly on lamina 1 neurons giving them an anatomical basis to act as an integrator of multimodal sensory inputs. It has also been well established that somatic or nerve injury produces a much wider nociceptive afferent input than the stimulated dermatome. Lissauer's tract (dorsolateral spinal cord) distributes the nociceptive input from dorsal root ganglion afferents at least two segments above and below the activated spinal cord segment. Synapses on nociceptive dorsal horn (DH) lamina I pain projecting neurons may be homosynaptic or heterosynaptic and are subject to maladaptive neuro-plasticity (central sensitization) that increases their excitability and response to different modalities of stimulation (A-beta afferences).

Recent experimental evidence derived from an in vitro intercostal T9 and greater splanchnic peripheral nerve preparation demonstrates that there is somatic and visceral thin-fiber (A delta and C-fiber) convergence onto a subset of lamina 1 neurons some of which are pain projecting and others are local circuit neurons. Synaptic input from both the somatic and visceral neurons is suprathreshold and evokes depolarization in a subset of pain projecting neurons. Thus these lamina I neurons are the first site in the CNS of so-maticvisceral convergence. Approximately 25% of the recorded lamina I neurons receive somatic and visceral inputs from converging monosynaptic C-fibers. The neurons are both pain projecting and local circuit. Lamina I neurons were also excited by either somatic or visceral afferents which is evidence for modality-specific pathways to the dorsal horn. As noted above, maladaptive neuroplasticity may occur in subthreshold stimulated pain projecting neurons (modality-specific sensitization) or in excitatory inter-neurons that mediate polysynaptic pathways. This may alter the processing of input in those neurons that receive converging input and determine the outcome of the somatovisceral integration. Other research has demonstrated that stimulation of intercostal afferents can inhibit the discharge of thoracic spinal neurons that are excited by noxious stimulation of visceral afferent nerves. Some lamina I neurons receive supra or subthreshold excitatory visceral projections as well as inhibitory somatic input that is the anatomical basis of this phenomenon. This may also be a mechanism to modulate visceral nociceptive activity in lamina I cells with somatovisceral convergence. In general, it requires strong somatic A-delta and C-fiber inhibition of lamina I convergent neurons to inhibit visceral pain.

The anatomy and physiologic function of lamina I neurons that receive inhibitory afferences from both somatic and visceral nerves is extremely complex. Inhibitory input occurs primarily in local circuit neurons that demonstrate a rhythmic pattern of intrinsic firing. A subset of these neurons is local circuit GABA-ergic neurons whose axons are immunoreactive for vesicular GABA transporter and project densely within lamina I and II. Inhibition of these cells would disinhibit their postsynaptic projections (double-disinhibition) that in turn would amplify excitation of pain projecting neurons. Some lamina I local circuit neurons are excitatory interneurons that directly target pain projecting neurons. Thus local circuit modulation of Aδ and C-fiber input from somatic or visceral afferents influences the physiologic activity of pain projecting neurons. This mechanism may be similar to the reciprocal inhibition demonstrated in somatic and visceral AB and Aδ afferent input to wide-dynamic neurons in both cat and monkey.

Present evidence supports the hypothesis that the neural substrate of referred pain is modulation of the somatic and visceral inputs to lamina I pain projecting neurons that receive converging somatic and visceral input.

Common Patterns of Referred Pain to the Chest, Back and Upper Extremity

1. Angina pectoris:
    a. Pain is often described as pressure, tightness, or heaviness in the substernal left chest wall and left upper arm (T2). Overwhelmingly does not radiate to the fingers
    b. Radiations to the neck, jaw, shoulders, back or one or both arms
    c. Associated indigestion or heart burn with nausea or vomiting
    d. Most often exercise (but not always) related
2. Pleuritic pain radiations:

a. Lancinating pain over the affected area of involved pleura
b. Referred pain to the shoulder and back that is exacerbated by inspiration and expiration or cough
c. Mechanical hyperalgesia or allodynia over the affected area of the chest wall

3. Gall bladder pain radiation:
   a. Severe colicky right upper abdominal pain
   b. Radiation to the interscapular areas, right scapula (sometimes to the tip at the T6 level) and shoulder
   c. Associated anorexia, nausea and vomiting
4. Liver disease pain radiations:
   a. Usually the pain is most severe in the right upper quadrant below the right costal margin
   b. Radiates to the back and right shoulder (less frequently)
5. Pancreatic pain radiations:
   a. Severe upper abdominal pain associated with nausea and vomiting; pain may be in the epigastrium
   b. Radiation is straight through to the back at times slightly relieved by sitting up and leaning forward with the knees flexed
   c. Less frequent radiations are to the chest, periumbilical area, back, lower abdomen and flanks
6. Spleen pain radiations:
   a. Pain discomfort or a feeling of fullness or heaviness in the upper left abdominal quadrant
   b. Pain radiation to the left shoulder and infrequently the back
7. Esophageal pain radiations
   a. Retrosternal chest pain that may radiate to the back
8. Stomach pain radiations:
   a. GERD radiates substernally
   b. Pain radiations are to the back particularly with posterior penetrating ulcers

Central Pain Syndromes That Affect the Axial Skeleton

Overview

After CNS lesions pain may be perceived in a specific body region or become widespread. In general, it is constant and moderate to severe in intensity. It is exacerbated by mechanical and thermal stimuli (most often cold) and emotional upset. Its quality is usually burning, although various dysesthetic sensations, "pins and needles", ache, and deep pressure are common. There may be spontaneous episodes of lancinating pain or sharp excruciating unrelenting pain. Patients frequently have decreased mechanical sensitivity in the areas affected by pain. The burning sensation and loss of mechanical sensitivity are usually most severe distally. During exacerbations, there may be associated vomiting, tachycardia, hypertension, and hyperventilation.

A major mechanism underlying central pain is central sensitization. Early studies demonstrated that nociceptive afferent activity from a peripheral injury could trigger a long lasting increased excitability of spinal cord neurons, an alteration of the usual stimulus-response relationship. In essence a change in the gain of the somatosensory system. Woolf and colleagues demonstrated that a 10-20 second low frequency (1-10 Hz) electrical or natural activation of peripheral nociceptors increased synaptic transmission (efficacy) in dorsal horn spinal cord neurons that lasted for minutes after cessation of the conditioning stimulus. This phenomenon differs from windup that causes a progressive neuronal discharge during continual identical stimuli (homosynaptic potentiation). Central sensitization induces facilitation after the conditioning stimulus that can be autonomous or requires a low level of nociceptive afference to maintain it. Central sensitization also produces heterosynaptic potentiation. In this situation, one type of nociceptor sensory fibers that are stimulated amplifies the response of other non-stimulated non-nociceptor or nociceptor fibers.

An underlying tenet of central sensitization is that in most central circuits, the receptive fields of dorsal horn neurons are only partially determined by the firing of an action potential. Most synaptic input to neurons is subthreshold; either not sufficient to depolarize the target neuron or the membrane excitability of the neuron is decreased by tonic inhibition. Normally subthreshold synaptic inputs can be amplified by:

1. A presynaptic increase in neurotransmitter release
2. Increased responsiveness of the postsynaptic membrane
3. Or decreased inhibition

These mechanisms raise subthreshold synaptic input sufficiently to produce action potentials and thus alter the functional properties of the target neuron. Central sensitization is also maintained by:

1. Activation of microglia (release cytokines, chemokines and neurotransmitters)
2. Astrocytes (more important in maintenance than induction)
3. Gap junctions
4. Membrane excitability
5. Gene transcription

The clinical features of central sensitization include:

1. Pain hypersensitivity
2. Dynamic tactile allodynia

3. Secondary punctate or pressure hyperalgesia
4. After sensations (the pain is not stimulus bound)
5. Enhanced temporal summation ("wind up")

On a molecular level, central sensitization is similar to activity-dependent synaptic plasticity. This is a complex process that involves synaptic modulation and excitatory amino acids, alterations in the kinetics and physiology of ion channels, increased synaptic density of ionotropic receptors and activation of pre and post synaptic threonine and serine kinases. These processes lead to increased calcium influx through NMDA receptors that induce multiple intracellular enzymatic cascades that increase neuronal membrane excitability and induce gene transcription that in turn increases synaptic strength (efficacy). These changes enable subthreshold nociceptive inputs to depolarize nociceptive neurons, reduce their threshold to fire, expand the size of their receptive fields, and enhance their responsiveness. A significant aspect of the process is that low threshold afferents (AB fibers) are able to depolarize nociceptive neurons and that afferences outside of the injury site can elicit pain.

Neuropathic pain is caused by lesions of the somatosensory nervous system that alter its anatomy and function. It manifests spontaneously and responses to both noxious and innocuous stimuli are pathologically amplified. It is a consequence of maladaptive neuroplasticity of the nociceptive system at many levels. Its underlying mechanisms include:

1. Ectopic generation of action potentials
2. Facilitation and disinhibition of synaptic transmission
3. Disrupted synaptic connectivity
4. Formation of new synaptic circuits
5. Neuroimmune activation of microglia and astrocytes

Genetic predisposition and polymorphisms, age, gender are important factors that determine risk of developing neuropathic pain. The pain is maladaptive as it does not alert the individual to a tissue destructive stimulus or participate in repair.

The following are central neuropathic pain disorders that affect the axial skeleton.

Central Post Stroke Pain (CPSP)

General Characteristics

1. The disease affects approximately 8% of all stroke patients: there are approximately 700,0000 new and recurrent strokes per year in the USA which would cause 56,000 patients with CPSP
2. It is a particularly devastating condition that is frequently refractory to medical, surgical and deep brain stimulation modalities of treatment
3. CPSP is a persisting neuropathic pain of central origin that cannot be attributed to peripheral, nociceptive, or inflammatory processes.
4. Possible criteria for post stroke pain:

a. A clear cerebrovascular accident
b. The onset of pain at some point after the stroke
c. Alteration primarily of the spinothalamic pathways

Clinical Manifestations

1. CPSP I is primarily associated with spinothalamic tract disruption irrespective of stroke type
2. Thalamic pain:
    a. The P1 component of the posterior cerebral artery may be infarcted or ischemic lesions of the thalamogeniculate and less frequently, the thalamoperforate arteries are involved.
    b. Thalamic hemorrhage in the ventrobasilar complex is well described
    c. Pain on the contralateral side of the body may be in a hemisensory pattern or primarily affect the extremities, face or axillary body surface
    d. Most CPSP patients present within one to six months of the stroke. However, some patients develop the pain from 1 to 6 years after the ictus
    e. There is loss of thermal sensibility that accompanies and may precede the onset of pain. There may be distorted cold or heat sensations as well as paradoxical reactions to painful stimuli
    f. Allodynia to cold or dysesthesia to cold is not infrequent
    g. Allodynia to mechanical stimuli is seen in approximately 75% of patients
    h. Pain is usually confined to regions of altered pinprick sensation. Painful areas may be smaller than the borders of sensory dysfunction
    i. Some studies have demonstrated that cold hypoesthesia may be associated with burning cold continuous pain but may not have associated cold allodynia
    j. Normal tactile mechanical sensibility may be associated with tactile allodynia
    k. The quality of pain varies. It may be:
        i Continuous or paroxysmal
        ii Lancinating
        iii Cramping
        iv Grueling
        v Burning
    l. The predominant pain may be continuous or evokes
    m. Evoked pains:
        i Are brief and last only for the duration of the stimulus
        ii Rarely, they are not stimulus bound and can last for minutes to hours (after sensations). Extremely rare after sensations last for days.
    n. Evoked and spontaneous pains may be predominant in deep tissue
    o. Movement induced allodynia and pain may be seen in approximately 20 % of patients

p. The most consistent abnormality is abnormal temperature and pain sensitivity but all patients have some loss of somatic sensory modalities (may be difficult to discern)

Neuropathology

1. Thalamic pain may be seen following ischemic infarction from thrombosis or emboli to the P1 area of the posterior cerebral artery, the thalamogeniculate or thalamoperforate arteries
2. Hemorrhage into the ventrobasilar complex
3. Lesions within the ventrocaudal nuclei of the thalamus, particularly the ventroposterior inferior nucleus are most commonly associated with CPSP
4. The pathogenesis of CPSP is incompletely understood. Possible mechanisms include:
   a. Hyperexcitability of thalamic pain projecting neurons following disruption of ascending spinothalamic pathways:
      i Release of inhibition from a lesion of lemniscal pathways or the spinothalamic pathway
      ii Release of inhibition due to degeneration of corticothalamic neurons that project to the reticular nucleus that activate GABAergic inhibitory neurons that regulate the excitability of somatosensory relay thalamic nuclei
      iii Loss of normal cold inhibition from lamina I projecting neurons to the insula cortex and thalamus. The lateral cool projecting (spinothalamic system) normally inhibits the medical system whose origins are heat-pinch-cold neurons. These neurons project from lamina I to the medical thalamus. A lesion of the lateral spinothalamic system disinhibits this system that causes cold allodynia, burning continuous pain from disruption of thermal modality integration inhibition of nociceptive neurons. An alternate view is that cold fiber projections drive pain-projecting neurons in the thalamus.
      iv The ventroposterior medial intralaminar and reticular nuclei are essential components of post stroke pain. It has been posited that an imbalance between spinothalamic and reticulothalamic pathways may be a component of post stroke pain.

Neuroimaging

1. MRI to delineate structural involvement of thalamic nuclei
2. MRA to evaluate the vertebral, posterior cerebral, thalamogeniculate and thalamoperforate arteries
3. CT to evaluate the location and volume of thalamic hemorrhage

Wallenberg Syndrome

General Characteristics

1. The incidence of pain has been reported in one series to be as high as 25% which is higher than in most series
2. The incidence of chronic post stroke pain (CPSP) has been estimated to be approximately 17% with vascular lesions of the ventroposterolateral complex in the thalamus

Clinical Manifestations

1. Burning spontaneous dysesthetic pain which may appear prominently in the chest as the sensory loss abates
2. Mechanical and static allodynia can be evoked in painful areas
3. Abnormalities of thermal sensation and hyperalgesia similar to those seen with thalamic lesions

Neuropathology

1. Thrombosis of the vertebral or posterior inferior cerebellar artery that infarcts the spinothalamic tract within the lateral medulla

Laboratory Evaluation

1. Neurophysiologic studies:
   a. Hyperexcitability of thalamic pain projecting neurons with burst firing
2. Central pain mechanisms:
   a. Increased regional cerebral blood flow in the thalamus with both Wallenberg and CPSP of cortical origin

Neuroimaging

1. MRI to delineate the structural damage in the lateral medulla
2. MRA to evaluate the vertebral and PICA arteries

Spinal Cord Injury Pain (SCI)

General Characteristics

1. Due to the large variation in culture, motor vehicles, social situations and accidents prevalence and incidence of spinal cord injury is difficult to obtain
2. The global incidence of SCI has been estimated to be 23 patients per one million persons (2007). True incidence is dependent on regional factors. In the USA prevalence has been estimated to be 4187 per million of the population

Clinical Manifestations

1. As a general rule:
   a. Neuropathic pain above the level of injury may be caused by compressive radiculopathies or complex regional pain syndrome
   b. Neuropathic pain at the level of injury may be caused by nerve root compression, involvement of the dorsal horns or syringomyelia

   c. Neuropathic pain below the level may be due to the trauma itself or other disorders
2. A prospective study of 90 patients with SCI evaluated at 1, 6 and 12 months revealed:
   a. 80% of patients reported pain at all interval evaluations
   b. Neuropathic pain increased with time
   c. Musculoskeletal pain slightly decreased
   d. Both neuropathic and musculoskeletal pain were present in 59% of patients concomitantly
   e. Other neuropathic pain that was not related to SC1 or visceral pain was seen in 1 to 3% of patients
   f. Sensory changes, particularly cold-evoked dysesthesia, predicted the development of neuropathic pain below the level of the injury
   g. Neuropathic pain may be localized at or below the level of injury and is manifested by mechanical and thermal allodynia and hyperalgesia in addition to severe at level sensory deficits
   h. There is no exacerbation of neuropathic pain with movement
   i. The development of central type neuropathic pain that is delayed a long time from the injury may be due to the development of post-traumatic syringomyelia. Concomitantly there may be loss of one to two segments of motor function above the area of injury
   j. Pain above the level of the injury may be due to carpal tunnel syndrome or musculoskeletal disorders due to wheelchair use and is usually not due to the SCI
   k. The pain fluctuates day to day due to activities and the patient's affect
   l. The pattern of pain develops in approximately 30% of spinal cord injured patient. Its major manifestations are:
      i Delayed development: months to years following injury
      ii Spontaneous and diffuse but may be evoked below the injury level
      iii Burning, aching, lancinating and may be associated with hyperalgesia
      iv The pain fluctuates with emotional state, activity, and infections. It may be triggered by unexpected loud noises or movement
      v Burning pain is associated with complete and incomplete lesions. If lemniscal modalities are spared, patients may suffer mechanical allodynia
      vi Non-painful phantom sensations occur in more than 90% of patients

Neuropathology

1. Spinal cord injury causes complex changes to damaged tissue at the molecular level that include alterations of:
   a. Sodium ion channels
   b. Voltage gated calcium channels

c. Glutamate and GABAergic metabolism
d. Serotonergic, noradrenergic, NMDA and opioid receptor physiology
e. Recent interest has been directed toward the GABAergic system in SC1 neuropathic pain:
   i Normal function of GABAergic systems is dependent on the activity of the cation chloride cotransporters Na^{+}- K^{+} - Cl^{-} cotransporter 1 (NKCC1)
   ii NKCC1 controls Cl^{-} influx and cotransporter 2 (KCC2) regulates Cl^{-} efflux
   iii Activation of NKCC1 and its regulatory pathway are associated with altered Cl^{-} regulation and chronic pain. The KCC2 cotransporter decreases the concentration of Cl^{-} in a pain projecting neuron. GABA release from an inhibitory interneuron onto the pain projecting neuron under physiologic conditions (higher extracellular chloride equilibrium potential) would hyperpolarize the cell, as the Cl^{-} concentration would increase intracellularly. If the KCC2 cotransporter is nonfunctional (less Cl^{-} efflux) or the NKCC1 transporter is upregulated, the intracellular Cl^{-} concentration is increased which reverses the normal chloride equilibrium potential. GABA opens the Cl^{-} channels with a resulting decrease of the concentration of Cl^{-} within the PPN that decreases its threshold to depolarize. In this instance, GABA would increase excitability of the PPN.

2. WNK1 (with no lysine K) is a serine / threonine kinase (encoded by the WNK gene). WNK, through intermediate kinases phosphorylates the Na-K-Cl-cotransporter 1 (NKCC1) and KCC2 and activates and deactivates the channels thus regulating inhibitory tone in dorsal horn pain projecting neurons. NKCC1 is essential in maintaining ionic homeostasis that is also critical for osmotic and GABAergic homeostasis.

Neuroimaging

1. MRI:
   a. This is the best modality to evaluate parenchymal injury, edema and associated soft tissue and visceral images
   b. CT of the spine:
      i This is the most effective imaging modality to evaluate bone pathology after SCI
      ii Somatosensory evoked potentials:
         1. A method to evaluate physiologic function of ascending spinal pathways
      iii Transcranial magnetic stimulation:

1. A method to evaluate spinal cord conduction time and functional connections

Transverse Myelitis (Complete and Incomplete)

General Characteristics

1. Complete transverse myelopathy is rare other than with high impact motor vehicle accidents or from falls and military combat
2. Spinal cord lesions that affect the cord transversely are most often incomplete and irregular, the neurologic examination reflecting the localization and extent of the lesion
3. T4-T6 is a spinal cord watershed area and conditions of a vascular nature affect this level. T4 is also frequently the level of involvement with embolic disease (drug abuse as well as autoimmune disease)
4. Acute transverse myelopathy is most often due to trauma, demyelinating disease, lymphoma, metastatic disease or vascular disorders

Clinical Manifestations

1. Complete cord transection disrupts all ascending pathways from below the lesion as well as all descending pathways from above the lesion. If acute, there is spinal shock with below level paralysis, complete sensory loss, absent reflexes and bowel and bladder incontinence
2. In complete lesions, particularly from extramedullary lesions, the sensory level may be dropped, many levels below the level of the lesion. High thoracic lesions may cause a sensory level at an upper lumbar level. This finding is due to the somatotopic organization of the spinothalamic tract. The lower spinal segments are represented more superficially and laterally
3. A band-like pain radiation or segmental paresthesias may occur at the level of the lesion
4. Localized vertebral pain, particularly to mechanical stimuli (over the vertebral spinous process) such as percussion occurs with destructive lesions, primarily malignancy or infection
5. Pain more severe with recumbency and relieved to a degree with sitting or standing is suggestive of intraparenchymal spinal lesions. Patients that have to sleep sitting up are very suspicious for intrinsic spinal cord tumor (blockade of venous return that increases spinal cord pressure)
6. In general, thoracic level lesions are characterized by root pain and paresthesias that mimic intercostal neuralgia, paraplegia, sensory loss blow the affected level and dysfunction of bowel, bladder and sexual function
7. Lesions above T5 may also have autonomic dysregulation with postural hypotension

Neuropathology

1. The differential diagnosis of transverse myelitis is extremely wide:
   a. Acute transverse myelitis:
      i Trauma
      ii Autoimmune disease (particularly multiple sclerosis and neuromyelitis optica)
      iii Malignancy, primarily metastasis and lymphoma
      iv Rarely arterial and venous infarction
2. Chronic transverse myelitis:
   a. Autoimmune disorders
   b. Metabolic diseases
   c. Blood dyscrasias
   d. Syphilis
   e. B12 deficiency
   f. Arachnoid cysts
   g. Benign tumors

Laboratory Evaluation

1. Medical evaluation to delineate the category of disease

Neuroimaging

1. MRI:
   a. A new classification to characterize acute transverse myelitis has been proposed:
      i Segmental with rash
      ii Polio-like
      iii Granulomatous nodular
      iv Longitudinally extensive transverse myelitis
      v Short-segment-ovoid or peripherally located
   b. The pattern of spinal cord involvement:
      i Posterior column predominant:
         1. B12 deficiency
         2. Sjogren's syndrome
         3. Syphilis
      ii Anterior 2/3 of the spinal cord:
         1. Anterior spinal artery
      iii Extramedullary:
         1. Malignancy
         2. Disc disease
         3. Cysts
         4. Degenerative disease of the vertebrae and discs
      iv Central cord:
         1. Syrinx

2. Trauma
3. Primary tumor

v Brown-Sequard (vertical hemisection):

1. Trauma
2. Radiation treatment
3. Rare autoimmune or vascular disease
4. Syringomyelia
5. Disc

Brown-Sequard Syndrome

General Characteristics

1. This is a functional hemisection of the spinal cord
2. Can be categorized as traumatic or non-traumatic

Clinical Manifestations

1. The thoracic spine is most commonly involved (75%); cervical spine (17%) and lumbar spine (8%)
2. Most patients are between 15 to 50 years of age
3. Loss of pain and temperature sensation contralateral to the hemisection:
   a. The sensory level is usually "dropped" – one or two segments below the level of the lesion
4. Ipsilateral loss of proprioception and vibration modalities:
   a. Tactile sensation may be normal or only minimally affected
5. Ipsilateral weakness below the lesion level due to disruption of the descending corticospinal tract
6. Segmental lower motor neuron and sensory loss at the level of the lesion

Neuropathology

1. Traumatic causes are the most common and include:
   a. Penetrating injuries (most commonly stab wounds:
      i Gunshot injuries
      ii Blunt trauma
   b. Non-traumatic lesions:
      i Arachnoid cyst
      ii X-RT
      iii Syringomyelia
      iv Hematomyelia
      v Herniated disc
      vi Neoplasms
      vii Demyelinating disease
      viii Infective / inflammatory disease
   c. Unusual causes:

   i Spinal cord herniation (transdural)
   ii Fibrocartilage embolization
   iii Decompression sickness

Laboratory Evaluation

1. Medical evaluation for causes of blood dyscrasia (if hematomyelia is present), autoimmune disease or infection

Neuroimaging

1. MRI:
   a. MRI with and without contrast to delineate structural parenchymal lesions
2. CT evaluation of bony structures

Central Cord Syndrome

General Characteristics

1. The central cord syndrome is most commonly seen with hyperextension injury of the neck. Underlying spinal cord degenerative disease such as spondylosis or posterior longitudinal ligament calcification are risk factors in elderly patients

Clinical Manifestations

1. Acute central spinal cord injury:
   a. Severe hyperextension injury of the neck:
      i Patients may be acutely quadriplegic; the legs most often recover within hours or occasionally within minutes
      ii There is patchy sensory loss below the lesion which may involve the thorax
      iii Bladder dysfunction with urinary retention is frequent
      iv Weakness is most severe in the arms and is predominate distally
2. Chronic central cord syndrome:
   a. Syringomyelia:
      i The clinical course is slowly progressive
      ii Syringomyelia is frequently associated with Chiari type I or II or Dandy-Walker malformations or follows spinal cord trauma
      iii The decussating fibers of the spinothalamic tract may be affected initially that cause lack of pain and temperature in a cape-like distribution (cervical syrinx) which frequently involves the upper thorax
      iv The pain and temperature loss is often in a suspended distribution and is most often bilateral
      v There is preservation of tactile, vibratory, and proprioceptive modalities that causes a dissociated sensory loss. If the syrinx is asymmetrical

it may involve the cervical thalamic tract and alter vibration sensibility

vi Anterior horn cells are destroyed at the level of the lesion that causes atrophy, paresis, and areflexia. There may be a Horner's syndrome from involvement of the ciliospinal center of Budge (C8-T2)

vii Kyphoscoliosis occurs from destruction of the paraspinal muscle innervating neurons of the ventromedian motor nuclei

viii Spastic paraparesis below the level of the lesion occurs from corticospinal tract involvement. In cervical syrinxes, the biceps and triceps reflexes are lost in association with hyperactive knee and ankle reflexes. Babinski sign is usually elicitable.

ix In the somatotopic lamination of the spinothalamic tract, cervical sensation is dorsomedial and sacral modalities are ventrolateral. This produces "sacral sparing" as the cervical fibers are affected initially being closer to the central cord

x Neuropathic pain may be severe in approximately 50% of patients

xi Neuropathic arthropathy may be seen, particularly in the shoulder, from denervated joints that suffer repeated minor trauma

Neuropathology

1. Chronic central cord syndrome is primarily caused by syringomyelia, hydromyelia, hematomyelia and intramedullary spinal cord tumors
2. Acute central cord syndrome is most often due to severe hyperextension injury of the neck

Neuroimaging

1. MRI to delineate the structural lesions
2. CT to evaluate bone pathology

Pain in the Thorax from Specific Nerve Injury

Intercostal Neuralgia

General Characteristics

1. The intercostal nerves are most often affected or injured during the course of thoracic surgery

Clinical Manifestations

1. The pain is usually constant and burning in quality in a specific thoracic dermatome
2. Pain may be lancinating
3. Usually the pain begins at the posterior axillary line and radiates anteriorly into the distribution of the injured nerve; it may radiate from front to back

4. In general patients do not splint
5. Patients may have decreased sensation or mechanical hyperalgesia and allodynia in the distribution of the affected nerve

Neuropathology

1. Most often intercostal neuralgia is due to a neuropractic injury during the course of retraction with thoracic surgery
2. The dorsal root ganglion and nerve are frequently involved by Herpes zoster that produces hemorrhagic necrosis of the dorsal root ganglia of thoracic segments

Herpes Zoster

General Characteristics

1. Herpes zoster is caused by reactivation of the Varicella zoster virus (VZV)
2. The risk of HZ increases with age. The virus persists asymptomatically in sensory ganglia of the cranial nerves and dorsal root ganglia. It reactivates with a decline in cellular immunity or with immunosuppression
3. The virus travels along the sensory nerves to the skin to cause prodromal pain and then the vesicular rash
4. Possibly one out of three individuals will develop HZ
5. The most common dermatomal involvement is in thoracic dermatomes

Clinical Manifestations

1. Classically HZ is unilateral. It does not cross the midline and is localized to one dermatome of a single sensory ganglion. In 20% of patients, adjacent dermatomes are involved.
2. Approximately 70% of patients with complications are older than 50 years of age
3. Prodromal symptoms in the involved dermatome are pruritus, dysesthesia and pain
4. Rarely, nerve pain is not associated with a skin rash
5. The skin rash is composed of grouped vesicles on an erythematous base. The rash begins as red macules and papules that over 7 to 10 days evolve into vesicles, pustules and then scabs. Healing may take more than a month

Post Herpetic Neuralgia (PHN)

1. PHN risk increases with age (90 days after the onset of pain); 5% in patients <60, 10% in patients 60 to 69 years of age and 20% in patients older than 80 years of age
2. The pain is neuropathic; it may be intermittent and not correlated with external stimuli
3. Frequently the affected dermatome may have decreased mechanical sensitivity

but demonstrates dynamic mechanical allodynia

Neuropathology

1. In general, one dorsal root ganglion is most severely involved; adjacent ganglia may show less severe pathology
2. Acutely, the maximally affected ganglion is swollen and congested
3. Microscopically there is lymphocytic and mononuclear cell inflammation
4. Necrosis of the walls of small blood vessels with thrombosis
5. Sensory neurons demonstrate loss of Nissl substance, cytoplasmic eosinophilia and neuronophagia

Laboratory Evaluation

1. Detection of viral DNA by polymerase chain reaction
2. Herpes zoster lesions contain high concentrations of VZV

Chest Wall Tumors that Involve Thoracic Segmental Nerves

General Characteristics

1. Primary chest wall tumors are 5% of all thoracic tumors and 0.04% of all primary tumors
2. Approximately 50% are metastatic or direct invasion from adjacent malignancies

Clinical Manifestations

1. Intercostal nerve pain as the nerves are infiltrated by tumor
2. Dull boring pain in the area of the primary tumor that evolves into lancinating pain with intercostal nerve involvement
3. Mesothelioma usually invades locally into the chest wall but has been described as causing intercostal neuralgia

Neuropathology

1. Metastatic lesions from any cancer but primarily breast, lung, prostate
2. Lymphoma and multiple myeloma
3. Adjacent malignant invasion from:
   a. Breast and lung cancer
   b. Mesothelioma
   c. Mediastinal tumors

Laboratory Evaluation

1. Medical evaluation to rule out a metastatic lesion
2. Biopsy of the tumor

Neuroimaging

1. CT and MRI to delineate boundaries of the tumor and detection of its invasion of nerves and vessels

2. ^{18}F-FDG accumulation on PET / CT

Medial and Lateral Pectoral Nerves

General Characteristics

1. The medial pectoral nerve takes origin from the medial cord of the brachial plexus or as a variant from the anterior division of the inferior trunk
2. It is derived from C8 and T1 roots
3. The nerve lies behind the axillary artery, courses between the axillary artery and vein and anastomoses anterior to the artery from a filament of the lateral pectoral nerve
4. The nerve enters the deep surface of the pectoralis minor muscle to supply the muscle
5. Branches of the nerve terminate in the sternocostal head of the pectoralis major muscle
6. It carries nociceptive and proprioceptive sensory fibers that project to the T1 areas of the anterior chest wall
7. The lateral pectoral nerve takes origin from the lateral cord of the brachial plexus; its roots are C5-C7
8. It courses across the axillary artery and vein, pierces the coracoclavicular fascia and terminates in the deep surface of the pectoralis major muscle
9. It anastomoses with the medial pectoral nerve to form a loop anterior to the proximal part of the axillary artery
10. It splits into 4 to 7 branches that pierce the clavipectoral fascia to innervate the pectoralis major muscle
11. It carries pain fibers to the upper anterior chest wall

Clinical Manifestations

1. Breast augmentation surgery is a common procedure with the great majority of implants being placed submuscularly
2. Tissue expansion is a commonly utilized technique for reconstruction of a breast that has undergone surgery for carcinoma
3. Submuscular implant placement causes anterior chest wall pain from stretching of the pectoralis major muscle and resulting muscle spasm
4. Pain may also be perceived in components of the medial and lateral pectoral muscle insertions which include:
    a. Insertion of the pectoralis major muscle:
        i Superolaterally into the proximal humerus
        ii Superiorly into the inferior clavicle
        iii Medially into the sternum (extending inferiorly to the seventh rib)
        iv The pectoralis minor muscle inserts superolaterally into the coracoid process of the anterior scapula and inferomedially into the 3-5th ribs

Neuropathology

1. The medial and lateral pectoral nerves may be injured with high impact motor vehicle or other forms of blunt trauma (avulsion)
2. They are frequently involved by neuropraxis during the course of submuscular device or tissue expansion reconstructive or breast augmentation surgery

Laboratory Evaluation

1. EMG
   a. To delineate the degree of muscle denervation

Neuroimaging

1. MRI:
   a. To delineate structural lesions in associated traumatic injuries
   b. Ultrasound evaluation of the nerves

Intercostobrachial Nerve (ICBN)

General Characteristics

1. The intercostobrachial nerve is a pure sensory nerve. It arises primarily from the second intercostal nerve and may receive variant contributions from intercostal nerves T1-T4
2. The major anatomical variants of the nerve (100 adult human formalin-fixed cadavers):
   a. Type I variant: 45% of patients had a branch from the nerve to the posterior antebrachial cutaneous nerve, a branch to the anterior and lateral areas of the axilla, a branch to the medial aspect of the arm and a branch to the medial antebrachial cutaneous nerve
3. Type II variant: in 25% of patients, the nerve arises from T2 and gives a branch to the brachial plexus
4. Type III variant: in 10% of patients, the lateral cutaneous branches of T2 and T3 fuse as a common trunk and then split after their exit from the intercostal space to form an ICBN
5. Type IV-VII are variants of T2 and T4 recombinations
6. Its extra-thoracic course runs parallel to the axillary vein for approximately 1.5cm in the vertical plane to innervate the axilla, upper medial arm and upper lateral chest wall
7. Most important of its pain radiations when the nerve is stimulated is under the breast to the sternum in the midline

Clinical Manifestations

1. The ICBN is most commonly injured during radical mastectomy with axillary lymph node dissection
2. Pain in the sensory distribution of the nerve is described as burning,

lancinating or a pressure sensation
3. Complex regional pain syndrome type II has been described primarily affecting the chest wall. It is associated with neurogenic edema, erythema and autonomic dysregulation

Neuropathology

1. The nerve is most often damaged during a neuropraxic injury (stretch injury leaving the axon intact); it may be transected as well.
2. The nerve may be damaged from high impact motor vehicle accidents, concomitantly with avulsion of the brachial plexus or severe blunt chest trauma from blast injuries

Neuroimaging

1. MRI neurography to evaluate the brachial plexus as well as the primary T2 root
2. Ultrasonography to delineate the nerve (ICBN)

Post-Mastectomy Syndrome

General Characteristics

1. Post-mastectomy pain syndrome (PMPS) is a chronic pain disorder, most often neuropathic, which occurs following breast surgery
2. Chronic pain occurs after breast procedures that include:
   a. Lumpectomy
   b. Breast reconstruction
   c. Augmentation
   d. Reduction
3. Chronic pain persists beyond the normal healing time of 3 months
4. The incidence of the disorder varies from 4-56% described in the past. At present, the incidence of post mastectomy pain is approximately 40%. The risk of PMPs may be increased in younger women. Body mass index does not appear to be a risk factor. Axillary dissection with the removal of 15 nodes is a risk factor

Clinical Manifestations

1. The descriptors for pain from the McGill pain questionnaire are stabbing, shooting, aching, gnawing, nagging, tiring and a sensation of tightness
2. The intensity of the pain is variable and most often moderate
3. Sleep is most often unaffected but a subgroup of patients have sleep interruption 2-3 nights / week
4. Pain is exacerbated by straining, lying down, cold weather, mechanical stimuli of the area and getting out of bed. Stretching aggravates the pain
5. Relieving factors in some patients are sitting, while for others it may be

recumbency

6. A review of neuropathic pain after breast surgery divided it into four syndromes:
   a. Phantom breast pain
   b. Intercostobrachial neuralgia
   c. Neuroma pain
   d. Other nerve pain

Neuropathology

1. Primary neuropractic injury or transection of the intercostobrachial nerve
2. Neuromas in the surgical scar

Neuroimaging

1. MRI neurography to evaluate the ICBN
2. Ultrasonography of ICBN and pectoral nerves

Phantom Breast Syndrome (PBS)

General Characteristics

1. Phantom breast syndrome is a disorder in which patients who have had removal of a breast retain the sensation of residual breast tissue. These include non-painful and painful sensations
2. The incidence varies widely and has been reported to affect between 30 to 90% of patients following mastectomy

Clinical Manifestations

1. The highest incidence occurs with combined mastectomy and reconstruction
2. Two risk factors for development of phantom breast pain are severe acute postoperative pain and greater postoperative use of analgesics
3. Patients may have pain and discomfort, itching, pins and needles, tingling pressure, burning and throbbing
4. The syndrome may be delayed up to a year after surgery
5. The pain and sensory alterations are localized to the axilla, medial upper arm and anterior chest wall

Neuropathology

1. Most often there is neuropractic damage or severance of the branches or complete section of the intercostobrachial nerve

Neuroimaging

1. Ultrasonography of the intercostobrachial nerve and its branches

Abdominal Wall Pain

Anterior Cutaneous Nerve Entrapment Syndrome (ANES)

General Characteristics

1. Terminal branches of thoracic intercostal nerves are entrapped in abdominal muscles that causes severe neuropathic pain

Clinical Manifestations

1. The site of abdominal wall tenderness is $< 2cm^2$ that is situated within the lateral boundaries of the rectus abdominis muscle
2. A positive Carnett's sign in which there is an exacerbation of pain during palpation with contraction of the abdominal musculature. The patient lies flat and flexes the head against resistance
3. Rarely there is hyperalgesia and allodynia to mechanical stimuli of the painful area

Neuropathology

1. Entrapment of the anterior cutaneous branches of intercostal nerves from structures of the abdominal wall that include the parietal peritoneum, subcutaneous tissue, aponeurosis and the abdominal muscles

Laboratory Evaluation

1. Normal laboratory analysis

Neuroimaging

1. MRI and / or CT to rule out other abdominal pathology

Iliohypogastric Nerve

General Characteristics

1. The iliohypogastric nerve is mixed and arises from the anterior rami of T12 and L1 nerve roots
2. It courses across the psoas muscle, behind the kidney, crosses the quadratus lumborum muscle to reach the iliac crest. It pierces the internal oblique and transversus abdominis muscles which it innervates
3. Its lateral cutaneous branch innervates the skin over the outer buttock and hip; its anterior cutaneous branch supplies the anterior abdominal wall above the pubis

Clinical Manifestations

1. There is little motor deficit

2. Hypoesthesia or mechanical hyperalgesia in the distribution of the anterior or lateral cutaneous branches of the nerve

Neuropathology

1. The nerve may be crushed or undergo neuropractic injury from severe pelvic trauma
2. The lateral branch is often injured during iliac crest bone marrow harvesting
3. The nerve is most commonly injured in the lumbar plexus, at the posterior or anterior abdominal wall or distally near the inguinal ring
4. The nerve may be injured during hernia repair

Neuroimaging

1. Ultrasonography of the nerve

Ilioinguinal Nerve

General Characteristics

1. The ilioinguinal nerve is mixed and takes origin from the anterior ramus of the first lumbar root. It courses laterally and downwards in parallel with the iliohypogastric nerve to the iliac crest. It supplies the internal oblique and transversus abdominis muscles
2. After innervating these two muscles it enters the inguinal canal, courses to the superficial inguinal ring from which its sensory fibers emerge
3. The sensory innervation is to the medial thigh below the inguinal ligament and the skin of the symphysis pubis and external genitalia

Clinical Manifestations

1. Hyper or hypoesthesia of the skin along the inguinal ligament with radiation to the lower abdomen
2. Pain may be localized to the medial groin, the labia majora or the scrotum
3. In approximately 75% of patients there is pain and tenderness with mechanical stimuli applied to the areas where the nerve exits the inguinal canal
4. Symptoms are exacerbated by hip extension
5. Patients may walk with the trunk forward flexed
6. Pain may be elicited by palpation medial to the anterior superior iliac spine

Neuropathology

1. Neuropractic or direct injury to the nerve occurs in the lumbar plexus, at the posterior or anterior abdominal wall or within the inguinal canal.
2. The nerve may be injured with herniorrhaphy or appendectomy
3. The nerve is usually entrapped as it passes through the muscles of the abdominal wall medial to the anterior superior iliac spine
4. The nerve may be stretched during pregnancy
5. Trauma to the external oblique muscle and aponeurosis has been described

in professional athletes which entraps the nerve in the injured muscle (one form of "sports" hernia)

Laboratory Evaluation

1. EMG to evaluate denervation in the external oblique muscle

Neuroimaging

1. Ultrasonography of the nerve

Genitofemoral Nerve (GFN)

General Characteristics

1. The genitofemoral nerve is primarily sensory
2. It arises from the first and second lumbar segments within the psoas muscle. It courses through the psoas muscle and divides near the inguinal ligament into the genital branch and femoral branch (lumboinguinal branch)
3. The external spermatic or genital branch (composed of fibers from L1) enters the deep inguinal ring courses through the inguinal canal and terminates in the cremaster muscle and skin of the scrotum or labia majoris and medial thigh
4. The lumboinguinal or femoral branch arises primarily from L2, courses behind the femoral artery to innervate the skin of the upper thigh and the femoral triangle

Clinical Manifestations

1. Pathology of the femoral branch of the nerve causes hypoesthesia over the anterior thigh below the inguinal ligament which distinguishes the nerve from the iliohypogastric or ilioinguinal nerves
2. Groin pain, paresthesias and burning sensation may be perceived from the lower abdomen to the medial thigh
3. There is overlapping sensory innervation with the ilioinguinal and ilio hypogastric nerves
4. Pain can be exacerbated by internal or external rotation of the hip, prolonged walking and mechanical stimuli (if hyperalgesia or allodynia has developed)
5. Loss of the cremasteric reflex

Neuropathology

1. The nerve can be injured during inguinal and femoral herniorrhaphy using both open and laparoscopic techniques
2. The nerve may be injured in the lumbar plexus, within the abdomen or in the femoral or inguinal region

Laboratory Evaluation

1. Nerve conduction velocity

Neuroimaging

1. Ultrasonography of the nerve

Postherniorrhaphy Inguinal Pain (CPIP)

General Characteristics

1. Inguinal hernia repair is one of the most common operations worldwide. Chronic postherniorrhaphy inguinal pain is its most feared complication
2. Approximately 800,000 inguinal repairs are performed annually in the USA; possibly the lifetime risk for men is 27% and 3% for women
3. The usual definition of chronic postherniorrhaphy inguinal pain (CPIP) is 3-6 months. The estimate of moderate to severe pain following surgery is 10-12%
4. The possible etiologies of this inguinal pain are:
    a. Hernia recurrence
    b. Tissue inflammation
    c. Meshoma
    d. Inguinal nerve injury or entrapment
5. The risk factors are:
    a. Female sex
    b. Young age
    c. High pre and postoperative pain levels
    d. CPIP (chronic postsurgical inguinal pain) is independent of technique
    e. Preoperative experimental stimuli (response to pain tests) have been shown to predict 4% to 54% of the postoperative pain experience
    f. Genetic susceptibility

Clinical Manifestations

1. Clinical symptomatology of CPIP has been categorized into:
    a. Neuropathic pain
    b. Somatic pain
    c. Visceral pain
2. Neuropathic pain:
    a. Spontaneous pain
    b. Hypoesthesia
    c. Hyperesthesia and allodynia to mechanical stimuli
    d. Burning paresthesia
    e. Stabbing, burning, pulling, throbbing, lancinating, sharp and prickling are the most common descriptors
    f. The most common sites of pain radiation are the scrotum, labium, and upper thigh
    g. Rarely a trigger point can be elicited that produces the pain radiations

   h. The pain is exacerbated by walking, twisting or stretching the torso, stooping or sitting, hyperextension of the hip and sexual intercourse
   i. A few male patients describe painful ejaculation
   j. Relieving factors are recumbency with flexion of the hip and thigh
3. Non-neuropathic pain (inflammatory pain):
   a. Dull ache, that is constant and perceived over the entire groin area
   b. No trigger points and no pain radiation
   c. Descriptors of the pain are: gnawing, tender, pounding or pulling
4. Nociceptive pain:
   a. Usually localized to the pubic tubercle
5. Visceral pain:
   a. Generally related to sexual dysfunction or ejaculatory pain (usually burning) which is perceived in the region of the superficial ring of the inguinal canal or the testicular or labial region
   b. Patients that have had their surgery from an anterior approach may have a tender spermatic cord
   c. Abdominal wall laxity from partial denervation of the oblique musculature

Neuropathology

1. Entrapment or injury of the iliohypogastric, ilioinguinal, and genital femoral nerves are common causes of CPIP. Operative neurectomy of the three nerves is a common mode of surgical therapy. The entrapment is frequently caused by sutures or fixating devices
2. There is significant anatomical variation of the IHN, IIN and GFN with cross innervation in the retroperitoneum and inguinal canal
3. Meshoma:
   a. The mesh is implanted in front of or behind the transversalus fascia; in the latter approach this is done through an open or laparoscopic technique
   b. The mesh is implanted without fixation or is fixed by sutures, metallic staples and tacks or various tissue glues
   c. Non or insufficient fixation or inadequate dissection for the prosthesis leads to folding and wrinkling of the mesh that continues until the mesh forms a ball, the meshoma
   d. Meshomas cause neuropathic pain from nerve entrapment, direct contact with mesh or compression of contiguous tissue which may cause both nociceptive pain or a foreign body feeling

Neuroimaging

1. Ultrasonography is the best initial modality to detect hernia recurrence or meshoma
2. Cross-sectional computed tomography (CT) and MRI of the abdominal wall are useful to exclude other pathologies and to validate meshoma and recurrent hernia as causative

Differential Diagnosis of Abdominal Referred Pain by Location

Right Upper Quadrant

1. Cholecystitis:
   a. Radiation to T6 (tip of the scapula)
2. Cholangitis
3. Pancreatitis:
   a. Radiation straight through to the back
4. Hepatitis
5. Budd-Chiari syndrome
6. Subdiaphragmatic abscess

Epigastric Referred Pain

1. Peptic ulcer
2. Gastritis
3. GERD-radiations into the chest and pharynx
4. Pancreatitis
5. Esophagitis-radiation as well into the chest

Left Upper Quadrant Referred Pain

1. Splenic infarct and rupture:
   a. Radiation to the ipsilesional side shoulder
2. Gastritis and gastric ulcer:
   a. Diffuse
3. Pancreatitis
4. Subdiaphragmatic abscess

Right Lower Quadrant

1. Appendicitis
2. Inguinal hernia
3. Nephrolithiasis
4. Inflammatory bowel disease
5. Mesenteric lymphadenitis
6. Typhlitis (recurrent appendiceal infection)

Periumbilical Referred Abdominal Pain

1. Early appendicitis

2. Gastroenteritis
3. Bowel obstruction

Left Lower Quadrant Referred Abdominal Pain

1. Diverticulitis
2. Inguinal hernia
3. Nephrolithiasis
4. Irritable bowel syndrome
5. Inflammatory bowel disease

Pelvic Pain

Pudendal Nerve

General Characteristics

1. The pudendal nerve is a mixed sensory nerve that arises from the lumbosacral plexus. It arises from the ventral rami of S2, S3 and S4 nerve roots.
2. The trunk passes between the coccygeus and pyriformis muscles and exits the pelvis at the lower border of the greater sciatic foramen. At this level it gives off its inferior rectal branch
3. The nerve re-enters the pelvis through the lesser sciatic foramen and traverses distally through the pudendal canal (Alcock's canal) concomitantly with internal pudendal vessels.
4. Alcock's canal is located along the lateral wall of the ischiorectal fossa. Its outer covering is the obturator fascia
5. At the level of the perineum, it gives off the perineal nerves and the dorsal nerve of the penis or clitoris.
6. Variants of this classic anatomy are frequent and include:
    a. Two pudendal nerve trunks that traverse the sacrotuberous ligament
    b. There may be two exits from Alcock's canal: one for the dorsal branch and one for the perineal branch of the nerve
    c. The pudendal nerve may originate from the sciatic nerve. Rarely dorsal rami of the first sacral nerve contribute to the pudendal nerve. Extremely rarely there is a contribution from S5
    d. The sensory innervation of the pudendal nerve serves:
        i The penis and clitoris through the dorsal nerve of the penis and dorsal clitoral branches
        ii The posterior scrotal nerves and posterior labial nerves give sensory innervation to the posterior scrotum and the labia respectively
        iii The anal canal
        iv Branches innervate the muscles of the perineum and pelvic floor which include the bulbospongiosus and ischiocavernosus muscles,

the levator ani muscle, the iliococcygeus, pubococcygeus, puborectalis, pubovaginalis (females) or the pubourethralis (males), the external anal sphincter and the external urethral sphincter

Clinical Manifestations (Pudendal Neuralgia)

1. Pain is localized to the vulva, vagina, perineum and rectum in females
2. In males pain is perceived in the glans penis, scrotum (excluding the testicles) perineum and rectum
3. The pain is spontaneous, most often a dull ache or burning, superimposed lancinating pain
4. Mechanical hyperalgesia and allodynia
5. Entrapment of the nerve is characterized by exacerbation of pain with sitting and relief of pain with standing. Pain is usually absent with recumbency or when sitting on a toilet seat
6. Associated signs and symptoms include:
    a. Urinary hesitancy and frequency
    b. Constipation and painful defection
    c. Fecal incontinence
    d. Numbness of the penis / scrotum or vulva
    e. Altered sensation of ejaculation
    f. Impotence in men

Neuropathology

1. In entrapment the compression points are:
    a. Compression between the sacrotuberous and sacrospinous ligament
    b. The falciform process
    c. The pudendal canal (Alcock's canal)
2. Neuropractic injury (the nerves are stretched but the axon is intact). This type of injury occurs with compression of the pelvic floor during childbirth or with chronic straining from severe constipation
3. The nerve may be injured with prolonged cycling (a numb penis or vulva)
4. Removal of pelvic tumors (surgical trauma)
5. Pelvic trauma from high impact injuries
6. Hip surgery

Laboratory Evaluation

1. Nerve latency testing in muscles supplied by the pudendal nerve

Neuroimaging

1. Ultrasound cannot identify small areas of scarring in the pelvis along the course of the nerve
2. Magnetic resonance neurography

Dysmenorrhea

General Characteristics

1. Primary dysmenorrhea is defined as painful menses, primarily cramping, in the lower abdomen often accompanied by hyperhidrosis, headache, nausea, vomiting, diarrhea and tremulousness
2. There is wide variance of prevalence rates with estimates that 2% of adolescent girls have severe pain

Clinical Manifestations

1. Cramping pain in the abdomen that occurs just before or during menstruation
2. Some reported prevalence rates are as high as 90%
3. Primary dysmenorrhea usually presents during adolescence or within three years of menarche
4. It is unusual for symptoms to begin prior to six months of menarche
5. Patients have sharp, cramping and intermittent pain that is usually located suprapubically
6. Radiations are to the back of the legs or the lower back
7. Associated symptoms most commonly are nausea, vomiting, fatigue and headache
8. Pain usually starts within hours of the start of menstruation and is most severe with the heaviest flow during the first two days of the cycle
9. The physical examination is normal
10. Symptoms suggestive of a secondary cause of dysmenorrhea:
    a. Dysmenorrhea that develops during the first one or two cycles of menarche:
        i Congenital outlet obstruction
    b. Dysmenorrhea that develops after 25 years of age
    c. Late onset of dysmenorrhea after previous painless menstruation
    d. Pelvic anomalies on examination

Neuropathology

1. Normal examination with primary dysmenorrhea
2. Causes of secondary dysmenorrhea:
    a. Adenomyosis
    b. Pelvic inflammatory disease
    c. Cervical stenosis and polyps
    d. Fibroids (intracavitary or intramural)
    e. Endometriosis
    f. Inflammation and scarring (surgery with adhesions)
    g. Functional ovarian cysts
    h. Benign or malignant tumors of the ovary, bowel or bladder

3. Release of prostaglandins may cause abnormal uterine contractions which cause pain

Laboratory Evaluation

1. Gynecologic ultrasonography
2. Medical evaluation for specific causes of secondary dysmenorrhea
3. Possible laparoscopy

Endometriosis

General Characteristics

1. Endometriosis is the presence of normal endometrial mucosa abnormally implanted in locations other than the uterine cavity. This tissue has the same steroid receptors as the normal endometrium and responds to the normal cyclic hormonal milieu
2. Typically the ectopic implants are located in the pelvis – the ovaries, fallopian tubes, vagina, cervix or the uterosacral ligaments and rectovaginal septum
3. Risk factors include:
   a. Family history of endometriosis
   b. Early age of menarche
   c. Short menstrual cycles (< 27 days)
   d. Long duration of menstrual flow (> 7 days)
   e. Heavy bleeding during menses
   f. Inverse relationship to parity
   g. Delayed childbearing
   h. Defects in the uterus or fallopian tubes
   i. Possible iron deficiency
   j. Genetic predisposition
   k. CYPIA1 polymorphism has been associated with an increased risk of endometriosis (particularly in Asian women)
   l. A patient with a first degree relative with endometriosis has a lifetime risk approximately 10 times that of women without an affected family member
   m. If the products of cystic sloughing of endometriotic implants become entrapped by cyst formation, the mass is called an endometrioma. These may occur in any location but are most commonly encountered on one or both ovaries

Clinical Manifestations

1. A significant number of patients are asymptomatic (approximately 1/3)
2. Midline implantation may be more painful than lateral disease
3. The location of the pain may be pelvic, lower abdominal or in the back
4. Inguinal pain

5. Patients often present with increasing pelvic pain and/ or secondary dysmenorrhea
6. Painful bowel movements associated with diarrhea in association with menses when endometriosis involves the rectosigmoid colon
7. Flank pain, dysuria or hematuria may occur if the bladder or uterus are affected
8. Depending on the site of implantation cyclic pain with menstruation may involve the bladder, bowel (painful defecation) or bleeding at uncommon sites such as the umbilicus, abdominal wall or perineum
9. The average onset of cyclic or noncyclic pain was 2.9 years after menarche (one large series)
10. Rarely, there can be a cyclically expanding mass in a pelvic surgery scar which is painful
11. Acute exacerbations of pain can occur from rupture of an endometriotic cyst (chemical peritonitis) or implantation in peripheral spinal nerves
12. Deep dyspareunia may occur particularly in the premenstrual phase of the cycle. This pain may be due to scarring of the uterosacral ligaments, nodularity of the rectovaginal septum, cul-de-sac obliteration
13. The most common physical finding is nonspecific pelvic tenderness
14. Pelvic examination may reveal tender nodular masses along thickened uterosacral ligaments, the posterior uterus or the posterior cul-de-sac
15. Pain may be exacerbated by exercise, micturition and defecation

Neuropathology

1. Ectopic endometrial tissue is most commonly encountered in the dependent areas of the pelvis which include the anterior and posterior cul-de-sac, the uterosacral ligaments, fallopian tubes and ovaries
2. The sloughed endometrial tissue and release of cytokines and prostaglandins induce an inflammatory response characterized by neovascularization and fibrosis
3. There is evidence of altered T and B cell function, complement deposition and increased IL-6 production
4. In endometriosis, there may be an aberrantly expressed factor SF-1 that induces the expression of aromatase. Aromatase converts C19 steroids to estrogen. Estrogen increases the synthesis of prostaglandin E2 that stimulates the uterus and induces aromatase.
5. Recent studies have demonstrated increased expression of neurotrophic factors and nerve fibers in endometriotic lesions, eutopic endometrium and the peritoneum which may be related to endometriosis pain

Laboratory Evaluation

1. Pelvic ultrasonography, CT and MRI are only useful in advanced disease

2. Laparoscopy to directly visualize endometrial implants

Vulvodynia

General Characteristics

1. Vulvodynia is a chronic pain condition that affects the vulvar area. The condition must last for at least 3 months to meet diagnostic criteria
2. It has been estimated to affect as many as 16% of women

Clinical Manifestations

1. Pain is the most disabling symptom
2. There is burning, stinging or lancinating pain that can be continuous or occurs only with mechanical stimuli
3. Symptoms may be localized or affect the entire vulvar area
4. It can occur during or after sexual activity or when prolonged pressure is applied to the area from activities of daily living
5. Vulvar vestibulitis syndrome (VVS) is pain localized to the vestibular area
6. It is the most common subtype of vulvodynia and has been estimated to affect 10 to 15% of premenstrual women that present to gynecologists
7. The pain is usually described as neuropathic in quality

Neuropathology

1. The cause of vulvodynia is incompletely understood. At present, it appears to be heterogeneous.
2. Proposed mechanisms include:
   a. Infections that include yeast, bacterial vaginosis, HPV, HSV
   b. Genetic predisposition to inflammation
   c. An autoimmune disorder
   d. Injury
   e. Possible use of hormonal contraceptives that contain low-dose estrogen prior to age 16
   f. Pelvic floor dysfunction
   g. Recent experimental evidence has demonstrated:
      i Site-specific inflammatory responses
      ii Fibroblasts isolated from the vestibule in patients are sensitive to proinflammatory stimuli and release inflammatory mediators that include IL-6 and PGE_2.

Laboratory Evaluation

1. Wet mount of vaginal secretions, vaginal pH, fungal culture and Gram stain

Differential Diagnosis

1. Candidiasis, herpes and HPV
2. Lichen planus

3. Paget's disease and vulvar carcinoma
4. Neuralgia secondary to herpes virus

Dyspareunia

General Characteristics

1. Dyspareunia is painful sexual intercourse that is multifactorial and is due to medical or psychological causes
2. It has recently been proposed that the diagnosis of vaginismus and dyspareunia be combined into the diagnostic entity of genito-pelvic-pain / penetration disorder with the following criteria:
   a. Percentage success of vaginal penetration
   b. Pain with vaginal penetration
   c. Fear of vaginal penetration or of genito-pelvic pain during vaginal penetration
   d. Pelvic floor muscle dysfunction
   e. Medical co-morbidity

Clinical Manifestations

1. Pain on attempted intercourse is described as superficial when perceived at the entrance to the vagina or surface of the genitalia and deep when initiated from the vault of the vagina
2. A proportion of women experience pain in more than one area
3. A subset of patients have had pain with intercourse from their first experiences while others develop it after an injury, infection or cyclically with menstruation
4. Pain is increased when the vagina in dry or undilated
5. Fear of pain exacerbates the discomfort
6. External genitalia may demonstrate lesions, thin skin, ulceration or discharge from vulvovaginal infections
7. Internal pelvic exam may demonstrate cervical lesions and anatomical variations of the uterus

Neuropathology

1. Conditions that affect the surface of the vulva include:
   a. Lichen sclerosus et atrophicus
   b. Xerosis (particularly after menopause)
   c. Sjogren's syndrome (dryness)
2. Infections that primarily affect the labia, vagina or lower urinary tract and include:
   a. Yeast infections
   b. Chlamydia
   c. Trichomoniasis

   d. Urinary tract infection
   e. Herpes
3. The above conditions cause surface genitalia primarily neuropathic pain often with mechanical hyperalgesia and less frequently allodynia
4. Infection of the cervix or fallopian tubes from pelvic inflammatory disease (PID) cause deeper pain
5. Pain from tissue injury occurs after surgery, childbirth or pelvic trauma
6. Associated anatomic variants that may be a component of pain include:
   a. Hymenal remnants
   b. Vaginal septa
   c. Thickened undilatable hymen
   d. Hypoplasia of the introitus, retroverted uterus or prolapse
7. Hormonal effects:
   a. Endometriosis and adenomyosis
   b. Estrogen deficiency that is associated with lubrication inadequacy
8. Deep vaginal pain can be caused by ovarian cysts, tumors and uterine fibroids
9. Interstitial cystitis:
   a. May cause pain during or after sex in women
   b. In men with interstitial cystitis pain occurs with ejaculation and radiates to the tip of the penis
   c. In females with interstitial cystitis pain is usually felt the following day and is thought to occur from spasm of the pelvic floor musculature

Laboratory Evaluation

1. Medical evaluation to rule out infection, hormonal deficiency and autoimmune causes

Neuroimaging

1. MRI
   a. To delineate anatomical variants and pathologies such as ovarian tumor or endometriosis

Differential Diagnosis of Dyspareunia

1. Superficial dyspareunia:
   a. Infection
   b. Inflammation
   c. Anatomic variants
   d. Tissue damage
   e. Psychosocial factors
   f. Pelvic floor muscle dysfunction
2. Deep dyspareunia:
   a. Endometriosis
   b. Ovarian cysts

c. Pelvic inflammatory disease
d. Psychosocial factors

Sexual Pain Disorders in Males

Prostatitis Chronic Pelvic Pain Syndrome (CP / CPPS)

General Characteristics

1. Prostodynia or chronic pelvic pain syndrome is utilized for unexplained chronic pelvic pain in men
2. The National Institutes of Health designation of categories of prostatitis is:
   a. Type I - Acute bacterial prostatitis
   b. Type II - Chronic bacterial prostatitis
   c. Type III - Chronic abacterial prostatitis
      i IIIa – inflammatory
      ii IIIb – noninflammatory
   d. Type IV - Asymptomatic inflammatory prostatitis
3. The majority of chronic prostatitis patients are type III (approximately 90-95%), without infection but with chronic pelvic pain. The chronic pelvic pain symptoms last for at least three to six months without a cause related to urinary tract infection or malignancy.
4. Worldwide it is estimated that 2 to 14% of men have CP / CPPS

Clinical Manifestations

1. The usual patient is a young to middle-aged man
2. The pain is localized:
   a. Between the rectum and testicles
   b. In the testicles
   c. In the tip of the penis
   d. Below the waist
3. The pain is usually moderate but can be severe and is usually a dull ache
4. The sensation of not emptying the bladder completely
5. Irritative and obstructive bladder symptomatology
6. Erectile dysfunction; pain with sitting
7. Anal sphincter tone may be increased
8. The prostate may have moderate to severe mechanical hyperalgesia
9. The gland may be slightly congested

Neuropathology

1. In the past infection, immunologic dysfunction and psychosocial issues have been proffered as causative
2. Organic and morphological pathology does not explain the chronic pelvic pain

3. Present theories for cause include:
    a. Stress-driven hypothalamic-pituitary-adrenal axis dysfunction
    b. Neurogenic inflammation
    c. Myofascial pain syndrome

Laboratory Evaluation

1. There are no definitive diagnostic tests for CP / CPPS
2. Categorization as IIIa (inflammatory) or non-inflammatory IIIb is based on levels of leukocytes in expressed prostatic secretions
3. TGFB 1 and IFN-γ have been shown to be increased in some patients with IIIa and IIIb disease
4. There is some evidence that nerve growth factor could be a biomarker of the disorder
5. Semen and prostatic fluid evaluation have shown elevated cytokines, myeloperoxidase and chemokines
6. Flexible cystoscopy (rule out bladder conditions)
7. Urodynamic tests to rule out bladder neck hypertrophy and urethral stricture

Interstitial Cystitis

General Characteristics

1. The de facto definition of the disease has been the modified National Institute of Diabetes and Digestive and Kidney Diseases NIDDK criteria which has been used and include:
    a. 2 inclusion criteria and 1 exclusion criterion
    b. At least 1 subjective symptom and 1 cystoscopic finding
2. Subjective symptoms:
    a. Pain associated with the bladder
    b. Urinary urgency
3. Cystoscopic criteria include:
    a. Glomerulations in at least 3 quadrants of the bladder and at least 10 glomerulations per quadrant (a glomerulation is a petechial hemorrhage of the bladder wall)
    b. Classic Hunner ulcer:
        i Distinctive areas of inflammation on the bladder wall
        ii Glomerulations cannot be along the path of the cystoscope
4. Exclusion criteria for interstitial cystitis:
    a. Cystometric bladder capacity > than 350 ml
    b. Absence of an urge to void when the bladder has been filled with 100ml of liquid
    c. Phasic involuntary bladder contractions at a fill rate of 30-100ml
        i Detrussor instability occurs in 14% of patients with IC

   d. Symptom duration of less than 9 months
   e. Nocturia
   f. Symptoms are relieved by antimicrobials, antiseptics, anticholinergics or antispasmodics
   g. Micturition frequency of less than 8 times daily

Clinical Manifestations

1. Day and night time frequency
2. Pelvic pain or pressure
3. Suprapubic pain related to bladder filling

Neuropathology

1. Findings in cystoscopy under anesthesia:
   a. Inflammatory infiltrate
   b. Granulation tissue
   c. Detrusor mastocytosis
   d. Intrafascicular fibrosis
   e. Hunner's ulcer (patches of reddened mucosa with small vessels radiating from a central pale scar)
   f. Nonulcer IC:
      i Multiple strawberry-like petechial hemorrhages ("glomerulations")

Laboratory Evaluation

1. Inflammatory mediators as urinary markers of IC / BPS syndrome (bladder pain syndrome) include:
   a. Mast cells, histamine and methylhistamine
   b. NGF
   c. IL-6, CRP, CXCL10 (chemokine), CXCR3, TNIFSF14
2. Elevated proliferative factors have been demonstrated and include:
   a. PD-ECGF, UEGF, NGF, EGF and HB-EGF
   b. Antiproliferative factor (APF):
      i Possibly the most promising biomarker
      ii It is a sialogy copeptide and inhibits endothelial proliferation
      iii Moderates the cell cycle by G2 blockage
      iv Has been detected in the urine of 95% of IC patients
3. Cystoscopy

Scrotal Pain

Overview

Scrotal pain is a common condition in urologic practice. It can present acutely or more commonly in chronic form. The more common urological problems are testicular torsion, epididymitis, postvasectomy pain, varicocele, and chronic orchalgia. Nonurological causes of scrotal pain are peritonitis, incarcerated hernia, ruptured abdominal aortic aneurysm, and referred scrotal pain.

The sensory innervation of the upper ureter and testes traverse spinal cord levels T11 and T12. Upper ureteral distension (stone or malignancy) refers pain to the testis (somatic-visceral convergence at these dorsal root ganglia). Lower ureteral distension causes ipsilateral scrotal pain. Less frequent causes of scrotal pain are Henoch-Schonlein purpura, testicular tumors and referred pain from disc or other vertebral pathologies (T10-L1 segments). Extremely rarely, it may be caused by a partial complex seizure that involves the cortical genital area. Testicular tumors primarily present as a painless scrotal mass. A rapidly growing tumor may have internal bleeding or infarction that presents as scrotal pain.

Testicular Torsion

General Characteristics

1. Testicular torsion is a medical emergency. The incidence is 1 in 4000 males < than 25 years of age

Clinical Manifestations

1. The classic presentation is the acute onset of intense unilateral scrotal pain often associated with nausea and vomiting
2. Patients may have a history of prior scrotal pain that resolved spontaneously (ischemic episodes)
3. "High riding" testicle due to shortening of the cord; the testicle may be transverse in the scrotum
4. Loss of the cremasteric reflex is common in pediatric patients
5. Testicular torsion usually occurs around puberty while epididymitis affects sexually active men after the age of 20
6. Patients with torsion of a testicular appendage such as an appendix testis or appendix epididymis have:
    a. Rare systemic complaints
    b. Gradual onset, less intense, unilateral scrotal pain that is localized to the superior pole of the testis
    c. The scrotal skin may reveal the "blue dot" sign from the nonviable appendage

Neuropathology

1. Testicular torsion may be intravaginal or extravaginal that typically occurs in neonates and in adolescents prior to complete testicular descent and scrotal wall fusion
    a. Intravaginal torsion:
        i The testicle can rotate within the tunica vaginalis due to the congenital

bell clapper anomaly. This anomaly is due to failure of a posterior anchor for the gubernaculum (the scrotal ligament, which secures the testis to the most inferior portion of the scrotum), epididymis and testis; this allows the testis to rotate within the tunica vaginalis

b. Extravaginal torsion:
   i The testis rotates within the scrotum due to inadequate fusion of the testicle to the scrotal wall
   ii The torsion is caused by rotation of the spermatic cord and causes ischemia
   iii Torsion of testicular appendages:
      1. Occurs in 7-13 year-old children
      2. Similar clinical presentation to testicular torsion
      3. Accounts for 24-46% of acute scrotal presentations

Laboratory Evaluation

1. Urinalysis:
   a. Hematuria or leukocytosis is more typical of epididymo-orchitis rather than torsion
   b. Doppler ultrasonography
      i Assess testicular blood flow

Epididymitis

General Characteristics

1. Epididymitis may cause acute scrotal pain that must be differentiated from testicular torsion
2. A painful parenchymal inflammatory process that causes epididymal swelling

Clinical Manifestations

1. Primarily encountered in men between 18-50 years of age; in pediatric patients, the peak incidence is during puberty
2. Infantile epididymitis is associated with other urogenital anomalies
3. Epididymitis presents with gradually increasing dull unilateral scrotal pain
4. Vasa involvement may be associated with exquisite pain that localizes to the entire hemiscrotum and the spermatic cord
5. The epididymis is swollen and tender; the cremasteric reflex is intact
6. There has often been a recent GU procedure or sexual activity

Neuropathology

1. If the swelling affects the testicles the disorder is defined as epididymo-orchitis
2. The most common organisms are dependent on age and sexual activity

3. The pathophysiology of the disorder is the spread of microorganisms from the urethra, prostate or seminal vesicles or rarely hematogenous spread (tbc) that causes a painful inflammatory process in the epididymis
4. Sexually active men <35 years of age are usually infected with Chlamydia Trachomatis and Neisseria gonorrhoeae
5. Older patients, those that have undergone recent genitourinary surgery or those with anatomical anomalies are usually infected with gram negative enterococci

Laboratory Evaluation

1. Urinalysis, urine cultures and urethral cultures to identify causative organisms
2. Color Doppler ultrasound or nuclear scintigraphy to assess scrotal blood flow (increased blood flow due to inflammation)

Post-Vasectomy Pain

General Characteristics

1. Chronic scrotal pain affects up to 15% of patients after vasectomy

Clinical Manifestations

1. Patients have scrotal pain and discomfort
2. Pain may be exacerbated or initiated during intercourse, pain with ejaculation and epididymal pain
3. Physical examination reveals:
    a. Tender epididymides
    b. Swollen epididymides
    c. Tender vasectomy site
    d. Palpable nodule

Neuropathology

1. The pathophysiology is not known but putative mechanisms include:
    a. Tender sperm granuloma
    b. Nerve entrapment
    c. Nerve proliferation at the operative vasectomy site
    d. Perineural fibrosis
    e. Mechanical duct obstruction with epididymal congestion
1. Histological evaluation:
    a. Epididymal engorgement
    b. Complex cystic disease
    c. Chronic epididymides

Laboratory Evaluation

1. Ultrasonography with Doppler may demonstrate:
    a. Epididymal thickening

b. Epididymal tubular ectasia
c. Blood flow

Varicocele

General Characteristics

1. Definition:
   a. A varicocele is an abnormal dilation of the spermatic veins due to an anatomical anomaly
   b. The incidence is 10-20% in the general male population and 2 to 15% in adolescents
   c. Varicoceles are associated with male infertility possibly due to increased temperature, stasis induced hypoxia and reflux of renal and adrenal metabolites

Clinical Manifestations

1. The pain associated with a varicocele is dull and aching in quality and less frequently throbbing
2. The pain is localized to the scrotum. There are no lancinating or referred components
3. The pain is exacerbated by long episodes of standing (causes increased hydrostatic pressure in the valveless veins of the pampiniform plexus)
4. Physical examination of the scrotum reveals a "bag of worms" on palpation
5. Classification of varicoceles:
   a. Grade 0: No palpable varicocele
   b. Grade 1: Palpable during a Valsalva maneuver
   c. Grade 2: Visible in the standing position during a Valsalva maneuver
   d. Grade 3: Visible in the standing position through scrotal skin without a Valsalva maneuver

Neuropathology

1. The putative mechanism is thought to be absent or malfunction of vein valves that allow retrograde flow into the pampiniform plexus. The plexus is located in the spermatic cord and scrotum that is derived from the internal spermatic and cremasteric veins. There may be lack of valves proximal to the renal veins and absent or incomplete valves along the internal spermatic vein. Varicoceles may be more frequent on the left side as the left gonadal vein is longer than the right (resulting in greater hydrostatic pressure) and it inserts into the left renal vein

Laboratory Evaluation

1. Evidence of venous dilation and reflux during a Valsalva maneuver by color Doppler

2. Vein diameter of 2.45mm at rest and 2.95mm during Valsalva maneuver can be demonstrated in grade 1-3 varicoceles.

Chronic Orchialgia

General Characteristics

1. It is defined as intermittent or constant testicular pain of at least 3 months duration that interferes with daily activities
2. 50% of patients present with an idiopathic etiology
3. In the USA it may affect up to 100,000 men /year

Clinical Manifestations

1. Moderate to severe dull aching pain in the testicle
2. In patients with a neuropathic etiology there may be mechanical hyperalgesia

Neuropathology

1. The causal spectrum of chronic orchialgia is wide and includes:
   a. Vasectomy
   b. Inguinal hernia surgery
   c. Recurrent epididymitis
   d. Varicocele and hydrocele
   e. Prior scrotal or abdominal surgery
   f. Trauma
   g. Idiopathic
2. Less frequent pathologies are:
   a. Diabetic neuropathy
   b. Retroperitoneal tumor
   c. Abdominal aortic aneurysm
   d. Polyarteritis nodosa
3. The ilioinguinal, genital branch of the genitofemoral or pudendal nerves are the most commonly affected nerves. They have been hypothesized to have undergone maladaptive neuroplasticity to produce neuropathic pain
4. Contralateral pain phenomena can occur due to decussation of the nerves in the pelvic plexus
5. An anatomical study has demonstrated a high density of nerve fibers undergoing Wallerian degeneration (that induced an immune response from neutrophils, macrophages and cytokines) in the spermatic cord:
   a. Cremasteric muscle fibers
   b. Perivasal tissues and vasal sheath
   c. Posterior peri-arterial lipomatous tissue

Laboratory Evaluation

1. Medical evaluation to rule out diabetes mellitus, periarteritis, inguinal hernia

and possible referred pain

Neuroimaging

1. Abdominal MRI to delineate possible sources of referred pain (ureteral stones, hernia, disc)
2. Scrotal Doppler

Pelvic Floor Dysfunction

General Characteristics

1. The pelvic floor or pelvic diaphragm is composed of the muscle fibers of the levator ani and the coccygeus muscle and associated connective tissue
2. The levator ani are horizontal in the floor of the pelvis; and are divided into three divisions:
   a. The pubococcygeus is the major portion of the levator and courses from the body of the pubis to the coccyx. There is some insertion into the prostate, urethra and vagina
   b. The two sides of the puborectalis muscles merge behind the anorectal junction to form a muscular sling. It has been proposed that these muscles are part of the sphincter ani externus
   c. The iliococcygeus muscle is the most posterior portion of the levator ani and may be poorly developed
3. The pelvic cavity is delineated by:
   a. The pelvic floor is the inferior boundary
   b. The pelvic brim is the superior border
   c. The perineum's superior border is the pelvic floor
   d. Posteriorly the pelvic floor extends into the anal triangle
   e. The hiatuses of the pelvic floor are:
      i The urogenital hiatus is anterior through which the urethra and vagina pass
      ii The rectal hiatus is posterior through which the anal canal traverses
   f. The pelvic floor is essential in the support of pelvic viscera and continence as it is a component of the urinary and anal sphincters. During childbirth, it is important in resisting descent of the presenting part which rotates the fetus forward and enables it to pass the pelvic girdle
   g. Pelvic floor dysfunction is extremely common and has been estimated to affect 50% of women at some time during their lifetime.

Clinical Manifestations

1. Patients complain of pelvic pain, heaviness and aching
2. Pain may be exacerbated by exertion, defecation, sitting and coitus
3. Postcoital pain may be long-lasting and persist for hours to days
4. Pain may radiate to the hip or lower back

5. Physical examination (intravaginal) may demonstrate banding, spasm or tenderness
6. Spasm of a portion of the levator ani is a palpable band
7. In healthy control patients, palpation of the levator ani and piriformis muscle is perceived as pressure. In patients with pelvic floor myalgia this maneuver causes hyperalgesia
8. Examination often reveals asymmetry between the right and left pelvic diaphragm. Spasm and contracture is ipsilateral to the patient's pain
9. In men with chronic prostatitis / chronic pelvic pain syndrome, myofascial trigger points in pelvic musculature have been identified

Neuropathology

1. The major mechanisms of pelvic floor dysfunction are widening of the pelvic floor hiatus and descent of the pelvic floor below the pubococcygeal line
2. Co-morbidities include obesity, menopause, pregnancy and difficult childbirth
3. Myofascial pain / pelvic floor hypertonia often co-exist with other illnesses thought to have a component of central sensitization and include:
    a. Endometriosis
    b. Painful bladder syndrome / interstitial cystitis
    c. Vulvodynia
    d. Irritable bowel syndrome
    e. Primary dysmenorrhea
4. The levator muscles and their nerve supply can be damaged in pregnancy and childbirth. They may also be damaged during hysterectomy
5. The perineal approach for pelvic surgery, between the anus and coccyx may damage the pelvic floor
6. Rarer causes of damage to the perineum and pelvic floor have been described with water-skiing, bicycle racing and equestrian sports
7. Damage to the pelvic floor that is severe causes urinary incontinence and pelvic organ prolapse in which the vagina, bladder, rectum or uterus protrude into or outside of the vagina

Neuroimaging

1. Grading of pelvic floor dysfunction by MRI:
    a. The pubococcygeal line connects the inferior margin of the pubic symphysis at the midline with the junction of the first and second coccygeal elements on a sagittal image
    b. The second landmark is the puborectalis muscle sling
    c. A perpendicular line between the pubococcygeal line and muscle sling is a measurement of pelvic floor descent
    d. A descent greater than 2cm is mild and 6cm is severe

e. A line from the pubic symphysis to the puborectalis muscle sling is a measurement of the pelvic floor hiatus. Greater than 6cm is mild and 10cm is severe. The degree of organ prolapse is measured relative to the hiatus. Any organ prolapse relative to the hiatus is abnormal and greater than 4cm is severe

Chronic Pelvic Pain

General Characteristics

1. Chronic pelvic pain lasts for at least 6 months and is of sufficient intensity to disrupt activities of daily living and requires medical or surgical treatment
2. Chronic cyclic pelvic pain (CCPP) is considered to be a subset of chronic pelvic pain that most often occurs with the menstrual cycle. Cyclic chronic pelvic pain also occurs with disorders that have a cyclic pattern that are not related to menstruation or hormonal fluctuations and include:
   a. Coital pain
   b. Pelvic floor myalgia
   c. Provoked vestibulodynia
   d. Pudendal neuralgia
   e. Ovulation that cause mittelschmerz pain
3. Interstitial cystitis and irritable bowel syndrome occur without a specific pattern but can be exacerbated by menstruation

Clinical Manifestations

1. The quality of the pain in the pelvis is usually a dull ache. There may be intermittent lancinating pains: cramping, pressure or heaviness deep in the pelvis are also descriptors
2. Pain may be exacerbated during intercourse, defecation, or micturition. It may be increased by sitting
3. Less frequently pain may be exacerbated by standing or relieved with recumbency

Neuropathology

1. Endometriosis
2. Endosalpingiosis
3. Pelvic adhesions
4. Ovarian remnant syndrome
5. Interstitial cystitis
6. Adenomyosis
7. Uterine leiomysis
8. Endometriosis affects approximately 50% of women with CPP:
   a. This diagnosis requires visual confirmation of the lesion during laparoscopy and histologic evidence of endometrial glands and stroma

9. Interstitial cystitis is often associated with CPP whose pathology is thought to be bladder epithelial dysfunction, mast cell activation, and peripheral sensitization of bladder nociceptive afferents. There may be increased permeability of the bladder epithelium that can be demonstrated by the Potassium Sensitivity Test. A large proportion of patients with IC may have concomitant endometriosis
10. After adjusting for age and education, women in all subgroups of chronic pelvic pain were found to have lower pain thresholds (increased pressure pain) than healthy controls. This supports the concept that central pain amplification may be a component of CPP

Laboratory Evaluation

1. Urinalysis and urine cytology
2. Urine and genital cultures
3. Mycoplasma and urealyticum (genital mycoplasma organism) cultures of the vaginal fornix
4. Bladder potassium sensitivity test
5. Laparoscopy
6. Cystoscopy (if IC symptoms are present)
7. MRI of the pelvis to delineate any structural lesions

Sexual Pain Disorders in Females

Ovarian Cysts

General Characteristics

1. The vast majority of ovarian cysts are benign and asymptomatic. They are detected incidentally by ultrasonography or on routine pelvic examination

Clinical Manifestations

1. Pain or discomfort in the lower abdomen or pelvis:
    a. Severe pain occurs with torsion or rupture that is characterized by:
        i Sudden onset
        ii Unilateral pelvic pain
        iii Lancinating sharp quality
        iv Associated peritoneal signs and abdominal distension
2. Moderate to large cysts:
    a. Dyspareunia particularly with deep penetration
    b. Increased urge to defecate (pressure on the bowel or rectum)
    c. Frequent micturition (bladder pressure)
    d. Abnormalities of the menstrual cycle:
        i Irregularity
        ii Abnormal vaginal bleeding

        iii Prolongation of the intermenstrual interval followed by menorrhagia
    e. Abdominal fullness and bloating
    f. Indigestion, symptoms of esophageal reflux and early satiety
    g. Endometriomas:
        i Associated with endometriosis
        ii Heavy menstrual bleeding
        iii Dyspareunia
    h. Polycystic ovarian syndrome:
        i Hirsutism
        ii Infertility
        iii Oligomenorrhea
        iv Obesity
        v Acne
    i. Dull bilateral pelvic pain:
        i Theca-lutein cysts
    j. Hyperpyrexia – due to ovarian torsion
    k. Adnexal or cervical motion tenderness
    l. Malignant disease:
        i Cachexia
        ii Weight loss
        iii Lymphadenopathy in the neck
        iv Shortness of breath
        v Pleural effusion
    m. Symptoms of early ovarian cancer may include:
        i Unexplained pelvic or abdominal pain
        ii Unexplained bloating
        iii Early satiety

Neuropathology

1. Features of an ovarian mass that suggest malignancy are:
    a. Large mass with irregularity
    b. Complexity and projections
    c. Projections and septations
    d. Bilaterality
2. Benign cysts:
    a. The most common is a functional cyst that forms during ovulation:
        i Either the egg is not released or the follicle in which the egg forms does not dissolve after the egg is released
    b. Polycystic ovaries:
        i The follicles fail to open and cysts form
    c. Endometriosis:
        i Endometrial tissue attaches to the ovary

d. Cystadenoma:
    i Form on the surface of the ovary and are often fluid-filled
e. Dermoid cysts:
    i Contain skin, hair and rarely teeth
f. Malignant tumors of the ovary:
    i Ovarian carcinomas:
        1. Serous
        2. Clear cell
        3. Mucinous
        4. Endometriotic
    ii Germ cell tumors
    iii Stromal tumors

Laboratory Evaluation

1. Complete blood count
2. Urinalysis
3. Urinary pregnancy test
4. Rh status
5. Cancer antigen 125 (CA125), HE4 markers (upregulated gene in epithelial ovarian carcinoma) may be more sensitive than 125CA
6. ROMA (Risk of Ovarian Malignancy Algorithm):
    a. Utilizes the combination of human epididymis protein 4 (HE4) and CA125 values to predict the risk of epithelial ovarian cancer in post-menopausal women but not in pre-menopausal women
7. Matrix metalloproteinase III (MM3) is good to differentiate benign ovarian cysts from ovarian cancer in post-menopausal women

Neuroimaging

1. Transvaginal ultrasonography is the first imaging choice
2. CT / MRI of the pelvis and abdomen if the mass is larger than 6cm or if there are extraadnexal symptoms or signs

Ectopic Pregnancy

General Characteristics

1. An ectopic pregnancy is the implantation of a fertilized egg outside of the uterine cavity
2. The most common locations are:
    a. The fallopian tubes (98%)
    b. Cervix, ovary, cornual region of the uterus and abdominal cavity
    c. In tubal pregnancies the most common sites of implantation are:
        i Ampulla (80%)
        ii Isthmus (12%)

        iii Cornua (2%)
        iv Interstitia (2-3%)
        v Fimbrial (5%)
3. Ectopic pregnancy is estimated to occur in 1 of 40 pregnancies or 25 patients / 1000 pregnancies in the USA

Clinical Manifestations

1. The classic clinical triad is abdominal or pelvic pain, amenorrhea, and vaginal bleeding.
    a. Approximately 50% of patients present with the entire triad.
2. 40 to 50% of patients have vaginal bleeding
3. 50% have a palpable adnexal mass
4. 75% have abdominal tenderness
5. Patients may present with symptoms of early pregnancy that include:
    a. Nausea
    b. Breast fullness
    c. Fatigue
    d. Low abdominal pain
    e. Shoulder pain
    f. Severe cramping
    g. Dyspareunia
6. Unruptured patients:
    a. Peritoneal signs
    b. Cervical motion tenderness
    c. Unilateral or bilateral abdominal or pelvic tenderness worse on the affected side
    d. Painful fetal movement (in advanced pregnancy)
    e. Dizziness and weakness
    f. Fever
    g. Flu-like symptoms
    h. Vomiting
    i. Syncope
    j. Cardiac arrest
7. Ruptured ectopic pregnancy
    a. A surgical emergency:
        i Hypovolemic shock with orthostatic hypotension and tachycardia
        ii Abdominal rigidity, guarding and severe tenderness
        iii Uterine or cervical motion tenderness
        iv May be difficult to delineate an abdominal mass

Neuropathology

1. Uterine contents in the vagina from shedding of the endometrial lining

Laboratory Evaluation

1. The B-HCG levels doubles every 48-72 hours in a normal pregnancy until it reaches 10,000-20,000mIU/ml. Mean serum B-HCG levels are lower with ectopic pregnancy
2. The discriminatory zone of B-HCG:
    a. Defined as the level of B-HCG that should be attained when an imaging scan demonstrates a gestational sac within the uterus:
        i 1500-1800mIU/ml with transvaginal ultrasonography; up to 2300 mIU/ml with multiple gestates
        ii 6000-6500mIU/ml with abdominal ultrasonography
3. Ultrasonography
4. Laparoscopy:
    a. Most often used for patients in pain or for those that are hemodynamically unstable

Uterine Leiomyoma (Fibroids)

General Characteristics

1. Fibroids are benign smooth muscle tumors of the uterus
2. Genetic influence in the pathogenesis of fibroids is demonstrated by:
    a. The daughter of a mother with fibroids has a three times higher incidence of fibroids than the average woman
3. Familial leiomyomata (Reed's syndrome):
    a. Caused by a mutation located on the long arm of chromosome 1q42.3-43 in the gene FH that encodes fumarate hydratase which is transmitted in an autosomal dominant manner: also associated with renal cell cancer
4. One form of uterine leiomyoma (UL) is due to fusion between an isoform of the recombinational repair gene RAD51B and the high mobility group protein gene HMG1C that maps to chromosome 12q14.3
5. Uterine leiomyomas are associated with other fusion partners of the HMG1C gene that include:
    a. ALDH2
    b. COX6C
    c. HEI10
6. Gene wide association studies have recently revealed loci in chromosome 10q24.33, 22q13.1 and 11p15.5 that are associated with uterine fibroids
7. Locations include:
    a. Intramural
    b. Subserosal
    c. Submucosal

   d. Cervical
   e. Rarely in the round ligament or uterosacral ligament
8. Most fibroids start in the wall of the uterus and may grow outwardly or toward the uterine cavity
9. Extrauterine fibroids of uterine origin occur rarely:
   a. Fibroids that metastasize:
      i Invade the vasculature
      ii Intravenous leiomyomata grow in veins with uterine fibroids
      iii Benign metastasizing fibroids have been demonstrated in the lungs and lymph nodes
      iv Disseminated intraperitoneal leiomyomatosis:
         1. The source is uterine fibroids
         2. The leiomyomata grow diffusely on the peritoneal and omental surfaces

Clinical Manifestations

1. Small fibroids are often asymptomatic; symptoms depend on the location and size of the leiomyoma
2. Abnormal uterine bleeding
3. Heavy or painful menstrual periods
4. Abdominal discomfort and bloating
5. Painful defecation
6. Frequency of micturition and rarely urinary retention
7. Dyspareunia and pelvic pain
8. Miscarriage, bleeding, premature labor
9. Infrequent cause of infertility (location is primarily submucosal)

Neuropathology

1. Leiomyomas demonstrate karyotypical chromosomal defects in approximately 40 to 50% of patients.
2. Mutations of the MED12 protein are commonly characterized
3. Genetic predisposition, prenatal hormone exposure and hormone growth factors and xenoestrogens are postulated as factors in their growth
4. Significant risk factors are:
   a. African ethnicity
   b. Obesity
   c. Polycystic ovary syndrome
   d. Diabetes mellitus
   e. Hypertension
   f. Never having given birth
5. Estrogen and progesterone have a mitogenic effect on leiomyomata as well as interacting with growth factors, cytokines and apoptotic factors and

hormones

6. It has been hypothesized that estrogen induces leiomyoma growth by up-regulating IGF1, EGFR, TGF-beta 1, TGF-beta 3 and PDGF
7. Estrogen may sustain survival or aberrant leiomyoma by down-regulating:
    a. P53
    b. Increasing expression of the anti-apoptotic factor PCP4,
    c. Blocking PPAR-gamma signaling
8. Progesterone influences leiomyoma growth by upregulating EGF, TGE-beta 1 and TGF-beta 3:
    a. Influences survival by up-regulating Bcl-2 expression and down-regulating TNF-alpha
9. Secondary changes that may develop within fibroids are:
    a. Hemorrhage
    b. Necrosis and cystic changes
    c. Calcify after menopause

Neuroimaging

1. Gynecologic ultrasonography is the standard imaging techniques and demonstrates:
    a. Leiomyomas as focal masses with a heterogeneous texture
    b. Shadowing of the ultrasound beam
    c. Location and dimensions of the mass can be determined
2. Other imaging techniques that may be used to evaluate the uterine cavity are:
    a. MRI
    b. Hysterosalpingography
    c. Sonohysterography
3. Imaging modalities cannot discriminate between benign uterine leiomyoma and malignant leiomyosarcoma. Distinguishing characteristics are:
    a. Fast or unexpected growth, as the usual pattern of growth is slow and associated with extracellular matrix
    b. Enlargement of a lesion after menopause
    c. Local invasion

Pathologies that Cause Pain in Any Area of the Body Surface

Surgically-Induced Neuropathic Pain (SNPP)

General Characteristics

1. Surgically induced neuropathic pain is estimated to occur in 10 to 50% of patients that have undergone common surgical procedures
2. SNPP occurs in:

a. 60% of patients after limb amputation
b. 20 to 40% of patients after mastectomy
c. 20 to 40% after thoracotomy
d. 20% following hernia repair

Clinical Manifestations

1. Some patients develop SNPP almost immediately after their procedure while it develops in others weeks or months following injury
2. Spontaneous pain that is burning or aching in quality
3. The pain may be lancinating on a background of burning or a dull aching sensation
4. There may be hypoesthesia in an area of nerve injury or mechanical and thermal hyperalgesia
5. Complex regional pain syndromes type I and II have been described from almost all surgical procedures and demonstrate:
   a. Severe spontaneous pain that spreads out of a dermatomal and nerve distribution. A mirror distribution of pain is common and in some patients, the pain becomes generalized. Dynamic and static mechanoallodynia and hyperalgesia are prominent as are thermal hyperalgesia particularly to cold.
   b. Autonomic dysregulation is prominent with earlier stages most often producing a warm extremity that evolves over time to a cold discolored extremity with livedo reticularis and cyanosis:
      i Neurogenic edema is present in the great majority of patients
   c. A motor syndrome is seen in which patients have difficulty initiating movement, are weak and may develop tremor, atrophy and dystonia
   d. Dystrophic changes evolve in hair, muscle, subcutaneous tissue and bone

Neuropathology

1. During surgical procedures nerves may be completely transected or undergo neuropractic injury in which the axon may be injured but remains intact
2. The nerve injury causes peripheral sensitization in which the threshold to discharge nociceptive afferents is lowered and central sensitization is produced. In this state, there are major changes in the pain matrix (those areas of the CNS that process pain) which lead to:
   a. Enlargement of nociceptive pain projecting neuron receptive fields
   b. Loss of inhibition at all levels of the pain matrix
   c. Spontaneous and evoked pain
   d. Emotional and motivational changes

Laboratory Evaluation

1. Imaging to delineate any structural lesion that may be maintaining a peripheral drive on central sensitization. Examples include:

   a. A poorly healed fracture, a meshoma (herniorrhaphy), entrapment of a peripheral nerve or a neuroma (in scar tissue)
2. Quantitative sensory testing
3. EMG and nerve conduction velocities to evaluate affected nerves

Neuroma

General Characteristics

1. A neuroma is a tangled mass of connective tissue in which are imbedded distally sprouting regenerating axons. There are both myelinated and unmyelinated axons in a neuroma
2. Neuromas may form in any tissue in which there is transection of a peripheral nerve
3. They are extremely common following traumatic amputation of a limb and in this instance may cause incapacitating pain in up to 10% of patients

Clinical Manifestations

1. Mechanical stimulation of a neuroma may induce minor dysesthesia to extreme pain
2. It is typically a painful or tender nodule
3. Usually they occur post-surgically but may occur following minor trauma
4. If they occur in a nerve plexus multiple neuromas can form
5. They may fire spontaneously and have extremely low mechanical thresholds for discharge. In some instances they are responsive to alpha adrenergic stimuli
6. Scar neuromas may form at any surgical site
7. Neuroma-in-continuity:
   a. May cause a dysfunctional nerve:
      i Tinel's sign (local tenderness over the injured nerve site that causes distal radiating tingling or paresthesia)
      ii Denervation atrophy of the innervated muscles, sensory loss and trophic changes in the territory of the injured nerve

Neuropathology

1. Traumatic neuromas are usually bulbous in shape
2. They consist of an unorganized network of connective tissue intermingled with regenerating nerve fibers, Schwann cells, macrophages, fibroblasts and myofibroblasts
3. Myofibroblasts may be a contributor to pain by causing the collagen matrix to contract around nerve fibers. Alpha smooth muscle actin (α-SMA) has been demonstrated in neuromas from patients that caused neuropathic pain
4. Electrophysiological studies demonstrate basal spontaneous discharge which is enhanced by mechanical stimuli that show that neuromas may act as an

ectopic generator of action potentials

5. There is experimental support for ephaptic transmission of efferent autonomic fibers to afferent sensory fibers within neuromas
6. Neuroma-in-continuity:
   a. Usually involves both myelin, axon and perineurial injury within a scarred nerve. The proximal injured nerve fascicles sprout but are unable to reunite correctly due to lattice disruption, dysfunctional regeneration, hypertrophy of nerve fascicles and fibrosis.
   b. Neuromas-in-continuity are divided into two forms:
      i Spindle neuromas with intact perineurium
      ii Lateral neuromas that occur after partial disruption of the perineurium or after nerve repair
   c. End-bulb neuromas:
      i May occur in any location; a nerve is completely divided and is unopposed by another neural tissue
      ii They are seen in nerves that have been completely severed and in amputations. They are also encountered in lacerations in which the nerve is not repaired or in post-operative patients in which the nerves have been severed

Neuroimaging

1. High-resolution ultrasound can distinguish neuromas in injured peripheral nerves
2. MRI:
   a. Microneurography utilizing fat-suppressed fluid-sensitive sequences in association with T1-weighted sequences demonstrate changes in nerve size, signal intensity and location
3. MRI in neuropraxia and axonometmesis:
   a. Enlarged and T2 hyperintense nerves are demonstrated possibly due to proximally obstructed axoplasmic flow and distal Wallerian degeneration
4. Neuroma-in-continuity:
   a. A round mass with nerve continuity on either side (may be similar in appearance to a neurofibroma or Schwannoma)
   b. Distinguishing features from nerve sheath tumors are:
      i Surrounding scarring
      ii Lack of a split fat or target sign
      iii Absence of abnormal enhancement
5. End bulb neuroma:
   a. Occurs in a completely severed nerve and demonstrates:
      i A T2 sequence nerve that terminates in a round mass that may resemble a balloon on a string or a green onion
      ii MRI of traumatic neuromas:

1. Some are neuromas-in-continuity and others are end-bulb neuromas
2. Mean size is usually 1.5cm (range 0.6 to 4.8cm)
3. Almost all have indistinct margins and may have a capsule
4. Approximately 80% will enhance
5. Most have a tail sign
6. There is a moderate correlation between the size of the affected nerve and the size of the neuroma

Phantom Pain

General Characteristics

1. The amputation of a limb causes an almost immediate experience of phantom sensations in 90 to 98% of patients. Approximately 75% of patients experience the phantom upon awakening from anesthesia and the remaining patients experience phantom sensations within days or weeks
2. Phantom pain is pain in the body part that is no longer present

Clinical Manifestations

1. Phantom sensations include:
    a. Feeling of the continued presence of the limb
    b. Feeling of a specific position, (often twisted), shape (often distorted and too small) or movement of the missing limb
    c. Sensations of warmth or cold, itch, tingling or lancinating (electric-like) sensations
    d. Sensations related to length and volume or that the phantom is behaving as the normal limb
    e. A feeling that the phantom limb is gradually shortening which is defined as "telescoping"
    f. In most patients that experience innocuous sensations also report pain
    g. Phantom pain:
        i May be related to a specific position or movement of the phantom
        ii The pain may be exacerbated by changes in the barometric pressure, stress (emotional) and mechanical stimuli
        iii The pain is more severe in the distal portion of the phantom
        iv The quality of the pain includes:
            1. Stabbing
            2. Throbbing
            3. Burning
            4. Cramping
            5. An unusual distorted posture
            6. Squeezing

v Phantom body pain occurs with spinal cord injury
vi Phantom pain is less frequent if the amputation occurs at a very young age. Older children have an adult pattern of pain
vii Phantom sensations occur in patients with congenital absence of a limb but pain under this circumstance is very rare
viii The stump of the amputated extremity may demonstrate mechanical allodynia particularly adjacent to the skin flap scar or near neuromas
ix Exacerbation of both painful and non-painful sensations by emotional stimuli, micturition or yawning
x Exacerbation of both painful and non-painful phantom limb sensations by noxious or innocuous stimuli at the stump or from distal body areas

Neuropathology

1. There is a correlation between pain in the residual stump and phantom limb pain
2. Ectopic discharge from stump neuromas are a component of the nociceptive input to the pain matrix
3. The rapid onset of phantom pain may be initiated from end bulbs of the severed nerves prior to the formation of neuromas
4. Another site of ectopic discharge following amputation is the dorsal root ganglia (DRG); ectopia here can also summate with that from neuromas in the residual stump
5. As noted earlier, increased sympathetic discharge and circulating epinephrine can exacerbate ectopic firing of neuromas (sympathetic – sensory coupling). This phenomena can occur both at the level of the neuroma and the DRG
6. Decreased near-surface blood flow to the skin has been suggested as predictive of burning phantom limb pain
7. Cramping and squeezing descriptions of phantom pain have been associated with muscle tension in the residual stump
8. Sympathetic-efferent and somatic-afferent mechanisms appear to be a component of a peripheral mechanism of phantom pain
9. Central mechanisms of phantom pain:
   a. Central sensitization at the spinal level of pain projecting neurons and at other levels of the pain matrix has been demonstrated experimentally:
      i A major component of this sensitization is due to increased efficacy of transmission of NMDA receptors to glutamate
      ii As part of central sensitization, mechanoreceptive A-beta fibers have input to the ascending pain projecting system. In neuropathic conditions, this may be a mechanism of mechanohyperalgesia and allodynia. In the instance of phantom pain, low threshold mechano

afferents may contribute to hyperexcitability and ectopic discharge of dorsal horn pain projecting neurons. Although controversial, it has been demonstrated that nociceptive afferents may degenerate and vacate lamina I of the dorsal horn. Deeper synapsing low-threshold afferents of lamina III-IV may sprout and synapse with the deafferented pain projecting neurons in lamina I

10. Other putative mechanisms that have been postulated to contribute to phantom pain:
    a. Down-regulation of opioid receptors in primary nociceptive afferents and intrinsic spinal neurons in addition to reduced GABAergic and glycinergic inhibition
    b. There is a phenotypic switch in which substance P is secreted by A-beta low threshold mechano afferents that renders them similar to nociceptors. Substance P is the ligand for NK1 receptors on lamina I pain projecting nociceptive neurons
    c. In injured tissue, cholecystokinin, an endogenous inhibitor of the mu opioid receptor is upregulated
    d. At the spinal cord level, descending inhibition from supraspinal levels may be lost as well as that from local intersegmental inhibitory mechanisms
    e. Brain level changes with phantom pain:
        i Cortical reorganization occurs in which the cortical representation of the amputated extremity is annexed by neighboring representational zones in both the primary somatosensory and motor cortex. This is the operational definition of maladaptive plasticity in which afferented areas enlarge or shift their activation into somatotopically deafferented brain areas. In some instances, the greater the shift the more severe the pain. There are inconsistencies with this construct as a mirror movement task has demonstrated reduced activity in patients with phantom pain (in the deafferented areas) which was correlated with decreased pain severity. In addition, other cortical brain areas including the supplementary motor cortex may be incorporated into maladaptive plasticity

Laboratory Evaluation

1. Ultrasound and MRI to identify stump neuromas that may contribute to the peripheral maintenance of phantom pain

Activated microglia have altered expression of genes that upregulate cell-surface receptors (P2X4R being primary) and intracellular signaling molecules (p38 MAPK as primary) that produce and secrete diffusible factors that include BDNF and proinflammatory cytokines that modulate pain processing in the dorsal horn of the spinal cord.

CHAPTER 8

NEUROPATHIC VISCERAL PAIN

Overview

Visceral pain results from the activation of nociceptors in the thoracic, pelvic, or abdominal organs. Studies have demonstrated a prevalence rate of 25% for intermittent abdominal pain and 20% for chest pain among adults. Approximately 25% of women suffer pelvic pain at some point in time.

Clinical Manifestations of Visceral Pain

Visceral pain has a temporal course and clinical characteristics that vary with the different phases of its evolution. In general, it commences as a diffuse and poorly defined midline body sensation in the lower sternum or upper abdomen. Different visceral organs project pain to specific somatic territories as exemplified by bladder pathologies to the perineum, the heart to the left arm, jaw, and neck, the left ureter to the left lower quadrant and groin. The diffuse nature of visceral pain and its consequent difficulty in localization has been ascribed to a low density of visceral sensory innervation and divergence of visceral nociceptive input within the central nervous system. As the pain evolves, pain may be referred to parietal structures within the same metameric field somewhat analogous to sclerotomal pain that occurs within the somatic system. As noted earlier, visceral somatic convergence of nociceptive input to dorsal horn pain projecting neurons and interneurons is a major mechanism of referred pain. Spatial discrimination of visceral pain entails referral to superficial (somatic) structures that produces secondary hyperalgesia of either superficial or deep body wall tissue. Referred pain may be sharper, better localized, and less often associated with autonomic manifestations than somatic pain.

Visceral pain is often associated with autonomic signs and symptoms that include:

1. Pallor
2. Hyperhidrosis

3. Nausea and vomiting
4. Alterations in temperature
5. Changes in heart rate and blood pressure.

Peripheral Visceral Innervation

The afferent fibers that innervate the viscera course to the CNS by autonomic sympathetic and parasympathetic nerves. A proportion of spinal afferents course with hypogastric, lumbar, colonic and splanchnic nerves and traverse prevertebral and paravertebral sympathetic ganglia to synapse in the thoracolumbar dorsal horn of the spinal cord.

Vagal afferents terminate in the brainstem and pelvic afferents synapse in the lumbosacral cord. These are major components of the parasympathetic innervation. Some visceral afferent fibers evoke conscious sensation while other afferences regulate autonomic functions and are not consciously perceived. These afferences are exemplified by hepatic chemoreceptors or pulmonary stretch receptors. Sensory afferents that innervate the GI tract and urinary tract have regulatory functions and contribute to evoked sensations of pain and fullness.

Visceral sensory afferents are primarily A-delta thinly myelinated (1-4μ) fibers and unmyelinated (1μ) C-fibers. There is a functional division of mechanosensitive visceral receptors into two physiological subgroups. High-threshold receptors that are in the heart, esophagus, colon, ureter, and uterus are only activated by noxious mechanical stimuli. Low-threshold receptors encode intensity and respond to a spectrum of innocuous to noxious stimuli. Under normal conditions, low-threshold AB-fibers only transmit innocuous mechanical modalities of sensation. Visceral organs are innervated by mechanically insensitive afferents that acquire mechanosensitivity following inflammation. They have been well characterized in rodent pelvic and splanchnic innervations as well as in cutaneous C-afferents by microneurography.

The convergence of visceral and somatic afferent inputs to the dorsal root ganglia and spinal cord dorsal horn pain transmitting neurons causes the referral of visceral pain to specific somatic sites on the body surface. It has been posited that viscerosomatic convergence may occur because of the low density of visceral afferent fibers that account for less than 10% of the total dorsal horn spinal cord afferent input. There is extensive divergence and intraspinal segmental distribution of visceral afferent terminals compared to cutaneous C-afferents that are usually restricted to one or two above or below segments due to their projections through Lissauer's tract. Viscerosomatic convergence may also cause maladaptive neuroplasticity of central nociceptive processing in both the spinal cord and other components of the pain matrix. The convergence of nociceptive visceral and somatic inputs is one mechanism that causes concomitant visceral and somatic pain. There may also be viscero-visceral convergence in which pain from one organ can be referred to another organ.

Brain-Gastrointestinal Interaction

There is bidirectional neuronal connectivity between cognitive, affective, and autonomic nuclei in the brain and neuro-endocrine nuclei, the enteric nervous system and the immune system. Visceral functions require complex regulation that involves CNS integration with the peripheral and enteric nervous system.

Vagal afferents project to the nucleus tractus solitarius in the medulla whose cell bodies are in the nodose ganglion. Convergent spinal visceral afferents synapse in the dorsal horn with second order pain transmitting neurons that project to higher centers via spinothalamic, parabrachial, and dorsal column pathways.

Lesion studies in animal models demonstrate:

1. Dorsal column lesions cause suppressed inhibition of exploratory behavior induced by noxious visceral stimulation and inhibition of potentiated visceromotor reflexes induced by colorectal distention after bowel inflammation;
2. The spinoparabrachial pathway is formed by projections from the superficial dorsal horn and is associated with autonomic and affective responses to painful stimuli.

The spinoparabrachial and nucleus tractus solitarious projections from vagal afferents synapse in the amygdala, hypothalamus and periaqueductal grey nuclei that are important in limbic and cognitive function. Spinothalamic projections from the deep dorsal horn along with a subset of lamina I neurons project to the contralateral ventroposterior lateral and ventroposterior medial thalamic nuclei. They in turn project to the insular and somatosensory cortices for sensory discrimination. Medial thalamic nuclei are primary for the affective and motivational components of pain processing projecting to the prefrontal and anterior cingulate cortex (ACC).

Descending modulation (descending nociceptive inhibitory controls in experimental protocols) is a neuronal system primarily from the periaqueductal grey of the midbrain and the rostral ventral medullary nuclei that has both inhibitory and facilitatory actions on the pain transmission neurons of the spinal dorsal horn. This modulatory system activates specific neurons of the RVM that can facilitate or suppress ascending nociceptive transmission. In animal pain models, it has been demonstrated that RVM neurons respond divergently to visceral and cutaneous stimuli. Dorsal horn pain transmission neurons that are depolarized by somatic stimuli can be inhibited by visceral inputs and vice versa. Human functional MRI studies demonstrate cortical activation after subliminal visceral stimulation and that cortical and subcortical circuitry can modulate brainstem pain processing.

Visceral Hyperalgesia

Peripheral sensitization of visceral nociceptors occurs from persistent stimulation from inflammatory mediators (cytokines, chemokines, and prostanoids) which produces ectopic activity and lowered discharge thresholds. The chemical milieu at the site of injury is an "inflammatory soup" composed of immune cells (that secrete cytokines, chemokines and prostaglandins), mast cells, enzymes and protons all of which act upon nociceptive receptors. An important mechanism for peripheral sensitization of visceral nociceptors may be lowered firing thresholds of voltage-gated sodium channels of visceral pain afferents. Tetrodotoxin-resistant currents are present on small nociceptive afferents and have been identified on DRG neurons that innervate the colon. $Na_v1.8$ channels have also been shown to be important in the sensitization of visceral nociceptors. The TRPV1 nociceptor is a non-selective cation channel that is gated by noxious heat, low pH and endogenous lipids and is widely expressed in visceral afferents. TRPV1 channels are upregulated in tissue samples from patients with irritable bowel syndrome (IBS) which has been correlated with pain intensity.

As occurs with somatic pain processing, persistent nociceptive drive causes central sensitization of pain transmission neurons in the visceral pain matrix. In patients with chronic visceral pain, secondary hyperalgesia in specific dermatomes has been demonstrated. Central sensitization has been clearly demonstrated in patients with esophageal and colon pathologies. Central changes derived from the affective-emotional and motivational circuitry, a top-down mechanism, is very important in the production of visceral hyperalgesia.

Some Aspects of the Neuroanatomy of Lower Gastrointestinal Pain Disorders

Chronic abdominal pain often arises from a local inflammatory process in the lower gastrointestinal tract that occurs with inflammatory bowel disease. Approximately 50 to 70% of patients with ulcerative colitis (UC) and Crohn's disease (CD) present with abdominal pain.

Intrinsic Innervation of the Enteric Nervous System

The intestinal wall of the esophagus, stomach, small intestine, and colon are innervated by a dense neuronal network, the enteric nervous system. This intrinsic network is composed of enteric nerve cell bodies (sensory, motor, and interneurons) and their processes that form plexuses characterized by the myenteric plexus (Auerbach's plexus) and the submucosal plexus (Meissner's plexus). The enteric nervous system (ENS) regulates the functions of the gut that include:

1. Motility
2. Mucosal secretion
3. Absorption
4. Mucosal growth
5. Local blood flow
6. Immune function

There are bidirectional connections between the CNS and the ENS. Intrinsic enteric afferents release serotonin, substance P, and calcitonin gene related peptide (CGRP) that can initiate or exacerbate neurogenic inflammation that may sensitize gut nociceptive afferents.

The vagal nerve innervates the entire gut except for the transverse and distal portion of the colon. Its cell bodies are in the nodose ganglion whose central afferents synapse in the nucleus tractus solitarius of the dorsal medulla. Vagal afferents regulate feeding by modulation of upper gut reflexes that include gastric accommodation, gastric emptying, pancreatic secretion, and emesis as well as the perceptions of hunger, fullness, bloating, and nausea.

Experimental studies in rodents demonstrate three types of vagal fibers:

1. Mechanoreceptors
2. Tension receptors
3. Chemoreceptors that are activated by bile

Intramuscular vagal mechanical afferents are parallel to either the longitudinal or circular muscle layers and respond to muscle stretch. Intraganglionic laminar afferents innervate the connective tissue surrounding the myenteric ganglia and convey afferences that signal distention and muscle contraction. Tension-sensitive afferents are activated maximally at distensions within the physiologic range and respond to peristaltic contractions. It is posited that vagal afferents code the physiologic perception of mechanical stimuli while pain from distension of the upper GI tract is carried by splanchnic nociceptive afferents. Vagal nociceptors may be a component of pain from gastric acid. There is evidence that low intensity stimulation of vagal nociceptors may facilitate pain and high intensity stimulation may be inhibitory. The vagal nerve may regulate the cholinergic tone of the immune response of macrophages and immunocytes that is anti-inflammatory.

The pelvic nerves innervate the colorectum, the bladder, and the reproductive organs. Pelvic nerves contain afferents from serosal, mucosal, intralaminar, and intramuscular arrays that project to the DRG of spinal segments L5-S2. These afferences primarily detect circular stretch generated by low-intensity colorectal distension. The pelvic nerves are posited to be a component of normal physiology similar to the vagal afferent system (physiologic sensations such as urinary urgency and the desire to defecate) as well as acute rather than inflammatory pain that is the domain of splanchnic afferents.

Splanchnic nerves innervate the entire GI tract and visceral afferents in splanchnic nerves (demonstrated in rodents) from the colorectum synapse in T10-L2 spinal segments. Splanchnic afferent fibers traverse the celiac, superior, and inferior mesenteric ganglia where they form "en passant" synapses with efferent sympathetic neurons. Splanchnic afferents are posited to convey the major proportion of nociceptive afferences from the gut and signal different modalities of mechanosensibility. In the upper GI tract, splanchnic afferents code gastric mechano-nociception while gastric chemo-nociception is mediated by vagal pain transmission neurons. Splanchnic afferents mediate abdominal pain from the lower GI tract. In rodents, splanchnic afferents of the colon are located in the serosa (36%) and mesenteric membranes (50%) often associated with the mesenteric blood supply. Mucosal spinal afferents are found associated with submucosal blood vessels where they form varicose branching axons. The naked nerve endings of submucosal and mesenteric afferents respond to gut distortion during stretch or contraction at tissue destructive levels.

Ascending Visceral Pathways from the Lower GI Tract

Extrinsic primary afferents that innervate the lower GI tract synapse with DH neurons of the thoraco- and lumbosacral spinal cord primarily in laminae I and II but also in laminae V and X. Ascending pathways of the contralateral anterior quadrant are composed of the spinoreticular, spinomesencephalic, spinohypothalamic and spinothalamic tracts. The spinoreticular tract synapses in the dorsal reticular nucleus and is thought to be involved in the affective-motivational components of visceral pain. The spinomesencephalic tract synapses in the PAG (periaqueductal grey) and other midbrain areas, which is extremely important in descending pain modulation. The spinohypothalamic tract in conjunction with the amygdala, medial thalamus, anterior cingulate cortex, locus coeruleus, and PAG modulate arousal, emotional and autonomic components of pain. Much of the sensory information conveyed by these pathways does not reach consciousness. The spinothalamic tract mediates pain, cold, heat, and a component of light touch. The posterolateral nucleus of the thalamus processes visceral innocuous and noxious inputs. The thalamic relays project to the pregenual anterior cingulate cortex (pACC), the midcingulate cortex, the insula, and the somatosensory cortex. Visceral sensation has a heavy representation in the secondary somatosensory cortex (SII). There is evidence from functional MRI studies that the cerebellum is activated during visceral nociception (as it is with painful somatic stimuli).

Recent studies support a role of the dorsal columns in visceral sensory transmission and nociception. The human limited midline myelotomy surgical procedure for intractable pelvic cancer pain is effective. The dorsal columns receive collateral branches of primary afferent fibers that arise from the dorsal root entry zone en route to the medulla as well as to the projecting axons from the deep lamina of the dorsal horn both of which synapse in the dorsal column nuclei. In experimental animals, there is input from the colon, the ureter, the pancreas, and the epigastric structures to dorsal column nuclei.

Descending Modulatory Pathways

Visceral pain is modulated by descending projections from the nucleus magnus raphus, the PAG and the periventricular grey of the hypothalamus. In the cortex, the anterior cingulate area projects to the amygdala and the PAG. These descending projections can be either facilitatory or inhibitory to visceral ascending pain transmission. As is true of the somatic pain system the major circuitry of this system is from the PAG to the rostral ventromedial medulla (RVM) to the dorsal horn. Endogenous opioids are the major transmitter of this circuitry. Other well-characterized neurotransmitters of the system include:

1. Noradrenaline
2. Dopamine
3. Serotonin

The pACC projects to the pontomedullary networks that are posited to be inhibitory due to their high content of opioids. In contrast, stimulation of the RVM that projects to the dorsal horn includes the raphe magnus nucleus that is serotonergic increases dorsal horn excitability.

Visceral pain has many of the same underlying mechanisms that have been characterized for somatic pain. These include peripheral sensitization of nociceptors, central sensitization, and descending pain modulation. The specificity of segmental organization and its innervation density by nociceptors is less than that of the somatic system.

Angina Pectoris

General Characteristics

1. Approximately ten million Americans are estimated to suffer angina annually. There are approximately 500,000 new patients per year.
2. Angina is more often the presenting symptom of coronary artery disease in women than men with a female-to-male ratio of 1.7:1
3. Angina pectoris is caused by an imbalance between myocardial blood supply and oxygen demand
4. Definitions:
   a. Stable angina:
      i Classic angina related to myocardial ischemia
      ii Chest pain or discomfort that is precipitated by a physical activity. There are minimal or no symptoms with rest. Symptoms recur with physical activity
      iii Precipitants of stable angina are cold weather, large meals and emotional stress
   b. Unstable angina ("crescendo angina"):
      i Angina pectoris that is exacerbated by or occurs:
         1. At rest or with minimal exertion and lasts for more than 10 minutes
         2. It is severe and of recent onset
         3. It has a crescendo pattern with more severe, prolonged or increase in frequency
      ii The pathophysiology is reduction of coronary blood flow due to transient platelet aggregation on normal endothelium, coronary artery spasm or thrombosis
      iii The process is initiated by atherosclerosis, evolves through an inflammatory stage to produce an active unstable plaque which may thrombose to cause myocardial ischemia
      iv Approximately 60% of unstable angina attacks occur between 10pm and 8am
   c. Microvascular angina (cardiac syndrome X):
      i Microvascular angina is manifest by angina-like chest pain with

normal epicardial coronary arteries

ii Possible pathogenic mechanisms are endothelial dysfunction and decreased blood flow in heart small resistance blood vessels

Clinical Manifestations

1. In general, angina is seen in a man older than 50 years of age or a woman older than 60.
2. The chief complain is most often of chest discomfort rather than frank pain. It is described most often as pressure, heaviness, tightness, squeezing, burning, or a choking sensation.
3. Patients may localize the pain to the sternum with a clenched fist (Levine's sign).
4. The pain is usually crescendo – decrescendo and most often lasts for two to five minutes.
5. Radiations are to either shoulder or both arms: most often medially to the humerus and to the medial forearm. Angina pain rarely crosses the wrist but if it does, it affects the ulnar side of the hand.
6. Less frequent radiations are to the interscapular areas, epigastrium, neck, jaw, teeth, back shoulder, and left medial humerus.
7. Rarely radiates below the umbilicus or above the mandible
8. Radiations to the trapezius muscle are more typical of pericarditis. Angina does not radiate to the trapezius muscles.
9. Typically angina is triggered by exercise, sexual activity, emotional stress, specific tasks, cold, or a large meal; it also occurs with rest and while the patient is recumbent (angina decubitus). The patient may be awakened from sleep with chest discomfort and dyspnea.
10. Angina equivalents are symptoms of myocardial ischemia that are more frequent in diabetic patients and the elderly. They include dyspnea, fatigue, hyperhidrosis, nausea, pallor, and presyncope.

Neuropathology:

1. Major angina risk factors:
   a. Age > than 45 years for men and > 55 for women
   b. Cigarette smoking
   c. Diabetes mellitus
   d. Dyslipidemia
   e. Family history of premature cardiovascular disease
   f. Hypertension
   g. Kidney disease (microalbuminuria or GFR < 60 ml/min)
   h. BMI > 30 kg /m^2
   i. Nonphysical life style
   j. Severe emotional stress (prolonged)

2. Myocardial ischemia may be caused by:
   a. Stenosis, spasm or acute occlusion of coronary vessels by emboli
   b. Increased resistance of coronary and microvessels: blood flow is proportional to the radius of the artery to the fourth power
   c. Reduced oxygen-carrying capacity of the blood from decreased oxygen tension and hemoglobin concentration
   d. Rheological factors that increase blood viscosity and decrease arterial blood flow
3. Angina pain:
   a. The extrinsic autonomic nerves access the heart via arterial routes and extend from the atria into the ventricular epicardium
   b. In addition to the ganglia around the coronary sinus and nodal areas, extrinsic nerves synapse with cell bodies of intrinsic cardiac nerves. The majority of intrinsic nerve cell bodies are located on the epicardial surface and within epicardial fat pads. Their axons are connected to adjacent neurons that form networks delineated as "ganglionic plexuses" (GPs). There are both afferent and efferent neurons within the intrinsic cardiac nervous system the majority of whose neurons may be local circuit neurons. Integration of sensory inputs from the heart occurs both in the intrinsic cardiac nervous system as well as in mediastinal, middle cervical and stellate ganglia. Cardiac afferent receptors have their cell bodies in the dorsal root, the nodose ganglia, and the intrathoracic ganglia. There is no topographic spatial representation of the myocardium in these ganglia. It is proposed that during myocardial ischemia ATP is degraded to adenosine that diffuses into the extracellular space. There it causes both arterial dilatation and also pain by stimulating A1 receptors of the cardiac nociceptive afferents. If adenosine is given as an intravenous bolus to healthy volunteers and patients with ischemic heart disease, it provokes angina-like pain in the absence of EKG changes. Patients with asymptomatic myocardial ischemia are less sensitive to adenosine while those with Syndrome X are more sensitive. Intra-arterial adenosine provokes pain in the corresponding vascular bed.

Laboratory Evaluation

1. Graded exercise stress testing

Neuroimaging

1. Chest radiography:
   a. Is usually normal with angina but may demonstrate cardiomegaly in patients with cardiomyopathy, prior myocardial infarction, pericardial effusion
   b. Myocardial perfusion scintigraphy

c. Coronary artery calcium (CAC) scoring by fast CT; electron-beam CT (EBCT) and multidetector CT (MDCT)

Pericarditis

General Characteristics

1. Acute pericarditis is seen in 1 per thousand hospital admissions
2. Chronic pericarditis occurs in approximately 6-10% of patients with advanced renal failure
3. Malignant disease is the most common cause of pericardial effusion with tamponade in Western countries. Tuberculosis is commonly causative in endemic areas
4. Acute pericarditis is more common in men than women and adolescents are affected more than young adults
5. The pericardium is composed of the parietal pericardium, its outer fibrous layer, and the visceral pericardium, an inner serous membrane that is composed of a single layer of mesothelial cells.
6. The fibrous layer attaches to the diaphragm, sternum and the costal cartilage
7. The visceral layer is adjacent to the heart and is attached to the epicardial fat. It reflects on itself to form the parietal pericardial layer
8. The pericardium contains between 20-50 ml of an ultrafiltrate of plasma. During tamponade there may be an additional 90-120 ml of pericardial fluid after which there is increased pericardial pressure which reduces stroke volume and cardiac output with consequent hypotension

Clinical Manifestations of Acute Pericarditis

1. Acute pericarditis is the most common pathological process in a wide spectrum of diseases
2. It's cardinal manifestations are:
   a. Pain
   b. A pericardial friction rub
   c. A pericardial effusion
   d. Tamponade and paradoxical pulse
3. Chest pain:
   a. Present in acute infection and autoimmune etiologies
   b. Pain may be absent in insidious development of tubercular, post radiation, neoplastic and uremic forms
   c. The pain is severe and typically retrosternal and left precordial. It is referred to the root of the neck, arms left shoulder and trapezius ridge.
   d. It has a pleuritic component due to concomitant pleural inflammation that is sharp and exacerbated by coughing and change of position. Less frequently, the pain may be steady and constricting with bilateral medial

arm radiations

e. The pain is relieved by sitting up and leaning forward and is made worse by lying down
f. An audible pericardial friction rub is present in 85% of patients. It is heard throughout the respiratory cycle.
g. Associated signs and symptoms include:
    i Low grade intermittent fever
    ii Dyspnea and tachypnea
    iii If tuberculosis is etiologic, fever, night sweats and weight loss occur in 80% of patients

Clinical Manifestations by Etiology

1. Rheumatoid arthritis:
    a. Pericarditis is associated with arthritis and pleuritis
    b. Often while the patient is being treated with anti-inflammatory agents that include corticosteroids, gold and antimalarials
2. Chronic patients:
    a. The heart rate may be bradycardic in association with tamponade, fever and hypotension that are due to autonomic involvement
3. Malignant pericarditis:
    a. Symptoms develop over days to weeks
    b. Dyspnea is often the most prominent symptom
4. Cardiac tamponade:
    a. May present subacutely with:
        i Anxiety
        ii Dyspnea
        iii Fatigue
        iv Altered mental status
    b. A waxing and waning course occurs with intermittently decompressing tamponade
    c. Traumatic tamponade
        i Presents with acute dyspnea and altered mental status
5. Physical signs with pericardial inflammation of any cause which are:
    a. Pericardial friction rub
    b. Dyspnea and tachycardia (usually with associated effusion)
    c. Ewart sign (dullness and bronchial breathing between the tip of the left scapula and the vertebral column)
    d. Cyanosis
    e. Altered mental status (if there is hypotension from tamponade)
    f. Rare hepatomegaly and ascites
    g. Tachycardia and cardiac arrhythmia

Neuropathology

1. Acute pericarditis:
    a. Serous pericarditis is most often caused by rheumatoid arthritis and systemic lupus erythematosus
    b. Rarely these processes are associated with fibrous adhesions
    c. Fibrous and non-fibrous pericarditis are the most frequent causes of pericarditis and include:
        i Myocardial infarction
        ii Post infarction
        iii Dressler's syndrome:
            1. Persistent low-grade fever
            2. Pleuritic chest pain
            3. Pericarditis often with a friction rub and or a pericardial effusion
            4. Signs and symptoms occur 2-3 weeks following a myocardial infarction but may be delayed for several months
            5. Usually subside in several days and is not often associated with pericardial tamponade
            6. Posited to be an autoimmune inflammatory process (may be associated with an elevated sed rate)
2. Purulent pericarditis:
    a. May arise from direct extension from an inflammatory chest process, hematogenous seeding or by lymphatic spread of infection
    b. Infection during cardiotomy procedures particularly in immunosuppressed patients
    c. Clinical manifestations include fever, chills and spiking temperatures
3. Specific causes of pericarditis include:
    a. Infections (viral, bacterial and tuberculous)
    b. Autoimmune disorders (RA, SLE, scleroderma, rheumatic fever)
    c. Metabolic disorders (hypothyroidism, uremia and hypercholesterolemia)
    d. Acute myocardial, Dressler's syndrome and aortic dissection
    e. Neoplasm
    f. Drugs
    g. Irradiation
    h. Trauma
    i. Cardiac surgical procedures
    j. Idiopathic
4. The pericardium is acutely inflamed and is infiltrated with polymorphonuclear leukocytes associated with vascularization
5. There is an associated fibrous reaction with exudates and adhesion. There may also be a serious or hemorrhagic effusion

Laboratory Evaluation

1. CBC, serum electrolytes, blood urea nitrogen and creatinine, erythrocyte sedimentation rate and C-reactive protein
2. Cardiac biomarkers
3. Lactate dehydrogenase
4. SGOT and AST
5. EKG:
   a. Typically demonstrates ST elevation in all leads
6. Echocardiography
7. Chest radiograph is helpful in patients with effusions larger than 250 ml

Acute Aortic Syndrome

1. Definition:
   a. Acute aortic syndrome (AAS) is the acute presentation of patients with "aortic pain" that includes:
      i Aortic dissection
      ii Intramural hematoma
      iii Penetrating atherosclerotic ulcer
      iv Aneurysmal leak
      v Traumatic transection

Aortic Dissection

General Characteristics

1. Evidence of aortic dissection is seen in 1 to 3% of autopsies
2. The incidence is estimated to be 5 to 30 patients per 1 million of the population
3. Aortic dissection is more frequent in black than white patients and males than females
4. Approximately 75% of dissections are seen in patients 40 to 70 years of age, the peak incidence is between 50 to 65 years; patients with connective tissue disorders present at an earlier age

Clinical Manifestations

1. Medical:
   a. Hypertension:
      i A catecholamine surge or underlying hypertension
   b. Hypotension:
      i Excessive vagal tone
      ii Cardiac tamponade
      iii Rupture of the dissection
   c. Blood pressure inter arm differential of more than 20 mmHg
   d. Signs of cardiac tamponade:

- i Distant or soft heart sounds
- ii Hypotension
- iii Pulsus paradoxus
- iv Jugular venous distension
- v Kussmaul sign (paradoxical rise in jugular venous pressure on inspiration)
- vi Superior vena cava syndrome (compression from a large distorted aorta)
- vii Right coronary artery ostial dissection may cause acute myocardial infarction

2. Neurologic deficits:
   a. Neurologic signs and symptoms occur in approximately 20% of patients and include:
      - i Syncope and altered mental status
      - ii Chest pain that is described as severe, acute, ripping and in some patients migratory
      - iii Radiation to the anterior chest or neck from the ascending aorta; rarely to the face and jaw
      - iv Pain radiates to the back when the pathology is in the descending aorta; flank pain with renal artery involvement
      - v There is no pain in approximately 10% of patients
      - vi Ascending aorta dissection into the great vessels causes a cerebrovascular accident with:
        1. Hemispheric symptoms of hemiplegia, hemianesthesia and aphasia (if left carotid artery is involved)
        2. Horner's syndrome with carotid involvement
        3. Dysphagia
        4. Syncope
        5. Difference in upper extremity blood pressure
        6. Pulse deficits
        7. Anxiety
        8. Feelings of impending doom
        9. Paraparesis (descending aortic dissection)

Neuropathology

1. An intimal tear that penetrates the aortic media
2. The entry tear occurs at the sites of greatest wall tension which is usually a few centimeters close to the aortic valve on the right lateral wall of the ascending aorta (type A dissection); it may also occur where the aorta is fixed near the ligamentum arteriosum of the descending aorta
3. Blood under high pressure dissects through the media to form a second or false channel that parallels the true lumen

4. The re-entrance tear allows blood to circulate through the false lumen
5. Organ ischemia occurs when the dissection flap occludes an aortic branch artery
6. Many aortic dissections are not associated with atherosclerosis as the fibrosis and calcification of that process may limit the progression of the dissection
7. Associated or underlying medical conditions include:
   a. Marfan syndrome
   b. Ehlers-Danlos type IV
   c. Adult polycystic disease
   d. Turner syndrome
   e. Osteogenesis imperfecta
   f. Bicuspid aortic valve
   g. Noonan syndrome
   h. Coarctation of the aorta
   i. Homocystinuria
   j. Familial hypercholesterolemia
   k. Familial aortic dissection
   l. Annuloaortic ectasia
   m. Cystic medial necrosis
8. Acquired causes of aortic dissection:
   a. Surgical procedures:
      i Aortic and mitral valve replacement
         1. Coronary artery bypass graft surgery
         2. Cardiac catheterization
         3. Percutaneous transluminal coronary angioplasty
      ii Syphilitic aortitis
      iii Deceleration injury with related blunt chest trauma
      iv Cocaine

Laboratory Evaluation

1. Leukocytosis and decreased hemoglobin
2. Elevated BUN and creatinine (renal artery involvement)
3. Elevated myocardial creatine kinase, myoglobin and troponin I and T levels (myocardial infarctions)
4. Lactate dehydrogenase (hemolysis of RBCs in the false lumen)
5. Smooth muscle myosin heavy-chain (90% sensitive and 97% specific) in the first 24 hours
6. Fibrin degradation products

Neuroimaging

1. Chest radiography:
   a. Widened mediastinum is the classic finding:
2. Other radiographic features include:
   a. Pleural effusion
   b. Left apical cap
   c. Tracheal deviation to the right
   d. Depression of the left mainstem bronchus
   e. Esophageal deviation
   f. Loss of paratracheal stripe
3. Spiral (helical) CT has a higher rate of detection and better resolution than incremental CT scanning
4. CT angiography delineates detailed anatomic definition of the dissection as well as plaque formation
5. MRI and transesophageal echocardiography are often limited by expense, availability and the need for MR compatible monitoring equipment
6. In many institutions contrast enhanced CT is utilized as the imaging procedure of choice as it is capable of providing 3D reconstructed images and assesses other thoracic structures

Penetrating Atherosclerotic Ulcer (PAU)

General Characteristics

1. Definition:
   a. PAU is a focal defect or lesion that occurs at the site of an intimal atherosclerotic plaque
   b. Patients are older and often have significant cardiovascular and pulmonary comorbidities. The most common patient profile is an elderly man with hypertension, coronary artery disease who smokes

Clinical Manifestations

1. Most often PAU involves the descending aorta (rarely it occurs in the ascending aorta) and may cause intramural hemorrhage, aortic aneurysm, pseudoaneurysm or dissection
2. It may be asymptomatic and is often incidentally diagnosed usually when confined to the intimal layer
3. The second stage of the lesion is when the atheromatous ulcer penetrates through the elastic lamina into the media
4. The major symptom is severe acute chest pain that radiates to the interscapular area

Neuropathology

1. The most common location is in the descending aorta
2. Progressive intimal erosion leads to pulsatile blood that enters the media that

results in hemorrhage

3. Erosion of the aortic vasa vasorum by the ulcer causes intramural hemorrhage, aortic dissection and aortic rupture
4. PAU represents 2 to 7% of acute aortic syndrome

Laboratory Evaluation

1. Spiral computed tomography CT provides two- and three-dimensional image reconstruction
2. Penetration into the adventitia causes:
   a. Pseudoaneurysm
   b. Aneurysm
   c. Aneurysm rupture

Intramural Hematoma (IMH)

General Characteristics

1. Intramural hematomas are approximately 10 to 30% of all patients with acute aortic syndrome
2. By definition it is a variation of dissection in which blood collects within the aortic media without an intimal flap
3. If the IMH involves the aortic arch and ascending aorta, its complications and mortality rates are high and are similar to type A aortic dissections. Type B IMH are more benign
4. Symptomatic IMH has an incidence of rupture at presentation of up to 38%

Clinical Manifestations

1. The natural history of IMH and its rate of progression are not well delineated but demonstrate that they may rupture, stabilize, regress or progress to dissection or aneurysm formation
2. Risk factors that predict IMH type A progression to dissection include:
   a. A dilated aorta
   b. An ascending aorta diameter of >5cm
   c. Less frequently PAU causes pleural and pericardial effusion, aortic regurgitation and mediastinal hematoma
3. Chest pain that is severe, ripping and acute:
   a. Radiates to the anterior chest or neck if in the ascending aorta
   b. If in the descending aorta the pain radiates to the interscapular area of the back
   c. Progression is unpredictable and sudden and may present as an acute aortic dissection

Neuropathology

1. Blood collects within the aortic media due to rupture of the vasa vasorum

which are located in the media
2. IMH may also occur from hemorrhage within an atherosclerotic plaque
3. IMH occurs close to the adventitia which causes its high rate of rupture (35%) compared to aortic dissection
4. The hemorrhage may extend toward the lumen to cause a dissection
5. Associated pleural, pericardial and mediastinal hemorrhage are posited to occur from increased aortic wall permeability

Laboratory Evaluation

1. Contrast enhanced computed tomography
2. The concept of "a micro-tear" that cannot be visualized with conventional imaging modalities is controversial
3. "Echo-free space" demonstrated by TEE and "focal contrast enhancement" on ultra-fast CT are being evaluated
4. C-reactive protein may be a method to predict adverse complications with acute aortic intramural hematoma

Other Causes of Acute Aortic Syndrome

1. Aortic aneurysm leak:
   a. The acute aortic syndrome can be caused by an acute expansion of an aneurysm
   b. Progressive vessel dilatation causes increasing vessel wall tension (LaPlace's Law) with more rapid dilatation and risk of rupture
2. Traumatic aortic transection:
   a. The aortic transection is caused by rapid deceleration forces or direct chest blunt trauma
   b. Most patients succumb immediately
   c. The location of the transection is just distal to the left subclavian artery of the aortic isthmus where the aorta is fixed by the ligamentum arteriosum
   d. Rarely patients present with an incomplete rupture that causes dissection, IMH or pseudo-aneurysm formation
   e. The pain is dependent on location of the pathology

Pulmonary Embolism

General Characteristics

1. The incidence in the USA is 1 per 1000 persons per year; it is the third commonest cause of death in hospitalized patients
2. An acute pulmonary embolus is situated centrally within the vascular lumen or if it occludes a vessel (vessel cut off sign). It often causes distention of the involved vessel
3. Chronic emboli are eccentric and are contiguous with the vessel wall. It reduces the arterial diameter more than 50% and there is evidence of recanalization

within the thrombus; an arterial web is present

4. A pulmonary embolus is characterized as central or peripheral depending on the branch occlusion. It is massive when it involves both pulmonary arteries or when it causes severe hemodynamic compromise

Clinical Manifestations

1. The classical presentation is the abrupt onset of pleuritic chest pain, dyspnea and hypoxia
2. Commonly patients have complained of bothersome symptoms prior to sudden death
3. Most often clinical signs and symptoms are non-specific and include dyspnea, tachypnea and /or chest pain
4. A cramp in the calf several days prior to an embolic event; clinical signs and symptoms of deep vein thrombosis
5. Heart rate > 100 beats / minute
6. Immobilization > 3 days; surgery within 4 weeks
7. Prior DVT or pulmonary embolus
8. Hemoptysis
9. Cancer
10. Pain:
    a. Pleuritic chest pain is more common with small peripheral emboli
    b. Patients with pleuritic pain may have mechanical hyperalgesia and allodynia in the somatic innervation over the area of lung peripheral infarction
11. Atypical signs and symptoms include:
    a. Seizure
    b. Syncope
    c. Abdominal pain
    d. New onset atrial fibrillation
    e. Flank pain
    f. Delirium in elderly patients

Neuropathology

1. Gas exchange abnormalities include hypoxemia (decreased arterial pO_2) and increased alveolar-arterial O_2 tension
2. Increased anatomic dead space
3. Increased pulmonary vascular resistance due to obstruction or platelet release of serotonin and other vasoactive mediators

Laboratory Evaluation

1. Blood screen:
    a. A hypercoagulable workup if there is no obvious cause for an embolus
    b. D-dimer testing
    c. Arterial blood gas
    d. Serum troponin levels
    e. Brain natriuretic peptide

Neuroimaging

1. Multidetector-row CTA (MDCTA):
    a. MDCTA is the criterion standard
    b. Pulmonary angiography if MDCTA is unavailable
2. MRI:
    a. Gated spin-echo techniques reveal increased signal intensity within the pulmonary artery

Pneumothorax

Overview

1. A pneumothorax is air or gas that accumulates in the pleural cavity
2. A pneumothorax may be spontaneous or is caused by trauma to the lung or chest wall. It is also divided into tension and non-tension subgroups. Non-tension pneumothorax is divided into open or closed (partial) type
3. Spontaneous pneumothorax is classified as either primary or secondary:
    a. Primary spontaneous pneumothorax is seen in young thin males and is caused by ruptured pleural blebs or bullae
    b. Secondary spontaneous pneumothorax occurs in older patients who have emphysema, asthma, chronic infections, lung cancer, and congenital diseases. These include cystic fibrosis, catamenial pneumothorax, and lymphangioleiomyomatosis.

Primary Spontaneous Pneumothorax (PSP)

General Characteristics

1. The age-adjusted incidence of PSP is between 7.4 to 18 patients per 100,000 of the population per year in males and from 1.2 to 6 patients per 100,000 of the population for females
2. It is primarily a disorder of tall, thin males who are between 10 and 30 years of age. It is rarely seen in patients over 40 years of age
3. Approximately 10% of patients have a family history
4. Some patients have been described with mutations of the FLCN gene that maps to chromosome 17p11.2 that causes Hogg-Dube syndrome (hair follicle hamartomas, kidney tumors, and spontaneous pneumothorax)

5. Smoking is a precipitating factor

Clinical Manifestations

1. PSP usually occurs at rest
2. Presents with the acute onset of local pleuritic chest pain:
    a. The pain may be mild to severe
    b. Its quality may be sharp or it has been described as a steady ache. It often resolves within 24 hours while the pneumothorax persists
    c. The pain is associated with shortness of breath
    d. The physical examination of large pneumothorax reveals:
        i Decreased breath sounds
        ii Decreased chest wall movement
        iii Hyper-resonance with percussion
        iv Decreased tactile fremitus

These findings are seen if free air occupies more than 15%-20% of the hemithorax. There may be associated reflex tachycardia.

1. Tension pneumothorax causes severe tachycardia, cold hyperhidrosis, hypotension and/or cyanosis

Neuropathology

1. It is posited that most patients have had the spontaneous rupture of a subpleural bleb or bulla
2. An alternative mechanism may be an increase in pleural porosity that occurs with inflammation. Only a subgroup of patients are found with blebs or bullae at surgery
3. Spontaneous hemopneumothorax are 0.5% to 2.6% of patients with spontaneous pneumothorax. It consists of air and blood > 400 ml. It is posited that the bleeding is caused by aberrant blood vessels that arise from the chest wall and grow into the pleural lesions

Laboratory Evaluation

1. Upright posteroanterior chest radiograph which demonstrates a pleural line with or without an air-fluid level
2. CT of the chest is utilized to delineate a small pneumothorax (less than 15% of the hemithorax area). It may also delineate the number, size and location of bullae / blebs, pleural adhesions, fluid and underlying pulmonary disease

Pleurodynia

General Characteristics

1. Pleurodynia is a rare complication of coxsackievirus B infection. It may also occur with ECHO viruses
2. Coxsackievirus B is an RNA Enterovirus that usually causes an asymptomatic

or short duration upper respiratory or gastrointestinal infection. It rarely causes meningitis and carditis

Clinical Manifestations

1. Pain:
    a. The onset of chest pain is acute
    b. Attacks cause severe, intense pain that is paroxysmal, lasts seconds to a minute that occur as attacks. They are associated with dyspnea
    c. The thoracic pain is usually located over the lower ribs and is unilateral. It can also occur over the back or substernally
    d. Between attacks patients may suffer a constant, dull, pleuritic type chest pain
    e. Attacks last for 3 to 5 days and rarely persist longer than a month. There may be remissions and exacerbations
2. Associated signs and symptoms:
    a. Constitutional symptoms that include headache (50%) of patients, fever and malaise
    b. Gastrointestinal symptoms of nausea, vomiting and diarrhea occur in 50% of patients
    c. Abdominal pain, primarily epigastric particularly in children
    d. Testicular pain (orchitis) in 10% of males

Neuropathology

1. Striated muscle is the primary target of the Coxsackie B virus and is the cause of the severe chest pain. A minority of patients have pleuritis
2. In patients with pleurodynia, the intercostal muscles are involved which is associated with increases in the serum creatine kinase
3. The virus has an incubation time of 1 week in the GI tract and then spreads hematogenously
4. The major target of the virus is skeletal muscle but it also can infect the CNS (meningitis or encephalitis) or the myocardium and pericardium

Laboratory Evaluation

1. The virus can be recovered from the stool or pharynx for up to 2 weeks following resolution of symptoms
2. Reverse transcriptase (PCR) is now replacing viral culture and neutralization assays

Tumors of the Lung and Pleura that are Associated with Chest Pain

Superior Sulcus Tumors (Pancoast Tumors)

General Characteristics

Superior sulcus tumors have a wide spectrum that are often painful as they invade the apical chest wall, the lower portion of the brachial plexus, the first rib, vertebrae, subclavian vessels or stellate ganglion. In general, they cause severe and unrelenting shoulder and arm pain in addition to C8, T1 and T2 thoracic spinal nerve involvement. If the tumor invades the intercostobrachial nerve (that arises from the medial cord of the brachial plexus), there is pain in the axilla which radiates to the anterior chest wall and sternum.

The anatomy of the region that is involved by Pancoast tumors is delineated by the thoracic inlet that is divided into three compartments. The first rib is the base of the thoracic inlet that is defined anteriorly by the sternum and posteriorly by the attachment of the anterior scalene muscle on the first rib. The compartment contains the sternocleidomastoid and omohyoid muscles, the subclavian and jugular veins and the scalene fat pad. The middle compartment lies between the anterior and middle scalene muscles and is crossed by the subclavian artery, phrenic nerve, and trunks of the brachial plexus. The posterior compartment is located behind the middle scalene muscle and contains the posterior scalene muscle, posterior scapular artery, stellate ganglion, sympathetic chain, long thoracic nerve, accessary nerve, neural foramina and vertebral bodies

Clinical Manifestations

1. Shoulder pain is often the initial symptom
2. Progression of the growth causes paresthesias and burning pain in C8, T1 distributions often accompanied by weakness of ulnar innervated muscles and atrophy of intrinsic hand muscles (primarily T1 root)
3. A Horner's syndrome is seen in 15-50% of patients (ptosis, meiosis, anhidrosis and apparent enophthalmos)
4. If the medial cord is involved, there is frequent invasion of the intercostobrachial nerve with axillary and anterior chest pain

Neuropathology

1. A wide spectrum of disorders cause Pancoast syndrome and include primary neoplasms of the lung and pleura, metastases, hematologic malignancies, inflammatory and infectious processes
2. The definition of a Pancoast tumor as proffered by the American College of Chest Physicians is:
    a. A lung cancer that arises from the apex of the lung that invades structures of the apical chest wall at the level of the first rib or above. A Horner's syndrome or arm pain is not required. The lesions frequently invade the brachial plexus, subclavian vessels, or spine.
3. The great majority of Pancoast tumors are bronchogenic carcinomas with adenocarcinoma the histologic type
4. Small cell bronchogenic tumors in this location are rare (less than 5%)
5. Pancoast tumors often demonstrate different biology than other non-small

cell lung tumors as demonstrated by local invasion rather than lymphatic or hematogenous metastasis

Laboratory Evaluation

1. Routine CBC, liver enzymes, coagulation parameters and electrolytes
2. Elevated oncofetal carcinoembryonic antigen and beta-2 microglobulins are often associated with small cell lung cancers and are related to the stage of the disease
3. Molecular analysis:
    a. Oncogenes associated with lung cancers include:
        i K-ras
        ii C-myc
        iii TP53
        iv HER-2/neu
4. Tumor markers that include bombesin, neuron-specific enolase and other peptides occur with small cell cancers and are related to the stage of the disease and its state of differentiation
5. Percutaneous transthoracic needle biopsy is definitive for diagnosis
6. Rarer tumors that may involve the thoracic inlet include:
    a. Askin tumor
    b. Ewing sarcoma and neurectodermal tumors of the mediastinum
    c. Giant solitary fibrous tumor of the pleura
    d. Langerhans cell histiocytosis

Neuroimaging

1. Chest radiographs may demonstrate a mass or pleural thickening at the apex of the lung that is associated with invasion or destruction of ribs or vertebrae
2. CT of the chest delineates the apical mass and its invasion of the bony thorax and the other structures of the thoracic inlet
3. MRI is the best modality to characterize the brachial plexus, subclavian vessels, spine and the neural foramina

Malignant Pleural Mesothelioma

General Characteristics

1. The incidence of malignant mesothelioma reported from Germany is 20 patients per million of the population
2. Due to extensive removal of asbestos the incidence is expected to decrease between 2015-2030
3. Greater than 80% of mesotheliomas arise from the mesothelial or submesothelial cells of the pleura
4. Approximately 80% of pleural mesotheliomas occur in men
5. It is a disease caused by occupational asbestos exposure

6. Asbestos is the commercial term for:
   a. Different forms of naturally occurring mineral fibers that include:
      i "White asbestos" and amphibole asbestos (crocidolite, amosite, anthophyllite, actinolite and tremolite)
7. Non-asbestos-related mesothelioma comprises 10% to 20% of afflicted patients. Mesotheliomas may be caused by zeolite, an asbestos-like mineral fiber. Other possible etiologic factors include SV-40 viruses, genetic predisposition, and recurrent infection.

Clinical Manifestations

1. Dyspnea is the first symptom in 90% of patients
2. It is a disease of the elderly with a median age of 74 years:
   a. Approximately 15% of patients are younger than 40 years of age
   b. Other series demonstrate a smaller percentage of 2% to 5.8% of patients under the age of 40 years
   c. There is no sex difference in younger patients.
3. Patients usually develop mesothelioma 20 to 40 years after asbestos exposure
4. Non-pleuritic chest wall pain is a common early complaint. It is thought to arise from irritation of the intercostal nerves or by infiltration of the malignancy into the chest wall
5. A proportion of patients are asymptomatic diagnosed by a pleural effusion by x-ray or physical examination
6. Rarer manifestations of malignant pleural mesothelioma include:
   a. Phrenic nerve involvement
   b. Irritative cough
   c. Paraneoplastic signs and symptoms
   d. Spontaneous pneumothorax
   e. Rare to have symptomatic metastasis

Neuropathology

1. Mesothelioma is subdivided into epitheliod, biphasic and sarcomatoid subtypes by their histomorphological growth pattern
2. The pleural surfaces are seeded with malignant mesothelioma cells that form nodules. As the disease progresses the pleural space is covered and the malignancy invades the chest wall, mediastinum and diaphragm
3. Approximately 90% of patients present with a pleural effusion. Only 32% are diagnostic. Thoracoscopically guided biopsy is diagnostic in 98% of patients.

Laboratory Evaluation

1. A new marker is serum mesothelin protein (SMRP) which is elevated in 84% of patients. Megakaryocyte potentiating factor may also be elevated

Neuroimaging

1. Chest CT:
   a. Obliteration of the diaphragm
   b. Nodular pleural thickening
   c. Decreased size of the involved thorax
   d. Radiolucent sheetlike encasement of the pleura
   e. A loculated effusion with opacification of the pleura

Rare Causes of Pleural Disease that May be Associated with Chest Pain

1. Pleural vasculitides:
   a. Asbestos exposure is associated with the onset of microscopic polyangiitis that has been described in the pleura
2. Severe chest wall toxicity from cryo ablation in the setting of prior ablative radiotherapy:
   a. A consequence of focal therapy for metastatic cancers
3. Pleuritic chest pain from portal hypertensive gastropathy (PHG):
   a. PHG may present with chest pain and hematemesis

Gastrointestinal Pain

Gastroesophageal Reflux Disease

General Characteristics

1. The esophagus is divided into cervical, thoracic and abdominal sections
2. Its body is composed of an inner circular and an outer longitudinal array of muscular layers. The proximal esophagus is composed of striated muscle that transitions to smooth muscle in its distal 2/3s. The proximal esophagus contains the upper esophageal sphincter which is composed of the cricopharyngeus muscle (cranial nerve IX) and the thyropharyngeus muscle (from the cervical plexus)
3. The distal esophagus is located to the left of the midline and, through the esophageal hiatus in the diaphragm, passes into the abdomen. The right crus of the diaphragm forms a sling around the esophagus from right and left pillars that narrow it when the diaphragm contracts
4. The phrenoesophageal ligament is the reflection of the subdiaphragmatic fascia onto transversalis fascia of the anterior abdominal wall that also encircles the esophagus. The phrenoesophageal ligament marks the esophogastric junction that lies in the abdomen and forms the angle of His. This angle and the length of the intra-abdominal portion of the esophagus determine the closure of the esophagus when there is increased intragastric or abdominal pressure
5. The lower esophageal sphincter or the distal esophageal high-pressure zone is

the most distal segment of the esophagus (3.5 cm in adults) and is crucial in preventing GERD. GERD can be caused by malfunction of any of the above structures

6. It is estimated that 25 to 40% of Americans have symptomatic GERD at some time during their lifetime
7. GERD occurs in all age groups, has no sex preference and increases in people over 40 years of age

Clinical Manifestations

1. Burning pain in the lower sternal area after eating
2. Regurgitation
3. Dysphagia
4. An acidic taste in the mouth
5. Increased salivation
6. Coughing
7. Hoarseness

Neuropathology

1. Major mechanisms for acid reflux include:
   a. Poor esophageal motility with decreased clearance of acidic material
   b. A dysfunctional lower esophageal sphincter which allows gastric juice to reflux upwards into the esophagus
   c. Delayed gastric emptying
2. Associated complications of GERD:
   a. Esophagitis:
      i Esophageal mucosal damage which occurs in approximately 50% of patients
      ii Stricture:
         1. An advanced form of esophagitis due to circumferential fibrosis. They are usually demonstrated in the mid-to-distal esophagus
      iii Barrett esophagus:
         1. The most serious complication of long-standing and severe GERD. It is defined by the metaplastic conversion of the normal distal squamous esophageal epithelium to columnar epithelium which may demonstrate dysplasia
         2. Barrett esophagus with intestinal type metaplasia has malignant potential risk for the development of esophageal adenocarcinoma (30-40 times that of normal individuals).

Laboratory Evaluation

1. Upper GI endoscopy and manometry

2. Manometry delineates lower esophageal sphincter pressure and determines motility disorders
3. Less frequently used studies:
   a. 24-hour pH probe test
   b. Upper GI series
   c. Nuclear medicine gastric emptying studies
4. Micro RNA expression of exfoliated tongue cells
   a. Validation demonstrates a sensitivity of miR-203 at 91% and a specificity of 87%

Esophageal Motility Disorder

General Characteristics

1. The esophagus is composed of two muscle types. It is 25cm in length and has an upper proximal and distal sphincter. The upper sphincter is composed of the cricopharyngeus and thyropharyngeus muscles. The lower esophageal sphincter is composed entirely of smooth muscle
2. The proximal esophagus is composed of striated muscle; the mid esophagus contains a graded transition of striated to smooth muscle while the distal esophagus is solely smooth muscle.
3. The longitudinal muscle shortens the esophagus and the circular muscle causes lumen-occluding ring contractions
4. Peristalsis is the sequential coordinated contraction wave that travels the length of the esophagus and propels the food bolus to the stomach
5. The lower esophageal sphincter is relaxed during swallowing and remains open until the peristaltic wave passes. It then contracts and resumes its basic tone
6. Primary peristalsis is defined as a peristaltic wave triggered by the swallowing center and travels at a speed of 2cm/s (correlates with manometry recorded contractions)
7. A secondary peristaltic wave is caused by esophageal distention from a retained food bolus, refluxed material or swallowed air
8. Tertiary contractions are simultaneous dysfunctional contractions that are not peristaltic. Their physiologic function is not known.

Achalasia

General Characteristics

1. The incidence of achalasia is approximately 1 per 100,000 persons per year
2. It is a primary esophageal motility disorder characterized by the absence of esophageal peristalsis and decreased relaxation of the lower esophageal sphincter
3. The incidence of achalasia in the USA is 1-3 patients per 100,000 of the

population per year

Clinical Manifestations

1. Progressive dysphagia for both liquids and solids
2. Chest pain characterized by a squeezing quality located retrosternally that may radiate to the neck, jaw, arms, or back. The chest pain may be exacerbated by food and may awaken the patient from sleep
3. A sensation of heart burn is reported by 30% of patients
4. Regurgitation of food retained in the proximal esophagus particularly at night. Patients may utilize multiple pillows or sleep upright in a chair
5. Symptoms may be present for a long time prior to diagnosis
6. Emotional stress and rapid eating exacerbate all symptoms
7. Slight weight loss is common

Neuropathology

1. The major cause of achalasia is the loss of ganglion cells from the wall of the esophagus that starts at the lower esophageal sphincter and progresses proximally. The degree of ganglion cell loss is concomitant with the disease duration. Immunohistochemical analysis reveals loss of nitric oxide synthase and vasoactive intestinal peptide (VIP) in inhibitory nerves. Inflammatory cells and inhibitory fiber loss are seen in the myenteric plexus. Acetylcholine intrinsic nerves are lost in the esophageal body. Wallerian degeneration may be demonstrated within the vagus nerve and dorsal motor nucleus. The circular muscle layer at the lower esophageal sphincter may be thickened. Physiologically, achalasia is most correlated with the loss of inhibitory nerves of the lower esophageal sphincter (LES) that decreases its ability to relax causing relative obstruction at the gastroesophageal junction.
2. Chagas disease secondary to Trypanosoma cruzi:
    a. Is transmitted by a reduviid bug bite
    b. Is endemic in Central and South America (rarely has been described as far north as Texas)
    c. Widespread ganglionic cell loss involves the esophagus, heart, gut, urinary and respiratory tract. Symptoms and signs may take years to develop
3. Rare causes of achalasia:
    a. Familial adrenal insufficiency with alacrima
    b. Pseudoachalasia from gastroesophageal junction obstruction:
        i Tumor
        ii Neurofibromatosis
        iii Pancreatic pseudocyst
    c. Infiltrative disorders causing pseudo-obstruction include:
        i Amyloidosis
        ii Sphingolipidosis

    iii Eosinophilic gastritis
    iv Sarcoid

d. A possible autoimmune mechanism has been suggested due to single nucleotide polymorphisms (SNPs) in the histocompatibility region of chromosome 6 that is associated with other autoimmune disorders

Neuroimaging

1. Chest radiographs:
    a. Dilated esophagus with a sigmoid shape
    b. An air-fluid level
    c. Widened mediastinum
    d. Absence of a gastric air-bubble
2. Esophagography:
    a. Tapering of the LES causing the "bird-beak" appearance
    b. Loss of peristalsis and transient stasis above the gastroesophageal junction
    c. Epiphrenic diverticula are noted (occasionally) above the LES

Laboratory Evaluation

1. Manometry:
    a. Elevated LES pressure greater than 40 mm Hg in > 60% of patients
    b. Aperistalsis with stasis of food and esophageal dilatation
    c. Nonperistaltic isolated contractions or low amplitude simultaneous contractions of the esophageal body
    d. High-amplitude >60 mmHg simultaneous contractions termed vigorous achalasia may be an early stage of the disorder

Esophageal Motility Disorders

Nutcracker Esophagus

General Characteristics

1. Nutcracker esophagus is a motility disorder of the esophagus in which contractions of its smooth muscle are normal in sequence but are too long or occur at increased amplitude
2. The disorder affects patients of all ages and is most common in the sixth and seventh decades
3. The disorder is not progressive and is not associated with complications

Clinical Manifestations

1. Chest pain is the hallmark symptom that is similar to that of achalasia and may mimic angina. The mechanism of the pain may be muscle ischemia, luminal distension or abnormal visceral sensation

2. Dysphagia for solids and liquids that may not be related to pain, is often intermittent and is not associated with weight loss
3. Patients may present with a sudden obstruction of the esophagus after eating food ("steakhouse syndrome")
4. The illness does not progress or have complications
5. A subgroup of patients are asymptomatic but may demonstrate the same motility findings as "nutcracker esophagus"

Neuropathology

1. There are no specific anatomical correlations but the disorder has been associated with the metabolic syndrome
2. The pathology may be related to alterations between excitatory and inhibitory transmitters in the distal esophagus

Laboratory Evaluation

1. Endoscopy is typically normal although abnormalities associated with GERD may be present
2. Manometry:
    a. Peristaltic contractions with an amplitude of greater that 180 mmHg taken 3 and 8 cm above the lower esophageal sphincter are demonstrated

Diffuse Esophageal Spasm (DES)

General Characteristics

1. Diffuse esophageal spasms are manifested by contractions that are of normal amplitude but are uncoordinated, simultaneous or too rapidly propagated
2. Hypertensive and nutcracker esophagus have coordinated sequential contractions whose amplitude is excessive (see above)
3. Jackhammer esophagus or hypercontractive esophagus is termed when contractions are of very high amplitude involve a major portion of the esophagus with a prolonged duration. It has a jackhammer appearance on high-resolution manometry

Clinical Manifestations

1. Esophageal spasm accounts for less than 10% of noncardiac chest pain:
    a. The pain is usually retrosternal and may radiate to the back, neck, arms and jaw
    b. It may be more severe than angina
2. Globus (a feeling that food or a object is trapped in the throat)
3. Dysphagia is seen in 33% to 66% of patients with diffuse esophageal spasm
4. Regurgitation
5. Heartburn is reported in approximately 20% of patients

6. Symptoms are intermittent and vary from day to day. They usually last for minutes to hours
7. As noted, patients with nutcracker esophagus usually present with chest pain. Only 10% have dysphagia

Neuropathology

1. The pathophysiology of DES has not been determined
2. It has been posited that there is increased release of or sensitivity to acetylcholine
3. Body mass index and total cholesterol may be predictive; BMI and glucose may be predictive of LES function
4. DES occurs when there is alteration of the sequential propagation of contractions

Laboratory Evaluation

1. The classic esophagram is a "cork screw" or "rosary bead" esophagus

Scleroderma Esophagus

General Characteristics

1. Scleroderma involves the esophagus in greater than 75% of patients in both progressive systemic sclerosis or the CREST syndrome

Clinical Manifestations

1. Symptoms usually reflect the severity of acid reflux
2. Heartburn, regurgitation and dysphagia
3. The severity of esophageal involvement does not correlate with involvement of other organs and may be the presenting complaint

Neuropathology

1. Erosive esophagitis is seen in approximately 60% of patients
2. The incidence of Barrett esophagus and adenocarcinoma of the esophagus are increased
3. Esophageal dysmotility develops when the smooth muscle of the distal 2/3 of the esophagus is replaced by fibrosis and scar tissue. Motility is preserved in the striated muscle of the proximal esophagus

Laboratory Evaluation

1. Esophageal manometry which demonstrates loss of peristalsis in the distal 2/3 of the esophagus
2. Endoscopy in patients with symptoms suggestive of erosive esophagitis

Other Causes of Esophageal Dysmotility

1. Spinal cord injury

2. Anorexia nervosa
3. After several endoscopic sclerotherapy procedures (for esophageal varices)
4. Diabetes mellitus
5. Alcoholism
6. Presbyesophagus

Gastric Pain

Acute Gastritis

General Characteristics

1. Acute gastritis is caused by entities that induce inflammatory changes in the gastric mucosa
2. In general, acute gastritis is divided into erosive and non-erosive forms
3. There is poor correlation between microscopic inflammation and abdominal pain, nausea and vomiting
4. The estimated prevalence is 6.3 patients per 100,000 of the population

Clinical Manifestations

1. The pain is often described as gnawing or burning and is located in the epigastrium
2. The pain may be exacerbated or relieved by eating
3. Associated symptoms include: nausea, vomiting, belching and bloating
4. Rarely acute abdominal pain is a presenting symptom which occurs with gangrene of the stomach (usually accompanied by vomiting of purulent gastric contents), fever, chills and hiccups
5. The physical examination is usually normal other than mild epigastric tenderness

Neuropathology

1. Acute gastritis is caused by specific drugs, alcohol, bacterial, viral and fungal infection
2. Less frequent causes are shock, radiation therapy, allergy and food poisoning, bile, ischemia and direct trauma
3. Histologic examination of a biopsy establishes the diagnosis in the majority of patients

Laboratory Evaluation

1. CBC (to assess for anemia from gastric bleeding)
2. Liver and kidney function tests
3. Pregnancy test
4. Stool evaluation for blood

Imaging

1. The radiologic signs are usually constant regardless of the etiology and include:
   a. Thick gastric folds
   b. Inflammatory nodules
   c. Erosions
   d. Coarse area gastrica
2. Endoscopy
3. H. pylori evaluation that is classified as nonendoscopy or endoscopy based

Helicobacter Pylori Infection

General Characteristics

1. Helicobacter pylori is ubiquitous and infects approximately 50% of the world's population
2. Caucasian patients comprise approximately 29% of cases and Hispanic patients 60%. There is no sex predilection but females have a higher incidence of reinfection
3. Infection may be acquired at any age but some studies suggest infection occurs in childhood

Clinical Manifestations

1. Approximately 30% to 35% of patients are asymptomatic
2. No specific signs and symptoms have been described
3. Symptomatic patients may have:
   a. Abdominal pain (similar to that of gastritis)
   b. Nausea and vomiting
   c. Heartburn
   d. Diarrhea
   e. Hunger in the morning
   f. Halitosis

Neuropathology

1. The disorder has been staged to follow:
   a. Chronic gastritis
   b. Atrophic gastritis
   c. Intestinal metaplasia that may evolve into dysplasia
   d. Gastric adenocarcinoma
   e. Gastric MALTomas:
      i Mucosa-associated lymphatic tissue lymphomas

Laboratory Evaluation

1. EGD (esophagogastroduodenoscopy) in patients with symptoms of peptic ulcer disease

2. EGD plus biopsy from the gastric antrum
3. Echography plus EGD is mandatory in patients with positive biopsy results for MALTomas
4. H. pylori antigen test
5. Carbon 13 urea breath test
6. H. pylori serology

Gastric Ulcer

General Characteristics

1. Anatomy of the vagal nerve innervation of the abdominal viscera:
    a. The left (anterior) and the right (posterior) branches of the vagus nerve descend along the distal esophagus to enter the lower thoracic cavity. They communicate by means of the esophageal plexus
2. Below the plexus, the trunks separate and the anterior trunk branches to form the hepatic, pyloric, and anterior gastric branches. The posterior trunk branches to form the posterior gastric and the celiac branch
3. The terminal branches of the anterior and posterior nerves innervate the parietal cells in a segmental fashion
4. In the USA the lifetime prevalence is approximately 11% to 14% in men and 8% to 11% in women
5. In patients infected with H. pylori the lifetime prevalence is approximately 20% with about 10% in younger patients

Clinical Manifestations

1. Gastric and duodenal ulcers are difficult to differentiate by history
2. Epigastric pain is the most common symptom for both conditions.
3. It is manifest by:
    a. Gnawing or burning quality which occurs shortly after meals with gastric ulcer and 2 to 5 hours after eating with duodenal ulcer
    b. Food and antacids relieve duodenal ulcer pain, but are usually ineffective for gastric ulcers
    c. Duodenal ulcer pain may awaken the patient from sleep
    d. 50 to 80% of patients with duodenal ulcers experience pain at night while only 30 to 40% of patients with gastric ulcers suffer this symptom
    e. Pain often follows an individual pattern for each patient
    f. If the pain radiates straight through to the back a posterior penetrating gastric ulcer may be causative due to concomitant pancreatitis
    g. Patients with gastric outlet obstruction due to chronic duodenal ulcer often complain of:
        i Fullness and bloating with nausea and vomiting several hours after

eating

ii Less frequent clinical manifestations include:
   1. Dyspepsia with belching, bloating, distention after fatty food
   2. Heart burn
   3. Chest pain
   4. Hematemesis or melena
   5. Symptoms due to anemia (fatigue and dyspnea)
   6. Sudden onset of symptoms is a sign of perforation
   7. NSAID-induced gastritis may be asymptomatic particularly in elderly patients
   8. The physical examination of uncomplicated peptic ulcer disease:
      a. Mild epigastric tenderness
      b. Rarely right upper quadrant tenderness which is more suggestive of biliary disease
      c. Perforated PUD:
         i. The sudden onset of severe, sharp abdominal pain sometimes in the epigastrium:
            1. Movement exacerbates the pain
            2. Fetal position
            3. Generalized tenderness, rebound tenderness, guarding and rigidity
            4. Signs of septic shock (tachycardia, hypotension and anuria)

Neuropathology

1. Peptic ulcers of the gastric or duodenal mucosa extend through the muscularis mucosa
2. The epithelial cells of the gastric and duodenal mucosa secrete mucus from acetylcholine release or stimulation of the epithelial lining which forms a protective gel layer that is impermeable to acid and pepsin
3. Gastric and duodenal cells secrete bicarbonate that buffers acid near the mucosa. Prostaglandin E is secreted which increases the production of both bicarbonate and mucus
4. Ion pumps located in the basolateral cell membrane of the epithelium are a component of the regulation of intracellular pH by removing excess hydrogen ion
5. If there is injury to the barrier, healthy cells migrate to the area in a process called restitution for repair. Mucosal blood flow is restorative by removing acid that had diffused through the mucosa in the area of injury and increases the concentration of bicarbonate
6. Under physiologic conditions there is a balance between gastric acid secretion and mucosal defense mechanisms that prevents injury and include:

a. Tight intercellular junctions
b. Mucus
c. Mucosal blood flow
d. Cellular restitution
e. Epithelial cell renewal

7. NSAIDs, H. pylori, alcohol, bile salts, acid and pepsin allow the back diffusion of hydrogen ions which causes epithelial cell injury
8. H. pylori, acid and pepsin are a major part of the triad that cause peptic ulcer disease
9. H. pylori is able to colonize the gastric mucosa and causes inflammation of the gastric mucosa. Under these circumstances, high levels of gastrin and pepsinogen and reduced levels of somatostatin occur which exposes the duodenum to high levels of acid
10. H. pylori also causes impaired secretion of duodenal bicarbonate which in combination with increased gastric acid secretion lowers the duodenal pH and promotes ulcer formation

Laboratory Evaluation

1. CBC, liver, amylase and lipase
2. Tests for H. pylori
   - i Biopsy:
   - ii Urease test
   - iii Histopathology
   - iv Culture
   - v Rapid urease tests are the endoscopic diagnostic test of choice

Imaging

1. Radiograph of the chest if perforation is suspected to detect free abdominal air
2. Upper GI endoscopy

Gastric Tumors

General Characteristics

1. Gastric cancer is the fourth leading cause of cancer mortality in the world
2. Gastric cancer is the 15th most common cancer in the USA

Clinical Manifestations

1. There are no associated symptoms in early disease; almost all signs, symptoms and complications are seen in late disease
2. Rare diffuse abdominal pain or pain from an associated gastric ulcer
3. Indigestion, nausea and vomiting
4. Dysphagia

5. Melena and hematemesis
6. Weight loss
7. Enlarged stomach with succession splash
8. Enlarged lymph nodes; Virchow's node in the left supraclavicular fossa and Irish node in the anterior axilla

Pathology

1. The frequency of gastric malignancies:
   a. Adenocarcinoma – 90% to 95%
   b. Lymphoma – 1-5%
   c. Stromal tumors (leiomyoma or leiomyosarcoma) – 2%
   d. Carcinoids – 1%
   e. Adenocanthoma – 1%
   f. Squamous cell carcinoma – 1%

Laboratory Evaluation

1. CBC, electrolytes, liver function tests
2. Tumor markers:
   a. Elevation of CEA is seen in 40-50% of patients
   b. Elevation of CA-19-9 occurs in 20% of patients

Imaging

1. Esophagogastroduodenoscopy (EGD):
   a. Evaluates the gastric wall and lymph nodes
   b. Double-contrast upper GI series
   c. Chest radiography (metastatic involvement)
2. CT or MRI of the chest, abdomen and pelvis to assess spread
3. Endoscopic ultrasonography
   a. Assess the depth of penetration of the tumor

Other Causes of Gastric Pain

1. Abdominal abscess
2. Abdominal angina
3. Abdominal hernia
4. Acute intermittent porphyria:
   a. Hereditary coproporphyria
   b. Doss porphyria
5. Acute mesenteric ischemia
6. Acute pancreatitis and pyelonephritis
7. Adrenal crisis
8. Appendicitis
9. Aortic dissection
10. Biliary disease

11. Cholecystitis
12. Chronic pelvic pain
13. Colonic obstruction
14. Diverticulitis
15. Lead poisoning
16. Esophageal disease
17. Familial Mediterranean fever
18. Gall bladder disease
19. Intestinal motility disorders
20. Ovarian cysts
21. Portal vein obstruction

Liver pain

General Characteristics

1. The usual patterns of liver disease are characterized as:
   a. Hepatocellular
   b. Cholestatic (obstructive)
   c. Mixed
2. Hepatocellular disease as exemplified by viral hepatitis or alcohol inflammation and necrosis are the predominant features
3. Cholestatic diseases (gall stone, malignant obstruction, primary biliary cirrhosis and drug induced liver disease) with inhibition of bile flow dominate the symptomatology
4. In mixed pattern both hepatocellular and cholestatic clinical features are manifest

Clinical Manifestations

1. Right upper quadrant discomfort or pain ("liver pain") is demonstrated in many liver diseases
2. Tenderness over the liver area
3. The pain is due to stretch of Glisson's capsule that encases the liver and is densely innervated with nociceptive afferent receptors
4. Associated signs and symptoms include:
   a. Nausea occurs with severe liver disease and may be induced by food odors or eating fatty food
   b. Fatigue is the commonest and most characteristic symptom of liver disease. The fatigue arises after exercise and is rare in the morning. It is variable from hour to hour or day to day
   c. Itching is seen with acute liver disease particularly in obstructive jaundice and later with hepatocellular disease
   d. Jaundice is the hallmark sign of liver disease and is a marker of its severity.

Jaundice is usually detectable at a bilirubin level of 2.5 mg/dl

e. Pain radiation to the right upper quadrant, the back and less frequently, to the right shoulder

Neuropathology

1. Dependent on the pathology of the liver disease
2. Pain behavior is mediated by vagal afferents. The hepatic branch innervates the liver in addition to the proximal duodenum, pancreas and pylorus
3. Pain behavior mediated by vagal afferents that are activated by lipopolysaccharides or inflammatory cytokines induces the sickness response that is manifested (experimentally in rodents) by:
    a. Immobility
    b. Decreased social interaction
    c. Decreased food intake
    d. Anorexia
    e. Fever
    f. Increased sleep
    g. Activation of the hypothalamic-pituitary-adrenal axis
4. A mechanism for the sickness response is that liposaccharides (a component of bacterial cell walls) activate hepatic macrophages (Kupffer cells), dendritic cells and leukocytes that release IL-B and TNF-α that in turn activate vagal afferents. The proinflammatory cytokines either activate vagal afferents directly or through glomus cells in the abdominal paraganglia:
    a. Pain behavior mediated by the sickness response may be responsible for the extreme fatigue seen in many patients with visceral pain
    b. Many of the cellular changes induced by the sickness response are abrogated by vagotomy
    c. Vagal abdominal afferents carried by the hepatic branch of the abdominal vagus nerves may serve as an interface between the immune system and the brain as proinflammatory cytokines trigger brain stem and hypothalamic illness responses

Laboratory Evaluation

1. Serum alanine and aspartate aminotransferases (ALT and AST), alkaline phosphatase, direct and total serum bilirubin, albumin and prothrombin time:
    a. The pattern of alterations delineates hepatocellular versus cholestatic disease
    b. If the process is acute or chronic
    c. The degree of hepatic dysfunction
2. Gamma-glutamyl transpeptidase (GGT) which defines if alkaline phosphatase elevations are due to liver disease

3. Hepatitis serology (type of viral hepatitis)
4. Autoimmune biomarkers (antimitochondrial antibody) for primary biliary cirrhosis, P-ANCA for sclerosing cholangitis, and antinuclear, smooth muscle and liver-kidney antibodies to delineate autoimmune hepatitis
5. Liver biopsy:
   a. The gold standard for the evaluation of chronic liver disease

Diagnostic Imaging

1. Ultrasound and CT:
   a. Biliary tract dilatation
   b. Obstructive jaundice
   c. Fatty liver
2. Magnetic resonance cholangiopancreatography (MRCP)
3. Endoscopic retrograde cholangiopancreatography (ERCP):
   a. Imaging of the biliary tree
4. Doppler ultrasound and MRI:
   a. Assess hepatic vasculature and hemodynamics
5. CT and MRI:
   a. Hepatic masses
6. Ultrasound elastography:
   a. Measures hepatic stiffness
   b. Monitoring fibrosis

Gallbladder Disease

General Characteristics

1. Anatomy:
   a. Bile formed in hepatic lobules is secreted into canaliculi, ductules and larger bile ducts that accompany lymphatics and branches of the portal vein and hepatic artery in portal tracts between hepatic lobules
   b. The interlobular bile ducts form larger septal ducts that in turn join and form the right and left hepatic ducts
   c. The common bile duct is formed from the hepatic and cystic duct of the gallbladder which enters the duodenum through the ampulla of Vater

Clinical Manifestations

1. Gallstone disease:
   a. Gallstones migrate into the cystic duct or common bile duct that causes inflammation or obstruction
   b. Biliary colic:
      i Begins suddenly and may persist for 30 minutes to 5 hours to subside gradually or rapidly
      ii It is a steady pain; if it lasts more than 5 hr it may be cholecystitis

iii Nausea and vomiting are frequent with painful episodes
iv The pain is a steady ache or fullness in the epigastrium or right upper quadrant of the abdomen
v Radiation of pain is to the interscapular area (often T6 tip of the scapula), right scapula or shoulder
vi Associated fever or chills suggests cholecystitis, pancreatitis or cholangitis
vii Precipitants of biliary colic include:
1. A fatty meal
2. A large meal followed by a period of fasting
3. Biliary colic may be nocturnal

2. Acute cholecystitis:
   a. Acute inflammation of the gallbladder walls most often is a consequence of cystic duct obstruction by a stone
   b. Clinical manifestation:
      i Often acute cholecystitis is initiated by an attack of biliary colic that progressively increases in intensity
      ii 60-70% of patients have had spontaneous similar attacks that resolved
      iii Pain becomes more generalized in the right upper abdomen as the attack evolves. The radiations are to the interscapular area, the right scapula and shoulder
      iv Peritoneal signs that include pain with movement or deep inspiration may be associated
      v Patients are anorectic, suffer nausea and vomiting, and become dehydrated. Jaundice can occur when edematous inflammation involves bile ducts
      vi A low-grade fever is common. It may be accompanied by shaking chills or rigors
      vii There is tenderness in the RUQ of the abdomen. In approximately 25 to 50% of patients, an enlarged tense gallbladder can be palpated
      viii Murphy's sign can be induced by a cough or deep inspiration (exacerbates the pain and causes an inspiratory arrest)
      ix Localized rebound tenderness in the RUQ, abdominal distention, and hypoactive bowel sounds are present. Generalized peritoneal signs and rigidity are absent unless there is perforation

Neuropathology

1. The great majority of patients with acute cholecystitis have an obstruction of the cystic duct by a stone
2. Inflammation of the GB wall is caused by:
   a. Increased intraluminal pressure and distention that causes ischemia of the GB mucosa and wall

b. The release of lysolecitin from the action of phospholipase on lecithin
c. Bacterial inflammation that occurs in 50-85% of patients. The most frequent organisms are Escherichia coli, Klebsiella, Streptococcus and rarely Clostridium

3. Complications of cholecystitis:
   a. Empyema
   b. Gangrene and perforation
   c. Fistula and gallstone ileus
   d. Bile and porcelain gallbladder

Laboratory Evaluation

1. Gallbladder ultrasound:
   a. Procedure of choice for GB stones
2. Radioisotope scans (HIDA, DIDA):
   a. Delineates cystic duct obstruction and evaluates bile ducts
3. Elevated serum bilirubin and or alkaline phosphatase supports the diagnosis of a common duct stone

Pancreatic Pain

General Characteristics

1. The pancreas secretes 1500-3000 ml of isosmotic alkaline (pH >8.0) fluid per day that contains approximately 20 enzymes and zymogens that effect the major digestive functions of the gastrointestinal tract
2. Gastric acid stimulates pancreatic secretion of water and electrolytes
3. Cholecystokinin release from the duodenum and jejunum is triggered by long chain fatty acids, tryptophan, phenylalanine, valine, methionine and gastric acid
4. CCK induces the secretion of enzymes from the pancreas
5. The vagus nerve significantly regulates pancreatic secretion via secretin and CCK that depend on permissive function of a vagal afferent and efferent pathway. This is particularly important for the enzyme secretin
6. Water and bicarbonate pancreatic secretions are primarily regulated by secretin and CCK
7. Vagal stimulation affects the release of vasoactive intestinal peptide (VIP) a secretin agonist
8. Bile salts stimulate pancreatic secretion which integrates the physiology of the biliary tract, pancreas and small intestine
9. Pancreatic exocrine secretion is also regulated by inhibitory neuropeptides
10. Bicarbonate is the most important ion in pancreatic secretions as it helps to neutralize gastric acid and provides the necessary pH for the activity of pancreatic enzymes

Clinical Manifestations of Acute Pancreatitis

1. Abdominal pain is the major symptom of acute pancreatitis:
   a. The pain may vary from mild discomfort to overwhelming distress
   b. The quality of the pain is steady and boring
   c. It is located in the epigastrium and periumbilical area and most often radiates straight through to the back. Less frequently it radiates to the chest, flank and lower abdomen
   d. Pain may be more intense in recumbency and patients' position of comfort is sitting with the trunk flexed and the knees flexed
   e. Associated signs and symptoms include:
      i Nausea and vomiting
      ii Abdominal distention that is due to ileus and chemical peritonitis
   f. Physical examination demonstrates:
      i An anxious patient in severe distress
      ii Low grade fever
      iii Tachycardia and hypotension
      iv Shock in some patients
      v Abdominal tenderness and rigidity are present to a variable degree but are much less prominent than the severe pain
      vi Bowel sounds are decreased or absent
      vii Rarely an enlarged pancreas or one with a pseudocyst may be palpated in the upper abdomen
      viii In severe necrotizing pancreatitis:
         1. Cullen's sign may be seen as a faint blue discoloration surrounding the umbilicus due to hemoperitoneum
         2. Turner's sign from blood breakdown products (blue-red, purple or green-brown) may be visible in the flank
      ix Systemic effects of pancreatitis occur in all systems
      x Erythematous skin nodules occur in 10-20% of patients

Pathology

1. Shock may occur from:
   a. Hypovolemia due to exudation of blood and plasma proteins into the retroperitoneal space
   b. Increased formation and release of kinen peptides that cause increased vascular permeability
   c. Systemic effects of proteolytic and lipolytic enzymes
   d. Common causes of pancreatitis:
      i Gallstones
      ii Alcohol
      iii Hypertriglyceridemia
      iv Blunt abdominal trauma

v Abdominal and nonabdominal procedures
vi Endoscopic retrograde cholangiopancreatography (ERCP) particularly after biliary manometry
vii Drugs
viii Sphincter of Oddi dysfunction

e. Less frequent causes of pancreatitis:
i Vascular causes and vasculitis:
   1. Hypoperfusion after cardiac arrest
ii Connective tissue diseases
iii Thrombotic thrombocytopenic purpura
iv Cancer of the pancreas
v Periampullary diverticulum
vi Pancreas divisum
vii Cystic fibrosis
viii Renal failure

Laboratory Evaluation

1. Increased serum amylase; values of three times normal are very supportive of acute pancreatitis if salivary gland disease and gut perforation or infarction are ruled out
2. There is no correlation between the severity of pancreatitis and the degree of serum amylase elevation. Pancreatic isoamylase and lipase levels may remain elevated for 7 to 14 days while total serum amylase may return to normal after 2 to 3 days even in the face of active clinical disease
3. Leukocytosis of 15,000 to 20,000 /μL and hemoconcentration may be seen
4. Hyperglycemia due to decreased insulin release, increased glucagon release and excessive secretion of glucocorticoids and catecholamines
5. Hypocalcemia occurs in approximately 25% of patients that is not completely understood
6. Hyper bilirubinemia is demonstrated in approximately 10% of patients which returns to normal in 4 to 7 days
7. Serum alkaline phosphatase and AST are transiently elevated
8. Approximately 25% of patients are hypoxemic
9. The EKG may demonstrate ST segment and T wave abnormalities that simulate myocardial ischemia
10. CT evaluation delineates the severity of the disorder
11. Ultrasonography evaluates the gallbladder

Intestinal Disease and Pain

Mesenteric Vascular Insufficiency

General Characteristics

1. Intestinal vascular insufficiency is divided into:
    a. Arteriosclerotic mesenteric ischemia
    b. Non-occlusive mesenteric ischemia
    c. Mesenteric venous thrombosis
2. Acute ischemia is more common than chronic ischemia
3. The blood supply to the intestines includes:
    a. Celiac artery
    b. The superior and inferior mesenteric arteries and branches of the internal iliac artery
4. There is extensive collateralization between the major mesenteric trunks and branches of the mesenteric arcade
5. Collateral vessels within the small bowel anastomose with vessels in the duodenum and the pancreas
6. Collateral vessels of the colon anastomose with vessels at the splenic plexus and descending / sigmoid colon which are known as Griffiths point and Sudeck's point respectively which are the most common locations for colonic ischemia
7. This splanchnic circulation may receive up to 30% of the cardiac output
8. Occlusive ischemia occurs if there is blockage of blood flow in a major artery that supplies the intestine
9. Chronic ischemia requires the progressive occlusion of at least two major vessels that supply the intestine (chronic intestinal angina)
10. Non-occlusive ischemia is caused by vasospasm from severe dehydration or shock

Clinical Manifestations (Acute Mesenteric Ischemia)

1. The usual cause is an arterial embolus in a patient with atrial fibrillation, valvular heart disease, recent myocardial infarction or vascular catheterization
2. The pain is acute in onset (if embolic), is severe and nonremitting
3. The location is abdominal
4. A striking feature is the severity of the pain which is out of proportion to the physical examination
5. Associated signs and symptoms include:
    a. Nausea and vomiting
    b. Transient diarrhea
    c. Bloody stools
6. There may be early abdominal distention and hypoactive bowel sounds
7. As the process evolves there are signs of peritonitis and vascular collapse

Neuropathology

1. The embolus is usually found just proximal to the origin of the middle colic

artery. The proximal jejunum may be spared while the remainder of the small bowel to the transverse colon is ischemic

Laboratory Evaluation

1. CBC, serum chemistries, coagulation profile, arterial blood gas, amylase, lactic acid and cardiac enzymes
2. EKG

Imaging

1. Abdominal radiographs
2. CT of the abdomen
3. Mesenteric angiography
4. Mesenteric duplex scan:
    a. High peak velocity of flow in the superior mesenteric artery is correlated with approximately 80% prediction of mesenteric ischemia
    b. Laparotomy is the "gold standard" for diagnosis

Non-Occlusive or Vasospastic Mesenteric Ischemia

General Characteristics

1. Usually encountered in circumstances of severe physiologic stress that is seen with severe dehydration or shock

Clinical Manifestations

1. Generalized abdominal pain
2. Anorexia
3. Bloody stools
4. Abdominal distention
5. A subgroup of patients present with obtundation

Pathology

1. Early intestinal ischemia is often associated with sequestration of fluid within the bowel wall that causes loss of interstitial volume
2. Decreased mucosal integrity is associated with nonocclusive mesenteric ischemia and less frequently with loss of inferior mesenteric arterial blood flow

Laboratory Evaluation

1. CBC, electrolytes, amylase, CPK, lactic acid
2. D-dimer, glutathione S-transferase, platelet activating factor (PAF) and mucosal pH monitoring

Imaging

1. Mesenteric ultrasound
2. Abdominal radiograph
3. CT of the abdomen

4. Mesenteric angiography

Ischemic Colitis

General Characteristics

1. Ischemic colitis is the most common form of acute ischemia of the intestine other than strangulated small bowel obstruction
2. It is the most frequent form of acute intestinal ischemia that complicates cardiovascular surgery
3. Vascular anatomic features:
    a. An index arterial lesion is unusual although many elderly patients have risk factors for atherosclerosis
    b. There may be narrowing of small vessels and increased tortuosity of long colic arteries
    c. In a great number of instances there is an acute self-limited decrease in intestinal blood flow from diffuse disease of small segmental vessels
    d. The colon has a relatively low blood flow that may predispose it to ischemic compromise
    e. The blood flow may also be affected by motor activity particularly during straining at stool. Experimental distension of the colon increases intraluminal pressure, reduces total blood flow and decreases the arteriovenous oxygen gradient in the colonic wall
    f. The microvasculature plexus is less well developed and is embedded in a thicker wall as compared to the small intestine
    g. The end-vessels to the bowel wall (vasa recta) are less developed in the right than left colon
    h. The vasa recta are sensitive to vasospasm and there is poor collateral circulation at this level
    i. As noted above, the watershed areas of the colon are at the splenic flexure and the rectosigmoid junction

Clinical Manifestations

1. Acute onset of a mild crampy abdominal pain with tenderness over the affected bowel segment
2. After 24 hours, there is usually bright red or maroon blood in the stool. There is minimal blood loss that is usually mixed with the stool. There is no hemodynamic compromise (may be seen with diverticulitis or vascular malformation)
3. Anorexia, nausea and vomiting may occur due to ileus
4. Approximately 15% of patients have rebound tenderness, rigidity and absent bowel sounds due to transmural infarction and necrosis

Pathology

1. Colonoscopy demonstrates:
   a. Mild ischemic change of the mucosa that causes minimal erythema
   b. Moderate ischemic change with pale mucosal ulcerations and extension to the muscular layer of the bowel wall
   c. Severe ischemic colitis presents with ulcerations that are deep and have a black or green discoloration of the mucosa. They represent full thickness bowel wall necrotic lesions
2. Local hypoperfusion and reperfusion injury are thought to be important mechanisms
3. The spectrum of injury includes:
   a. Reversible colopathy with subpial hemorrhage and edema
   b. Transient colitis
   c. Chronic colitis
   d. Stricture
   e. Gangrene
   f. Fulminant universal colitis
4. The distribution of the lesions are segmental:
   a. Left sided disease, the inferior mesenteric artery distribution, is more frequently involved than right-sided involvement (superior mesenteric artery)
5. Patients with isolated right colon ischemia have a worse prognosis

Laboratory Evaluation

1. Colonoscopy (the most accurate study)
2. Serum lactate, lactate dehydrogenase, alkaline phosphatase and systemic acidosis are markers of ischemia

Imaging

1. CT:
   a. The most common finding is segmental circumferential wall thickening
   b. May be positive in 89% of patients

Right Sided Colonic Ischemia

General Characteristics

1. In left-side colon ischemia, which is the more common type, "watershed" areas are usually the ischemic segments. The limited collateral flow is between the superior mesenteric (SMA) and inferior mesenteric (IMA) artery circulations. Less frequently there is ischemia between the territories of the superior hemorrhoidal artery and the IMA circulations that affect the descending and sigmoid colon
2. Rates of surgery and mortality are greater with right-side colon ischemia that

suggest a different pathophysiology in a subset of patients which has been posited to occur from large artery disease

Clinical Manifestations

1. Series of 49 patients:
    a. Presenting clinical features start less than 10 days prior to diagnosis
    b. The median age of patients was approximately 70 (with an 11 year range)
    c. Abdominal pain occurs in over 90% of patients:
        i Abdominal angina occurs in a subset of patients
        ii There is a predominance of pain over bleeding with RSCI (right sided colon ischemia)
        iii Higher rates of comorbidities which include:
            1. Coronary artery disease
            2. Atrial fibrillation
            3. Dialysis dependency
        iv Female predominance

Pathology

1. Role of large artery ischemia is posited to be significant with RSCI
2. The SMA supplies a great proportion of the small bowel and the proximal and transverse colon such that SMA hypoperfusion can cause extensive acute mesenteric ischemia
3. There are often poor collateral vessels in the mesentery of the right colon compared to the left. This is important when the IMA is sacrificed during abdominal aortic aneurysm repair or colon resection

Laboratory Evaluation

1. Colonoscopy
2. Mesenteric (SMA and IMA) angiography to R/O large vessel disease

Imaging

1. CT with contrast

Mesenteric Venous Thrombosis (MVT)

General Characteristics

1. As noted earlier, the blood flow to the intestines arises from the superior mesenteric artery whose origin is the abdominal aorta. It has branches to the pancreas and duodenum, supplies three branches to the proximal colon, and terminates in the arteriae rectae that supply the jejunum and ileum.
2. Venous blood drains into the venae rectae that then flow into the ileocolic, middle colic and right colic veins. These veins coalesce to form the superior mesenteric vein that merges with the splenic vein which forms the portal vein:

   a. The left gastric vein drains the lower part of the esophagus and upper part of the lesser curvature of the stomach via the left gastric vein that enters the portal vein at its origin.
   b. The fundus of the stomach is drained by short veins that drain into the splenic vein
   c. The left colon venous drainage is through the inferior mesenteric vein to the splenic vein
3. The incidence of MVT is 2.7 patients per 100,000 of the population. It is responsible for 6% to 9% of acute mesenteric ischemia
4. Risk factors for MVT include:
   a. Prothrombotic states
   b. Inflammatory bowel disease
   c. Malignancy
5. Thrombosis of the larger distal portion of the mesenteric veins is usually secondary to malignancy, pancreatitis and infection and is often associated with portal vein thrombosis
6. Thrombosis that originates from the venae rectae that causes MVT is most often related to a prothrombotic state and causes isolated MVT
7. Primary MVT accounts for approximately 21-49% of patients with MVT
8. JAK V16 mutation that maps to chromosome 9p24.1 is found in a subset of patients with MVT often associated with myeloproliferative disorders

Clinical Manifestations

1. Patients most commonly present with acute abdominal pain in 90 to 100% of cases
2. Common associations are nausea, vomiting and melena
3. The duration of symptoms before diagnosis is usually 1.5 to 2 days
4. The abdominal pain is out of proportion to the physical findings
5. Approximately 15% of patients have melena, hematemesis, or hematochezia (the passage of fresh blood through the anus). Occult blood is demonstrated in approximately 50% of patients
6. Fever and peritoneal signs signal progression of the infarction and may evolve to a blood pressure of less than 90 mmHg systolic with ascites
7. The physical examination often demonstrates abdominal distention with mild to moderate tenderness

Pathology

1. Malignancies particularly myeloproliferative disorders are the most common prothrombotic disorder with MVT
2. Oral contraceptive use is causative in 9 to 18% of young women
3. Antithrombin III, protein S, and protein C deficits have been associated with

MVT

4. Intra-abdominal surgery, particularly splenectomy, are risk factors for MVT
5. MVT and portal vein thrombosis are more common in patients with advanced cirrhosis
6. Patients awaiting liver transplantation may have portal vein thrombosis (15% of patients)
7. Possible association of MVT has been posited for hyperhomocysteinemia and methylene tetrahydrofolate reductase C677T mutations

Laboratory Evaluation

1. Serum lactate level does not initially correlate with intestinal infarction. At the time the process demonstrates lactic acidosis it is late in the course of the illness and mortality is 75%
2. Leukocytosis and hemoconcentration are commonly seen

Imaging

1. Plain abdominal radiographs are usually negative but are helpful in eliminating other disorders
2. Radiographic signs of bowel ischemia include:
    a. Thumb printing (semi-opaque indentations in the bowel lumen from edema)
    b. Air in the intestines
    c. Air in the portal vein and free peritoneal air
3. Contrast enhanced CT:
    a. A filling defect in the mesenteric vein is a diagnostic finding
    b. Bowel wall ischemia is suggested by:
        i Bowel wall thickening
        ii Portal vein air
        iii Persistent enhancement of the bowel wall
    c. The above findings are specific but have low sensitivity
4. Doppler ultrasound

Chronic Intestinal Ischemia

General Characteristics

1. Definition: Abdominal angina is postprandial pain that occurs in patients with mesenteric vascular occlusive disease in which blood flow cannot increase enough to meet visceral demands
2. The mean age of patients is slightly older than 60
3. Median arcuate ligament syndrome may be causative in young patients. It has a 3:1 female predominance

Clinical Manifestations

1. Abdominal pain that occurs a few minutes after eating and subsides within a few hours
2. Patients report cramping as the quality of the pain
3. Diarrhea may be associated
4. There may be a fear of eating with consequent weight loss
5. An abdominal bruit is occasionally auscultated although in one series it was reported in 60 to 90% of patients
6. The abdomen is scaphoid and soft even during episodes of pain
7. Peripheral vascular disease and smoking are co-morbidities

Pathology

1. The most common cause is atherosclerosis which most often involves the ostia of mesenteric vessels
2. There are collateral vessels between the celiac artery and the SMA (the pancreaticoduodenal arcades). Fewer collaterals are present between the IMA and SMA
3. Collateral circulation to the hind gut and midgut is also provided by the iliac arteries
4. There is significant increase of blood flow to the celiac and mesenteric arteries after eating under normal circumstances
5. Usually there is severe stenosis of at least two mesenteric vessels
6. Rarely the median arcuate ligament can compress both the celiac axis and the mesenteric artery (the median arcuate ligament syndrome MALS).
7. Rare causes of intestinal angina include:
    a. Cardiomyopathy
    b. Acute acalculous cholecystitis

Laboratory Evaluation

1. An evaluation for malignancy and gastric ulcer should be undertaken if the history and examination are suggestive
2. A guiac positive stool occurs in 10% of patients

Imaging

1. Duplex ultrasound of the mesenteric vessels
2. Mesenteric angiography

Acute Intestinal Obstruction

General Characteristics

1. In approximately 75% of patients, acute intestinal obstruction occurs from previous abdominal surgery that has produced adhesive bands. Internal and external hernias are also major etiologies
2. The incidence of acute intestinal obstruction within the post-operative period

is falling; but has been reported as 5 to 25%. The incidence of obstruction is lower with laparoscopic surgery
3. Adynamic ileus and primary intestinal pseudo obstruction may simulate obstruction
4. After postsurgical and internal hernias, disorders of the intestinal wall cause approximately 25% of intestinal obstructions

Clinical Manifestations

1. Mechanical intestinal obstruction:
   a. The pain is cramping and located in the midabdomen
   b. It is worse the higher the obstruction
   c. The pain is paroxysmal and the patient is relatively comfortable between paroxysms
   d. Patients often note borborygmi concomitantly with episodes of pain
   e. The pain may decrease as distention increases (possibly due to decreased intestinal mobility from edema of the intestinal wall)
   f. If strangulation occurs, the pain is often more localized, may be steady and may lose its colicky paroxysmal character
   g. Vomiting is associated and is earlier and more severe the higher the level of the obstruction. The vomitus is composed of bile and mucus with high obstructions. In ileal obstruction, the vomitus may become feculent and malodorous due to bacterial overgrowth proximal to the obstruction. Singultus is common.
   h. If the obstruction is complete, there is obstipation and failure to pass gas by rectum. Diarrhea may occur with partial obstruction
   i. Blood in the stool is rare, but may occur with intussuception
   j. In both adynamic ileus and pseudo-obstruction (colonic), there is absence of paroxysmal colicky pain but pain does occur from distention. Vomiting does occur but is not as severe as with mechanical obstruction. Singultus commonly occurs.
   k. The physical examination demonstrates:
      i Abdominal distention (the predominant sign in all forms of obstruction)
      ii Distention is least with high obstructions in the small intestine and most severe with colonic obstruction
      iii Early obstruction of both the large and small intestine produce minimal tenderness and rigidity and the temperature is rarely > 100oF
      iv Perforation causes shock, tenderness, rigidity and fever from bacterial contamination of the peritoneum
      v Hernial orifices (if they are the cause of the obstruction) will demonstrate a mass
      vi Loud, high-pitched borborygmi are concomitant with paroxysms of

pain. This finding may be absent in patients who have strangulation or nonstrangulating lesions

vii A quiet abdomen may occur with obstruction and does not make the diagnosis of adynamic ileus

viii A palpable abdominal mass is often a closed-loop strangulating small-bowel obstruction. The palpable lesion is the tense fluid-filled loop

Pathology

1. The accumulation of gas and fluid proximal to the obstruction causes the abdominal distension. Approximately 70 to 80% of the intestinal gas is from swallowed air which is primarily nitrogen and is not absorbed well from the intestinal lumen
2. The accumulated proximal fluid is a combination of ingested food, saliva, gastric juice, biliary and pancreatic secretions and the failure of physiologic water and ion transport
3. There is an increase of intraluminal pressure from 2-4 cm H20 to 8-10 cm H20
4. Fluid shifts into the intestinal lumen and may be massive which causes systemic hypovolemia, renal failure and shock
5. There is edema of the intestinal wall and peritoneum from blockage of venous return from the intestine which also contributes to fluid and electrolyte loss
6. A closed loop obstruction occurs when the small intestine is occluded at two points by a fascial hernia or adhesive band, which may also compromise the segmental blood supply. If a closed loop is present, peristalsis may increase intraluminal pressure to 30-60 cm H_20
7. Decreased blood supply to the gastrointestinal tract is associated with bacterial invasion and peritonitis

Laboratory Evaluation

1. Leukocytosis with shift to the left is common with strangulation
2. Elevated amylase is seen in all forms of obstruction

Imaging

1. Roentgenographic studies demonstrate:
    a. Distention of fluid- and gas-filled loops of small intestines arranged in a "stepladder" pattern
2. Air-fluid levels are noted in the absence of colonic gas
3. A " coffee bean" mass may be demonstrated with a strangulating closed loop obstruction
    a. CT:
        i The modality of choice to evaluate post-operative patients as it can delineate a dynamic ileus, partial obstruction and complete obstruction

b. Abdominal roentgenograms:
   i May have characteristic features of colonic obstruction:
   i "Birds beak" sign with sigmoid volvulus
   ii An enlarged cecum with cecal torsion or bascule (folding of the cecum anteriorly over the ascending colon)
   iii Colonic obstruction with a competent ileocecal valve demonstrates gas distention which is confined to the colon

Intestinal Pseudo-Obstruction (Ogilvie Syndrome)

General Characteristics

1. Definition:
   a. A clinical syndrome characterized by clinical signs supportive of mechanical obstruction without obstruction in the intestine
   b. Pseudo-obstruction is divided into acute and chronic forms:
      i Acute colonic pseudo-obstruction (ACPO):
         1. The colon is dramatically dilated which may lead to perforation and peritonitis
         2. ACPO can recur
      ii Chronic pseudo-obstruction (CCPO):
         1. Symptoms of recurrent bowel obstruction within 6 months
         2. Abdominal bloating and / or pain within the previous 3 months
   c. Suggestive radiographs of bowel obstruction
   d. No evidence of anatomic structural lesions
   e. In burn and orthopedic patients the prevalence rate of acute colonic pseudo-obstruction (ACPO) is 0.29%
   f. ACPO is most often encountered in hospitalized patients:
      i The usual underlying disorders are:
         1. Trauma
         2. Pregnancy
         3. Caesarean delivery
         4. Sepsis
         5. Cardiothoracic, pelvic and orthopedic surgery
   g. This is generally a disease of elderly patients. The mean age is often reported to be in the sixth decade. It is very common in younger patients with spinal cord injury. More recent studies support the mean age to occur in the seventh and eighth decade

Clinical Manifestations

1. The usual setting is an elderly debilitated hospitalized patient with multiple medical issues who have undergone medical or surgical procedures
2. Presenting symptoms include:

a. Abdominal pain (80%)
b. Nausea and vomiting (80%)
c. Obstipation (40%)
d. Fever (37%)

3. Physical examination:
   a. Abdominal distention (90 to 100%)
   b. Abdominal tenderness (66%)
   c. Hypoactive high pitched or absent bowel sounds (60%); bowel sounds may be normal or hyperactive in 40% of patients
   d. Empty rectum on digital examination
   e. Abnormal tenderness in the abdomen occurs with perforation or ischemia but may also occur in patients with viable bowel

Pathology

1. The three most common causes of acute colonic pseudo-obstruction are:
   a. Trauma (particularly retroperitoneal)
   b. Systemic serious infections
   c. Myocardial infarction and congestive heart failure
   d. Commonly associated disorders include:
      i Old age (particularly hospitalized debilitated patients with multiple medical problems)
      ii Hypothyroidism
      iii Hyponatremia, hypokalemia, hypocalcemia, hypercalcemia and hypomagnesemia
      iv Renal failure
      v Medications (narcotics, tricyclic antidepressants, phenothiazines and anesthetics)
      vi Less frequent causes:
         1. Megacystis megacolon
         2. Amyloidosis
         3. GI carcinoma
         4. Guillain-Barre syndrome
         5. Multiple myeloma
         6. Alcohol abuse
         7. SLE
         8. Systemic sclerosis
2. Mechanisms posited for pseudo-obstruction include:
   a. Increased sympathetic tone concomitantly with decreased parasympathetic tone
   b. Disruption of sacral parasympathetic innervation to the distal colon
   c. Involvement of the transition zone (Tz) between the dilated and non-dilated bowel loops that causes proximal distention and smooth muscle

hypertrophy. This may be caused by deficiency of the myenteric plexus and ganglia neurons, particularly nitric oxide synthase positive neurons that affect the transitional zone

Laboratory Evaluation

1. Radiography of the abdomen
2. Contrast enema
3. CT to delineate perforation, obstruction and toxic megacolon
4. Colonoscopy

Acute Appendicitis

General Characteristics

1. Appendicitis is the most common abdominal surgical emergency in the USA
2. The peak incidence is between the second and third decade of life
3. Perforation is more common in infancy and in the elderly
4. Males and females are affected equally with the exception of the period between puberty and age 25

Clinical Manifestations

1. Pain is located periumbilically initially and then localizes to the right lower quadrant. This sequence occurs in approximately 2/3 of patients
2. The pain (visceral in quality) is usually mild, cramping and lasts 4-6 hours
3. When inflammation spreads to involve the parietal peritoneum (primarily somatic) it becomes steady, more severe and is aggravated by movement and cough
4. Anorexia is common; a hungry patient does not have appendicitis
5. Nausea and vomiting occur in 50 to 60% of patients and is usually self-limited
6. Urinary frequency and dysuria may occur if the inflamed appendix is adjacent to the bladder. Similarly, juxtaposition near the sigmoid colon may cause diarrhea. These symptoms may also occur from complex interactions of C-fiber and A-delta fiber interactions, at the level of the dorsal root ganglia or superficial dorsal horn of the spinal cord
7. Recurrent acute appendicitis may rarely recur with complete resolution of signs and symptoms between attacks; it may also recur if a long appendiceal stump is left from the initial operation
8. Physical examination:
    a. The signs vary with the time of the examination in relation to the onset of the inflammation and with the anatomical location of the appendix

b. Anatomical locations include:
   i Deep in the pelvic cul-de-sac
   ii In the right lower quadrant adjacent to the peritoneum, cecum and small intestine
   iii In the right upper quadrant particularly during pregnancy
   iv Rarely in the left lower quadrant
c. Tenderness may be absent in the initial stage of the disorder but evolves and is localized to the anatomical position of the appendix
d. The typical location for tenderness is McBurney's point (located in a line one-third of the way between the anterior iliac crest and the umbilicus).
e. Abdominal tenderness is often absent if the position of the appendix is retrocecal or deep in the pelvis. In these instances, tenderness may be in the flank, or demonstrated on rectal or pelvic examination. Referred rebound tenderness may be elicited
f. Flexion of the right hip and decreased right lower extremity movement are due to parietal peritoneal inflammation
g. Mechanical hyperesthesia of the skin over the right lower quadrant as well as positive psoas and obturator signs occur late in the course
h. The temperature is normal or slightly elevated; perforation is suggested if it is >38.3C (101°F). Tachycardia is concomitant with the elevated temperature
i. Abdominal rigidity and tenderness increase with evolution of the process to perforation with localized or diffuse peritonitis
j. Distension is rare unless there is diffuse peritonitis
k. An abdominal mass may be palpated if there is perforation but usually occurs three days after the event. Earlier detection of a mass is seen with Crohn's disease or carcinoma of the cecum
l. Perforation rarely occurs prior to 24 hr after onset but occurs commonly after 48 hours

Pathology

1. Appendicitis most often occurs from luminal obstruction due to a fecalith. This forms from accumulation and inspissation of fecal matter around vegetable fibers
2. Rarer causes of luminal obstruction of the appendix are:
   a. Enlarged lymphoid follicles associated with viral illness
   b. Pinworms, Ascaris and Taenia
   c. Tumors (carcinoid and adenocarcinoma)
   d. Barium contrast
3. If there is appendiceal ulceration. Luminal bacteria invade the appendiceal wall; there is an increase of luminal pressure with consequent decrease of arterial blood flow. If the process evolves slowly it may be walled off by the

terminal ileum, cecum, and omentum. If this occurs, there is a local abscess. Rupture of appendiceal abscesses may cause fistulas from the appendix to other abdominal organs

Laboratory Evaluation

1. Moderate leukocytosis (10,000-18,000 cells/μL) with a shift to the left is classic. Leukocytosis > 20,000 μ/L is evidence of perforation
2. Anemia with guiac positive stool suggests carcinoma of the cecum particularly in elderly patients
3. Urinalysis may reveal a few white or red cells without bacteria if the appendix is adjacent to the right ureter or bladder

Imaging

1. A fecalith in the right lower quadrant is seen in 5% of patients
2. CT demonstrates a thickened appendix, periappendicular stranding, and a fecalith. The sensitivity and specificity are over 90%

Pathological Correlates of Periumbilical and Right Lower Quadrant Pain

Periumbilical Pain

1. Appendicitis
2. Small bowel obstruction
3. Gastroenteritis
4. Mesenteric ischemia

Right Lower Quadrant Pain

1. Gastrointestinal etiologies:
    a. Appendicitis
    b. Inflammatory bowel disease
    c. Diverticulitis (unusual on the right side)
    d. Gastroenteritis
    e. Inguinal hernia
2. Gynecologic etiologies:
    a. Ovarian tumor or torsion
    b. Pelvic inflammatory disease
3. Renal etiologies:
    a. Pyelonephritis
    b. Perinephric abscess
    c. Nephrolithiasis

Acute Peritonitis

General Characteristics

1. Definition:
    a. Peritonitis is an inflammation of the peritoneum that may be localized or diffuse, acute or chronic and is due to infection or nonseptic causes
    b. Acute peritonitis is most often infectious and is related to a perforated viscus which is defined as secondary peritonitis
    c. If no intra-abdominal source is identified, infectious peritonitis is defined as primary or spontaneous

Clinical Manifestations

1. The cardinal sign and symptom of peritonitis is acute abdominal pain and tenderness most often associated with fever
2. The location of the pain is dependent on the underlying cause and whether the inflammation is localized or generalized
3. In localized peritonitis from appendicitis or diverticulitis both the pain and physical findings are restricted to the site of inflammation
4. Bowel sounds are most often absent
5. Tachycardia, hypotension and dehydration are common
6. In peritoneal dialysis patients in whom peritonitis is not infrequent approximately, 20% of patients do not have pain or fever. These patients are older than other patients undergoing dialysis

Pathology

1. A perforated viscus, penetrating wound of the abdominal wall or a foreign object in the abdomen are the main causes of infective peritonitis
2. The most common causes of peritonitis are:
    a. Ruptured appendix
    b. Ruptured diverticulum
    c. Perforated peptic ulcer
    d. Incarcerated hernia
    e. Gangrenous gall bladder
    f. Volvulus
    g. Bowel infarction
    h. Cancer
    i. Inflammatory bowel disease
    j. Intestinal obstruction
3. Bacterial peritonitis:
    a. May occur in the absence of an intraperitoneal source of bacteria. In 90% of instances, it occurs in a setting of ascites and liver cirrhosis in patients who have a protein concentration of < 1g/L
4. Aseptic peritonitis may be caused by peritoneal irritation from gastric juice, bile, pancreatic enzymes, blood, urine and sterile foreign bodies

5. Medical causes of aseptic peritonitis are SLE, familial Mediterranean fever and porphyria

Laboratory Evaluation

1. Leukocytosis and marked acidosis are expected
2. Paracentesis with a cell count of >250 neutrophils is usual in the peritoneal fluid. Protein and lactate dehydrogenase may be elevated

Imaging

1. Plain abdominal radiographs:
   a. Dilation of both the small and large intestines with edema of the bowel wall
   b. Free air under the diaphragm is almost always diagnostic of a perforated viscus
2. CT:
   a. May demonstrate free fluid or an abscess

Inflammatory Bowel Diseases

Crohn's Disease (CD)

General Characteristics

1. The incidence of CD is 3.1 to 14.6 patients per 100,000 person years
2. Prevalence of CD is 37-246 patients per 100,000 person years
3. The peak age of onset is between 15 and 30 years. A second peak is seen between 60-80 years of age
4. The male to female ratio for CD is 1.1 to 1.8:1

Clinical Manifestations

1. Most often presents as acute or chronic bowel inflammation; it evolves toward:
   a. A fibrostenotic-obstructive pattern or a penetrating fistulous pattern. The site of the disease determines clinical features

Ileocolitis

1. The commonest site of inflammation is the terminal ileum
2. Patients complain of right lower quadrant pain and diarrhea
3. The presentation may mimic that of acute appendicitis with severe right lower quadrant pain, a palpable mass with fever and leukocytosis
4. Pain is colicky and is relieved by defecation and is associated with a low grade fever
5. A high-spiking fever is more consistent with an abscess
6. Weight loss occurs from diarrhea, anorexia and fear of eating and may reach 10 to 20% of normal body weight

7. An enlarged mass may be palpated in the right lower quadrant that consists of inflamed bowel, adherent and indurated mesentery and enlarged lymph nodes
8. The mass may extend to obstruct the right ureter or irritate the bladder which is associated with dysuria and fever
9. Early in the disease course, there may be intermittent obstruction from bowel wall edema and spasm that cause postprandial pain. If the process continues over years it evolves into fibrostenotic narrowing and stricture
10. If there is a stricture, diarrhea decreases and is replaced by chronic bowel obstruction. Acute episodes of obstruction are precipitated by bowel inflammation, spasm or impaction of undigested food
11. Severe inflammation of the ileocecal area may lead to fistula with the adjacent bowel, skin, urinary bladder, or abscess within the mesentery. Enterovesicle fistulas are associated with:
    a. Dysuria
    b. Recurrent bladder infections
    c. Pneumaturia (rare)
    d. Fecaluria (rare)
12. Enterocutaneous fistulas often drain through abdominal surgical scars
13. Enterovaginal fistulas present as dyspareunia or feculent foul-smelling painful discharge

Jejunoileitis

1. Associated with a loss of digestive and absorptive surface that may manifest as malabsorption or steatorrhea
2. The intestinal malabsorption may be associated with hypoalbuminemia, hypocalcemia, hypomagnesemia, coagulopathy, hyperoxalurea
3. Secondary disorders from the malabsorption are B12 deficiency, vertebral fractures (vitamin D deficiency), hypocalcemia, and steroid use. Pellagra from niacin deficiency has been reported

Colitis and Perianal Disease

1. The clinical manifestations of colitis are:
    a. Crampy abdominal pain
    b. Low grade fever
    c. Hematochezia
2. Gross bleeding is not as common as that which occurs with ulcerative colitis and occurs in approximately 50% of patients with exclusive colitis
3. It is posited that pain occurs from irritation by fecal material in inflamed segments of the large bowel
4. Decreased rectal compliance may be another cause of diarrhea
5. Massive gross bleeding and toxic megacolon are rare occurrences

6. Bowel obstruction from strictures occurs in 4 to 16% of patients
7. Fistulas occur into the stomach and duodenum that cause vomiting, and in the proximal and midbowel that are associated with malabsorption
8. Approximately 10% of women develop a rectovaginal fistula
9. Perianal disease is seen in approximately 1/3 of patients and is characterized by:
    a. Incontinence
    b. Hemorrhoidal tags
    c. Strictures
    d. Anorectal fistulae
    e. Perirectal abscesses

Gastroduodenal Disease

1. The symptom and signs of patients that develop upper gastrointestinal tract disease are:
    a. Epigastric pain
    b. Nausea
    c. Vomiting
2. These patients often have H. pylori–negative gastritis.
3. Disease is usually more severe in the second portion of the duodenum rather than the bulb.
4. Patients may develop fistulae from the large and small bowel and may develop gastric outlet obstruction.

Pathology

1. Early lesions are aphthoid ulcerations and focal crypt abscesses associated with aggregations of macrophages. These form non caseating granulomas in all layers of the bowel wall as well as in lymph nodes, mesentery, peritoneum, liver and pancreas
2. Granulomas are seen in approximately 50% of patients but are rarely demonstrated by mucosal biopsy
3. Submucosal or subserosal lymphoid aggregates, skip areas, and transmural inflammation are other characteristic microscopic features of CD
4. CD can affect the entire GI tract from the mouth to the anus. The terminal ileum is affected in 90% of patients with small-intestinal disease
5. The inflammation in Crohn's disease and other inflammatory bowel disorders has been linked to a loss of tolerance to self-antigens which would support the existence of specific autoantibodies in disease phenotypes
6. Genome wide association studies have demonstrated immune-related susceptibility loci
7. Emerging evidence suggests that there is an innate immune response to a low-diversity and altered gut microbiota that initiates and perpetuates the

chronic inflammation seen in IBD

Laboratory Evaluation

1. Elevated ESR and CRP
2. Hypoalbuminemia, anemia and leukocytosis occur in severe patients
3. Endoscopy:
    a. Aphthous ulcers, fistulae, and skip areas with rectal sparing. Important for biopsy of affected areas
    b. Wireless capsule endoscopy allows visualization directly; visualizes the entire small bowel mucosa
4. Biomarkers:
    a. Autoantigenic targets:
        i The major zymogen granule membrane glycoprotein 2 (GP2) is evaluated in CD

Imaging

1. Radiographic evaluation:
    a. Thickened folds and aphthous ulcers in early disease. Strictures, fistulas, inflammatory masses and abscesses are seen in long standing disease
    b. The "string sign" is due to long areas of circumferential inflammation
2. CT enterography demonstrates mural enhancement, stratification, engorged vasa recta and perienteric pathology

Ulcerative Colitis

General Characteristics

1. The incidence of UC is 2.2 to 14.3 patients per 100,000 person-years
2. The prevalence is 37 to 246 patients per 100,000 person-years
3. The male to female ratio is 1:1
4. There is increased frequency of both CD and UC in patients of Jewish ancestry

Clinical Manifestations

1. Crampy abdominal pain
2. Diarrhea and rectal bleeding
3. Tenesmus
4. Passage of mucus
5. The disorder may present acutely but most often there is an insidious onset over weeks to months
6. Tenesmus (urgency with a feeling of incomplete evacuation) but rarely have severe abdominal pain
7. In patients with distal disease, proctitis or proctosigmoiditis, intestinal transit time slows which may cause constipation

8. Blood mixed stools or grossly bloody diarrhea may occur if the disease spreads beyond the rectum. There is usually increased transit time due to inflammation
9. Diarrhea may be nocturnal or postprandial
10. A subgroup of patients have vague lower abdominal discomfort or mild central abdominal cramping which may be exacerbated by active disease
11. Anorexia, nausea, vomiting, fever and weight loss may be associated

Physical Examination

1. Proctitis causes a tender anal canal with blood
2. Extensive disease is associated with abdominal tenderness over the colon
3. Toxic colitis causes severe abdominal pain and bleeding
4. Megacolon patients have hepatic tympany
5. Peritonitis occurs with perforation

Pathology

1. The disorder is restricted to the mucosa and superficial submucosa. The deeper layers are unaffected other than in fulminant disease
2. The crypt architecture of the colon is disrupted becoming bifid and decreased in number with a gap between the crypt base and the muscularis mucosa
3. A subgroup of patients have plasma cells and basal lymphoid aggregates
4. The mucosa demonstrates vascular congestion, edema, focal hemorrhage and an inflammatory cell infiltrate
5. There is neutrophilic cryptitis and in time cryptic abscess formation

Laboratory Evaluation

1. Active disease is associated with an increased ESR, C-reactive protein, platelet count and decreased hemoglobin
2. Fecal calprotectin is increased (released by activated neutrophils) and correlates with inflammation
3. Endoscopy

Imaging

1. Single contrast barium enema:
   a. Earliest change is fine mucosal granularity
   b. As the disease evolves the mucosa thickens and develops superficial ulcers
   c. When the ulcers have penetrated the mucosa they are called "collar-button ulcers"
   d. The haustral folds become thickened and edematous and the colon becomes shortened and narrowed
   e. There may be post-inflammatory or pseudopolyps, adenomatous polyps as well as carcinoma in long standing disease
   f. CT scanning is not as diagnostic as endoscopy or barium enema

Diverticulitis

General Characteristics

1. In some studies of western populations, diverticulosis may affect 50% of the populations > 60 years of age but only 20% of patients with diverticulosis develop symptomatic disease
2. The mean at presentation of the disease is 59 years of age
3. The prevalence between males and females is equal

Clinical Manifestations

1. Acute uncomplicated diverticulitis presents with:
   a. Left lower quadrant abdominal pain
   b. Anorexia
   c. Fever
   d. Obstipation
2. Perforation:
   a. Less than 25% of patients present with generalized peritonitis from diverticular perforation
   b. Physical examination reveals abdominal distention and localized or generalized peritonitis

Pathology

1. The two types of diverticula that occur in the intestines are true or pseudodiverticula
2. A true diverticulum is the herniation of the entire bowel wall while a pseudodiverticulum is the protrusion of only the mucosa through the muscularis propria of the colon. Pseudodiverticula are the most common type that affects the colon
3. The protrusion occurs where the nutrient artery (vasa recti) enters the muscularis propria. The sigmoid colon is most commonly affected
4. The location of the diverticula is posited to be the result of high pressure generated by the muscular sigmoid colon
5. Diverticulitis is inflammation of a diverticulum from material within the protruded diverticular sac and the formation of a fecalith. The vasa recti are either compressed or eroded that causes perforation or bleeding
6. Most bleeds are self-limited, occur in patients > 60 years of age who are hypertensive, atherosclerotic and regularly use nonsteroidal anti-inflammatory drugs
7. The low fiber content of the Western diet is associated with decreased intestinal content and size of the lumen that may cause transmission of muscular contraction pressure to the wall of the colon. Other factors that may be important in pathogenesis are low grade inflammation, altered intestinal microbiota, visceral hypersensitivity and abnormal colonic motility

Laboratory Evaluation

1. Barium enema and colonoscopy should not be obtained during acute attacks due to the risk of perforation
2. Fever with associated leukocytosis is associated with complicated diverticular disease which includes perforation or abscess formation

Imaging

1. CT:
   a. Sigmoid diverticula
   b. Thickened colonic wall (>4mm)
   c. Inflammation of the pericolic fat
   d. An abscess may be detected in 16% of patients

Differential Diagnosis of Left Lower Quadrant Abdominal Pain

1. Diverticulitis
2. Salpingitis
3. Inguinal hernia
4. Ectopic pregnancy
5. Nephrolithiasis
6. Irritable bowel syndrome
7. Inflammatory bowel disease

Irritable Bowel Disease (IBS)

General Characteristics

1. Definition:
   a. IBS is a disorder with complex symptoms that manifest as abdominal pain or discomfort associated with altered bowel patterns
   b. There is an estimated prevalence of 5.8 to 17.5% of the population
   c. The Rome III criteria have categorized the disorder into subgroups:
      i IBS with constipation
      ii IBS with diarrhea
      iii Mixed type IBS
      iv IBS unsubtyped
   d. Approximately 10% of patients with infective gastroenteritis may develop IBS

Clinical Manifestations

1. Abdominal pain:
   a. Variable in intensity and location
   b. Its location is the hypogastrium in 25%, the right side in 20%, the left side in 20% and the epigastrium in 10% of patients

   c. It is episodic and crampy in quality but may be superimposed on a chronic ache. It varies greatly in intensity
   d. Pain is usually present only during wakefulness, although severely affected patients have sleep disruption
   e. Pain may be exacerbated by eating or emotional distress and may be relieved by defecation or passing flatus
   f. Menstrual and premenstrual periods may exacerbate symptoms
2. Altered bowel habits:
   a. A change in bowel pattern is the most consistent manifestation of IBS. The most common pattern is constipation that alternates with diarrhea; constipation increases and becomes intractable over time. Many patients suffer tenesmus (a feeling of incomplete evacuation)
   b. Diarrhea may be predominant in a subgroup of patients and is characterized by a small volume of loose stools (<200 ml). There is no nocturnal diarrhea. It may be exacerbated by emotional stress or eating. The stool may be associated with a large amount of mucus.
   c. Bleeding, malabsorption and weight loss are not features of IBS
   d. Abdominal distension and belching are frequent. Many patients have impaired transit and tolerance of an intestinal gas load
   e. Approximately 25% of patients have dyspepsia, heartburn, nausea and vomiting

Pathology

1. IBS is considered to be a multifactorial and heterogeneous disease
2. Possible mechanisms:
   a. Inflammation
   b. Immunity
   c. Infection
   d. The gut microbiota
   e. Psychosocial factors
   f. Stress
   g. An abnormal brain-gut axis
3. Recent studies support:
   a. Genetic susceptibility
   b. Diet / drug intolerance
   c. Environmental pollutants as possible associations of IBS
4. Serotonin (5-HT) mediates intercellular signal transmission in the gut; it is synthesized by enterochromaffin (EC) cells (90%) and the serotonergic neurons of the myenteric plexus. EC cells are the primary source of enteric 5-HT

in the gastrointestinal tract and 5-HT inactivation may be as important as its release in maintaining gut homeostasis

5. Enteric 5-HT is essential for secretion, motility and bowel sensation; the involvement or alteration of the metabolism of this neurotransmitter is critical in the pathogenesis of IBS. Higher concentrations of 5-HT are found in IBS patients as compared to healthy controls that is associated with depressed serotonin transporter (SERT) mRNA. The regulation of SERT in IBS pathogenesis is under intense investigation as it is now postulated that 5-HT signaling is an essential component of this disorder

Pain Mechanisms in IBS

1. The bidirectional Brain-Gut Axis:
    a. Brain-gut interaction is critical in modulation of gut function. Afferent information from the lumen of the gut is transmitted from enteric, spinal, and vagal inputs to the CNS that trigger homeostatic reflexes in response to physiologic and pathologic visceral stimuli:
        i These reflexes are affected at the level of the:
            1. Enteric nervous system
            2. Spinal cord
            3. Pontomedullary nuclei
            4. Limbic CNS areas
        ii Vagal visceral afferent input is a component of modulation of:
            1. Emotion
            2. Pain sensitivity
            3. Satiety
            4. Immune response
        iii Descending cortico-limbic modulation can set the gain of enteric reflexes. This top down modulation may occur during:
            1. Sleep
            2. Stress response
            3. Fear
            4. Anger

Visceral Hypersensitivity

The clinical observations of abdominal pain during palpation of the sigmoid colon and during endoscopic evaluation suggested that IBS patients have visceral hypersensitivity. Barostat controlled balloon distention of the colorectum demonstrates:

1. Lowered mechanical thresholds for perception
2. Increased sensory ratings and viscerosomatic referral patterns.

These findings support:

1. Up-regulation of the sensitivity of visceral afferent pathways,

2. Spinal or brainstem alterations in sensitivity to visceral afferents
3. CNS amplification of visceral input

Peripheral Up-Regulation of Visceral Afferent Sensitivity

Evidence supports mucosal immune activation in maintaining a chronic state of visceral afferent sensitization possibly by spino-bulbo-spinal pain amplification through the rostral ventromedullary nucleus (RVM). However a large number of patients with inflammatory bowel disease who suffer similar symptomatology do not have visceral hypersensitivity.

Spinal and Supraspinal Up-Regulation of Visceral Afferent Sensitivity

In a subset of IBS patients, there is evidence that enhanced stress responsiveness is important in the development of IBS. In response to emotional or physiologic stress, there is activation of the emotional motor system that includes:

1. Ascending monoaminergic pathways
2. The autonomic system
3. The hypothalamic-pituitary adrenal axis as well as endogenous pain modulatory systems
4. Corticotropin-releasing factor (CRF), a neuropeptide, integrates these outputs in response to stress
5. There are long-term consequences in this system from early aversive events
6. Central stress circuits have been demonstrated to alter visceral nociceptive responses
7. Mild stress associated with anxiety states may cause hyperalgesia
8. Alteration of central pain modulation has been suggested from functional MRI paradigms:
   a. IBS patients demonstrate increased activation of the anterior cingulate cortex in response to rectal stimulation; this region is responsive to emotional and attentional stimuli
   b. The dorsal ACC also projects to major components of the endogenous pain modulating system. There may be facilitation of pain circuits to a visceral stimulus
   c. Some fMRI studies have demonstrated decreased activation of the PAG which suggests less activation of inhibitory pain circuitry
   d. IBS patients have also demonstrated increased activation of limbic and paralimbic areas that include the amygdala, hypothalamus, ventral and rostral ACC and dorsomedial prefrontal cortex than ulcerative colitis patients or healthy controls
   e. Other fMRI studies have demonstrated that IBS patients have hypervigilance for visceral afferences

Laboratory Evaluation

1. In patients greater than 40 years of age:

   a. Air-contrast barium enema
   b. Colonoscopy
2. The diagnostic evaluation suggested by the American Gastroenterological Association is determined by:
   a. The duration of symptoms
   b. The change in symptoms over time
   c. The age and sex of the patient
   d. Prior diagnostic studies
   e. A family history of colorectal cancer
   f. Psychological dysfunction

Differential Diagnosis of Pain in IBS

1. Epigastric or periumbilical pain:
   a. Biliary tract disease
   b. Peptic ulcer
   c. Intestinal ischemia
   d. Carcinoma of the stomach or pancreas
2. Pain in the lower abdomen:
   a. Colon diverticular disease
   b. Inflammatory bowel disease
   c. Ulcerative colitis and Crohn's disease
   d. Carcinoma of the colon
3. Postprandial pain with bloating, nausea and vomiting:
   a. Gastroparesis
   b. Partial intestinal obstruction
   c. Intestinal infestation Giardia lamblia
4. Acute intermittent porphyria (painful constipation)
5. Lead poisoning (painful constipation)

Spleen Disease

Spleen Pain

General Characteristics

1. The spleen is located in the left upper quadrant (LUQ) and is attached to the stomach by the gastrolienal ligament and to the kidney by the lienorenal ligament
2. Accessary spleens are seen in approximately 20% of patients
3. The major functions of the spleen are:
   a. Quality control of erythrocytes performed in the red pulp by removal of defective and senescent RBCs
   b. Synthesis of antibodies in the white pulp

   c. Removal of antibody tagged bacteria and RBCs from the circulation
4. The spleen enlarges from:
   a. Increased demand of its basic functions,
   b. Abnormal splenic or portal blood flow, and
   c. Infiltration

Clinical Manifestations

1. The most common symptoms of diseases of the spleen are pain and a heavy sensation in the left upper quadrant
2. Pain may occur from acute splenic swelling due to stretch of its capsule, infarction or inflammation
3. Occlusion of splenic blood flow from thromboembolism may cause LUQ and pleuritic chest pain
4. Vascular occlusion in children with sickle cell disease is painful. In the past it was felt that splenic infarction was painless
5. Rupture of the spleen:
   a. From trauma or infiltrative disease may cause a break in the capsule with intraperitoneal bleeding, shock and death
   b. Referred pain is often to the cap of the left shoulder (subdiaphragmatic C5 nerve root irritation)
6. A palpable spleen is the major physical finding in disorders of the organ. The normal spleen weighs less than 250 grams, decreases with age and lies entirely within the rib cage

Pathology

1. Reticuloendothelial cell hyperplasia
2. Immune hyperplasia
3. Disordered immunoregulation
4. Extramedullary hematopoiesis
5. Abnormal splenic or portal blood flow
6. Infiltration by benign and malignant disorders
7. Infectious agents (malaria)

Laboratory Evaluation (Splenomegaly)

1. The abnormalities are determined by the underlying systemic illness
2. Erythrocyte counts may be decreased with thalassemia major, SLE, cirrhosis with portal hypertension
3. Increased erythrocyte counts are seen with polycythemia vera
4. Granulocyte counts may be decreased with Felty's syndrome, congestive splenomegaly or leukemia, or increased with infectious or inflammatory diseases

Imaging

1. MRI or CT of the abdomen

Kidney Disease

Urinary Tract Obstruction

General Characteristics

1. Mechanical obstruction can occur at any level of the urinary tract from the renal calyces to the external urethral meatus
2. Areas of narrowing include:
   a. The ureteropelvic junction
   b. Ureterovesical junction
   c. The bladder neck
   d. Ureteral meatus
3. Blockage above the level of the bladder causes unilateral dilatation of the ureter and the renal pyelocalyceal system
4. In adults, urinary tract obstruction (UTO) is primarily acquired from pelvic tumors, calculi and urethral stricture

Clinical Manifestations

1. Pain is the most prominent symptom and is caused by distention of the collecting system or the renal capsule
2. The rate of distention rather than its degree determine the severity of pain
3. Ureteral stone pain:
   a. Is excruciating (10/10 on a visual analogue scale) and is known as renal colic
   b. The pain is continuous with little fluctuation in intensity
   c. Radiation is to the lower abdomen, testes, tip of the penis and labia
   d. In contrast, chronic narrowing of the ureteropelvic junction may be painless but can destroy the affected kidney
   e. Flank pain with micturition is strong evidence for vesicoureteral reflux
   f. Associated azotemia develops with:
      i Bladder outlet obstruction
      ii Acute renal failure and anuria should be suspected with bilateral obstruction
      iii Polyuria and nocturia are seen with partial obstruction
      iv Fluctuation in urine output in a patient with azotemia is suggestive of intermittent or partial obstruction
      v Obstruction at or below the level of the bladder is associated with hesitancy and difficulty with initiating micturition, post void dribbling, urinary frequency and incontinence

Pathology

1. UTO is associated with urinary tract infection and urolithiasis
2. Hypertension may occur with acute and subacute unilateral obstruction (due to release of renin by the affected kidney)
3. Prostatic enlargement
4. Congenital lesions
5. Intra-abdominal mass lesions

Laboratory Evaluation

1. Urinalysis may reveal hematuria, pyuria and bacteriuria

Imaging

1. Abdominal scout film may demonstrate nephrocalcinosis or a radio-opaque stone
2. Abdominal ultrasonography to evaluate renal and bladder size and pyelocalyceal contour; ultrasonography is approximately 90% specific and sensitive for hydronephrosis
3. Intravenous urography; retrograde or antegrade urography in azotemic patients
4. Voiding cystourethrography is used for the diagnosis of vesicoureteral reflux, bladder neck and urethral obstruction
5. CT is used to evaluate intra-abdominal and retroperitoneal causes of obstruction

Atheroembolic Renovascular Disease

General Characteristics

1. Renal infarctions are rare. In one large series of 250,000 patients seen in an emergency department 1.4% had an infarction
2. The etiology of acute renal infarction is usually an embolus that arises from the heart or the aorta. The most common underlying disorder is atrial fibrillation

Clinical Manifestations

1. Acute flank pain is most typical that is associated with tenderness
2. The pain is continuous
3. Pain may be experienced in lumbar areas; abdominal pain is common
4. Associated symptoms and signs:
    a. Acute elevation of blood pressure (renin release in the peri-infarction zone)
    b. Nausea and vomiting
    c. Elevated temperature > 37.5oC
    d. Urinary symptoms

Pathology

1. Thrombi from the suprarenal aorta
2. Renal artery dissection
3. Hypercoagulable states
4. Endovascular studies
5. Cocaine
6. Sickle cell disease
7. A predilection for infarction of the upper pole

Laboratory Evaluation

1. Elevated C-reactive protein
2. Elevated lactate dehydrogenase
3. Leukocytosis
4. Microscopic hematuria and proteinuria
5. Elevated serum creatinine and alkaline phosphatase

Imaging

1. CT angiography
2. Renal angiography
    a. A wedge-shaped zone of peripheral hypodensity that does not enhance

Urinary Tract Infections

Overview

1. Urinary tract infections are divided into lower tract that includes the ureters and bladder and the upper tract that includes:
    a. Acute pyelonephritis
    b. Prostatitis
    c. Intrarenal and perinephric abscess
2. Urethral and bladder infections are considered mucosal while tissue invasion occurs with prostatitis, pyelonephritis and renal abscess
3. The infections are categorized as catheter-associated (nosocomial) and non-catheter-associated
4. The majority of acute symptomatic infections occur in young women
5. UTIs are unusual in male patients <50 years of age

Cystitis

General Characteristics

1. Urinary tract infections are extremely common in females and cystitis is the major cause of these infections

Clinical Manifestations

1. Dysuria
2. Urgency and frequency
3. A sensation of bladder fullness
4. Suprapubic tenderness to palpation
5. Flank pain and costovertebral angle tenderness is more suggestive of upper tract UTI but may be seen with cystitis
6. Rarely there are fever, chills and malaise; these symptoms are much more common with upper UTI

Pathology

1. Escherichia is the cause of the majority of uncomplicated bladder infections.
2. Other pathogens are:
   a. Staphylococcus saprophyticus
   b. Proteus mirabilis
   c. Klebsiella pneumonia
   d. Enterococcus faecalis

Laboratory Evaluation

1. Urinalysis for pyuria:
   a. Positive leukocyte esterase dipstick test
   b. Leukocytes in unspun fresh urine (greater than 10 WBCs is abnormal)
   c. 50% of patients have microscopic hematuria
   d. Low grade proteinuria
2. Urine culture is the criterion standard for diagnosis

Urethritis

General Characteristics

1. Urethritis is documented in approximately 4 million Americans per year. There are over 700,000 new patients with gonococcal urethritis annually in the USA. The incidence of both gonococcal and non-gonococcal is increasing
2. Risk factors for contracting non-gonococcal urethritis secondary to a sexually transmitted disease are:
   a. Contraceptive use
   b. Age at first intercourse (younger age is associated with higher risk)
   c. Number of sexual partners
   d. Sexual preference
   e. Previous STDs

Clinical Manifestations

1. A large number of patients are asymptomatic and are diagnosed due to partner screening. Approximately 75% of women with Chlamydia trachomatis infections are asymptomatic

2. Symptoms start 4 days to 2 weeks after contact with an infected sexual partner
3. Urethral discharge of yellow, green, brown or blood-tinged material
4. Dysuria is usually localized to the distal penis or urethral meatus. It is most severe during the first morning void. It is exacerbated by alcohol
5. Urinary frequency and urgency are usually absent and suggest prostatitis or cystitis
6. Itching of the urethra or irritation may persist between voidings. Some patients report itching rather than pain or burning with urination
7. Orchialgia may occur in men expressed as heaviness in the genitals. Testicular pain may be epididymitis or orchitis
8. Symptoms may worsen during the menstrual period
9. Systemic symptoms are usually absent (fever, chills, hyperhidrosis, or nausea).
10. If systemic symptoms are present they may be from:
    a. Disseminated gonococcemia
    b. Pyelonephritis
    c. Arthritis
    d. Pneumonia
    e. Otitis media
    f. Reactive arthritis
    g. Iritis
    h. Rash that involves the palms and soles

Pathology

1. Neisseria gonorrhoeae
2. Chlamydia trachomatis
3. Ureaplasma urealyticum
4. Mycoplasma hominis
5. Mycoplasma genitalium
6. Trichomonas vaginalis
7. Multiple rare organisms
8. Post traumatic urethritis occurs in 2 to 20% of patients with intermittent catheterization

Laboratory Evaluation

1. Demonstration of a mucopurulent or purulent discharge
2. A urethral smear with 5 or more leukocytes per oil immersion field
3. A first voided specimen with leukocyte esterase on dipstick

4. More than 30% of patients with NGU have no leukocytes in their urine
5. PCR assays for gonococcal urethritis and Chlamydia infections

Pyelonephritis

General Characteristics

1. A population based study in the USA demonstrated a rate of 15-17 patients per 10,000 females and 3-4 male patients per 10,000 of the population
2. Some women who initially present with lower urinary tract symptomatology have pyelonephritis

Clinical Manifestations

1. The classic triad of acute pyelonephritis is fever, costovertebral angle pain, nausea, and vomiting. The signs and symptoms may not present concomitantly and all may not occur
2. Signs and symptoms develop rapidly usually over hours to a day. Rarely they are insidious and develop over weeks
3. Symptoms of cystitis may be concomitant
4. Pain:
    a. Pain may be mild to severe
    b. Flank pain is usually more severe over the affected kidney but may be bilateral
    c. Pain may radiate to the lower middle lumbar dermatomes as well as across the surapubic area
    d. Suprapubic radiations may be described as:
        i Discomfort
        ii Heaviness
        iii Pressure
    e. Upper abdominal pain is unusual
    f. Radiation of pain to the groin suggests a ureteral stone
5. Fever is not always present but if present may exceed 103oF (39.4oC). Patients may have rigor and chills without fever
6. Malaise is frequent and severe
7. Anorexia is common; nausea and vomiting vary and diarrhea is rare
8. Elderly patients may present with fever, alteration of mental status or decompensation in another organ system

Physical Examination

1. If fever is present it may be greater than 103°F (39.4°C); it may be subnormal in patients with gram negative sepsis
2. Tachycardia is frequent in association with dehydration and sepsis
3. Low blood pressure suggests shock from sepsis or perinephric abscess
4. There is suprapubic tenderness without rebound; there is no rigidity or

guarding. Bowel sounds are usually normally active

5. Pelvic examination:
   a. Cervical, adnexal and uterine tenderness should be absent

Renal Abscesses

Clinical Manifestations

1. Corticomedullary abscess:
   a. Patients present with chills, fever, flank and abdominal pain
   b. There is often dysuria and nausea and vomiting
   c. The abscess is usually associated with vesicoureteral reflux or obstruction

Perinephric Abscess

Clinical Manifestation

1. The abscess is located between the renal capsule and the renal fascia and is secondary to chronic or recurrent pyelonephritis, rupture of a suppurative process from the kidney, dissemination from the blood
2. The abscess is usually restricted to the perinephric space but can extend to the colon, flank, and groin. Unusual extension is to the lung, paracervical region, peritoneal cavity, psoas muscle, skin or the subphrenic space
3. Symptoms develop insidiously and may include:
   a. Fever and chills
   b. 70% have unilateral flank pain
   c. Dysuria (40% of patients)
   d. Nausea and vomiting
   e. Costovertebral angle tenderness
   f. Pain may be referred to the hip, thigh or knee
   g. A flank or abdominal mass may be palpated in less than 50% of patients
   h. Curvature of the spine away from the involved kidney

Renal Cortical Abscess

Clinical Manifestation

1. Patients present with chills, fever and flank or abdominal pain
2. Physical examination may demonstrate a flank or lumbar mass

Pathology

1. Complications occur in patients with diabetes mellitus, chronic renal disease, all forms of immunosuppression, renal transplantation and HIV infection
2. Complications include:
   a. Acute kidney injury
   b. Chronic hypertension and renal failure
   c. Sepsis (most often gram negative)

   d. Renal papillary necrosis
   e. Xanthogranulomatous pyelonephritis
3. Corticomedullary abscess:
   a. Usually associated with a urinary tract anomaly (vesicoureteral reflux or obstruction)
   b. The usual organism is Enterobacteriaceae
4. Perinephric abscess:
   a. The abscess is located between the renal capsule and the encompassing renal fascia
   b. The suppuration is usually from chronic pyelonephritis
5. Renal cortical abscess
   a. Usually caused by hematogenous spread of S. aureus; more common in men than women

Laboratory Evaluation

1. Urinalysis
2. Urine culture

Imaging

1. CT to delineate alteration in renal parenchymal perfusion, contrast excretion, perinephric fluid and nonrenal disease
2. MRI for evaluation of infection, masses, obstruction and vasculature
3. Ultrasonography
4. Scintigraphy

Pelvic Pain in Females

Ovary Cysts

General Characteristics

1. Ovarian cysts are demonstrated by ultrasound (transvaginal) in a large proportion of premenopausal women and up to 18% of post-menopausal women
2. Mature cystic dermoids are greater than than 10% of all ovarian neoplasms
3. Luteal cysts are seen after ovulation in reproductive-age women and most benign neoplastic cysts occur during this period

Clinical Manifestations

1. Most patients with ovarian cysts are asymptomatic and are found during routine pelvic examination or by ultrasonography
2. Malignant ovarian cysts often do not cause symptoms until they are advanced
3. Pain or discomfort in the lower abdomen
4. Discomfort (dyspareunia) with intercourse
5. Difficulty with defecation

6. Tenesmus and desire to defecate if the cyst puts pressure on the large bowel
7. Increased micturition from pressure on the bladder
8. Irregular menstrual periods with abnormal vaginal bleeding
9. Abdominal fullness and bloating
10. Early satiety, indigestion or heartburn
11. Associated with endometriosis
12. Dull bilateral pain (theca-lutein cysts)
13. Adnexal or cervical motion tenderness
14. Cyst rupture or torsion:
    a. Severe acute pain
    b. Sharp and unilateral pelvic pain that may be associated with trauma, exercise or coitus
    c. Abdominal distension
    d. Hyperpyrexia
    e. Abdominal rebound tenderness and guarding
    f. A large cyst may be palpable on abdominal examination

Pathology

1. An ovarian cyst is a fluid filled sac within the ovary
2. Most ovarian cysts are related to the ovulatory cycle and are either follicular or corpus luteum cysts
3. Other cysts include:
    a. Those due to endometriosis
    b. Dermoids
    c. Cystadenomas
    d. Pelvic inflammatory disease
    e. Rarely in association with pelvic cancer

Laboratory Evaluation

1. Urinary pregnancy test
2. CBC
3. Urinalysis
4. Cancer antigens CA125

Imaging

1. Ultrasonography
2. Definitive diagnosis is based on histologic analysis

Ovarian Cancer

General Characteristics

1. Ovarian cancer develops from germ cells, stromal cells or epithelial cells:
    a. Epithelial ovarian cancer is the most common and the leading cause of

death from gynecologic cancer in the USA

b. Epithelial cancers are uncommon prior to age 40 and have a higher incidence in women with a family history, those that have been exposed to asbestos or talc and those with disordered ovarian function

2. Familial cases cause approximately 10% of all ovarian cancer
3. Two types of autosomal dominant familial cancers have been delineated:
   a. Breast / ovarian cancer syndrome and
   b. Lynch type II cancer family syndrome
4. Two susceptibility genes have been identified in hereditary breast / ovarian cancer, BRCA1 located on chromosome 17q12-21 and BRCA2 that maps to chromosome 13q12-13. Both are tumor suppressor genes that synthesize nuclear proteins that interact with RAD51 that assists in the repair of DNA double strand breaks. RAD51 is overexpressed in many cancers

Clinical Manifestations

1. Approximately 70% of patients are diagnosed after the cancer has spread beyond the pelvis
2. Abdominal pain, bloating and urinary symptoms are indications of advanced disease
3. Localized ovarian cancer is most often asymptomatic. If symptomatic, patients complain of:
   a. Progressive enlargement of an ovarian tumor may produce urinary frequency or constipation
   b. Rarely torsion of the mass causes an acute abdomen
   c. There is rare vaginal bleeding
   d. Physical examination may reveal a palpable adnexal mass
   e. The mass is solid, irregular and fixed; other adnexal masses include:
      i Pedunculated uterine fibroid
      ii Endometriosis
      iii Benign ovarian neoplasms
      iv Inflammatory bowel disease

Pathology

1. Epithelial tumors account for 85% of ovarian neoplasms, approximately 1/3 of which are malignant. Epithelial tumors of malignant potential have cytological features of malignancy but have not invaded the stroma
2. The other two types of malignancies of the ovary are stromal and germ cell tumors
3. Metastases to the ovary occur from the breast, colon, pancreas, and stomach. The Krukenberg tumor is a bilateral ovarian metastasis from a mucin secreting gastrointestinal cancer

Laboratory Evaluation

1. CA-125 is relatively insensitive

Imaging

1. Abdominal CT or MRI scans delineate the tumor and the extent of its spread
2. Ultrasonography of the abdomen and pelvis are useful screening procedures. Transvaginal sonography is frequently used but is associated with significant false-positives

Uterine Cancer

General Characteristics

1. Carcinoma of the endometrium is the most common female pelvic malignancy. Approximately 75% of these tumors are restricted to the body of the uterus at the time of diagnosis and are curable
2. It is a disease of postmenopausal women. Approximately 25% of women are affected prior to fifty years of age
3. Risk factors include:
   a. Obesity
   b. Low fertility index
   c. Early menarche
   d. Late menopause
   e. Chronic anovulation
4. Chronic unopposed estrogen replacement and tamoxifen use have increased risk

Clinical Manifestations

1. The cancer occurs most frequently in the sixth and seventh decades
2. Abnormal vaginal discharge (90%), abnormal postmenopausal bleeding (80%), and leucorrhea (10%)
3. Rarely there is pain with micturition, intercourse and in the pelvis
4. Uterine papillary, serous or clear cell cancers may present with abdominal pain and bloating or with symptoms from metastasis
5. Uterine sarcomas present similarly to endometrial carcinomas with vaginal bleeding or pelvic pressure
6. Leiomyosarcoma present most commonly in the sixth decade with irregular menses or postmenopausal bleeding, pelvic pain or pressure and a rapidly expanding pelvic mass. There is a similar presentation for endometrial stromal carcinoma
7. Weight loss, anorexia, pelvic pain or pressure associated with difficulties with micturition and defecation are signs and symptoms of advanced uterine cancer

Pathology

1. Approximately 80% of endometrial carcinomas are endometrial adenocarcinomas
2. Less frequent tumors include:
   a. Clear cell
   b. Papillary serous carcinoma
3. Sarcomas account for less than 9% of uterine corpus malignancies and include:
   a. Mixed homologous mullerian tumors (40-50%)
   b. Leiomyosarcomas (40%)
   c. Endometrial stromal tumors (sarcomas) (8-10%)

Laboratory Evaluation

1. Endometrial biopsy is often the first procedure performed and the degree of malignancy often determines the extent of imaging

Imaging

1. Ultrasonography helps to exclude other pelvic pathologies
2. Chest radiographs to rule out metastatic disease
3. CT of the chest, abdomen and pelvis in all patients with high grade cancer and those with sarcoma of the uterine body

Uterine Leiomyoma (Fibroids)

General Characteristics

1. Definition:
   a. Leiomyomas of the uterus are benign growths that arise from the smooth muscle and connective tissue of the uterus
   b. Rarely a uterine leiomyoma undergoes malignant transformation to a leiomyosarcoma. The incidence of this occurrence is less than 1% and may be as low as 0.2%
   c. Approximately 20%-30% of women develop fibroids by the age of 50. They have a genetic tendency

Clinical Manifestations

1. Small fibroids are usually asymptomatic. Signs and symptoms depend on both the location and the size of the growth
2. Abnormal uterine bleeding
3. Heavy or painful menstrual periods
4. Abdominal discomfort or bloating
5. Painful defecation
6. Low back pain
7. Urinary frequency or retention
8. Rarely infertility (possibly 3%)

9. Dyspareunia

Pathology

1. Fibroids are round, well circumscribed but not encapsulated growths
2. Histologically the cells are elongated, spindle-shaped with a cigar-shaped nucleus in a whorled pattern
3. Most fibroids arise in the muscular wall of the uterus. They may be single or multiple
4. Secondary changes in a fibroid include hemorrhage, necrosis, calcification and cyst formation
5. Rarely fibroids metastasize; they enlarge in a benign fashion but cause symptoms due to their location. Extrauterine metastasizing leiomyomas grow in the lungs and lymph nodes. They may invade blood vessels and grow diffusely on the peritoneal and omental surfaces
6. Fibroids are monoclonal tumors and 40-50% demonstrate chromosomal abnormalities
7. In 70% of patients there are specific mutations of the MED12 protein
8. Estrogen and progesterone have a mitogenic influence on leiomyoma cells

Laboratory Evaluation

1. In palpable growths on pelvic examination gynecologic ultrasound is the standard screening tool that demonstrates focal masses that are heterogenous with shadowing of the ultrasound beam
2. MRI delineates the size and location of the fibroids within the uterus

Cervical Cancer

General Characteristics

1. The mortality rate of cervical cancer has declined by 50% over the last 40 years due to the widespread screening with the Pap smear
2. It is more common in women from lower socioeconomic groups, in those with early initial sexual activity and or multiple sexual partners and in smokers

Clinical Manifestations

1. Most patients are asymptomatic. The disease is detected on pelvic examination
2. Other presentations are abnormal bleeding or postcoital bleeding or spotting that becomes more profuse intermenstrually or during menstruation
3. Lumbosacral back pain
4. Lower extremity edema
5. Urinary symptoms
6. Yellowish vaginal discharge

Pathology

1. HPV (human papilloma virus) is an important pathogenic viral infection in cervical cancer. Greater than 66 variants of HPV have been identified and many are associated with genital warts
2. HPV types associated with cervical cancer are 16, 18, 31, 33, 52, and 58; approximately 70% of patients are associated with HPV-16 and HPV-18:
   a. The protein product of HPV-16 is the E7 protein which binds and inactivates the tumor-suppressor gene Rb
   b. The E6 protein from HPV-18 binds to and inactivates the tumor suppressor gene p53
3. Uncomplicated HPV infection can progress to CIN (cervical intraepithelial neoplasia) which precedes invasive cervical carcinoma
4. Carcinoma in situ demonstrates histologic evidence of neoplasia but does not invade through the basement membrane. It can remain stable for 10 years but usually progresses to invasive carcinoma

Laboratory Evaluation

1. The Pap smear is 90 to 95% accurate for detecting cervical intraepithelial neoplasia but is less effective in detecting invasive cancer or a fungating mass
2. Colposcopic biopsy is required to evaluate any lesion visible on the cervix

Imaging

1. Chest x-ray, intravenous pyelograms, and CT are required for staging
2. MRI is important for delineating extracervical extension

Abdominal Pain in the Elderly

Biliary Tract Disease in the Elderly

General Characteristics

1. Biliary tract disease includes active cholelithiasis, choledocholithiasis, calculus and acalculous cholecystitis and ascending cholangitis
2. Approximately 30 to 50% of patients older than 65 years of age have gallstones. Cholecystitis affects approximately 10% of patients with gallstones
3. Biliary disease is one of the most common conditions of elderly patients that present with abdominal pain
4. Diagnostic difficulties occur in the 25% of elderly patients that have no significant right upper quadrant pain, less than 50% have fever, vomiting or leukocytosis
5. The major complications of biliary tract disease include:
   a. Gallbladder perforation with consequent peritonitis
   b. Emphysematous cholecystitis:
      i An acute infection of the gallbladder caused by Clostridium or Escherichia coli (gas forming organisms)

ii It is rare, but causes a rapidly progressive acute cholecystitis characterized by early gangrene, perforation of the gallbladder wall

iii Develops in approximately 1% of all patients with acute cholecystitis and is associated with a mortality of 15 to 25%

c. Symptomatic cholelithiasis

d. Choledocholithiasis

e. Calculus and acalculous cholecystitis

f. Ascending cholangitis

g. Gallstone ileus

i Associated with approximately 2% of small bowel obstructions in elderly patients

Appendicitis in the Elderly

General Characteristics

1. Approximately 10% of patients with appendicitis are 60 years of age or older. Fifty percent of deaths from appendicitis occur in this subgroup of patients.
2. The rate of perforation is approximately 5x higher in this group than in younger patients because 75% of elderly patients wait more than 24 hours before seeking medical attention
3. Approximately 50% of patients have no fever or leukocytosis at presentation
4. Approximately 1/3 of patients do not have right lower quadrant pain and 25% do not have tenderness or peritoneal signs in the right lower quadrant
5. Only 20% of elderly patients present with the classic signs of acute appendicitis (fever, anorexia and RLQ pain)

Diverticulitis in the Elderly

General Characteristics

1. Diverticulitis is rare in patients younger than 40 years of age. Diverticula occur in 50-80% of patients older than 65 years of age. Diverticulitis causes microperforation of the colon.
2. Approximately 85% of patients have the disease in the left colon
3. Right-sided diverticulitis is a more benign disorder
4. Elderly patients may be afebrile, the white count is only elevated in 50% and only 25% have a guaiac positive stool

Mesenteric Ischemia in the Elderly

General Characteristics

1. Mesenteric ischemia causes approximately less than 1% of abdominal pain in elderly patients.
2. Patients have severe abdominal pain but have minimal tenderness on

examination

3. Associated vomiting and diarrhea are common
4. Risk factors are important to make this diagnosis and include severe atherosclerosis, atrial fibrillation and a low cardiac ejection fraction
5. Recurrent postprandial abdominal pain (intestinal angina) is rare

Bowel Obstruction in the Elderly

General Characteristics

1. Bowel obstruction causes approximately 12% of abdominal pain in elderly patients.
2. Cecal volvulus is rare and usually presents as small bowel obstruction.
3. Sigmoid volvulus is more common and distention of the colon greater than 9cm is a sign of impending perforation. Major risk factors for sigmoid volvulus are inactivity and laxative use.

Abdominal Aortic Aneurysm (AAA) in the Elderly

General Characteristics

Approximately 5% of men older than 65 years of age have an AAA. The disorder is much more common in males than females with a ratio of 7:1. If the patient is hemodynamically stable at presentation, the mortality is 25% whereas presentation in shock carries a mortality of 80%.

1. Patients may present with clinical features of renal colic or back pain (often at the T10 level)

Peptic Ulcer Disease (PUD) in the Elderly

General Characteristics

1. The incidence of peptic ulcer disease is increasing in elderly patients possibly due to the use of nonsteroidal anti-inflammatory agents. If NSAIDs are used consistently, there is 5 to 10 times an increased incidence of PUD.
2. Approximately 35% of elderly patients with PUD present with no pain
3. The most common presentation is with melena
4. Perforation in elderly patients may be painless
5. Free abdominal air may be absent on abdominal radiographs in more than 68% of patients

Gastroenteritis in the Elderly

General Characteristics

Gastroenteritis is a diagnosis of exclusion in elderly patients who present with vomiting and diarrhea.

Urinary Tract Infections in the Elderly

General Characteristics

The usual symptoms of dysuria, frequency, and urgency are less common in elderly patients. Patients may present with alterations of mental status with or without fever.

Unusual Causes of Abdominal Pain in Elderly Patients

General Characteristics

Both myocardial infarction and pneumonia may rarely present as vague abdominal pain.

CHAPTER 9

SUGGESTED REFERENCES FOR CLINICAL PAIN

Master List – Alphabetically Ordered

ABDOMINAL AORTIC ANEURYSM

Azhar, B. et al., 2014. Misdiagnosis of Ruptured Abdominal Aortic Aneurysm: Systematic Review and Meta-Analysis. Journal of Endovascular Therapy, 21(4), pp.568–575. http://dx.doi.org/10.1583/13-4626mr.1.

Hernesniemi, J.A., Vänni, V. & Hakala, T., 2015. The prevalence of abdominal aortic aneurysm is consistently high among patients with coronary artery disease. Journal of Vascular Surgery, 62(1), pp.232–240.e3. http://dx.doi.org/10.1016/j.jvs.2015.02.037.

ABDOMINAL PAIN IN THE ELDERLY

Coulie, MD, PhD, B. & Camilleri, MD, M., 1999. Intestinal Pseudo-obstruction. Annual Review of Medicine, 50(1), pp.37–55.
http://dx.doi.org/10.1146/annurev.med.50.1.37.

Esses, D. et al., 2004. Ability of CT to alter decision making in elderly patients with acute abdominal pain. The American Journal of Emergency Medicine, 22(4), pp.270–272. http://dx.doi.org/10.1016/j.ajem.2004.04.004.

Huang, Q. et al., 2015. Predictors of intestinal pseudo-obstruction in systemic lupus erythematosus complicated by digestive manifestations: data from a Southern China lupus cohort. Lupus, 25(3), pp.248–254. http://dx.doi.org/10.1177/0961203315605366.

Kizer, K.W. & Vassar, M.J., 1998. Emergency department diagnosis of abdominal disorders in the elderly. The American Journal of Emergency Medicine, 16(4), pp.357–362. http://dx.doi.org/10.1016/s0735-6757(98)90127-9.

Lewis, L.M. et al., 2005. Etiology and Clinical Course of Abdominal Pain in Senior Patients: A Prospective, Multicenter Study. The Journals of Gerontology Series A: Biological Sciences and Medical Sciences, 60(8), pp.1071–1076. http://dx.doi.org/10.1093/gerona/60.8.1071.

Saunders, M.D., 2007. Acute colonic pseudo-obstruction. Best Practice & Research Clinical Gastroenterology, 21(4), pp.671–687. http://dx.doi.org/10.1016/j.bpg.2007.03.001.

Vanek, V.W. & Al-Salti, M., 1986. Acute pseudo-obstruction of the colon (Ogilvie's syndrome). Diseases of the Colon & Rectum, 29(3), pp.203–210. http://dx.doi.org/10.1007/bf02555027.

ABSENCE OF C2

Baumgart, M. et al., 2016. Morphometric study of the neural ossification centers of the atlas and axis in the human fetus. Surgical and Radiologic Anatomy, 38(10), pp.1205–1215. http://dx.doi.org/10.1007/s00276-016-1681-2.

Chau, A.M.T., Wong, J.H.-Y. & Mobbs, R.J., 2009. Cervical Myelopathy Associated With Congenital C2/3 Canal Stenosis and Deficiencies of the Posterior Arch of the Atlas and Laminae of the Axis. Spine, 34(24), pp.E886–E891. http://dx.doi.org/10.1097/brs.0b013e3181b64f0a.

Hosalkar, H.S. et al., 2008. Congenital Osseous Anomalies of the Upper Cervical Spine. The Journal of Bone and Joint Surgery-American Volume, 90(2), pp.337–348. http://dx.doi.org/10.2106/jbjs.g.00014.

Srivastava, S.K. et al., 2016. Congenital Absence of Posterior Elements of C2 Vertebra with Atlanto-Axial Dislocation and Basilar Invagination: A Case Report and Review of Literature. Asian Spine Journal, 10(1), p.170. http://dx.doi.org/10.4184/asj.2016.10.1.170.

ACUTE APPENDICITIS

Gorter, R.R. et al., 2016. Diagnosis and management of acute appendicitis. EAES consensus development conference 2015. Surgical Endoscopy, 30(11), pp.4668–4690. http://dx.doi.org/10.1007/s00464-016-5245-7.

Katagiri, H. et al., 2016. Barium appendicitis: A single institution review in Japan. World Journal of Gastrointestinal Surgery, 8(9), p.651. http://dx.doi.org/10.4240/wjgs.v8.i9.651.

Segev, L. et al., 2016. Appendectomy in Pregnancy: Appraisal of the Minimally Invasive Approach. Journal of Laparoendoscopic & Advanced Surgical Techniques, 26(11), pp.893–897. http://dx.doi.org/10.1089/lap.2016.0280.

ACRYLAMIDE

Wei, X. et al., 2015. Neuroprotective Effect of Calpeptin on Acrylamide-Induced Neuropathy in Rats. Neurochemical Research, 40(11), pp.2325–2332. Available at: http://dx.doi.org/10.1007/s11064-015-1722-y.

Perez-Saad, H. et al., 2017. Neuroprotective effect of epidermal growth factor in experimental acrylamide neuropathy: an electrophysiological approach. Journal of the Peripheral Nervous System, 22(2), pp.106–111. Available at: http://dx.doi.org/10.1111/jns.12214.

ACUTE PERITONITIS

Abdalla, S.M., Kalra, G. & Moshiree, B., 2016. Motility Evaluation in the Patient with Inflammatory Bowel Disease. Gastrointestinal Endoscopy Clinics of North America, 26(4), pp.719–738. http://dx.doi.org/10.1016/j.giec.2016.06.010.

Asicioglu, E. et al., 2010. Unusual presentation of peritonitis with persistent clear aspirate: a case report. Journal of Medical Case Reports, 4(1). http://dx.doi.org/10.1186/1752-1947-4-383.

Blevrakis, Evangelos et al., 2016. Primary bacterial peritonitis in a previously healthy adolescent female: A case report. International Journal of Surgery Case Reports, 28, pp.111–113. http://dx.doi.org/10.1016/j.ijscr.2016.09.009.

Hirata, Y., Ihara, S. & Koike, K., 2016. Targeting the complex interactions between microbiota, host epithelial and immune cells in inflammatory bowel disease. Pharmacological Research, 113, pp.574–584. http://dx.doi.org/10.1016/j.phrs.2016.09.044.

Law, S.-T. & Li, K.K., 2013. Age-related differences in the clinical course of Crohn's disease in an asian population: A retrospective cohort review. Indian Pediatrics, 50(12), pp.1148–1152. http://dx.doi.org/10.1007/s13312-013-0301-z.

Lobo, L.A., Benjamim, C.F. & Oliveira, A.C., 2016. The interplay between microbiota and inflammation: lessons from peritonitis and sepsis. Clinical & Translational Immunology, 5(7), p.e90. http://dx.doi.org/10.1038/cti.2016.32.

Lopez, R.N. et al., 2016. Faecal Biomarkers in Inflammatory Bowel Disease. Journal of Gastroenterology and Hepatology. http://dx.doi.org/10.1111/jgh.13611.

Roggenbuck,D.,Reinhold,D., Baumgart,D.C., Schierack,P., Conrad,K., Laass, M.W. 2016. Autoimmunity in Crohn's Disease—A Putative Stratification Factor of the Clinical Phenotype, 77, pp.77-101. https://www.ncbi.nlm.nih.gov/pubmed/27717419

Ştefănescu, D. et al., 2016. Advanced Endoscopic Imaging Techniques for the Study of Colonic Mucosa in Patients with Inflammatory Bowel Disease. Romanian Journal Of Internal Medicine, 54(1). http://dx.doi.org/10.1515/rjim-2015-0050.

ACUTE POLYNEUROPATHY CYTOSINE ARABINOSIDE

Nevill, T.J., Benstead, T.J., McCormick, C.W. and Hayne, O.A., 1989. Horner's syndrome and demyelinating peripheral neuropathy caused by high-dose cytosine arabinoside. American journal of hematology, 32(4), pp.314-315. https://doi.org/10.1002/ajh.2830320414

Openshaw, H., et al., 1996, Acute polyneuropathy after high dose cytosine arabinoside in patients with leukemia. Cancer, 78(9), pp. 1899-1905. https://www.ncbi.nlm.nih.gov/pubmed/8909309

ADHESIVE ARACHNOIDITIS

Carlswärd, C. et al., 2016. Chronic Adhesive Arachnoiditis After Repeat Epidural Blood Patch. Obstetric Anesthesia Digest, 36(2), pp.112–113. http://dx.doi.org/10.1097/01.aoa.0000482649.39000.84.

Idris, Z., Ghazali, F. & Abdullah, J., 2014. Fibromyalgia and arachnoiditis presented as an acute spinal disorder. Surgical Neurology International, 5(1), p.151. http://dx.doi.org/10.4103/2152-7806.143364.

Petty, P.G., Hudgson, P. & Hare, W.S.C., 2000. Symptomatic lumbar spinal arachnoiditis: fact or fallacy? Journal of Clinical Neuroscience, 7(5), pp.395–399. http://dx.doi.org/10.1054/jocn.1999.0223.

Riley, C.A. & Spiegel, J.E., 2009. Complications following large-volume epidural blood patches for postdural puncture headache. Lumbar subdural hematoma and arachnoiditis: initial cause or final effect? Journal of Clinical Anesthesia, 21(5), pp.355–359. http://dx.doi.org/10.1016/j.jclinane.2008.08.028.

AGE RELATED PAIN DIFFERENCES

Briggs, A.M. et al., 2016. Musculoskeletal Health Conditions Represent a Global Threat to Healthy Aging: A Report for the 2015 World Health Organization World Report on Ageing and Health. The Gerontologist, 56(Suppl 2), pp.S243–S255. Available at: http://dx.doi.org/10.1093/geront/gnw002.

Oosterman, J.M. & Veldhuijzen, D.S., 2016. On the interplay between chronic pain and age with regard to neurocognitive integrity: Two interacting conditions? Neuroscience & Biobehavioral Reviews, 69, pp.174–192. Available at: http://dx.doi.org/10.1016/j.neubiorev.2016.07.009.

Molton, I.R. & Terrill, A.L., 2014. Overview of persistent pain in older adults. American Psychologist, 69(2), pp.197–207. Available at: http://dx.doi.org/10.1037/a0035794.

Gagliese, L., 2009. Pain and Aging: The Emergence of a New Subfield of Pain Research. The Journal of Pain, 10(4), pp.343–353. Available at: http://dx.doi.org/10.1016/j.jpain.2008.10.013.

ALCOHOL

Zeng, L., Alongkronrusmee, D. & van Rijn, R.M., 2017. An integrated perspective on diabetic, alcoholic, and drug-induced neuropathy, etiology, and treatment in the US. Journal of Pain Research, Volume 10, pp.219–228. Available at: http://dx.doi.org/10.2147/jpr.s125987.

Wöhrle, J.C. et al., 1998. Alcohol-Related Acute Axonal Polyneuropathy. Archives of Neurology, 55(10), p.1329. Available at: http://dx.doi.org/10.1001/archneur.55.10.1329.

Koike, H. et al., 2001. Painful alcoholic polyneuropathy with predominant small-fiber loss and normal thiamine status. Neurology, 56(12), pp.1727–1732. Available at: http://dx.doi.org/10.1212/wnl.56.12.1727.

Chopra, K. & Tiwari, V., 2012. Alcoholic neuropathy: possible mechanisms and future treatment possibilities. British Journal of Clinical Pharmacology, 73(3), pp.348–362. Available at: http://dx.doi.org/10.1111/j.1365-2125.2011.04111.x.

ALTERNATING HEMIPLEGIA OF CHILDHOOD

Heimer, G. et al., 2015. CAOS--Episodic Cerebellar Ataxia, Areflexia, Optic Atrophy, and Sensorineural Hearing Loss: A Third Allelic Disorder of the ATP1A3 Gene. Journal of Child Neurology, 30(13), pp.1749–1756. http://dx.doi.org/10.1177/0883073815579708.

Holm, T.H. & Lykke-Hartmann, K., 2016. Insights into the Pathology of the α3 Na+/K+-ATPase Ion Pump in Neurological Disorders; Lessons from Animal Models. Frontiers in Physiology, 7. http://dx.doi.org/10.3389/fphys.2016.00209.

Sweney, M.T., Newcomb, T.M. & Swoboda, K.J., 2015. The Expanding Spectrum of Neurological Phenotypes in Children With ATP1A3 Mutations, Alternating Hemiplegia of Childhood, Rapid-onset Dystonia-Parkinsonism, CAPOS and Beyond. Pediatric Neurology, 52(1), pp.56–64.

http://dx.doi.org/10.1016/j.pediatrneurol.2014.09.015.

Swoboda, K.J. et al., 2004. Alternating hemiplegia of childhood or familial hemiplegic migraine?: A novelATP1A2 mutation. Annals of Neurology, 55(6), pp.884–887. http://dx.doi.org/10.1002/ana.20134.

AMIODARONE

Niimi, N. et al., 2016. Involvement of oxidative stress and impaired lysosomal degradation in amiodarone-induced schwannopathy M. Watanabe, ed. European Journal of Neuroscience, 44(1), pp.1723–1733. http://dx.doi.org/10.1111/ejn.13268.

Rosseti, N. et al., 2010. Amiodarone-related pneumonitis and peripheral neuropathy in an elderly patient. Aging Clinical and Experimental Research, 22(5-6), pp.466–469. http://dx.doi.org/10.1007/bf03324945.

Ankylosing Spondylitis Blair, H.A. & Dhillon, S., 2016. Secukinumab: A Review in Ankylosing Spondylitis. Drugs, 76(10), pp.1023–1030.

http://dx.doi.org/10.1007/s40265-016-0598-8.

Braun, J. & Sieper, J., 2007. Ankylosing spondylitis. The Lancet, 369(9570), pp.1379–1390. http://dx.doi.org/10.1016/s0140-6736(07)60635-7.

Hung, Y.-M. et al., 2016. Midlife Ankylosing Spondylitis Increases the Risk of Cardiovascular Diseases in Males 5 Years Later. Medicine, 95(18), p.e3596. http://dx.doi.org/10.1097/md.0000000000003596.

Nuki, G., 1998. Ankylosing spondylitis, HLA B27, and beyond. The Lancet, 351(9105), pp.767–769. http://dx.doi.org/10.1016/s0140-6736(05)78922-4.

Osman, M.S. & Maksymowych, W.P., 2016. An update on the use of tumor necrosis factor alpha inhibitors in the treatment of ankylosing spondylitis. Expert Review of

Clinical Immunology, pp.1–7. http://dx.doi.org/10.1080/1744666x.2016.1218761.

Toussirot, E., 2012. The IL23/Th17 Pathway as a Therapeutic Target in Chronic Inflammatory Diseases. Inflammation & Allergy-Drug Targets, 11(2), pp.159–168. http://dx.doi.org/10.2174/187152812800392805.

Weiss, B.G. et al., 2015. Whole Body Magnetic Resonance Imaging Features in Diffuse Idiopathic Skeletal Hyperostosis in Conjunction with Clinical Variables to Whole Body MRI and Clinical Variables in Ankylosing Spondylitis. The Journal of Rheumatology, 43(2), pp.335–342. http://dx.doi.org/10.3899/jrheum.150162.

ANTERIOR CUTANEOUS NERVE

Chrona, E. et al., 2017. Anterior cutaneous nerve entrapment syndrome: management challenges. Journal of Pain Research, Volume 10, pp.145–156. Available at: http://dx.doi.org/10.2147/jpr.s99337.

Applegate, W., 2002. Abdominal Cutaneous Nerve Entrapment Syndrome (ACNES): A Commonly Overlooked Cause of Abdominal Pain. The Permanente Journal, 6(3), pp 20-27. Available at:
https://www.thepermanentejournal.org/files/Summer2002/acnes.pdf

Van Assen, T. et al., 2015. Incidence of abdominal pain due to the anterior cutaneous nerve entrapment syndrome in an emergency department. Scandinavian Journal of Trauma, Resuscitation and Emergency Medicine, 23(1), p.19. Available at: http://dx.doi.org/10.1186/s13049-015-0096-0.

Applegate, W., 1997. Microanatomy of the structures contributing to abdominal cutaneous nerve entrapment syndrome. J Am Board Fam Pract.,10(5), pp. 329-32. Abstract available at: https://www.ncbi.nlm.nih.gov/pubmed/9297657

ANTERIOR CUTANEOUS NERVE ENTRAPMENT

Glissen Brown, J.R. et al., 2016. Chronic Abdominal Wall Pain. Journal of Clinical Gastroenterology, 50(10), pp.828–835. http://dx.doi.org/10.1097/mcg.0000000000000636.

Rivero Fernández M, Moreira Vicente V, Riesco López JM, Rodríguez Gandía MA, Garrido Gómez E, Milicua Salamero JM. [Pain originating from the abdominal wall: a forgotten diagnostic option]. Gastroenterol Hepatol. 2007 Apr;30(4):244-50. Review. Spanish. http://europepmc.org/abstract/med/17408555

Roumen RM, Scheltinga MR. [Abdominal intercostal neuralgia: a forgotten cause of abdominal pain]. Ned Tijdschr Geneeskd. 2006 Sep 2;150(35):1909-15. Dutch. https://www.ncbi.nlm.nih.gov/pubmed/16999272

Rozen, W.M. et al., 2008. Refining the course of the thoracolumbar nerves: A new understanding of the innervation of the anterior abdominal wall. Clinical Anatomy, 21(4), pp.325–333. http://dx.doi.org/10.1002/ca.20621.

Van Assen, T. et al., 2015. Incidence of abdominal pain due to the anterior cutaneous nerve entrapment syndrome in an emergency department. Scandinavian Journal of Trauma, Resuscitation and Emergency Medicine, 23(1), p.19. http://dx.doi.org/10.1186/s13049-015-0096-0.

ANTERIOR INTEROSSEOUS NERVE

Komaru, Y. & Inokuchi, R., 2017. Anterior interosseous nerve syndrome. QJM, 110 (4), pp. 243. Available at: http://dx.doi.org/10.1093/qjmed/hcw227.

Kowalska, B. et al., 2012. Ultrasound assessment on selected peripheral nerve pathologies. Part I: Entrapment neuropathies of the upper limb – excluding carpal tunnel syndrome. Journal of Ultrasonography, 12(50), pp.307–318. Available at: http://dx.doi.org/10.15557/jou.2012.0016.

Strohl, A.B. & Zelouf, D.S., 2017. Ulnar Tunnel Syndrome, Radial Tunnel Syndrome, Anterior Interosseous Nerve Syndrome, and Pronator Syndrome. Journal of the American Academy of Orthopaedic Surgeons, 25(1), pp.e1–e10. Available at: http://dx.doi.org/10.5435/jaaos-d-16-00010.

APERT SYNDROME

Breik, O. et al., 2016. Central nervous system and cervical spine abnormalities in Apert syndrome. Child's Nervous System, 32(5), pp.833–838. http://dx.doi.org/10.1007/s00381-016-3036-z.

Thompson, D.N. et al., 2008. Congenital Cervical Spinal Fusion; A Study in Apert Syndrome. Pediatric Neurosurgery, 25(1), pp.20–27. http://dx.doi.org/10.1159/000121091.

Arsenic Fowler, B.A. & Weissberg, J.B., 1974. Arsine Poisoning. New England Journal of Medicine, 291(22), pp.1171–1174. http://dx.doi.org/10.1056/nejm197411282912207.

Kuhn, M. et al., 2016. Severe acute axonal neuropathy following treatment with arsenic trioxide for acute promyelocytic leukemia: a case report. Mediterranean Journal of Hematology and Infectious Diseases, 8, p.2016023. http://dx.doi.org/10.4084/mjhid.2016.023.

Massey, E.W., 1981. Arsenic neuropathy. Neurology, 31(8), pp.1057–1057. http://dx.doi.org/10.1212/wnl.31.8.1057-a.

ATYPICAL ODONTALGIA

Baad-Hansen, L., 2008. Atypical odontalgia - pathophysiology and clinical management. Journal of Oral Rehabilitation, 35(1), pp.1–11. http://dx.doi.org/10.1111/j.1365-2842.2007.01813.x.

Balasubramaniam, R. Okeson, J.P., et al., 2011. Non-odontogenic toothache revisited. Open Journal of Stomatology, 01(03), pp.92–102. http://dx.doi.org/10.4236/ojst.2011.13015.

Marbach, J.J. et al., 1982. Incidence of phantom tooth pain: An atypical facial neuralgia. Oral Surgery, Oral Medicine, Oral Pathology, 53(2), pp.190–193. http://dx.doi.org/10.1016/0030-4220(82)90285-7.

Melis, M. et al., 2003. Atypical Odontalgia: A Review of the Literature. Headache: The Journal of Head and Face Pain, 43(10), pp.1060–1074. http://dx.doi.org/10.1046/j.1526-4610.2003.03207.x.

Okeson, J.P. et al., 2000 Non-odontogenic toothache. North-west Dent, 79, pp 37-44. https://www.ncbi.nlm.nih.gov/labs/articles/11413614/

Okeson, J.P. et al., 2000. Nonodentogenic Toothache. Tex. Dent J, 117:64-74 https://www.ncbi.nlm.nih.gov/pubmed/11858065

Sotorra-Figuerola, D. et al., 2016. Continuous neurophatic orofacial pain: A retrospective study of 23 cases. Journal of Clinical and Experimental Dentistry, 8(2), pp. e153-9. http://dx.doi.org/10.4317/jced.52560.

Vickers, E.R. et al., 1998. Analysis of 50 patients with atypical odontalgia. Oral Surgery, Oral Medicine, Oral Pathology, Oral Radiology, and Endodontology, 85(1), pp.24–32. http://dx.doi.org/10.1016/s1079-2104(98)90393-6.

Zakrzewska, J.M., 2013. Multi-dimensionality of chronic pain of the oral cavity and face. The Journal of Headache and Pain, 14(1), p.37. http://dx.doi.org/10.1186/1129-2377-14-37.

AVULSION INJURY

Chu, T.-H. & Wu, W., 2009. Neurotrophic Factor Treatment After Spinal Root Avulsion Injury. Central Nervous System Agents in Medicinal Chemistry, 9(1), pp.40–55. http://dx.doi.org/10.2174/187152409787601914.

Eggers, R. et al., 2015. Clinical and neurobiological advances in promoting regeneration of the ventral root avulsion lesion D. Kirik, ed. European Journal of Neuroscience, 43(3), pp.318–335. http://dx.doi.org/10.1111/ejn.13089.

Sporns, P.B., Fortmann, T., Zimmer, S., Zoubi, T. and Schwindt, W., 2015. Traumatic plexus lesion with cervicothoracic root avulsions and vertical laceration of the spinal cord. RöFo: Fortschritte auf dem Gebiete der Röntgenstrahlen und der Nuklearmedizin, 187(10), p.938. https://www.ncbi.nlm.nih.gov/pubmed/26019050

AXILLARY NERVE

Perlmutter, G.S., 1999. Axillary Nerve Injury. Clinical Orthopaedics and Related Research, 368, p.28-36. Available at: http://dx.doi.org/10.1097/00003086-199911000-00005.

Perlmutter, G.S. & Apruzzese, W., 1998. Axillary Nerve Injuries in Contact Sports. Sports Medicine, 26(5), pp.351–361. Available at: http://dx.doi.org/10.2165/00007256-199826050-00005

B6 (PYRIDOXINE) DEFICIENCY

Albin, R.L. et al., 1987. Acute sensory neuropathy-neuronopathy from pyridoxine overdose. Neurology, 37(11), pp.1729–1729. http://dx.doi.org/10.1212/wnl.37.11.1729.

Gandhi, A.K. et al., 2012. Crystal Structures of Human Pyridoxal Kinase in Complex with the Neurotoxins, Ginkgotoxin and Theophylline: Insights into Pyridoxal Kinase Inhibition I. Silman, ed. PLoS ONE, 7(7), p.e40954. http://dx.doi.org/10.1371/journal.pone.0040954.

Ghavanini, A.A. & Kimpinski, K., 2014. Revisiting the Evidence for Neuropathy Caused by Pyridoxine Deficiency and Excess. Journal of Clinical Neuromuscular Disease, 16(1), pp.25–31. http://dx.doi.org/10.1097/cnd.0000000000000049.

Lheureux, P., Penaloza, A. & Gris, M., 2005. Pyridoxine in clinical toxicology: a review. European Journal of Emergency Medicine, 12(2), pp.78–85. http://dx.doi.org/10.1097/00063110-200504000-00007.

BACKPACK PALSY

Mäkelä, J.P. et al., 2006. Brachial Plexus Lesions after Backpack Carriage in Young Adults. Clinical Orthopaedics and Related Research, 452, pp.205–209. http://dx.doi.org/10.1097/01.blo.0000229338.29277.29.

Nylund, T. et al., 2011. Recovery of brachial plexus lesions resulting from heavy backpack use: A follow-up case series. BMC Musculoskeletal Disorders, 12(1). http://dx.doi.org/10.1186/1471-2474-12-62.

BEHÇET'S DISEASE

Hatemi, G., Seyahi, E., Fresko, I., Talarico, R. and Hamuryudan, V., 2014. Behçet's syndrome: a critical digest of the 2013-2014 literature. Clin Exp Rheumatol, 32(4 Suppl 84), pp.S112-S122. https://www.ncbi.nlm.nih.gov/pubmed/26487500

Morton, L.T., Situnayake, D. & Wallace, G.R., 2016. Genetics of Behçet's disease. Current Opinion in Rheumatology, 28(1), pp.39–44. http://dx.doi.org/10.1097/bor.0000000000000234.

Noel N, Drier A, Wechsler B, Piette JC, De Paz R, Dormont D et al, 2014, Neurological manifestations of Behcet's disease. Rev Med Interne. 2014 Feb;35(2):112-20. http://dx.doi:10.1016/j.jcv.2016.03.003.

BORNHOLM'S DISEASE

Kenzaka, T. et al., 2016. A case of epidemic myalgia with symptoms resembling acute purulent spondylitis and discitis. BMC Musculoskeletal Disorders, 17(1). http://dx.doi.org/10.1186/s12891-016-1181-x.

Mizuta, K. et al., 2012. Epidemic Myalgia in Adults Associated with Human Parechovirus Type 3 Infection, Yamagata, Japan, 2008. Emerging Infectious Diseases, 18(11), pp.1787–1793. http://dx.doi.org/10.3201/eid1811.111570.

BORTEZOMIB

Abid, M.B. et al., 2016. Bortezomib-related neuropathy may mask CNS relapse in multiple myeloma: A call for diligence. Cancer Biology & Therapy, 17(7), pp.723–726. http://dx.doi.org/10.1080/15384047.2016.1178427.

Badros, A. et al., 2007. Neurotoxicity of bortezomib therapy in multiple myeloma: A single-center experience and review of the literature. Cancer, 110(5), pp.1042–1049. http://dx.doi.org/10.1002/cncr.22921.

Castro, T.B.M. et al., 2016. Pharmacovigilance of patients with multiple myeloma being treated with bortezomib and/or thalidomide. Brazilian Journal of Medical and Biological Research, 49(6). http://dx.doi.org/10.1590/1414-431x20165128.

Joh, T. et al., 2009. Dorsal Column Degeneration after Bortezomib Therapy in a Patient with Multiple Myeloma. Case Reports in Oncology, 2(3), pp.184–188. http://dx.doi.org/10.1159/000231996.

BRACHIAL PLEXUS IMAGING

Boulanger, X. et al., 2013. Imaging of the non-traumatic brachial plexus. Diagnostic and Interventional Imaging, 94(10), pp.945–956. http://dx.doi.org/10.1016/j.diii.2013.06.015.

Silbermann-Hoffman, O. & Teboul, F., 2013. Post-traumatic brachial plexus MRI in practice. Diagnostic and Interventional Imaging, 94(10), pp.925–943. http://dx.doi.org/10.1016/j.diii.2013.08.013.

BRACHIAL PLEXUS INJURY

Cho, A.B. et al., 2015. Intercostal nerve transfer to the biceps motor branch in complete traumatic brachial plexus injuries. Microsurgery, 35(6), pp.428–431. http://dx.doi.org/10.1002/micr.22453.

De Moraes, F.B. et al., 2015. Evaluation of elbow flexion following free muscle transfer from the medial gastrocnemius or transfer from the latissimus dorsi, in cases of traumatic injury of the brachial plexus. Revista Brasileira de Ortopedia (English Edition), 50(6), pp.660–665. http://dx.doi.org/10.1016/j.rboe.2015.09.007.

Giuffre, J.L. et al., 2010. Current Concepts of the Treatment of Adult Brachial Plexus Injuries. The Journal of Hand Surgery, 35(4), pp.678–688.

http://dx.doi.org/10.1016/j.jhsa.2010.01.021.

Miranda, G.E. and Torres, R.Y., 2016. Epidemiology of Traumatic Peripheral Nerve Injuries Evaluated with Electrodiagnostic Studies in a Tertiary Care Hospital Clinic. Puerto Rico health sciences journal, 35(2), pp.76-80. https://www.ncbi.nlm.nih.gov/pubmed/27232868

Sinha, S. et al., 2016. Adult brachial plexus injuries: Surgical strategies and approaches. Neurology India, 64(2), p.289. http://dx.doi.org/10.4103/0028-3886.177597.

BRACHIAL PLEXUS METASTATIC TUMOR

Arnold, W.D. et al., 2012. Electrodiagnostic Findings Heralding Neoplastic Brachial Plexopathy. PM&R, 4(3), pp.238–240. http://dx.doi.org/10.1016/j.pmrj.2011.12.002.

Lynch, A. & Peters, G., 2012. Brachial plexus tumor simulating an axillary metastasis from breast carcinoma. Radiology Case Reports, 7(3), p.712. http://dx.doi.org/10.2484/rcr.v7i3.712.

Maâroufi, M., Kamaoui, I., Boubbou, M., Sqalli, N. and Tizniti, S., 2013. [A rare cause of brachial plexopathy: a metastasis of breast cancer]. The Pan African medical journal, 18, pp.12-12. http://europepmc.org/articles/pmc4213524

Metter, I., Alkalay, D., Mozes, M., Geffen, D.B. and Ferit, T., 1995. Isolated metastases to peripheral nerves. Report of five cases involving the brachial plexus. Cancer, 76(10), pp.1829-1832. https://doi.org/10.1002/1097-0142(19951115)76:10<1829::aid-cncr2820761023>3.0.co;2-7

Yuh, E.L. et al., 2014. Diffusivity Measurements Differentiate Benign from Malignant Lesions in Patients with Peripheral Neuropathy or Plexopathy. American Journal of Neuroradiology, 36(1), pp.202–209. http://dx.doi.org/10.3174/ajnr.a4080.

BRACHIAL PLEXUS RADIATION-INDUCED PLEXOPATHIES

Belaid, A., Kanoun, S., Kallel, A., Ghorbel, I., Azoury, F., Heymann, S., Pichenot, C., Verstraet, R., Marsiglia, H. and Bourgier, C., 2010. [Breast cancer with axillary lymph node involvement]. Cancer radiotherapie: journal de la Societe francaise de radiotherapie oncologique, 14, pp.S136-46. http://europepmc.org/abstract/med/21129656

Dropcho, E.J., 2010. Neurotoxicity of Radiation Therapy. Neurologic Clinics, 28(1), pp.217–234. http://dx.doi.org/10.1016/j.ncl.2009.09.008.

Gosk, J., Rutowski, R., Reichert, P. and Rabczynski, J., 2007. Radiation-induced brachial plexus neuropathy-aetiopathogenesis, risk factors, differential diagnostics, symptoms and treatment. Folia Neuropathologica, 45(1), p.26. https://www.ncbi.nlm.nih.gov/pubmed/17357008

Jaeckle, K., 2010. Neurologic Manifestations of Neoplastic and Radiation-Induced Plexopathies. Seminars in Neurology, 30(03), pp.254–262. http://dx.doi.org/10.1055/s-0030-1255219.

BRACHIAL PLEXUS PRIMARY TUMORS

Binder, D.K., Smith, J.S. & Barbaro, N.M., 2004. Primary brachial plexus tumors: imaging, surgical, and pathological findings in 25 patients. Neurosurgical FOCUS, 16(5), pp.1–6. http://dx.doi.org/10.3171/foc.2004.16.5.12.

Chhabra, A. et al., 2012. High-Resolution 3T MR Neurography of the Brachial Plexus and Its Branches, with Emphasis on 3D Imaging. American Journal of Neuroradiology, 34(3), pp.486–497. http://dx.doi.org/10.3174/ajnr.a3287.

Siqueira, M.G., Martins, R.S. & Teixeira, M.J., 2009. Management of brachial plexus region tumours and tumour-like conditions: relevant diagnostic and surgical features in a consecutive series of eighteen patients. Acta Neurochirurgica, 151(9), pp.1089–1098. http://dx.doi.org/10.1007/s00701-009-0380-8.

BRACHIAL PLEXUS: GUNSHOT/LACERATION

Kim, D.H. et al., 2004. Mechanisms of injury in operative brachial plexus lesions. Neurosurgical FOCUS, 16(5), pp.1–8. http://dx.doi.org/10.3171/foc.2004.16.5.3.

Kim, D.H. et al., 2005. Lacerations to the Brachial Plexus: Surgical Techniques and Outcomes. Journal of Reconstructive Microsurgery, 21(07), pp.435–440. http://dx.doi.org/10.1055/s-2005-918895.

Kim, D.H. et al., 2006. Gunshot Wounds Involving the Brachial Plexus: Surgical Techniques and Outcomes. Journal of Reconstructive Microsurgery, 22(02), pp.067–072. http://dx.doi.org/10.1055/s-2006-932499.

BRAIN TUMOR HEADACHE

Alentorn, A., Hoang-Xuan, K. & Mikkelsen, T., 2016. Presenting signs and symptoms in brain tumors. Gliomas, pp.19–26. http://dx.doi.org/10.1016/b978-0-12-802997-8.00002-5.

Churchill, N. et al., 2016. Brain Structure and Function Associated with a History of Sport Concussion: A Multi-Modal Magnetic Resonance Imaging Study. Journal of Neurotrauma. http://dx.doi.org/10.1089/neu.2016.4531

Hoffer, M.E. et al., 2016. Neurosensory Symptom Complexes after Acute Mild Traumatic Brain Injury F. H. Kobeissy, ed. PLOS ONE, 11(1), p.e0146039. http://dx.doi.org/10.1371/journal.pone.0146039.

Lucas, S., 2015. Posttraumatic Headache: Clinical Characterization and Management. Current Pain and Headache Reports, 19(10). http://dx.doi.org/10.1007/s11916-015-0520-1.

Merritt, V.C., Ukueberuwa, D.M. & Arnett, P.A., 2016. Relationship between the apolipoprotein E gene and headache following sports-related concussion. Journal of Clinical and Experimental Neuropsychology, 38(9), pp.941–949. http://dx.doi.org/10.1080/13803395.2016.1177491.

Wright, A.D. et al., 2016. Myelin Water Fraction Is Transiently Reduced after a Single

Mild Traumatic Brain Injury – A Prospective Cohort Study in Collegiate Hockey Players F. de Castro, ed. PLOS ONE, 11(2), p.e0150215. http://dx.doi.org/10.1371/journal.pone.0150215.

Zhang, P. et al., 2016. Clinical, radiological, and pathological features of 33 adult unilateral thalamic gliomas. World Journal of Surgical Oncology, 14(1). http://dx.doi.org/10.1186/s12957-016-0820-x.

BROWN-SEQUARD SYNDROME

Beltran, M. 2016. Transdural spinal cord herniation: A rare cause of Brown-Sequard syndrome. Revue médicale de Bruxelles, 37(2):.101-103. https://www.ncbi.nlm.nih.gov/pubmed/27487695

Dlouhy, B.J., Dahdaleh, N.S. and Howard 3rd, M.A., 2013. Radiographic and intraoperative imaging of a hemisection of the spinal cord resulting in a pure Brown-Sequard syndrome: case report and review of the literature. Journal of neurosurgical sciences, 57(1), pp.81-86. https://www.ncbi.nlm.nih.gov/pubmed/23584224

Ranga, U. and Aiyappan, S.K., 2014. Brown-Séquard syndrome. The Indian journal of medical research, 140(4), p.572. https://www.ncbi.nlm.nih.gov/pmc/articles/PMC4277151/

BURNER/STINGER

Kelly, J.D., Aliquo, D., Sitler, M.R., Odgers, C. and Moyer, R.A., 2000. Association of burners with cervical canal and foraminal stenosis. The American journal of sports medicine, 28(2), pp.214-217. https://doi.org/10.1177/03635465000280021

Quong, W.L., Hynes, S.L. & Arneja, J.S., 2015. Pediatric Stinger Syndrome. Plastic and Reconstructive Surgery - Global Open, 3(11), p.e560.

http://dx.doi.org/10.1097/gox.0000000000000543.

Weinberg, J., Rokito, S. & Silber, J.S., 2003. Etiology, treatment, and prevention of athletic "stingers." Clinics in Sports Medicine, 22(3), pp.493–500. http://dx.doi.org/10.1016/s0278-5919(02)00057-1.

BURNING MOUTH SYNDROME

Beneng, K. et al., 2016. Pain Part 8: Burning Mouth Syndrome. Dent Update, 43(3):254-6.
http://www.exodontia.info/files/Dent_Update_2016._Pain_Part_8._Burning_Mouth_Syndrome.pdf

Nasri-Heir, C. et al., 2015. Burning mouth syndrome: Current concepts. The Journal of Indian Prosthodontic Society, 15(4), p.300.

http://dx.doi.org/10.4103/0972-4052.171823.

Shinozaki, T. et al., 2016. Spatial and Temporal Brain Responses to Noxious Heat Thermal Stimuli in Burning Mouth Syndrome. Journal of Dental Research, 95(10), pp.1138–1146. http://dx.doi.org/10.1177/0022034516653580.

Steele, J.C., 2016. The practical evaluation and management of patients with symptoms of a sore burning mouth. Clinics in Dermatology, 34(4), pp.449–457. http://dx.doi.org/10.1016/j.clindermatol.2016.02.017.

CALCIUM CHANNELS

Bourinet, E. et al., 2004. Silencing of the Cav3.2 T-type calcium channel gene in sensory neurons demonstrates its major role in nociception. The EMBO Journal, 24(2), pp.315–324. http://dx.doi.org/10.1038/sj.emboj.7600515.

Jacus, M.O. et al., 2012. Presynaptic CaV3.2 Channels Regulate Excitatory Neurotransmission in Nociceptive Dorsal Horn Neurons. Journal of Neuroscience, 32(27), pp.9374–9382. http://dx.doi.org/10.1523/jneurosci.0068-12.2012.

Jagodic, M.M. et al., 2007. Cell-Specific Alterations of T-Type Calcium Current in Painful Diabetic Neuropathy Enhance Excitability of Sensory Neurons. Journal of Neuroscience, 27(12), pp.3305–3316. http://dx.doi.org/10.1523/jneurosci.4866-06.2007.

Weiss, N. et al., 2011. A Cav3.2/Syntaxin-1A Signaling Complex Controls T-type Channel Activity and Low-threshold Exocytosis. Journal of Biological Chemistry, 287(4), pp.2810–2818. http://dx.doi.org/10.1074/jbc.m111.290882.

CARPEL TUNNEL SYNDROME

Hermiz, S.J. & Kalliainen, L.K., 2017. Evidence-Based Medicine. Plastic and Reconstructive Surgery, 140(1), p.120e–129e. Available at: http://dx.doi.org/10.1097/prs.0000000000003477.

Jaeschke, R. et al., 2017. Systematic review: hand activity and ultrasound of the median nerve. Occupational Medicine, 67(5), pp.389–393. Available at: http://dx.doi.org/10.1093/occmed/kqx059.

Tang, D.T. et al., 2015. Nerve Entrapment. Plastic and Reconstructive Surgery, 135(1), p.199e–215e. Available at: http://dx.doi.org/10.1097/prs.0000000000000828.

CAROTIDYNIA

Aydil, U., Kizil, Y. & Köybaşioğlu, A., 2011. Less known non-infectious and neuromusculoskeletal system-originated anterolateral neck and craniofacial pain disorders. European Archives of Oto-Rhino-Laryngology, 269(1), pp.9–16.

http://dx.doi.org/10.1007/s00405-011-1746-0.

Burton, B.S., Syms, M.J., Petermann, G.W. and Burgess, L.P., 2000. MR imaging of patients with carotidynia. American journal of neuroradiology, 21(4), pp.766-769. https://www.researchgate.net/publication/12533569_MR_Imaging_of_patients_with_carotidynia

Ellul, D. et al., 2007. Nasopharyngeal carcinoma presenting as carotidynia in an 18-year-old patient. The Journal of Laryngology & Otology, 122(02). http://dx.doi.org/10.1017/s0022215107007293.

Emmanuelli, J.L., Gutierrez, J.R., Chiossone, J.A. and Chiossone, E., 1998. Carotidynia: a frequently overlooked or misdiagnosed syndrome. Ear, nose & throat journal, 77(6), p.462. http://connection.ebscohost.com/c/articles/1092514/carotidynia-frequently-overlooked-misdiagnosed-syndrome

CATAMENIAL NEUROENDOMETRIOSIS

Cimsit, C., Yoldemir, T. & Akpinar, I.N., 2016. Sciatic neuroendometriosis: Magnetic resonance imaging defined perineural spread of endometriosis. Journal of Obstetrics and Gynaecology Research, 42(7), pp.890–894. http://dx.doi.org/10.1111/jog.12998.

Eric L. Zager, M.D. Mark J. Brown, M.D., 1999. Catamenial Mononeuropathy and Radiculopathy. Journal of Neurosurgery, 90(2). http://dx.doi.org/10.3171/jns.1999.90.2.0374.

Siquara De Sousa, A.C. et al., 2015. Neural involvement in endometriosis: Review of anatomic distribution and mechanisms. Clinical Anatomy, 28(8), pp.1029–1038. http://dx.doi.org/10.1002/ca.22617.

CATHETER ENTRAPMENT

Han, J.L., Loriaux, D.B., Tybout, C., Kinon, M.D., Rahimpour, S., Runyon, S.L., Hopkins, T.J., Boortz-Marx, R.L. and Lad, S.P., 2016. Thoracic Nerve Root Entrapment by Intrathecal Catheter Coiling: Case Report and Review of the Literature. Pain physician, 19(3), pp.E499-504. https://www.ncbi.nlm.nih.gov/pubmed/27008308

CAUDA EQUINA SYNDROME POST POST-RADIATION

Abraham, A. & Drory, V.E., 2013. Postradiation lower motor neuron syndrome: case series and literature review. Journal of Neurology, 260(7), pp.1802–1806. http://dx.doi.org/10.1007/s00415-013-6881-7.

Bowen, J. et al., 1996. The Post-irradiation lower motor neuron syndrome Neuronopathy or radiculopathy? Brain, 119(5), pp.1429–1439. http://dx.doi.org/10.1093/brain/119.5.1429.

Matsuda, N. et al., 2015. Cauda Equina Involvement in Post-Radiation Lower Motor Neuron Syndrome. Internal Medicine, 54(11), pp.1415–1419. http://dx.doi.org/10.2169/internalmedicine.54.4182.

Wohlgemuth, W.A. et al., 1998. Radiogene Amyotrophie. Der Nervenarzt, 69(12), pp.1061–1065. http://dx.doi.org/10.1007/s001150050383.

CENTRAL CORD SYNDROME

Douglas, J.D.M. & McIver, N.K.I., 2016. Re: Case report—Brown-Séquard syndrome: a rare manifestation of decompression sickness. Occupational Medicine, 66(4), pp.339–340. http://dx.doi.org/10.1093/occmed/kqw045.

Galgano, M. & Chin, L.S., 2015. Central Cord Syndrome in a Young Patient with Early Diffuse Idiopathic Skeletal Hyperostosis and Ossification of the Posterior Longitudinal Ligament after Minor Trauma: A Case Report and Review. Cureus. http://dx.doi.org/10.7759/cureus.284.

Schroeder, G.D. et al., 2016. The effect of increased T2 signal intensity in the spinal cord on the injury severity and early neurological recovery in patients with central cord syndrome. Journal of Neurosurgery: Spine, 24(5), pp.792–796. http://dx.doi.org/10.3171/2015.9.spine15661.

Stevenson, C.M. et al., 2016. Traumatic central cord syndrome: neurological and functional outcome at 3 years. Spinal Cord, 54(11), pp.1010–1015. http://dx.doi.org/10.1038/sc.2016.34

CERVICAL SPONDYLOLISTHESIS

Jiang, S.-D., Jiang, L.-S. & Dai, L.-Y., 2011. Degenerative cervical spondylolisthesis: a systematic review. International Orthopaedics, 35(6), pp.869–875. http://dx.doi.org/10.1007/s00264-010-1203-5.

Oichi, T. et al., 2016. Cervical Anterolisthesis. SPINE, 41(8), pp.E467–E473. http://dx.doi.org/10.1097/brs.0000000000001277.

Suzuki, A. et al., 2016. Clinical Outcome of Cervical Laminoplasty and Postoperative Radiological Change for Cervical Myelopathy With Degenerative Spondylolisthesis. SPINE, 41(23), pp.1808–1812. http://dx.doi.org/10.1097/brs.0000000000001706.

Woiciechowsky, C., Thomale, U.-W. & Kroppenstedt, S.-N., 2004. Degenerative spondylolisthesis of the cervical spine — symptoms and surgical strategies depending on disease progress. European Spine Journal, 13(8), pp.680–684. http://dx.doi.org/10.1007/s00586-004-0673-9.

CERVICAL CANCER

Akbar, S.A.M. et al., 2016. Papillary Squamotransitional Cell Carcinoma of the Uterine Cervix: A Case Report and Review of the Literature. Case Reports in Obstetrics and Gynecology, 2016, pp.1–3. http://dx.doi.org/10.1155/2016/7107910.

Benoulaid, M. et al., 2016. Skin metastases of cervical cancer: two case reports and review of the literature. Journal of Medical Case Reports, 10(1). http://dx.doi.org/10.1186/s13256-016-1042-0.

Kaur, A., 2013. Transitional Cell Carcinoma: A Case Report with Clinical, Histological and Cytological Findings. Journal of Clinical and Diagnostic Research, 7(12), 2954-2955 http://dx.doi.org/10.7860/jcdr/2013/6070.3804.

CERVICAL MYELOPATHY

Baba, S. et al., 2016. Risk Factor Analysis for C5 Palsy after Double-Door Laminoplasty for Cervical Spondylotic Myelopathy. Asian Spine Journal, 10(2), p.298. http://dx.doi.org/10.4184/asj.2016.10.2.298.

Nouri, A. et al., 2016. Magnetic resonance imaging assessment of degenerative cervical myelopathy: a review of structural changes and measurement techniques. Neurosurgical Focus, 40(6), p.E5. http://dx.doi.org/10.3171/2016.3.focus1667.

Patel, A.A. et al., 2012. Evidence of an Inherited Predisposition for Cervical Spondylotic Myelopathy. Spine, 37(1), pp.26–29. http://dx.doi.org/10.1097/brs.0b013e3182102ede.

Stoops, W.L. & King, R.B., 1962. Neural Complications of Cervical Spondylosis: Their Response to Laminectomy and Foramenotomy. Journal of Neurosurgery, 19(11), pp.986–999. http://dx.doi.org/10.3171/jns.1962.19.11.0986.

CERVICAL PERINEURAL CYST

Joshi, V.P. et al., 2014. Cervical Perineural Cyst Masquerading as a Cervical Spinal Tumor. Asian Spine Journal, 8(2), p.202. http://dx.doi.org/10.4184/asj.2014.8.2.202.

Kim, K., Chun, S.W. & Chung, S.G., 2011. A case of symptomatic cervical perineural (Tarlov) cyst: clinical manifestation and management. Skeletal Radiology, 41(1), pp.97–101. http://dx.doi.org/10.1007/s00256-011-1243-y.

Sen, R.K. et al., 2012. Tarlov Cysts: A Report of Two Cases. Journal of Orthopaedic Surgery, 20(1), pp.87–89. http://dx.doi.org/10.1177/230949901202000117.

CERVICAL SPINAL STENOSIS

Freedman, B.A. et al., 2015. A Comparison of Computed Tomography Measures for Diagnosing Cervical Spinal Stenosis Associated with Myelopathy: A Case-Control Study. Asian Spine Journal, 9(1), p.22. http://dx.doi.org/10.4184/asj.2015.9.1.22.

Morio, Y. et al., 2001. Correlation Between Operative Outcomes of Cervical Compression Myelopathy and MRI of the Spinal Cord. Spine, 26(11), pp.1238–1245. http://dx.doi.org/10.1097/00007632-200106010-00012.

Stafira, J.S., Sonnad, J.R., Yuh, W.T., Huard, D.R., Acker, R.E., Nguyen, D.L., Maley, J.E., Ramji, F.G., Li, W.B. and Loftus, C.M., 2003. Qualitative assessment of cervical spinal stenosis: observer variability on CT and MR images. American journal of neuroradiology, 24(4), pp.766-769. https://www.ncbi.nlm.nih.gov/pubmed/12695220

CHANGE IN MYELINATED FIBERS

Hökfelt, T. et al., 2006. Central consequences of peripheral nerve damage. Wall and Melzack's Textbook of Pain, pp.947–959. Available at: http://dx.doi.org/10.1016/b0-443-07287-6/50065-5.

Gillespie, C.S. et al., 2000. Peripheral Demyelination and Neuropathic Pain Behavior in Periaxin-Deficient Mice. Neuron, 26(2), pp.523–531. Available at: http://dx.doi.org/10.1016/s0896-6273(00)81184-8.

Inoue, M. et al., 2004. Initiation of neuropathic pain requires lysophosphatidic acid receptor signaling. Nature Medicine, 10(7), pp.712–718. Available at: http://dx.doi.org/10.1038/nm1060.

Mueller, B.K., Mack, H. & Teusch, N., 2005. Rho kinase, a promising drug target for neurological disorders. Nature Reviews Drug Discovery, 4(5), pp.387–398. Available at: http://dx.doi.org/10.1038/nrd1719.

Ueda, H. et al., 2013. Lysophosphatidic acid: Chemical signature of neuropathic pain. Biochimica et Biophysica Acta (BBA) - Molecular and Cell Biology of Lipids, 1831(1), pp.61–73. Available at: http://dx.doi.org/10.1016/j.bbalip.2012.08.014.

CHERIRALGIA

Chodoroff G, Honet JC., 1985. Cheiralgia paresthetica and linear atrophy as a complication of local steroid injection. Arch Phys Med Rehabil., 66(9), pp. 637-9. Available at: https://www.ncbi.nlm.nih.gov/pubmed/4038032

Lazzarino, L.G., Nicolai, A. & Toppani, D., 1983. A case of cheiralgia paresthetica secondary to diabetes mellitus. The Italian Journal of Neurological Sciences, 4(1), pp.103–106. Available at: http://dx.doi.org/10.1007/bf02043447.

Longfield, R.N., 1981. Cheiralgia Paresthetica After Necrotic Arachnidism. Archives of Neurology, 38(7), pp.470. Available at: http://dx.doi.org/10.1001/archneur.1981.00510070104030.

CHEST WALL TUMOR

Kobayashi, H. et al., 2015. Intercostal neuralgia as a symptom of an osteoblastoma in thoracic spine. BMJ Case Reports, p.bcr2015210720. http://dx.doi.org/10.1136/bcr-2015-210720.

Mori T, 2011, Chest Wall Tumor, rib tumor. Kyobu Geka. 2011 Jul;64(8 Suppl):725-32. https://www.ncbi.nlm.nih.gov/pubmed/21916185

Yaguchi, D. et al., 2015. An Autopsied Case of Malignant Sarcomatoid Pleural Mesothelioma in Which Chest Pain Developed Several Months Earlier without Abnormality on Imaging. Case Reports in Oncology, 8(3), pp.439–446. http://dx.doi.org/10.1159/000441468.

CHLORIDE CHANNELS

Andre, S., 2003. Axotomy-Induced Expression of Calcium-Activated Chloride Current in Subpopulations of Mouse Dorsal Root Ganglion Neurons. Journal of Neurophysiology, 90(6), pp.3764–3773. http://dx.doi.org/10.1152/jn.00449.2003.

Cho, H. et al., 2012. The calcium-activated chloride channel anoctamin 1 acts as a heat sensor in nociceptive neurons. Nature Neuroscience, 15(7), pp.1015–1021. http://dx.doi.org/10.1038/nn.3111.

Hartzell, C., Putzier, I. & Arreola, J., 2005. Calcium-activated chloride channels. Annu. Rev. Physiol., 67(1), pp.719–758. http://dx.doi.org/10.1146/annurev.physiol.67.032003.154341.

Kenyon, J.., 2000. The reversal potential of Ca2+-activated Cl– currents indicates that chick sensory neurons accumulate intracellular Cl–. Neuroscience Letters, 296(1), pp.9–12. http://dx.doi.org/10.1016/s0304-3940(00)01610-4.

Liu, B. et al., 2010. The acute nociceptive signals induced by bradykinin in rat sensory neurons are mediated by inhibition of M-type K+ channels and activation of Ca2+-activated Cl– channels. Journal of Clinical Investigation, 120(4), pp.1240–1252. http://dx.doi.org/10.1172/jci41084.

CHRONIC PELVIC PAIN

Abbott, J., 2010. Optimal management of chronic cyclical pelvic pain: an evidence-based and pragmatic approach. International Journal of Women's Health, p.263. http://dx.doi.org/10.2147/ijwh.s7991.

As-Sanie, S. et al., 2013. Increased Pressure Pain Sensitivity in Women With Chronic Pelvic Pain. Obstetrics & Gynecology, 122(5), pp.1047–1055. http://dx.doi.org/10.1097/aog.0b013e3182a7e1f5.

Chung MK, Chung RP, Gordon D. Interstitial cystitis and endometriosis in patients with chronic pelvic pain: The "Evil Twins" syndrome. JSLS. 2005 Jan-Mar;9(1):25-9.

https://www.ncbi.nlm.nih.gov/pmc/articles/PMC3015562/

CHRONIC PROSTATITIS/CHRONIC PELVIC PAIN SYNDROME

Dimitrakov, J. et al., 2008. Adrenocortical Hormone Abnormalities in Men with Chronic Prostatitis/Chronic Pelvic Pain Syndrome. Urology, 71(2), pp.261–266. http://dx.doi.org/10.1016/j.urology.2007.09.025.

Hu Y, Niu X, Wang G, Huang J, Liu M, Peng B. Chronic prostatitis/chronic pelvic pain syndrome impairs erectile function through increased endothelial dysfunction, oxidative stress, apoptosis, and corporal fibrosis in a rat model. Andrology. 2016 Aug 27. https://www.ncbi.nlm.nih.gov/pubmed/27565759

Pontari, M.A. & Ruggieri, M.R., 2008. Mechanisms in Prostatitis/Chronic Pelvic Pain Syndrome. The Journal of Urology, 179(5), pp.S61–S67. http://dx.doi.org/10.1016/j.juro.2008.03.139.

SHOSKES, D.A. et al., 2004. IMPACT OF POST-EJACULATORY PAIN IN MEN WITH CATEGORY III CHRONIC PROSTATITIS/CHRONIC PELVIC PAIN SYNDROME. The Journal of Urology, 172(2), pp.542–547. http://dx.doi.org/10.1097/01.ju.0000132798.48067.23.

CHURG-STRAUSS SYNDROME

Khoury, P. et al., 2012. Serum biomarkers are similar in Churg-Strauss syndrome and hypereosinophilic syndrome. Allergy, 67(9), pp.1149–1156. http://dx.doi.org/10.1111/j.1398-9995.2012.02873.x.

Kim, M. et al., 2012. Clinical Features And Prognostic Factors Of Churg-strauss Syndrome. Journal of Allergy and Clinical Immunology, 129(2), p.AB214. http://dx.doi.org/10.1016/j.jaci.2011.12.085.

CISPLATIN

Ewertz, M., Qvortrup, C. & Eckhoff, L., 2015. Chemotherapy-induced peripheral neuropathy in patients treated with taxanes and platinum derivatives. Acta Oncologica, 54(5), pp.587–591. http://dx.doi.org/10.3109/0284186x.2014.995775.

Huang, Z.-Z. et al., 2016. Cerebrospinal Fluid Oxaliplatin Contributes to the Acute Pain Induced by Systemic Administration of Oxaliplatin. Anesthesiology, 124(5), pp.1109–1121. http://dx.doi.org/10.1097/aln.0000000000001084.

Khattak, M.A., 2011. Calcium and Magnesium Prophylaxis for Oxaliplatin-Related Neurotoxicity: Is It a Trade-off Between Drug Efficacy and Toxicity? The Oncologist, 16(12), pp.1780–1783. http://dx.doi.org/10.1634/theoncologist.2011-0157.

Lin, H., Heo, B.H. & Yoon, M.H., 2015. A New Rat Model of Cisplatin-induced Neuropathic Pain. The Korean Journal of Pain, 28(4), p.236. http://dx.doi.org/10.3344/kjp.2015.28.4.236.

Taguchi, K., 2016. Role of Transient Receptor Potential Channels in Paclitaxel- and Oxaliplatin-induced Peripheral Neuropathy. YAKUGAKU ZASSHI, 136(2), pp.287–296. http://dx.doi.org/10.1248/yakushi.15-00214.

CLIOQUINOL

Saito, Y., Sakai, K. & Konagaya, M., 2016. The prevalence of dementia in subacute myelo-optico-neuropathy (SMON) patients who underwent medical checkups. Nippon Ronen Igakkai Zasshi. Japanese Journal of Geriatrics, 53(2), pp.152–157. Available at: http://dx.doi.org/10.3143/geriatrics.53.152.

Konagaya M1.2015. SMON: toxicity of clioquinol and the status quo. Brain Nerve., 67(1) pp. 49-62. Abstract available at: https://www.ncbi.nlm.nih.gov/pubmed/25585435. Article in Japanese. http://dx.doi.org/10.11477/mf.1416200086

Katsuyama, M. et al., 2012. Clioquinol induces DNA double-strand breaks, activation of ATM, and subsequent activation of p53 signaling. Toxicology, 299(1), pp.55–59. Available at: http://dx.doi.org/10.1016/j.tox.2012.05.013.

Tateishi, J., 2000. Subacute myelo-optico-neuropathy: Clioquinol intoxication in humans and animals. Neuropathology, 20(s1), pp.20–24. Available at: http://dx.doi.org/10.1046/j.1440-1789.2000.00296.x.

Fukui, T. et al., 2015. Histone deacetylase inhibitor attenuates neurotoxicity of clioquinol in PC12 cells. Toxicology, 331, pp.112–118. Available at: http://dx.doi.org/10.1016/j.tox.2015.01.013.

COCCYDYMIA

Grgić V., 2012. [Coccygodynia: etiology, pathogenesis, clinical characteristics, diagnosis and therapy]. Liječnički Vjesnik, 134(1-2), 49-55. https://www.ncbi.nlm.nih.gov/pubmed/22519253

Kim, N.H. & Suk, K.S., 1999. Clinical and radiological differences between traumatic and idiopathic coccygodynia. Yonsei Medical Journal, 40(3), p.215. http://dx.doi.org/10.3349/ymj.1999.40.3.215.

Maigne, J.-Y., Pigeau, I. & Roger, B., 2012. Magnetic resonance imaging findings in the painful adult coccyx. European Spine Journal, 21(10), pp.2097–2104. http://dx.doi.org/10.1007/s00586-012-2202-6.

Patijn, J. et al., 2010. Coccygodynia. Pain Practice, 10(6), pp.554–559. http://dx.doi.org/10.1111/j.1533-2500.2010.00404.x.

COMPARTMENT SYNDROME

McQueen, M.M. et al., 2013. The Estimated Sensitivity and Specificity of Compartment Pressure Monitoring for Acute Compartment Syndrome. The Journal of Bone and Joint Surgery, 95(8), pp.673–677. Available at: http://dx.doi.org/10.2106/jbjs.k.01731.

Ferlic, P.W. et al., 2012. The acute compartment syndrome following fractures of the lower leg in children. Injury, 43(10), pp.1743–1746. Available at: http://dx.doi.org/10.1016/j.injury.2012.06.025.

Braver, R.T., 2016. Chronic Exertional Compartment Syndrome. Clinics in Podiatric Medicine and Surgery, 33(2), pp.219–233. Available at: http://dx.doi.org/10.1016/j.cpm.2015.12.002.

CONDENSING OSTEITIS

Hsu, C. Y., F. Frassica, and E. G. McFarland. Condensing osteitis of the clavicle: case report and review of the literature. American journal of orthopedics (Belle Mead, NJ) 27.6 (1998): 445-447. http://dx.doi.org/europepmc.org.

Imran, M.B. & Othman, S., 2010. Bilateral condensing osteitis of clavicles: differential diagnosis of an unusual case. Rheumatology International, 32(9), pp.2921–2923. http://dx.doi.org/10.1007/s00296-010-1480-8.

Rand, T. et al., 1998. Condensing Osteitis of the Clavicle: MRI. Journal of Computer Assisted Tomography, 22(4), pp.621–624. http://dx.doi.org/10.1097/00004728-199807000-00021.

CONGENITAL DEFECTS (ABSENT PEDICLE)

Abduljabbar, F.H. et al., 2015. Misdiagnosing absent pedicle of cervical spine in the acute trauma setting. Orthopedic Reviews, 7(3). http://dx.doi.org/10.4081/or.2015.5889.

Goodwin, C.R. et al., 2016. Cervical Fusion for Absent Pedicle Syndrome Manifesting with Myelopathy. World Neurosurgery, 86, pp.515.e17–515.e22. http://dx.doi.org/10.1016/j.wneu.2015.09.017.

Oh, Y.-M. et al., 2009. Posterior arch defects of the cervical spine: a comparison between absent pedicle syndrome and spondylolysis. The Spine Journal, 9(7), pp.e1–e5. http://dx.doi.org/10.1016/j.spinee.2009.01.006.

CONGENITAL INSENSITIVITY TO PAIN

Eregowda, N.I., 2016. Girl with No Pain: Congenital Insensitivity To Pain and Anhidrosis (HSAN) Type IV - A Case Report. Journal of Clinical and Diagnostic Research [serial online] 2016 Feb [cited:2017 Jan 1] 02 ZL01 - ZL02 http://dx.doi.org/10.7860/jcdr/2016/16514.7317.

Kurth, I. et al., 2016. Whole exome sequencing in congenital pain insensitivity identifies a novel causative intronicNTRK1-mutation due to uniparental disomy. American Journal of Medical Genetics Part B: Neuropsychiatric Genetics, 171(6), pp.875–878. http://dx.doi.org/10.1002/ajmg.b.32458.

Pérez-López, L.M. et al., 2015. Update Review and Clinical Presentation in Congenital Insensitivity to Pain and Anhidrosis. Case Reports in Pediatrics, 2015, pp.1–7. http://dx.doi.org/10.1155/2015/589852.

Wang, Q.-L. et al., 2016. Phenotypes and Genotypes in Five Children with Congenital Insensitivity to Pain with Anhidrosis. Pediatric Neurology, 61, pp.63–69. http://dx.doi.org/10.1016/j.pediatrneurol.2016.04.006.

Zhang, S. et al., 2016. Clinical features for diagnosis and management of patients with PRDM12 congenital insensitivity to pain. Journal of Medical Genetics, 53(8), pp.533–535. http://dx.doi.org/10.1136/jmedgenet-2015-103646.

COSTOCHONDRITIS

Jindal, A. & Singhi, S., 2011. Acute Chest Pain. The Indian Journal of Pediatrics, 78(10), pp.1262–1267. http://dx.doi.org/10.1007/s12098-011-0413-1.

Oh, R.C. & Johnson, J.D., 2012. Chest Pain and Costochondritis Associated with Vitamin D Deficiency: A Report of Two Cases. Case Reports in Medicine, 2012, pp.1–3. http://dx.doi.org/10.1155/2012/375730.

COUGH HEADACHE

Allena, M. et al., 2010. Focus on therapy of the Chapter IV headaches provoked by exertional factors: primary cough headache, primary exertional headache and primary headache associated with sexual activity. The Journal of Headache and Pain, 11(6), pp.525–530. http://dx.doi.org/10.1007/s10194-010-0261-9.

Cordenier, A. et al., 2013. Headache associated with cough: a review. The Journal of Headache and Pain, 14(1), p.42. http://dx.doi.org/10.1186/1129-2377-14-42.

CRICOID CARTILAGE

Hoeve HJ. 1997, Malformation and Stenosis of the Cricoid Cartilage in Association With Larsen's Syndrome With Larsen's Syndrome. Laryngoscope 107(6) pp. 792 to

794. Available at: https://doi.org/10.1097/00005537-199706000-00013

Kunachak, S., 1995. Anterior cervical pain syndromes: hyoid, thyroid and cricoid cartilage syndromes and their treatment with triamcinolone acetonide. The Journal of Laryngology & Otology, 109(01). http://dx.doi.org/10.1017/s0022215100129214.

CRPS

Edinger, L., Schwartzman, R.J., Ahmad, A., Erwin, K. and Alexander, G.M., 2012. Objective sensory evaluation of the spread of complex regional pain syndrome. Pain physician, 16(6), pp.581-591. https://www.ncbi.nlm.nih.gov/pubmed/24284843

Maleki, J. et al., 2000. Patterns of spread in complex regional pain syndrome, type I (reflex sympathetic dystrophy). Pain, 88(3), pp.259–266. http://dx.doi.org/10.1016/s0304-3959(00)00332-8.

Schwartzman, R.J., Erwin, K.L. & Alexander, G.M., 2009. The Natural History of Complex Regional Pain Syndrome. The Clinical Journal of Pain, 25(4), pp.273–280. http://dx.doi.org/10.1097/ajp.0b013e31818ecea5.

CYSTITIS

Abrahamian, F.M., Moran, G.J. & Talan, D.A., 2008. Urinary Tract Infections in the Emergency Department. Infectious Disease Clinics of North America, 22(1), pp.73–87. http://dx.doi.org/10.1016/j.idc.2007.10.002.

Little, P. et al., 2010. Presentation, pattern, and natural course of severe symptoms, and role of antibiotics and antibiotic resistance among patients presenting with suspected uncomplicated urinary tract infection in primary care: observational study. BMJ, 340(feb05 1), pp.b5633–b5633. http://dx.doi.org/10.1136/bmj.b5633.

Mehnert-Kay, S.A., 2005. Diagnosis and management of uncomplicated urinary tract infections. Am Fam Physician, 72(3), pp.451-6. http://www.aafp.org/afp/2005/0801/p451.html

Molander, U. et al., 2000. A longitudinal cohort study of elderly women with urinary tract infections. Maturitas, 34(2), pp.127–131. http://dx.doi.org/10.1016/s0378-5122(99)00102-4.

DIABETIC NEUROPATHY

Albers, J.W. & Pop-Busui, R., 2014. Diabetic Neuropathy: Mechanisms, Emerging Treatments, and Subtypes. Current Neurology and Neuroscience Reports, 14(8). http://dx.doi.org/10.1007/s11910-014-0473-5.

Anon, 2014. Painful diabetic neuropathy. BMJ, 348(may20 12), pp.g3440–g3440. http://dx.doi.org/10.1136/bmj.g3440.

Coppini, D.V., 2016. Enigma of painful diabetic neuropathy: can we use the basic science, research outcomes and real-world data to help improve patient care and outcomes? Diabetic Medicine, 33(11), pp.1477–1482. http://dx.doi.org/10.1111/dme.13089.

Tesfaye, S. et al., 2016. Diabetic peripheral neuropathy may not be as its name suggests. PAIN, 157, pp.S72–S80. http://dx.doi.org/10.1097/j.pain.0000000000000465.

Tesfaye, S., 2016. PL37: a new hope in the treatment of painful diabetic neuropathy? Pain Management, 6(2), pp.129–132. http://dx.doi.org/10.2217/pmt.15.68.

Tran, C. et al., 2015. Acute painful diabetic neuropathy: an uncommon, remittent type of acute distal small fibre neuropathy. Swiss Medical Weekly. http://dx.doi.org/10.4414/smw.2015.14131.

Won, J.C. & Park, T.S., 2016. Recent Advances in Diagnostic Strategies for Diabetic Peripheral Neuropathy. Endocrinology and Metabolism, 31(2), p.230. http://dx.doi.org/10.3803/enm.2016.31.2.230.

Zhang, Y.P. et al., 2016. Acute Hypoglycemia Induces Painful Neuropathy and the Treatment of Coenzyme Q10. Journal of Diabetes Research, 2016, pp.1–7. http://dx.doi.org/10.1155/2016/4593052.

DIABETIC THORACIC POLYRADICULOPATHY

Brewer, R., 2003. Diabetic thoracic radiculopathy: an unusual cause of post-thoracotomy pain. Pain, 103(1), pp.221–223. http://dx.doi.org/10.1016/s0304-3959(02)00446-3.

Longstreth, G.F., 2005. Diabetic thoracic polyradiculopathy. Best Practice & Research Clinical Gastroenterology, 19(2), pp.275–281. http://dx.doi.org/10.1016/j.bpg.2004.09.003.

Massie, R. et al., 2012. Diabetic cervical radiculoplexus neuropathy: a distinct syndrome expanding the spectrum of diabetic radiculoplexus neuropathies. Brain, 135(10), pp.3074–3088. http://dx.doi.org/10.1093/brain/aws244.

DIFFUSE IDIOPATHIC SKELETAL HYPEROSTOSIS (DISH)

Kuperus, J.S. et al., 2016. Histological characteristics of diffuse idiopathic skeletal hyperostosis. Journal of Orthopaedic Research. http://dx.doi.org/10.1002/jor.23267.

Mazières, B. 2013. Diffuse idiopathic skeletal hyperostosis (Forestier-Rotes-Querol disease): What's new? Joint Bone Spine 80.5: 466-470.. https://doi.org/10.1016/j.jbspin.2013.02.011. Epub 2013 Apr 6. https://www.ncbi.nlm.nih.gov/pubmed/23566663

Weiss, B.G. et al., 2015. Whole Body Magnetic Resonance Imaging Features in Diffuse Idiopathic Skeletal Hyperostosis in Conjunction with Clinical Variables to

Whole Body MRI and Clinical Variables in Ankylosing Spondylitis. The Journal of Rheumatology, 43(2), pp.335–342. http://dx.doi.org/10.3899/jrheum.150162.

DIFFUSE NOXIOUS INHIBITORY CONTROLS (DNIC)

Bannister, K. et al., 2015. Diffuse noxious inhibitory controls and nerve injury. PAIN, 156(9), pp.1803–1811. http://dx.doi.org/10.1097/j.pain.0000000000000240.

Chebbi, R. et al., 2014. The nucleus raphe magnus OFF-cells are involved in diffuse noxious inhibitory controls. Experimental Neurology, 256, pp.39–45. http://dx.doi.org/10.1016/j.expneurol.2014.03.006.

Dogrul, A., Ossipov, M.H. & Porreca, F., 2009. Differential mediation of descending pain facilitation and inhibition by spinal 5HT-3 and 5HT-7 receptors. Brain Research, 1280, pp.52–59. http://dx.doi.org/10.1016/j.brainres.2009.05.001.

Honigman, L. et al., 2016. Nonpainful wide-area compression inhibits experimental pain. PAIN, 157(9), pp.2000–2011. http://dx.doi.org/10.1097/j.pain.0000000000000604.

Le Bars, D. et al., 1991. Diffuse Noxious Inhibitory Controls (DNIC) in animals and in man. Acupuncture in Medicine, 9(2), pp.47–56. http://dx.doi.org/10.1136/aim.9.2.47.

Meléndez-Gallardo, J. & Eblen-Zajjur, A., 2016. Noxious mechanical heterotopic stimulation induces inhibition of the spinal dorsal horn neuronal network: analysis of spinal somatosensory-evoked potentials. Neurological Sciences, 37(9), pp.1491–1497. http://dx.doi.org/10.1007/s10072-016-2613-y.

Torta, D.M. et al., 2015. The effect of heterotopic noxious conditioning stimulation on Aδ-, C- and Aβ-fibre brain responses in humans M. Barrot, ed. European Journal of Neuroscience, 42(9), pp.2707–2715. http://dx.doi.org/10.1111/ejn.13071.

2,4 - DINITROPHENOL

Grundlingh, J. et al., 2011. 2,4-Dinitrophenol (DNP): A Weight Loss Agent with Significant Acute Toxicity and Risk of Death. Journal of Medical Toxicology, 7(3), pp.205–212. Available at: http://dx.doi.org/10.1007/s13181-011-0162-6.

Suozzi, JC. et al., 2005. DNP 2,4 – Dinitrophenol: a deadly way to lose weight JEMS, 30 (1), pp. 82-89.Available on Pub Med: https://www.ncbi.nlm.nih.gov/pubmed/15662347

DISCITIS

Brinjikji, W., Everist, B.M., Wald, J.T., Lane, J.I. and Morris, J.M., 2015. Association between imaging findings and microbiological findings for image-guided biopsies for spine infections. Journal of neurosurgical sciences. Journal of Neurosurgical Sciences, 2016 Sep 9 [Epub ahead of print]. http://europepmc.org/abstract/med/26354188

Cottle, L. & Riordan, T., 2008. Infectious spondylodiscitis. Journal of Infection, 56(6), pp.401–412. http://dx.doi.org/10.1016/j.jinf.2008.02.005.

Hooten, W.M. et al., 2006. Discitis after Lumbar Epidural Corticosteroid Injection: A Case Report and Analysis of the Case Report Literature. Pain Medicine, 7(1), pp.46–51. http://dx.doi.org/10.1111/j.1526-4637.2006.00088.x.

Radcliff, K.E. et al., 2016. Distinguishing Pseudomeningocele, Epidural Hematoma, and Postoperative Infection on Postoperative MRI. Clinical Spine Surgery, 29(9), pp.E471–E474. https://dx.doi.org/10.1097/BSD.0b013e31828f9203.

DISULFIRAM NEUROPATHY

Filosto, M. et al., 2008. Disulfiram neuropathy: Two cases of distal axonopathy. Clinical Toxicology, 46(4), pp.314–316. http://dx.doi.org/10.1080/15563650701636390.

Tran, A.T., Rison, R.A. & Beydoun, S.R., 2016. Disulfiram neuropathy: two case reports. Journal of Medical Case Reports, 10(1).
http://dx.doi.org/10.1186/s13256-016-0865-z.

Vujisic, S. et al., 2012. Disulfiram-induced polyneurophaty. Military Medical and Pharmaceutical Journal of Serbia, 69(5), pp.453–475.
http://dx.doi.org/10.2298/vsp1205453v.

DIVERTICULITIS

Fernández, L.A., González, V.M., Martínez, S.N., Tamayo, R.M. and Albarracín, M.B.A., 2016. Acute abdomen from duodenal diverticulitis. A case report. Revista espanola de enfermedades digestivas: organo oficial de la Sociedad Espanola de Patologia Digestiva, 108(10), p.661. http://scielo.isciii.es/pdf/diges/v108n10/imagenes5.pdf

Feuerstein, J.D. & Falchuk, K.R., 2016. Diverticulosis and Diverticulitis. Mayo Clinic Proceedings, 91(8), pp.1094–1104. http://dx.doi.org/10.1016/j.mayocp.2016.03.012.

Scaioli, E. et al., 2015. Pathophysiology and Therapeutic Strategies for Symptomatic Uncomplicated Diverticular Disease of the Colon. Digestive Diseases and Sciences, 61(3), pp.673–683. http://dx.doi.org/10.1007/s10620-015-3925-0.

DORSAL HORN CIRCUITRY

Baron, R., Binder, A. & Wasner, G., 2010. Neuropathic pain: diagnosis, pathophysiological mechanisms, and treatment. The Lancet Neurology, 9(8), pp.807–819.
http://dx.doi.org/10.1016/s1474-4422(10)70143-5.

Benarroch, E.E., 2016. Dorsal horn circuitry. Neurology, 86(11), pp.1060–1069. http://dx.doi.org/10.1212/wnl.0000000000002478.

Braz, J.M. et al., 2005. Parallel "Pain" Pathways Arise from Subpopulations of Primary Afferent Nociceptor. Neuron, 47(6), pp.787–793. http://dx.doi.org/10.1016/j.neuron.2005.08.015.

Duan, B. et al., 2014. Identification of Spinal Circuits Transmitting and Gating Mechanical Pain. Cell, 159(6), pp.1417–1432. http://dx.doi.org/10.1016/j.cell.2014.11.003.

Foster, E. et al., 2015. Targeted Ablation, Silencing, and Activation Establish Glycinergic Dorsal Horn Neurons as Key Components of a Spinal Gate for Pain and Itch. Neuron, 85(6), pp.1289–1304. http://dx.doi.org/10.1016/j.neuron.2015.02.028.

Kim, Y.H. et al., 2012. TRPV1 in GABAergic Interneurons Mediates Neuropathic Mechanical Allodynia and Disinhibition of the Nociceptive Circuitry in the Spinal Cord. Neuron, 74(4), pp.640–647. http://dx.doi.org/10.1016/j.neuron.2012.02.039.

Knowlton, W.M. et al., 2013. A Sensory-Labeled Line for Cold: TRPM8-Expressing Sensory Neurons Define the Cellular Basis for Cold, Cold Pain, and Cooling-Mediated Analgesia. Journal of Neuroscience, 33(7), pp.2837–2848. http://dx.doi.org/10.1523/jneurosci.1943-12.2013.

Luo, C., Kuner, T. & Kuner, R., 2014. Synaptic plasticity in pathological pain. Trends in Neurosciences, 37(6), pp.343–355. http://dx.doi.org/10.1016/j.tins.2014.04.002.

Mendell, L.M., 2014. Constructing and deconstructing the gate theory of pain. Pain, 155(2), pp.210–216. http://dx.doi.org/10.1016/j.pain.2013.12.010.

Polgár, E. et al., 2013. A Quantitative Study of Inhibitory Interneurons in Laminae I-III of the Mouse Spinal Dorsal Horn S. D. Ginsberg, ed. PLoS ONE, 8(10), p.e78309. http://dx.doi.org/10.1371/journal.pone.0078309.

Prescott, S.A. & Ratté, S., 2012. Pain processing by spinal microcircuits: afferent combinatorics. Current Opinion in Neurobiology, 22(4), pp.631–639. http://dx.doi.org/10.1016/j.conb.2012.02.010.

Todd, A.J., 2010. Neuronal circuitry for pain processing in the dorsal horn. Nature Reviews Neuroscience, 11(12), pp.823–836. http://dx.doi.org/10.1038/nrn2947.

Von Hehn, C.A., Baron, R. & Woolf, C.J., 2012. Deconstructing the Neuropathic Pain Phenotype to Reveal Neural Mechanisms. Neuron, 73(4), pp.638–652. http://dx.doi.org/10.1016/j.neuron.2012.02.008.

Wang, X. et al., 2013. Excitatory Superficial Dorsal Horn Interneurons Are Functionally Heterogeneous and Required for the Full Behavioral Expression of Pain and Itch.

Neuron, 78(2), pp.312–324. http://dx.doi.org/10.1016/j.neuron.2013.03.001.

Zeilhofer, H.U., Wildner, H. & Yevenes, G.E., 2012. Fast Synaptic Inhibition in Spinal Sensory Processing and Pain Control. Physiological Reviews, 92(1), pp.193–235. http://dx.doi.org/10.1152/physrev.00043.2010.

Zhang, J. et al., 2013. The modality-specific contribution of peptidergic and non-peptidergic nociceptors is manifest at the level of dorsal horn nociresponsive neurons. The Journal of Physiology, 591(4), pp.1097–1110. http://dx.doi.org/10.1113/jphysiol.2012.242115.

DRY EYE SYNDROME

Kovács, I. et al., 2016. Abnormal activity of corneal cold thermoreceptors underlies the unpleasant sensations in dry eye disease. PAIN, 157(2), pp.399–417. http://dx.doi.org/10.1097/j.pain.0000000000000455.

Matossian, C. & Micucci, J., 2016. Characterization of the serological biomarkers associated with Sjögren’s syndrome in patients with recalcitrant dry eye disease. Clinical Ophthalmology, Volume 10, pp.1329–1334. http://dx.doi.org/10.2147/opth.s106973.

DYSMENORRHEA

Coco AS. Primary dysmenorrhea. Am Fam Physician. 1999 Aug;60(2):489-96. Review. https://www.ncbi.nlm.nih.gov/pubmed/10465224

De Sanctis V, Soliman A, Bernasconi S, Bianchin L, Bona G, Bozzola M, Buzi F, De Sanctis C, Tonini G, Rigon F, Perissinotto E. Primary Dysmenorrhea in Adolescents: Prevalence, Impact and Recent Knowledge. Pediatr Endocrinol Rev. 2015 Dec;13(2):512-20. Review. https://www.ncbi.nlm.nih.gov/pubmed/26841639

Dun, W. et al., 2016. Abnormal white matter integrity during pain-free periovulation is associated with pain intensity in primary dysmenorrhea. Brain Imaging and Behavior. http://dx.doi.org/10.1007/s11682-016-9582-x.

Jones, A.V. et al., 2016. Genome-wide association analysis of pain severity in dysmenorrhea identifies association at chromosome 1p13.2, near the nerve growth factor locus. PAIN, 157(11), pp.2571–2581. http://dx.doi.org/10.1097/j.pain.0000000000000678.

DYSPAREUNIA

Boardman, L.A. & Stockdale, C.K., 2009. Sexual Pain. Clinical Obstetrics and Gynecology, 52(4), pp.682–690. http://dx.doi.org/10.1097/grf.0b013e3181bf4a7e.

Graziottin, A., Gambini, D. & Bertolasi, L., 2015. Genital and sexual pain in women. Handbook of Clinical Neurology, pp.395–412. http://dx.doi.org/10.1016/b978-0-

444-63247-0.00023-7.

Melles, R.J. et al., 2016. Attentional Bias for Pain and Sex, and Automatic Appraisals of Sexual Penetration: Differential Patterns in Dyspareunia vs Vaginismus? The Journal of Sexual Medicine, 13(8), pp.1255–1262. http://dx.doi.org/10.1016/j.jsxm.2016.05.008.

Monforte M, Mimoun S, Droupy S. [Sexual pain disorders in females and males]. Prog Urol. 2013 Jul;23(9):761-70. Review. French. http://europepmc.org/abstract/med/23830271

EAGLE SYNDROME

Ho S. Styloid/C1 transverse process juxtaposition as a cause of Eagle's syndrome. Head & Neck volume 37 issue 11 on pages E153 to E156 .Available at https://doi.org/10.1002/hed.24024.

Kent DT et al., Conventional and 3-Dimensional Computerized Tomography in Eagle's Syndrome, Glossopharyngeal Neuralgia, and Asymptomatic Controls. Otolaryngol Head Neck Surg. 2015 Jul;153(1):41-7. Available at

http://10.1177/0194599815583047.

Mayrink, G. et al., 2011. Cervicofacial pain associated with Eagle's syndrome misdiagnosed as trigeminal neuralgia. Oral and Maxillofacial Surgery, 16(2), pp.207–210. http://dx.doi.org/10.1007/s10006-011-0276-7.

ECTOPIC PREGNANCY

Farquhar, C.M., 2005. Ectopic pregnancy. The Lancet, 366(9485), pp.583–591. http://dx.doi.org/10.1016/s0140-6736(05)67103-6.

Saito, M. et al., 1975. Site of Ovulation and Ectopic Pregnancy. Acta Obstetricia et Gynecologica Scandinavica, 54(3), pp.227–230. http://dx.doi.org/10.3109/00016347509157766.

Stein, J.C. et al., 2010. Emergency Physician Ultrasonography for Evaluating Patients at Risk for Ectopic Pregnancy: A Meta-Analysis. Annals of Emergency Medicine, 56(6), pp.674–683. http://dx.doi.org/10.1016/j.annemergmed.2010.06.563.

EHLERS-DANLOS

Bovet, C., Carlson, M. & Taylor, M., 2016. Quality of life, unmet needs, and iatrogenic injuries in rehabilitation of patients with Ehlers-Danlos Syndrome hypermobility type/Joint Hypermobility Syndrome. American Journal of Medical Genetics Part A, 170(8), pp.2044–2051. http://dx.doi.org/10.1002/ajmg.a.37774.

Cazzato, D. et al., 2016. Small fiber neuropathy is a common feature of Ehlers-Danlos syndromes. Neurology, 87(2), pp.155–159. http://dx.doi.org/10.1212/wnl.0000000000002847.

Grahame, R., 2016. Ehlers-Danlos syndrome. South African Medical Journal, 106(6), p.45. http://dx.doi.org/10.7196/samj.2016.v106i6.10991.

ENDOMETRIOSIS

Arafat, S. et al., 2016. Rare manifestation of endometriosis causing complete recto-sigmoid obstruction: A case report. International Journal of Surgery Case Reports, 26, pp.30–33. http://dx.doi.org/10.1016/j.ijscr.2016.07.004.

Fan, W. et al., 2016. The cytochrome P4501A1 gene polymorphisms and endometriosis: a meta-analysis. Journal of Assisted Reproduction and Genetics, 33(10), pp.1373–1383. http://dx.doi.org/10.1007/s10815-016-0783-4.

Miller, E.J. & Fraser, I.S., 2015. The importance of pelvic nerve fibers in endometriosis. Women's Health, 11(5), pp.611–618. http://dx.doi.org/10.2217/whe.15.47.

Morotti, M. et al., 2014. Peripheral changes in endometriosis-associated pain. Human Reproduction Update, 20(5), pp.717–736. http://dx.doi.org/10.1093/humupd/dmu021.

Yosef, A. et al., 2016. Multifactorial contributors to the severity of chronic pelvic pain in women. American Journal of Obstetrics and Gynecology, 215(6), pp.760.e1–760.e14. http://dx.doi.org/10.1016/j.ajog.2016.07.023.

ETHAMBUTOL

Cinici, E., 2016. Gene expression and histopathological evaluation of thiamine pyrophosphate on optic neuropathy induced with ethambutol in rats. International Journal of Ophthalmology. Available at: http://dx.doi.org/10.18240/ijo.2016.10.04.

Holdiness, M.R., 1987. Neurological Manifestations and Toxicities of the Antituberculosis Drugs. Medical Toxicology, 2(1), pp.33–51. Available at: http://dx.doi.org/10.1007/bf03259859.

Osaguona, V.B. et al., 2014. Optic Chiasm Involvement on MRI With Ethambutol-Induced Bitemporal Hemianopia. Journal of Neuro-Ophthalmology, 34(2), pp.155–158. Available at: http://dx.doi.org/10.1097/wno.0000000000000095.

Song, W. & Si, S., 2017. The rare ethambutol-induced optic neuropathy. Medicine, 96(2), p.e5889. Available at: http://dx.doi.org/10.1097/md.0000000000005889.

ETHYLENE OXIDE

Patch, P.C. & Hartlage, L.C., 2001. Neurological and Emotional Sequelae of Exposure to Ethylene Oxide. International Journal of Neuroscience, 106(1-2), pp.101–107. Available at: http://dx.doi.org/10.3109/00207450109149741.

Matsuoka, M. et al., 1990. Inhibition of creatine kinase activity by ethylene oxide. Occupational and Environmental Medicine, 47(1), pp.44–47. Available at: http://dx.doi.org/10.1136/oem.47.1.44.

Zampollo, A., Zacchetti, O. & Pisati, G., 1984. On ethylene oxide neurotoxicity: Report of two cases of peripheral neuropathy. The Italian Journal of Neurological Sciences, 5(1), pp.59–62. Available at: http://dx.doi.org/10.1007/bf02043971.

EPIDURAL ABSCESS

Al-Hourani, K., Al-Aref, R. & Mesfin, A., 2015. Upper Cervical Epidural Abscess in Clinical Practice: Diagnosis and Management. Global Spine Journal, 06(04), pp.383–393. http://dx.doi.org/10.1055/s-0035-1565260.

Darouiche, R.O., 2006. Spinal Epidural Abscess. New England Journal of Medicine, 355(19), pp.2012–2020. http://dx.doi.org/10.1056/nejmra055111.

Grewal, S., 2006. Epidural abscesses. British Journal of Anaesthesia, 96(3), pp.292–302. http://dx.doi.org/10.1093/bja/ael006.

Reihsaus, E., Waldbaur, H. & Seeling, W., 2000. Spinal epidural abscess: a meta-analysis of 915 patients. Neurosurgical Review, 23(4), pp.175–204. http://dx.doi.org/10.1007/pl00011954.

Sendi, P., Bregenzer, T. & Zimmerli, W., 2007. Spinal epidural abscess in clinical practice. QJM, 101(1), pp.1–12. http://dx.doi.org/10.1093/qjmed/hcm100.

Shweikeh, F. et al., 2014. An institutional series and contemporary review of bacterial spinal epidural abscess: current status and future directions. Neurosurgical Focus, 37(2), p.E9. http://dx.doi.org/10.3171/2014.6.focus14146.

Suppiah, S. et al., 2016. How Best to Manage the Spinal Epidural Abscess? A Current Systematic Review. World Neurosurgery, 93, pp.20–28. http://dx.doi.org/10.1016/j.wneu.2016.05.074.

EPOTHILONE

Argyriou, A.A. et al., 2011. Epothilone-Induced Peripheral Neuropathy: A Review of Current Knowledge. Journal of Pain and Symptom Management, 42(6), pp.931–940. http://dx.doi.org/10.1016/j.jpainsymman.2011.02.022.

Zhang, H. et al., 2014. Multiple Effects of a Novel Epothilone Analog on Cellular Processes and Signaling Pathways Regulated by Rac1 GTPase in the Human Breast Cancer Cells. The Korean Journal of Physiology & Pharmacology, 18(2), p.109.

http://dx.doi.org/10.4196/kjpp.2014.18.2.109.

ETOPOSIDE

Bruserud, Ø. et al., 2012. High-dose etoposide in allogeneic stem cell transplantation. Cancer Chemotherapy and Pharmacology, 70(6), pp.765–782. http://dx.doi.org/10.1007/s00280-012-1990-z.

Imrie, K.R., Couture, F., Turner, C.C., Sutcliffe, S.B. and Keating, A., 1994. Peripheral neuropathy following high-dose etoposide and autologous bone marrow transplantation. Bone marrow transplantation, 13(1), pp.77-79. https://www.ncbi.nlm.nih.gov/pubmed/8019457.

FABRY'S DISEASE

Bersano, A. et al., 2012. Neurological features of Fabry disease: clinical, pathophysiological aspects and therapy. Acta Neurologica Scandinavica, 126(2), pp.77–97. http://dx.doi.org/10.1111/j.1600-0404.2012.01661.x.

Burlina, A.P. et al., 2011. Early diagnosis of peripheral nervous system involvement in Fabry disease and treatment of neuropathic pain: the report of an expert panel. BMC Neurology, 11(1). http://dx.doi.org/10.1186/1471-2377-11-61.

Mehta, A. et al., 2004. Fabry disease defined: baseline clinical manifestations of 366 patients in the Fabry Outcome Survey. European Journal of Clinical Investigation, 34(3), pp.236–242. http://dx.doi.org/10.1111/j.1365-2362.2004.01309.x.

Ranieri, M. et al., 2016. Fabry Disease: Recognition, Diagnosis, and Treatment of Neurological Features. Current Treatment Options in Neurology, 18(7). http://dx.doi.org/10.1007/s11940-016-0414-5.

Schäfer, E. et al., 2005. Thirty-four novel mutations of the GLA gene in 121 patients with Fabry disease. Human Mutation, 25(4), pp.412–412. http://dx.doi.org/10.1002/humu.9327.

Schiffmann, R. et al., 2003. Enzyme replacement therapy improves peripheral nerve and sweat function in Fabry disease. Muscle & Nerve, 28(6), pp.703–710. http://dx.doi.org/10.1002/mus.10497.

Wani, M. et al., 2016. Fabry's disease: Case series and review of literature. Annals of Medical and Health Sciences Research, 6(3), pp193-197. https://doi.org/10.4103/2141-9248.183935

Wozniak, M.A. et al., 2009. Frequency of Unrecognized Fabry Disease Among Young European-American and African-American Men With First Ischemic Stroke. Stroke, 41(1), pp.78–81. http://dx.doi.org/10.1161/strokeaha.109.558320.

FACET SYNDROME

McCormick, Z.L. et al., 2015. Long-Term Function, Pain and Medication Use Outcomes of Radiofrequency Ablation for Lumbar Facet Syndrome. International journal of anesthetics and anesthesiology, 2(2). https://www.ncbi.nlm.nih.gov/pmc/articles/PMC4440581/

Oh, J. et al., 2016. Facetoplasty Using Radiofrequency Thermocoagulation for Facet Joint Hypertrophy. Pain Physician, 19(4), pp.E649–52. https://www.ncbi.nlm.nih.gov/pubmed/27228518

Pacetti, M., Fiaschi, P. & Gennaro, S., 2016. Percutaneous radiofrequency thermocoagulation of dorsal ramus branches as a treatment of "lumbar facet syndrome" - How I do it. Acta Neurochirurgica, 158(5), pp.995–998. http://dx.doi.org/10.1007/s00701-016-2759-7.

FAMILIAL EPISODE PAIN SYNDROME

Boukalova, S., Touska, F., Marsakova, L., Hynkova, A., Sura, L., Chvojka, S., Dittert, I. and Vlachova, V., 2014. Gain-of-function mutations in the transient receptor potential channels TRPV1 and TRPA1: how painful?. Physiol Res. 2014;63 Suppl 1:S205-13. Erratum in 2014;63(5), pp667. https://www.ncbi.nlm.nih.gov/pubmed/24564660

Bouklova S1, Touska F, Marsakova L, Hynkova A, Sura L, Chvojka S, Dittert I, Vlachova V. 2014. Ava Gain-of-function mutations in the transient receptor potential channels TRPV1 and TRPA1: how painful?, Physiol Res., 63(5):667. https://www.ncbi.nlm.nih.gov/pubmed/24564660

Okuda, H. et al., 2016. Infantile Pain Episodes Associated with Novel Nav1.9 Mutations in Familial Episodic Pain Syndrome in Japanese Families L. S. Premkumar, ed. PLOS ONE, 11(5), p.e0154827. http://dx.doi.org/10.1371/journal.pone.0154827.

Zhang, X.Y. et al., 2013. Gain-of-Function Mutations in SCN11A Cause Familial Episodic Pain. The American Journal of Human Genetics, 93(5), pp.957–966. http://dx.doi.org/10.1016/j.ajhg.2013.09.016.

Zíma, V. et al., 2015. Structural modeling and patch-clamp analysis of pain-related mutation TRPA1-N855S reveal inter-subunit salt bridges stabilizing the channel open state. Neuropharmacology, 93, pp.294–307. http://dx.doi.org/10.1016/j.neuropharm.2015.02.018.

FEMORAL NERVE

Moore, A.E. & Stringer, M.D., 2011. Iatrogenic femoral nerve injury: a systematic review. Surgical and Radiologic Anatomy, 33(8), pp.649–658. Available at: http://dx.doi.org/10.1007/s00276-011-0791-0.

Fox AJ1, Bedi A, Wanivenhaus F, Sculco TP, Fox JS, 2012. Femoral neuropathy following total hip arthroplasty: review and management guidelines. Acta Orthop Belg.,78(2), pp. 145-51. Abstract available at:
https://www.ncbi.nlm.nih.gov/pubmed/22696981

Kalita, J. et al., 2016. Sports induced femoral neuropathy: Review of literature. Neurology India, 64(6), p.1303. Available at:
http://dx.doi.org/10.4103/0028-3886.193823.

Abel, N.A. et al., 2017. Femoral nerve and lumbar plexus injury after minimally invasive lateral retroperitoneal transpsoas approach: electrodiagnostic prognostic indicators and a roadmap to recovery. Neurosurgical Review. Available at:
http://dx.doi.org/10.1007/s10143-017-0863-7.

FIBROMYALGIA

Caro, X.J. & Winter, E.F., 2014. Evidence of Abnormal Epidermal Nerve Fiber Density in Fibromyalgia: Clinical and Immunologic Implications. Arthritis & Rheumatology, 66(7), pp.1945–1954. http://dx.doi.org/10.1002/art.38662.

Caro, X.J. & Winter, E.F., 2014. Evidence of Abnormal Epidermal Nerve Fiber Density in Fibromyalgia: Clinical and Immunologic Implications. Arthritis & Rheumatology, 66(7), pp.1945–1954. http://dx.doi.org/10.1002/art.38662.

Caro, X.J. & Winter, E.F., 2015. The Role and Importance of Small Fiber Neuropathy in Fibromyalgia Pain. Current Pain and Headache Reports, 19(12).
http://dx.doi.org/10.1007/s11916-015-0527-7.

Fomberstein, K., Qadri, S. & Ramani, R., 2013. Functional MRI and pain. Current Opinion in Anaesthesiology, 26(5), pp.588–593.
http://dx.doi.org/10.1097/01.aco.0000433060.59939.fe.

Ichesco, E. et al., 2014. Altered Resting State Connectivity of the Insular Cortex in Individuals With Fibromyalgia. The Journal of Pain, 15(8), pp.815–826.e1.
http://dx.doi.org/10.1016/j.jpain.2014.04.007.

Momi, S.K. et al., 2015. Neuropathic pain as part of chronic widespread pain. PAIN, 156(10), pp.2100–2106. http://dx.doi.org/10.1097/j.pain.0000000000000277.

GALLBLADDER

Behar, J. et al., 2006. Functional Gallbladder and Sphincter of Oddi Disorders. Gastroenterology, 130(5), pp.1498–1509. http://dx.doi.org/10.1053/j.gastro.2005.11.063.

Dauer, M. & Lammert, F., 2009. Mandatory and optional function tests for biliary disorders. Best Practice & Research Clinical Gastroenterology, 23(3), pp.441–451.

http://dx.doi.org/10.1016/j.bpg.2009.04.001.

Halldestam, I., Kullman, E. & Borch, K., 2009. Incidence of and potential risk factors for gallstone disease in a general population sample. British Journal of Surgery, 96(11), pp.1315–1322. http://dx.doi.org/10.1002/bjs.6687.

Williams, T.P. et al., 2015. Hospital readmission after emergency room visit for cholelithiasis. Journal of Surgical Research, 197(2), pp.318–323.
http://dx.doi.org/10.1016/j.jss.2015.04.032.

GENERAL NEUROPATHIC PAIN

Denk, F., McMahon, S.B. & Tracey, I., 2014. Pain vulnerability: a neurobiological perspective. Nature Neuroscience, 17(2), pp.192–200.
http://dx.doi.org/10.1038/nn.3628.

Flores-Méndez, M., Mendez-Flores, O.G. & Ortega, A., 2016. Glia plasma membrane transporters: Key players in glutamatergic neurotransmission. Neurochemistry International, 98, pp.46–55. http://dx.doi.org/10.1016/j.neuint.2016.04.004.

Gracely, R.H., Lynch, S.A. & Bennett, G.J., 1992. Painful neuropathy: altered central processing maintained dynamically by peripheral input. Pain, 51(2), pp.175–194. http://dx.doi.org/10.1016/0304-3959(92)90259-e.

Kahle, K.T. et al., 2014. Therapeutic Restoration of Spinal Inhibition via Druggable Enhancement of Potassium-Chloride Cotransporter KCC2–Mediated Chloride Extrusion in Peripheral Neuropathic Pain. JAMA Neurol, 71(5), p.640.
http://dx.doi.org/10.1001/jamaneurol.2014.21.

Latremoliere, A. & Woolf, C.J., 2009. Central Sensitization: A Generator of Pain Hypersensitivity by Central Neural Plasticity. The Journal of Pain, 10(9), pp.895–926. http://dx.doi.org/10.1016/j.jpain.2009.06.012.

Li, L. et al., 2016. Chloride Homeostasis Critically Regulates Synaptic NMDA Receptor Activity in Neuropathic Pain. Cell Reports, 15(7), pp.1376–1383.
http://dx.doi.org/10.1016/j.celrep.2016.04.039.

Luo, X. et al., 2016. Crosstalk between astrocytic CXCL12 and microglial CXCR4 contributes to the development of neuropathic pain. Molecular Pain, 12(0).
http://dx.doi.org/10.1177/1744806916636385.

Maier, C. et al., 2010. Quantitative sensory testing in the German Research Network on Neuropathic Pain (DFNS): Somatosensory abnormalities in 1236 patients with different neuropathic pain syndromes. Pain, 150(3), pp.439–450.
http://dx.doi.org/10.1016/j.pain.2010.05.002.

Martínez-Lozada, Z. & Ortega, A., 2015. Glutamatergic Transmission: A Matter of Three. Neural Plasticity, 2015, pp.1–11. http://dx.doi.org/10.1155/2015/787396.

Prescott, S.A., Ma, Q. & De Koninck, Y., 2014. Normal and abnormal coding of somatosensory stimuli causing pain. Nature Neuroscience, 17(2), pp.183–191. http://dx.doi.org/10.1038/nn.3629.

Ringkamp, M., Raja, S.N., Campbell, J.N. and Meyer, R.A., 2013. Peripheral mechanisms of cutaneous nociception. Wall and Melzack's textbook of pain. Elsevier Saunders, pp.1-30. https://www.elsevier.com/books/wall-and-melzacks-textbook-of-pain/mcmahon/978-0-7020-4059-7#

Sandkuhler, J., 2009. Models and Mechanisms of Hyperalgesia and Allodynia. Physiological Reviews, 89(2), pp.707–758. http://dx.doi.org/10.1152/physrev.00025.2008.

Woolf, C.J. & Mannion, R.J., 1999. Neuropathic pain: aetiology, symptoms, mechanisms, and management. The Lancet, 353(9168), pp.1959–1964. http://dx.doi.org/10.1016/s0140-6736(99)01307-0.

Woolf, C.J., 2011. Central sensitization: Implications for the diagnosis and treatment of pain. Pain, 152(Supplement), pp.S2–S15. http://dx.doi.org/10.1016/j.pain.2010.09.030.

Yarnitsky, D., 2010. Conditioned pain modulation (the diffuse noxious inhibitory control-like effect): its relevance for acute and chronic pain states. Current Opinion in Anaesthesiology, 23(5), pp.611–615. http://dx.doi.org/10.1097/aco.0b013e32833c348b.

GENETIC INFLUENCES ON PAIN

Zubieta, J.-K., 2003. COMT val158met Genotype Affects micro-Opioid Neurotransmitter Responses to a Pain Stressor. Science, 299(5610), pp.1240–1243. Available at: http://dx.doi.org/10.1126/science.1078546.

Diatchenko, L., 2004. Genetic basis for individual variations in pain perception and the development of a chronic pain condition. Human Molecular Genetics, 14(1), pp.135–143. Available at: http://dx.doi.org/10.1093/hmg/ddi013.

Fillingim, R.B. et al., 2005. The A118G single nucleotide polymorphism of the μ-opioid receptor gene (OPRM1) is associated with pressure pain sensitivity in humans. The Journal of Pain, 6(3), pp.159–167. Available at: http://dx.doi.org/10.1016/j.jpain.2004.11.008.

Belfer, I. et al., 2013. Pain modality- and sex-specific effects of COMT genetic functional variants. Pain, 154(8), pp.1368–1376. Available at: http://dx.doi.org/10.1016/j.pain.2013.04.028.

Bjorland, S. et al., 2017. Genetic predictors of recovery in low back and lumbar radicular pain. PAIN, p.1. Available at: http://dx.doi.org/10.1097/j.pain.0000000000000934.

Parisien, M. et al., 2017. Effect of Human Genetic Variability on Gene Expression in Dorsal Root Ganglia and Association with Pain Phenotypes. Cell Reports, 19(9), pp.1940–1952. Available at: http://dx.doi.org/10.1016/j.celrep.2017.05.018.

De Gregori, M. et al., 2016. Human Genetic Variability Contributes to Postoperative Morphine Consumption. The Journal of Pain, 17(5), pp.628–636. Available at: http://dx.doi.org/10.1016/j.jpain.2016.02.003.

Nielsen, L.M. et al., 2017. Genetic Influences of OPRM1, OPRD1 and COMT on Morphine Analgesia in a Multi-Modal, Multi-Tissue Human Experimental Pain Model. Basic & Clinical Pharmacology & Toxicology, 121(1), pp.6–12. Available at: http://dx.doi.org/10.1111/bcpt.12757.

GIANT CELL ARTERITIS

Caselli, R.J. et al., 1988. Peripheral neuropathic syndromes in giant cell (temporal) arteritis. Neurology, 38(5), pp.685–685. http://dx.doi.org/10.1212/wnl.38.5.685.

Golbus, J. and McCune, W.J., 1987. Giant cell arteritis and peripheral neuropathy: a report of 2 cases and review of the literature. The Journal of rheumatology, 14(1), pp.129-134. https://www.ncbi.nlm.nih.gov/pubmed/3033236

Lensen, K.D.F., Voskuyl, A.E., Comans, E.F.I., van der Laken, C.J. and Smulders, Y.M., 2016. Extracranial giant cell arteritis: A narrative review. Light blue sclerae and normal bones: what is your diagnosis?, p.182. https://www.ncbi.nlm.nih.gov/pubmed/27323671

Nesher, G., 2014. The diagnosis and classification of giant cell arteritis. Journal of Autoimmunity, 48-49, pp.73–75. http://dx.doi.org/10.1016/j.jaut.2014.01.017.

Ness, T. et al., 2013 The Diagnosis and Treatment of Giant Cell Arteritis. Dtsch. Arztebl. Int., 110(21), pp.376-386. https://www.ncbi.nlm.nih.gov/pmc/articles/PMC3679627/

Ninan, J., Lester, S. & Hill, C., 2016. Giant cell arteritis. Best Practice & Research Clinical Rheumatology, 30(1), pp.169–188. http://dx.doi.org/10.1016/j.berh.2016.05.001.

Tan, B.L. et al., 2016. Diagnosing an atypical site of giant cell arteritis with magnetic resonance angiography: a case report. Journal of Medical Case Reports, 10(1). http://dx.doi.org/10.1186/s13256-016-0971-y.

Yates, M. et al., 2016. The prevalence of giant cell arteritis and polymyalgia rheumatica in a UK primary care population. BMC Musculoskeletal Disorders, 17(1). http://dx.doi.org/10.1186/s12891-016-1127-3.

GLIA AND PAIN

Batti, L. et al., 2016. TMEM16F Regulates Spinal Microglial Function in Neuropathic Pain States. Cell Reports, 15(12), pp.2608–2615. http://dx.doi.org/10.1016/j.celrep.2016.05.039.

Beggs, S. & Salter, M.W., 2013. The known knowns of microglia–neuronal signalling in neuropathic pain. Neuroscience Letters, 557, pp.37–42. http://dx.doi.org/10.1016/j.neulet.2013.08.037.

Berta, T. et al., 2016. Microglial Signaling in Chronic Pain with a Special Focus on Caspase 6, p38 MAP Kinase, and Sex Dependence. Journal of Dental Research, 95(10), pp.1124–1131. http://dx.doi.org/10.1177/0022034516653604.

Jin, X. et al., 2014. P2X4 receptor in the dorsal horn partially contributes to brain-derived neurotrophic factor oversecretion and toll-like receptor-4 receptor activation associated with bone cancer pain. Journal of Neuroscience Research, 92(12), pp.1690–1702. http://dx.doi.org/10.1002/jnr.23443.

Matsumura, Y. et al., 2016. A novel P2X4 receptor-selective antagonist produces anti-allodynic effect in a mouse model of herpetic pain. Scientific Reports, 6, p.32461. http://dx.doi.org/10.1038/srep32461.

Ohara, P.T. et al., 2009. Gliopathic Pain: When Satellite Glial Cells Go Bad. The Neuroscientist, 15(5), pp.450–463. http://dx.doi.org/10.1177/1073858409336094.

Shaqura, M. et al., 2016. Membrane-bound glucocorticoid receptors on distinct nociceptive neurons as potential targets for pain control through rapid non-genomic effects. Neuropharmacology, 111, pp.1–13. http://dx.doi.org/10.1016/j.neuropharm.2016.08.019.

Suter, M.R., 2016. Microglial role in the development of chronic pain. Current Opinion in Anaesthesiology, 29(5), pp.584–589. http://dx.doi.org/10.1097/aco.0000000000000373.

Taylor, A.M.W. et al., 2016. Topography of microglial activation in sensory- and affect-related brain regions in chronic pain. Journal of Neuroscience Research. http://dx.doi.org/10.1002/jnr.23883.

Tsuda, M. & Inoue, K., 2016. Neuron–microglia interaction by purinergic signaling in neuropathic pain following neurodegeneration. Neuropharmacology, 104, pp.76–81. http://dx.doi.org/10.1016/j.neuropharm.2015.08.042.

Tsuda, M., 2016. P2 receptors, microglial cytokines and chemokines, and neuropathic pain. Journal of Neuroscience Research. http://dx.doi.org/10.1002/jnr.23816.

Wen Y-R et al. Role of microglia in neuropathic pain. J Formosa Med Assoc 2014 110(8), pp.487-494. https://www.ncbi.nlm.nih.gov/pmc/articles/PMC3169792/

GLOSSOPHARYNGEAL NEURALGIA

Gaul, C. et al., 2011. Diagnosis and neurosurgical treatment of glossopharyngeal neuralgia: clinical findings and 3-D visualization of neurovascular compression in 19 consecutive patients. The Journal of Headache and Pain, 12(5), pp.527–534. http://dx.doi.org/10.1007/s10194-011-0349-x.

Liesegang, T., 2008. Herpes Zoster Ophthalmicus Natural History, Risk Factors, Clinical Presentation, and Morbidity. Ophthalmology, 115(2), pp.S3–S12. http://dx.doi.org/10.1016/j.ophtha.2007.10.009.

Marin, M. et al., 2016. Risk Factors for Herpes Zoster Among Adults. Open Forum Infectious Diseases, 3(3), p.ofw119. http://dx.doi.org/10.1093/ofid/ofw119.

Petersen, K.L. et al., 2010. Natural history of cutaneous innervation following herpes zoster. Pain, 150(1), pp.75–82. http://dx.doi.org/10.1016/j.pain.2010.04.002.

Schmader, K., 2016. Herpes Zoster. Clinics in Geriatric Medicine, 32(3), pp.539–553. http://dx.doi.org/10.1016/j.cger.2016.02.011.

Singh, P., Trikha, A. & Kaur, M., 2013. An uncommonly common: Glossopharyngeal neuralgia. Annals of Indian Academy of Neurology, 16(1), p.1. http://dx.doi.org/10.4103/0972-2327.107662.

Zhang, Y, Yu, B. et al, 2016. Microstructural Abnormalities in Gray Matter of Patients with Postherpetic Neuralgia: A Diffusional Kurtosis Imaging Study. Pain physician, 19, pp.E601-E611. https://pdfs.semanticscholar.org/522b/a07e4629cf5878a64bba6cfd6d81bd16b79e.pdf

GONYALGIA

Massey, E.W. et al., 1981. Letters to the Editor. Muscle & Nerve, 4(1), pp.80–84. Available at: http://dx.doi.org/10.1002/mus.880040115.

GRANULOMATOSIS WITH POLYANGIITIS

Asakura, K. and Muto, T., 2013. [Neurological involvement in Wegener's granulomatosis]. Brain and nerve= Shinkei kenkyu no shinpo, 65(11), pp.1311-1317. https://www.ncbi.nlm.nih.gov/pubmed/24200609.

Kubaisi, B., 2016. Granulomatosis with polyangiitis (Wegener's disease): An updated review of ocular disease manifestations. Intractable & Rare Disease Research, 5(2), pp 61-69. https://doi.org/10.5582/irdr.2016.01014

GREATER AURICULAR NERVE

Correia-Sá, I.B. et al., 2016. Eleven Years of Parotid Gland Surgery in a Plastic and Reconstructive Department. Journal of Craniofacial Surgery, 27(1), pp.e26–e33. http://dx.doi.org/10.1097/scs.0000000000002299.

Lefkowitz, T. et al., 2012. Anatomical Landmarks to Avoid Injury to the Great Auricular Nerve During Rhytidectomy. Aesthetic Surgery Journal, 33(1), pp.19–23. http://dx.doi.org/10.1177/1090820x12469625.

GREATER OCCIPITAL NERVE

Ashkenazi, A. & Levin, M., 2007. Greater occipital nerve block for migraine and other headaches: Is it useful? Current Pain and Headache Reports, 11(3), pp.231–235. http://dx.doi.org/10.1007/s11916-007-0195-3.

Cuadrado, M.L. et al., 2016. Short-term effects of greater occipital nerve blocks in chronic migraine: A double-blind, randomised, placebo-controlled clinical trial. Cephalalgia. http://dx.doi.org/10.1177/0333102416655159.

Janis, J.E., 2011. Reply: The Anatomy of the Greater Occipital Nerve: Part II. Compression Point Topography. Plastic and Reconstructive Surgery, 128(1), pp.322–323. http://dx.doi.org/10.1097/prs.0b013e318218fd86.

Shimizu, S., 2014. Scalp neuralgia and headache elicited by cranial superficial anatomical causes: supraorbital neuralgia, occipital neuralgia, and post-craniotomy headache. Rinsho Shinkeigaku, 54(5), pp.387–394. http://dx.doi.org/10.5692/clinicalneurol.54.387.

HANDL

Babi, M.-A. et al., 2016. Syndrome of transient headache and neurologic deficits with cerebrospinal fluid lymphocytosis presenting as acute neurological emergencies. Cephalalgia. http://dx.doi.org/10.1177/0333102416642733.

Filina, T., Feja, K.N. & Tolan, R.W., 2013. An Adolescent With Pseudomigraine, Transient Headache, Neurological Deficits, and Lymphocytic Pleocytosis (HaNDL Syndrome): Case Report and Review of the Literature. Clinical Pediatrics, 52(6), pp.496–502. http://dx.doi.org/10.1177/0009922813483358.

Rivero-Sanz, E., Pias-Peleteiro, L. & Gonzalez-Alvarez, V., 2016. HaNDL syndrome in a 14-year-old girl. BMJ Case Reports, p.bcr2015213018.

http://dx.doi.org/10.1136/bcr-2015-213018.

Stelten, B.M. et al., 2015. Syndrome of transient headache and neurological deficits with cerebrospinal fluid lymphocytosis (HaNDL): A case report with serial electroencephalography (EEG) recordings.. Is there an association with human herpes virus type 7 (HHV-7) infection? Cephalalgia, 36(13), pp.1296–1301. http://dx.doi.org/10.1177/0333102415618616.

Tada, Y. et al., 2005. A Patient of Migraine-like Headache with Amnesia, Pleocytosis and Transient Hypoperfusion of Cerebral Blood Flow. Internal Medicine, 44(7), pp.743–746. http://dx.doi.org/10.2169/internalmedicine.44.743.

HCN CHANNELS

Acosta, C. et al., 2012. HCN1 and HCN2 in Rat DRG Neurons: Levels in Nociceptors and Non-Nociceptors, NT3-Dependence and Influence of CFA-Induced Skin Inflammation on HCN2 and NT3 Expression Z. Zhang, ed. PLoS ONE, 7(12), p.e50442. http://dx.doi.org/10.1371/journal.pone.0050442.

Benarroch, E.E., 2013. HCN channels: Function and clinical implications. Neurology, 80(3), pp.304–310. http://dx.doi.org/10.1212/wnl.0b013e31827dec42.

Emery, E.C. et al., 2011. HCN2 Ion Channels Play a Central Role in Inflammatory and Neuropathic Pain. Science, 333(6048), pp.1462–1466. http://dx.doi.org/10.1126/science.1206243.

Wan, Y., 2008. Involvement of hyperpolarization-activated, cyclic nucleotide-gated cation channels in dorsal root ganglion in neuropathic pain. Sheng li xue bao:[Acta physiologica Sinica], 60(5), p.579. PMID: 18958363 https://www.ncbi.nlm.nih.gov/pubmed/18958363

Weng, X. et al., 2012. Chronic inflammatory pain is associated with increased excitability and hyperpolarization-activated current (Ih) in C- but not Aδ-nociceptors. Pain, 153(4), pp.900–914. http://dx.doi.org/10.1016/j.pain.2012.01.019.

HEADACHE: CERVICOGENIC

Antonaci, F. & Sjaastad, O., 2010. Cervicogenic Headache: A Real Headache. Current Neurology and Neuroscience Reports, 11(2), pp.149–155. http://dx.doi.org/10.1007/s11910-010-0164-9.

Becker, W.J., 2010. Cervicogenic Headache: Evidence That the Neck is a Pain Generator. Headache: The Journal of Head and Face Pain, 50(4), pp.699–705. http://dx.doi.org/10.1111/j.1526-4610.2010.01648.x.

Fredriksen, T.A., Antonaci, F. & Sjaastad, O., 2015. Cervicogenic headache: too important to be left un-diagnosed. The Journal of Headache and Pain, 16(1), p.6. http://dx.doi.org/10.1186/1129-2377-16-6.

Park, S.W. et al., 2011. The Effect of Radiofrequency Neurotomy of Lower Cervical Medial Branches on Cervicogenic Headache. Journal of Korean Neurosurgical Society, 50(6), p.507. http://dx.doi.org/10.3340/jkns.2011.50.6.507.

Sjaastad, O., 2008. Cervicogenic headache: comparison with migraine without aura; Vågå study. Cephalalgia, 28(s1), pp.18–20. http://dx.doi.org/10.1111/j.1468-2982.2008.01610.x.

Watson, D.H. & Drummond, P.D., 2016. The Role of the Trigemino Cervical Complex in Chronic Whiplash Associated Headache: A Cross Sectional Study. Headache: The Journal of Head and Face Pain, 56(6), pp.961–975. http://dx.doi.org/10.1111/head.12805.

HEADACHE: CLUSTER

Costa, A. et al., 2015. The Neuropharmacology of Cluster Headache and other Trigeminal Autonomic Cephalalgias. Current Neuropharmacology, 13(3), pp.304–323. http://dx.doi.org/10.2174/1570159x13666150309233556.

Curto, M. et al., 2016. Altered serum levels of kynurenine metabolites in patients affected by cluster headache. The Journal of Headache and Pain, 17(1). http://dx.doi.org/10.1186/s10194-016-0620-2.

Lainez, M.J. & Marti, A.S., 2016. Sphenopalatine ganglion stimulation in cluster headache and other types of headache. Cephalalgia, 36(12), pp.1149–1155. http://dx.doi.org/10.1177/0333102416644968.

Leone, M. & Proietti Cecchini, A., 2016. Advances in the understanding of cluster headache. Expert Review of Neurotherapeutics, pp.1–8. http://dx.doi.org/10.1080/14737175.2016.1216796.

Manzoni, G.C. et al., 2016. Age of onset of episodic and chronic cluster headache – a review of a large case series from a single headache centre. The Journal of Headache and Pain, 17(1). http://dx.doi.org/10.1186/s10194-016-0626-9.

HEADACHE: HYPNIC

Holle, D. & Obermann, M., 2012. Hypnic headache and caffeine. Expert Review of Neurotherapeutics, 12(9), pp.1125–1132. http://dx.doi.org/10.1586/ern.12.100.

Lisotto, C. et al., 2010. Focus on therapy of hypnic headache. The Journal of Headache and Pain, 11(4), pp.349–354. http://dx.doi.org/10.1007/s10194-010-0227-y.

Singh, N.N. & Sahota, P., 2013. Sleep-Related Headache and its Management. Current Treatment Options in Neurology, 15(6), pp.704–722.

http://dx.doi.org/10.1007/s11940-013-0258-1.

HEADACHE: LINEAR

Casas-Limón, J. et al., 2016. Pain Paroxysms With Coronal Radiation: Case Series and Proposal of a New Variant of Epicrania Fugax. Headache: The Journal of Head and Face Pain, 56(6), pp.1040–1044. http://dx.doi.org/10.1111/head.12821.

Cuadrado, M.L., Guerrero, A.L. & Pareja, J.A., 2016. Epicrania Fugax. Current Pain and Headache Reports, 20(4). http://dx.doi.org/10.1007/s11916-016-0557-9.

López-López, A. et al., 2016. Stress, Coping, and Personality in Patients with Epicrania Fugax, and Their Relation to the Clinical Characteristics of Pain. Pain Medicine, p.pnw130. http://dx.doi.org/10.1093/pm/pnw130.

Lu, Y.-N. et al., 2016. Linear headache: clinical characteristics of eight new cases. SpringerPlus, 5(1). http://dx.doi.org/10.1186/s40064-016-1991-1.

Pareja, J.A. & Bandrés, P., 2015. Linear interictal pain in Epicrania Fugax. The Journal of Headache and Pain, 16(1). http://dx.doi.org/10.1186/s10194-015-0507-7.

Wang, L. et al., 2016. A recurrent headache circumscribed in a coronal line-shaped area around the head: a coronal linear headache. SpringerPlus, 5(1). http://dx.doi.org/10.1186/s40064-016-1786-4.

HEADACHE: TENSION

Andersen, S. et al., 2015. Pressure pain thresholds assessed over temporalis, masseter, and frontalis muscles in healthy individuals, patients with tension-type headache, and those with migraine—a systematic review. PAIN, 156(8), pp.1409–1423. http://dx.doi.org/10.1097/j.pain.0000000000000219.

Ghadiri-Sani M, Silver N., 2016. Headache (chronic tension-type). Systematic review. BMJ Clinical Evidence, 1205 http://clinicalevidence.bmj.com/x/systematic-review/1205/overview.html

Moraska, A.F. et al., 2015. Myofascial Trigger Point-focused Head and Neck Massage for Recurrent Tension-type Headache. The Clinical Journal of Pain, 31(2), pp.159–168. http://dx.doi.org/10.1097/ajp.0000000000000091.

HEADACHE: THUNDERCLAP

Devenney, E., Neale, H. & Forbes, R.B., 2014. A systematic review of causes of sudden and severe headache (Thunderclap Headache): should lists be evidence based? The Journal of Headache and Pain, 15(1), p.49. http://dx.doi.org/10.1186/1129-2377-15-49.

Mortimer, A.M. et al., 2013. Thunderclap headache: Diagnostic considerations and neuroimaging features. Clinical Radiology, 68(3), pp.e101–e113. http://dx.doi.org/10.1016/j.crad.2012.08.032.

HEADACHE: TROCHLEAR

Smith, J.H., Garrity, J.A. & Boes, C.J., 2013. Clinical features and long-term prognosis of trochlear headaches. European Journal of Neurology, 21(4), pp.577–585. http://dx.doi.org/10.1111/ene.12312.

HEREDITARY AND IDIOPATHIC HNA

Bai, X. et al., 2013. Novel septin 9 repeat motifs altered in neuralgic amyotrophy bind and bundle microtubules. The Journal of Cell Biology, 203(6), pp.895–905. http://dx.doi.org/10.1083/jcb.201308068.

Chance, P.F., 2006. Inherited Focal, Episodic Neuropathies: Hereditary Neuropathy With Liability to Pressure Palsies and Hereditary Neuralgic Amyotrophy. NeuroMolecular Medicine, 8(1-2), pp.159–174. http://dx.doi.org/10.1385/nmm:8:1:159.

Fukushima, K. and Ikeda, S., 2014. [Neuralgic amyotrophy]. Brain and nerve= Shinkei kenkyu no shinpo, 66(12), pp.1421-1428. http://europepmc.org/abstract/med/25475029

Park, M.S., Kim, D.H. & Sung, D.H., 2014. Magnetic Resonance Neurographic Findings in Classic Idiopathic Neuralgic Amyotrophy in Subacute Stage: A Report of Four Cases. Annals of Rehabilitation Medicine, 38(2), p.286. http://dx.doi.org/10.5535/arm.2014.38.2.286.

Tjoumakaris, F.P. et al., 2012. Neuralgic Amyotrophy (Parsonage-Turner Syndrome). Journal of the American Academy of Orthopaedic Surgeons, 20(7), pp.443–449. http://dx.doi.org/10.5435/jaaos-20-07-443.

Van Alfen, N., 2011. Clinical and pathophysiological concepts of neuralgic amyotrophy. Nature Reviews Neurology, 7(6), pp.315–322. http://dx.doi.org/10.1038/nrneurol.2011.62.

Van Alfen, N., van Engelen, B.G. & Hughes, R.A., 2009. Treatment for idiopathic and hereditary neuralgic amyotrophy (brachial neuritis) N. van Alfen, ed. Cochrane Database of Systematic Reviews. http://dx.doi.org/10.1002/14651858.cd006976.pub2.

HEREDITARY NEUROPATHY WITH LIABILITY TO PRESSURE PALSY

Cortese, A. et al., 2016. Laryngeal and phrenic nerve involvement in a patient with hereditary neuropathy with liability to pressure palsies (HNPP). Neuromuscular Disorders, 26(7), pp.455–458. http://dx.doi.org/10.1016/j.nmd.2016.05.007.

Park, D., Ryu, J.S. & Kim, K.-J., 2016. Compression of Root Level in a Patient with Hereditary Neuropathy with Liability to Pressure Palsy Diagnosed by Magnetic Resonance Imaging. American Journal of Physical Medicine & Rehabilitation, 95(9), pp.e140–e144. http://dx.doi.org/10.1097/phm.0000000000000515.

Spagnoli, C. et al., 2016. Hereditary neuropathy with liability to pressure palsies in childhood: Case series and literature update. Neuromuscular Disorders, 26(6), p.394. http://dx.doi.org/10.1016/j.nmd.2016.04.007.

HERPES SIMPLEX VIRUS

Alstadhaug, Karl B., Hanne W. Kvarenes, Jan Prytz, and Christian Vedeler. "A Case of Relapsing–remitting Facial Palsy and Ipsilateral Brachial Plexopathy Caused by HSV-1." Journal of Clinical Virology 78 (May 2016): 62–65.
http://www.journalofclinicalvirology.com/article/S1386-6532(16)30031-2/abstract

Benjamin, Mina M., et al. "Herpes simplex virus meningitis complicated by ascending paralysis." Proceedings (Baylor University. Medical Center) 26.3 (2013): 265. https://www.ncbi.nlm.nih.gov/pmc/articles/PMC3684292/

Jaques, D.A. et al., 2016. Herpes simplex encephalitis as a complication of neurosurgical procedures: report of 3 cases and review of the literature. Virology Journal, 13(1). http://dx.doi.org/10.1186/s12985-016-0540-4.

Piedade, D. & Azevedo-Pereira, J., 2016. The Role of microRNAs in the Pathogenesis of Herpesvirus Infection. Viruses, 8(6), p.156. http://dx.doi.org/10.3390/v8060156.

Sili, U., Kaya, A. & Mert, A., 2014. Herpes simplex virus encephalitis: Clinical manifestations, diagnosis and outcome in 106 adult patients. Journal of Clinical Virology, 60(2), pp.112–118. http://dx.doi.org/10.1016/j.jcv.2014.03.010.

Steiner, I. & Benninger, F., 2013. Update on Herpes Virus Infections of the Nervous System. Current Neurology and Neuroscience Reports, 13(12).
http://dx.doi.org/10.1007/s11910-013-0414-8.

Steiner, I., 2013. Herpes virus infection of the peripheral nervous system. Peripheral Nerve Disorders, pp.543–558.
http://dx.doi.org/10.1016/b978-0-444-52902-2.00031-x.

HERPES ZOSTER / VARICELLA–ZOSTER VIRUS

Arvin, A., 2005. Aging, Immunity, and the Varicella–Zoster Virus. New England Journal of Medicine, 352(22), pp.2266–2267. http://dx.doi.org/10.1056/nejmp058091.

Cukic, V., 2016. The Uncommon Localization of Herpes Zoster. Medical Archives, 70(1), p.72. http://dx.doi.org/10.5455/medarh.2016.70.72-75.

Forbes, H.J. et al., 2016. Quantification of risk factors for postherpetic neuralgia in herpes zoster patients. Neurology, 87(1), pp.94–102. http://dx.doi.org/10.1212/wnl.0000000000002808.

Gilden, D.H. et al., 2000. Neurologic Complications of the Reactivation of Varicella–Zoster Virus. New England Journal of Medicine, 342(9), pp.635–645. http://dx.doi.org/10.1056/nejm200003023420906.

Gilden, D. et al., 2010. Neurological Disease Produced by Varicella Zoster Virus Reactivation Without Rash. Curr Topics Microbiol Immunol, pp.243–253. http://dx.doi.org/10.1007/82_2009_3.

Gnann, J.W., 2008. Vaccination to Prevent Herpes Zoster in Older Adults. The Journal of Pain, 9(1), pp.31–36. http://dx.doi.org/10.1016/j.jpain.2007.10.007.

Gnann, Jr., J.W., 2002. Varicella-Zoster Virus: Atypical Presentations and Unusual Complications. The Journal of Infectious Diseases, 186(s1), pp.S91–S98. http://dx.doi.org/10.1086/342963.

Ibrahim, W. et al., 2015. Varicella Zoster Aseptic Meningitis: Report of an Atypical Case and Literature Review. American Journal of Case Reports, 16, pp.594–597. http://dx.doi.org/10.12659/ajcr.894045.

Keating, G.M., 2016. Shingles (Herpes Zoster) Vaccine (Zostavax®): A Review in the Prevention of Herpes Zoster and Postherpetic Neuralgia. BioDrugs, 30(3), pp.243–254. http://dx.doi.org/10.1007/s40259-016-0180-7.

Kennedy, P.G.E. et al., 2015. A comparison of herpes simplex virus type 1 and varicella-zoster virus latency and reactivation. Journal of General Virology, 96(7), pp.1581–1602. http://dx.doi.org/10.1099/vir.0.000128.

Sampathkumar, P., Drage, L.A. & Martin, D.P., 2009. Herpes Zoster (Shingles) and Postherpetic Neuralgia. Mayo Clinic Proceedings, 84(3), pp.274–280. http://dx.doi.org/10.4065/84.3.274.

Steiner, I., Kennedy, P.G. & Pachner, A.R., 2007. The neurotropic herpes viruses: herpes simplex and varicella-zoster. The Lancet Neurology, 6(11), pp.1015–1028. http://dx.doi.org/10.1016/s1474-4422(07)70267-3.

Teo, H.K., Chawla, M. & Kaushik, M., 2016. A Rare Complication of Herpes Zoster: Segmental Zoster Paresis. Case Reports in Medicine, 2016, pp.1–3. http://dx.doi.org/10.1155/2016/7827140.

Wollina, U. & Machetanz, J., 2016. Herpes zoster und postzosterische Neuralgie. Der Hautarzt, 67(8), pp.653–665. http://dx.doi.org/10.1007/s00105-016-3834-y.

HIP ARTHROPLASTY AND PERIOPERATIVE NERVE INJURY

Chomiak, J. et al., 2015. Lesion of gluteal nerves and muscles in total hip arthroplasty through 3 surgical approaches. An electromyographically controlled study. Hip International, 25(2), pp.176–183. http://dx.doi.org/10.5301/hipint.5000199.

Jacob, A.K. et al., 2011. Perioperative Nerve Injury after Total Hip Arthroplasty. Anesthesiology, p.1. http://dx.doi.org/10.1097/aln.0b013e3182326c20.

Wettstein, M., Garofalo, R. & Mouhsine, E. Musculoskelet Surg (2010) 94(2), pp.77–80. http://dx.doi.org/10.1007/s12306-010-0078-3.

HUMAN IMMUNODEFICIENCY VIRUS (HIV)

Bhatia, N.S. & Chow, F.C., 2016. Neurologic Complications in Treated HIV-1 Infection. Current Neurology and Neuroscience Reports, 16(7). http://dx.doi.org/10.1007/s11910-016-0666-1.

Cherry, C.L., Wadley, A.L. & Kamerman, P.R., 2016. Diagnosing and treating HIV-associated sensory neuropathy: a global perspective. Pain Management, 6(2), pp.191–199. http://dx.doi.org/10.2217/pmt.15.65.

Panos, G. et al., 2016. Differential diagnosis and treatment of acute cauda equina syndrome in the human immunodeficiency virus positive patient: a case report and review of the literature. Journal of Medical Case Reports, 10(1). http://dx.doi.org/10.1186/s13256-016-0902-y.

Phillips, T.J.C. et al., 2010. Pharmacological Treatment of Painful HIV-Associated Sensory Neuropathy: A Systematic Review and Meta-Analysis of Randomised Controlled Trials N. P. Pai, ed. PLoS ONE, 5(12), p.e14433. http://dx.doi.org/10.1371/journal.pone.0014433.

HYOID BONE

Monceaux, G. et al., 1999. Osteoradionecrosis of the hyoid bone: A report of 3 cases. American Journal of Otolaryngology, 20(6), pp.400–404. http://dx.doi.org/10.1016/s0196-0709(99)90081-9.

Robinson, P.J., Davis, J.P. & Fraser, J.G., 1994. The hyoid syndrome: a pain in the neck. The Journal of Laryngology & Otology, 108(10). http://dx.doi.org/10.1017/s0022215100128324.

Stern, N., Jackson-Menaldi, C. & Rubin, A.D., 2013. Hyoid Bone Syndrome: A Retrospective Review of 84 Patients Treated with Triamcinolone Acetonide Injections.

Annals of Otology, Rhinology & Laryngology, 122(3), pp.159–162. http://dx.doi.org/10.1177/000348941312200303.

Zhang, I. et al., 2014. Chondrosarcoma of the hyoid bone: Case report and review of current management options P. Andersen, ed. Head & Neck, 36(7), pp.E65–E72. http://dx.doi.org/10.1002/hed.23373.

IDIOPATHIC PLEXOPATHY

Bradley, W.G. et al., 1984. Painful lumbosacral plexopathy with elevated erythrocyte sedimentation rate: A treatable inflammatory syndrome. Annals of Neurology, 15(5), pp.457–464. http://dx.doi.org/10.1002/ana.410150510.

Delaney, H., Bencardino, J. & Rosenberg, Z.S., 2014. Magnetic Resonance Neurography of the Pelvis and Lumbosacral Plexus. Neuroimaging Clinics of North America, 24(1), pp.127–150. http://dx.doi.org/10.1016/j.nic.2013.03.026.

Evans, B.A., Stevens, J.C. & Dyck, P.J., 1981. Lumbosacral plexus neuropathy. Neurology, 31(10), pp.1327–1327. http://dx.doi.org/10.1212/wnl.31.10.1327.

Imam, Y., Deleu, D. & Salem, K., 2012. Idiopathic lumbosacral plexitis. Qatar Medical Journal, 2012(2), p.20. http://dx.doi.org/10.5339/qmj.2012.2.20.

IFOSFAMIDE

Frisk, P. et al., 2001. Painful peripheral neuropathy after treatment with high-dose ifosfamide. Medical and Pediatric Oncology, 37(4), pp.379–382. http://dx.doi.org/10.1002/mpo.1210.

Sunela, K. and Bärlund, M., 2015. [Treatment and prevention of iphosphamide-induced encephalopathy]. Duodecim; laaketieteellinen aikakauskirja, 132(4), pp.314-317. https://www.ncbi.nlm.nih.gov/pubmed/27017785.

Turner, A.R., Duong, C.D. & Good, D.J., 2003. Methylene Blue for the Treatment and Prophylaxis of Ifosfamide-induced Encephalopathy. Clinical Oncology, 15(7), pp.435–439. http://dx.doi.org/10.1016/s0936-6555(03)00114-6.

ILIOHYPOGASTRIC/ILIOINGUINAL/GENITOFEMORAL

Reinpold, W. et al., 2015. Retroperitoneal anatomy of the iliohypogastric, ilioinguinal, genitofemoral, and lateral femoral cutaneous nerve: consequences for prevention and treatment of chronic inguinodynia. Hernia, 19(4), pp.539–548. Available at: http://dx.doi.org/10.1007/s10029-015-1396-z.

Geh, N. et al., 2015. Retroperitoneal course of iliohypogastric, ilioinguinal, and genitofemoral nerves: A study to improve identification and excision during triple neurectomy. Clinical Anatomy, 28(7), pp.903–909. Available at:

http://dx.doi.org/10.1002/ca.22592.

Grunert, P. et al., 2017. Injury to the Lumbar Plexus and its Branches After Lateral Fusion Procedures: A Cadaver Study. World Neurosurgery, 105, pp.519–525. Available at: http://dx.doi.org/10.1016/j.wneu.2017.06.027.

Cesmebasi, A. et al., 2014. Genitofemoral neuralgia: A review. Clinical Anatomy, 28(1), pp.128–135. Available at: http://dx.doi.org/10.1002/ca.22481.

ILIOLYMPHOGASTRIC, ILIOLINGUAL AND GENITOFEMORAL NERVES

Cesmebasi, A. et al., 2014. Genitofemoral neuralgia: A review. Clinical Anatomy, 28(1), pp.128–135. http://dx.doi.org/10.1002/ca.22481.

Hsu, W. et al., 2012. Preservation Versus Division of Ilioinguinal Nerve on Open Mesh Repair of Inguinal Hernia: A Meta-analysis of Randomized Controlled Trials. World Journal of Surgery, 36(10), pp.2311–2319. http://dx.doi.org/10.1007/s00268-012-1657-2.

Reinpold, W. et al., 2015. Retroperitoneal anatomy of the iliohypogastric, ilioinguinal, genitofemoral, and lateral femoral cutaneous nerve: consequences for prevention and treatment of chronic inguinodynia. Hernia, 19(4), pp.539–548. http://dx.doi.org/10.1007/s10029-015-1396-z.

Shin, J.H. & Howard, F.M., 2012. Abdominal Wall Nerve Injury During Laparoscopic Gynecologic Surgery: Incidence, Risk Factors, and Treatment Outcomes. Journal of Minimally Invasive Gynecology, 19(4), pp.448–453. http://dx.doi.org/10.1016/j.jmig.2012.03.009.

INFLAMMATORY NERVE ROOT DISORDER

Niino, M., Tsuji, S. & Tashiro, K., 1999. Chronic Inflammatory Demyelinating Polyneuropathy with Multiple Hypertrophic Nerves in Intracranial, and Intra- and Extra-Spinal Segments. Internal Medicine, 38(5), pp.445–449. http://dx.doi.org/10.2169/internalmedicine.38.445.

Norris, B., Gonzales, M. & Drummond, K.J., 2011. Solitary localised hypertrophic neuropathy of the cauda equina. Journal of Clinical Neuroscience, 18(5), pp.712–714. http://dx.doi.org/10.1016/j.jocn.2010.08.021.

Shah, J.R. & Lewis, R.A., 2003. Sarcoidosis of the cauda equina mimicking Guillain–Barré syndrome. Journal of the Neurological Sciences, 208(1-2), pp.113–117. http://dx.doi.org/10.1016/s0022-510x(02)00414-8.

INHERITED ERYTHROMELALGIA

Crunkhorn, S., 2016. Pain: Blocking pain in inherited erythromelalgia. Nature Reviews Drug Discovery, 15(6), pp.384–384. http://dx.doi.org/10.1038/nrd.2016.102.

Dabby, R., 2011. Pain Disorders and Erythromelalgia Caused by Voltage-Gated Sodium Channel Mutations. Current Neurology and Neuroscience Reports, 12(1), pp.76–83. http://dx.doi.org/10.1007/s11910-011-0233-8.

Yang, Y. et al., 2016. Nav1.7-A1632G Mutation from a Family with Inherited Erythromelalgia: Enhanced Firing of Dorsal Root Ganglia Neurons Evoked by Thermal Stimuli. Journal of Neuroscience, 36(28), pp.7511–7522. http://dx.doi.org/10.1523/jneurosci.0462-16.2016.

INTERCOSTOBRACHIAL NERVE

Loukas, M. et al., 2006. The gross anatomy of the extrathoracic course of the intercostobrachial nerve. Clinical Anatomy, 19(2), pp.106–111. http://dx.doi.org/10.1002/ca.20226.

Satija A, et al., 2014. Breast cancer pain management - A review of current & novel therapies. Indian J Med Res 2014 ;139:216-25. Available from: http://www.ijmr.org.in/text.asp?2014/139/2/216/130257

Silva, J.G. et al., 2014. Electrocortical Analysis of Patients with Intercostobrachial Pain Treated with TENS after Breast Cancer Surgery. Journal of Physical Therapy Science, 26(3), pp.349–353. http://dx.doi.org/10.1589/jpts.26.349.

Thallaj, A. et al., 2015. Ultrasound imaging accurately identifies the intercostobrachial nerve. Saudi Medical Journal, 36(10), pp.1241–1244. http://dx.doi.org/10.15537/smj.2015.10.11758.

INTERSTITIAL CYSTITIS

Chen, W. et al., 2016. Elevated level of nerve growth factor in the bladder pain syndrome/interstitial cystitis: a meta-analysis. SpringerPlus, 5(1). http://dx.doi.org/10.1186/s40064-016-2719-y.

Chiu, B. et al., 2016. Botulinum Toxin A for Bladder Pain Syndrome/Interstitial Cystitis. Toxins, 8(7), p.201. http://dx.doi.org/10.3390/toxins8070201.

Kim, H.-J., 2006. Update on the Pathology and Diagnosis of Interstitial Cystitis/Bladder Pain Syndrome: A Review. International Neurourology Journal, 20(1), pp.13–17. http://dx.doi.org/10.5213/inj.1632522.261.

INTERVERTEBRAL DISC

Ajayi, O. et al., 2016. Atypical Presentation of a Sequestered Posterolateral Disc Fragment. Cureus. http://dx.doi.org/10.7759/cureus.502.

Akhaddar, A., El-asri, A. & Boucetta, M., 2011. Posterior epidural migration of a lumbar disc fragment: a series of 6 cases. Journal of Neurosurgery: Spine, 15(1), pp.117–128. http://dx.doi.org/10.3171/2011.3.spine10832.

Jinkins, Whittemore, A. & Bradley, W., 1989. The anatomic basis of vertebrogenic pain and the autonomic syndrome associated with lumbar disk extrusion. American Journal of Roentgenology, 152(6), pp.1277–1289. http://dx.doi.org/10.2214/ajr.152.6.1277.

Kjaer, P. et al., 2016. Progression of lumbar disc herniations over an eight-year period in a group of adult Danes from the general population – a longitudinal MRI study using quantitative measures. BMC Musculoskeletal Disorders, 17(1). http://dx.doi.org/10.1186/s12891-016-0865-6.

Lin, Y. et al., 2015. Survivin is expressed in degenerated nucleus pulposus cells and is involved in proliferation and the prevention of apoptosis in vitro. Molecular Medicine Reports. http://dx.doi.org/10.3892/mmr.2015.4605.

Sarath Babu, N. et al., 2016. Quantitative proteomic analysis of normal and degenerated human intervertebral disc. The Spine Journal, 16(8), pp.989–1000. http://dx.doi.org/10.1016/j.spinee.2016.03.051.

Takahashi, K., Aoki, Y. & Ohtori, S., 2008. Resolving discogenic pain. European Spine Journal, 17(S4), pp.428–431. http://dx.doi.org/10.1007/s00586-008-0752-4.

Wang, Z. et al., 2015. Interleukin-2 is upregulated in patients with a prolapsed lumbar intervertebral disc and modulates cell proliferation, apoptosis and extracellular matrix metabolism of human nucleus pulposus cells. Experimental and Therapeutic Medicine. http://dx.doi.org/10.3892/etm.2015.2809.

INTESTINAL ANGINA

Hamaoka, T. et al., 2016. Intestinal angina in a patient with hypertrophic obstructive cardiomyopathy: a case report. Journal of Medical Case Reports, 10(1). http://dx.doi.org/10.1186/s13256-016-1055-8.

Melo, R. et al., 2016. Acute acalculous cholecystitis as a rare manifestation of chronic mesenteric ischemia. A case report. International Journal of Surgery Case Reports, 25, pp.207–211. http://dx.doi.org/10.1016/j.ijscr.2016.06.044.

O'Brien, K. & Ferral, H., 2016. Lessons learned from a case of multivessel median arcuate ligament syndrome in the setting of an Arc of Buhler. Radiology Case Reports, 11(3), pp.182–185. http://dx.doi.org/10.1016/j.radcr.2016.04.013.

INTESTINAL OBSTRUCTION

Barbosa, L. et al., 2016. Left paraduodenal hernia: a rare cause of small bowel obstruction in the elderly. BMJ Case Reports, p.bcr2015209678. http://dx.doi.org/10.1136/bcr-2015-209678.

Eskelinen, M., Ikonen, J. & Lipponen, P., 1994. Contributions of History-Taking, Physical Examination, and Computer Assistance to Diagnosis of Acute Small-Bowel Obstruction: A Prospective Study of 1333 Patients with Acute Abdominal Pain. Scandinavian Journal of Gastroenterology, 29(8), pp.715–721. http://dx.doi.org/10.3109/00365529409092499.

Kappus, M. et al., 2016. Intestinal Failure: New Definition and Clinical Implications. Current Gastroenterology Reports, 18(9). http://dx.doi.org/10.1007/s11894-016-0525-x.

Macina, S., Testa, T. & Losacco, C., 2016. Congenital internal hernia through defect in the falciform ligament in adult: A case report and review of the literature. International Journal of Surgery Case Reports, 26, pp.104–107. http://dx.doi.org/10.1016/j.ijscr.2016.05.003.

Ng, Y.S. et al., 2016. Pseudo-obstruction, stroke, and mitochondrial dysfunction: A lethal combination. Annals of Neurology, 80(5), pp.686–692. http://dx.doi.org/10.1002/ana.24736.

Udo, I., Abudu, E. & Uduma, F., 2016. Adult intussusception: An 8 years institutional review. Nigerian Medical Journal, 57(4), p.204. http://dx.doi.org/10.4103/0300-1652.188324.

INTRASPINAL HEMATOMA

Castillo, J.M. et al., 2015. Non-Traumatic Spontaneous Spinal Subdural Hematoma in a Patient with Non-Valvular Atrial Fibrillation During Treatment with Rivaroxaban. American Journal of Case Reports, 16, pp.377–381. http://dx.doi.org/10.12659/ajcr.893320.

Famularo, G., Sajeva, M.R. & Gasbarrone, L., 2014. Warfarin-associated Hematomyelia. Internal Medicine, 53(6), pp.623–626. http://dx.doi.org/10.2169/internalmedicine.53.1544.

Inamasu, J. et al., 2016. Warfarin-associated Intraspinal Hematoma. The Keio Journal of Medicine, 65(4), pp.74–77. http://dx.doi.org/10.2302/kjm.2015-0012-cr.

Leech, R.W., Pitha, J.V. & Brumback, R.A., 1991. Spontaneous haematomyelia: a necropsy study. Journal of Neurology, Neurosurgery & Psychiatry, 54(2), pp.172–174. http://dx.doi.org/10.1136/jnnp.54.2.172.

IRRITABLE BOWEL SYNDROME

Jin, D.-C. et al., 2016. Regulation of the serotonin transporter in the pathogenesis of irritable bowel syndrome. World Journal of Gastroenterology, 22(36), p.8137. http://dx.doi.org/10.3748/wjg.v22.i36.8137.

Quigley, E.M.M. et al., 2016. World Gastroenterology Organisation Global Guidelines Irritable Bowel Syndrome. Journal of Clinical Gastroenterology, 50(9), pp.704–713. http://dx.doi.org/10.1097/mcg.0000000000000653.

Sibelli, A, Chalder, T., Everitt, H., Workman, P., Windgassen, S. and Moss-Morris, R., A Systematic review with meta-analysis of the role of anxiety and depression in irritable bowel syndrome onset. 2016 Nov;46(15):3065-3080 https://www.ncbi.nlm.nih.gov/pubmed/27605134

Staudacher, H.M. & Whelan, K., 2016. Altered gastrointestinal microbiota in irritable bowel syndrome and its modification by diet: probiotics, prebiotics and the low FODMAP diet. Proceedings of the Nutrition Society, 75(03), pp.306–318. http://dx.doi.org/10.1017/s0029665116000021.

ISCHEMIC COLITIS

Feuerstadt, P. & Brandt, L.J., 2015. Update on Colon Ischemia: Recent Insights and Advances. Current Gastroenterology Reports, 17(12). http://dx.doi.org/10.1007/s11894-015-0469-6.

Lee, M.J. et al., 2016. Risk factors for ischaemic colitis after surgery for abdominal aortic aneurysm: a systematic review and observational meta-analysis. International Journal of Colorectal Disease, 31(7), pp.1273–1281. http://dx.doi.org/10.1007/s00384-016-2606-6.

Weaver, L.K. and Deru, K., 2015. Ischemic colitis associated with acute carbon monoxide poisoning--a case report. Undersea & hyperbaric medicine: Journal of the Undersea and Hyperbaric Medical Society, Inc, 43(2), pp.175-180. https://www.ncbi.nlm.nih.gov/pubmed/27265995

ISONAIZID

Nisar, M. et al., 1990. Exacerbation of isoniazid induced peripheral neuropathy by pyridoxine. Thorax, 45(5), pp.419–420. http://dx.doi.org/10.1136/thx.45.5.419.

Steichen, O., Martinez-Almoyna, L. & De Broucker, T., 2006. Neuropathie toxique induite par l'isoniazide : pensez à la prévention. Revue des Maladies Respiratoires, 23(2), pp.157–160. http://dx.doi.org/10.1016/s0761-8425(06)71480-2.

Jacobs, J.M., Miller, R.H. & Cavanagh, J.B., 1979. The distribution of degenerative changes in INH neuropathy. Acta Neuropathologica, 48(1), pp.1–9. Available at:

http://dx.doi.org/10.1007/bf00691784.

Verma, A.K. et al., 2015. Isoniazid prevents Nrf2 translocation by inhibiting ERK1 phosphorylation and induces oxidative stress and apoptosis. Redox Biology, 6, pp.80–92. Available at: http://dx.doi.org/10.1016/j.redox.2015.06.020.

ISCHEMIC MONOMELIC NEUROPATHY

Santilli, J et al., 1999. Chronic Critical Limb Ischemia:Diagnosis, Treatment, and prognosis. Am Fam Physician 59(7), pp.1899-1908 Available at: https://www.aafp.org/afp/1999/0401/p1899.html

Singh, V. et al., 2017. Ischemic monomelic neuropathy: a long-term follow-up of two cases. The Journal of Vascular Access, pp.0–0. Available at: http://dx.doi.org/10.5301/jva.5000743.

Weinberg, D.H. et al., 2001. Chronic ischemic monomelic neuropathy from critical limb ischemia. Neurology, 57(6), pp.1008–1012. Available at: http://dx.doi.org/10.1212/wnl.57.6.1008.

Jujo, K. et al., 2017. Pilot Cohort Study Assessing the Efficacy of Endovascular Revascularization in the Restoration of Peripheral Sensory Disturbance in Patients With Critical Limb Ischemia. Circulation Journal. Available at: http://dx.doi.org/10.1253/circj.cj-17-0405.

JOINT PAIN RADIATIONS

Boswell, M.V. et al., 2007. A systematic review of therapeutic facet joint interventions in chronic spinal pain. Pain Physician, 10(1), pp.229–253. https://www.ncbi.nlm.nih.gov/pubmed/17256032

Cohen, S.P. & Raja, S.N., 2007. Pathogenesis, Diagnosis, and Treatment of Lumbar Zygapophysial (Facet) Joint Pain. Anesthesiology, 106(3), pp.591–614. http://dx.doi.org/10.1097/00000542-200703000-00024

Datta, S. et al., 2009. Systematic assessment of diagnostic accuracy and therapeutic utility of lumbar facet joint interventions. Pain Physician, 12(2), pp.437–460. https://www.ncbi.nlm.nih.gov/pubmed/19305489

Patel, V.B., Wasserman, R. & Imani, F., 2015. Interventional Therapies for Chronic Low Back Pain: A Focused Review (Efficacy and Outcomes). Anesthesiology and Pain Medicine, 5(4). http://dx.doi.org/10.5812/aapm.29716.

KLIPPEL – FEIL SYNDROME

Bejiqi, R., 2015. Klippel – Feil Syndrome Associated with Congential Heart Disease Presentaion of Cases and a Review of the Current Literature. Open Access Macedonian Journal of Medical Sciences. http://dx.doi.org/10.3889/oamjms.2015.022.

Brokinkel, B. et al., 2013. Surgical treatment in a patient with Klippel–Feil syndrome and anterior cervical meningomyelocele: a case report and review of literature. European Spine Journal, 22(S3), pp.517–520.
http://dx.doi.org/10.1007/s00586-013-2769-6.

Kariki, E. et al., 2014. The Rare Sprengel Deformity: Our Experience with Three Cases. Journal of Clinical Imaging Science, 4(1), p.55.
http://dx.doi.org/10.4103/2156-7514.143407.

Samartzis, D. et al., 2006. Symptomatic Cervical Disc Herniation in a Pediatric Klippel-Feil Patient. Spine, 31(11), pp.E335–E338.
http://dx.doi.org/10.1097/01.brs.0000217628.32344.73.

LATERAL FEMORAL CUTANEOUS NERVE

Lee, S. et al., 2017. Anatomy of the lateral femoral cutaneous nerve relevant to clinical findings in meralgia paresthetica. Muscle & Nerve, 55(5), pp.646–650. Available at: http://dx.doi.org/10.1002/mus.25382.

Hanna, A.S., 2017. Lateral femoral cutaneous nerve transposition: Renaissance of an old concept in the light of new anatomy. Clinical Anatomy, 30(3), pp.409–412. Available at: http://dx.doi.org/10.1002/ca.22849.

Weng, W.-C. et al., 2017. Risk factor analysis for meralgia paresthetica: A hospital-based study in Taiwan. Journal of Clinical Neuroscience, 43, pp.192–195. Available at: http://dx.doi.org/10.1016/j.jocn.2017.04.024.

LATERAL RECESS SYNDROME

Bajek, G., Bajek, S., Zoričić Cvek, S., Bobinac, D., Splavski, B. and Šepić Grahovac, D., 2010. Histomorphological analysis of the osteophytic appositions in patients with lumbar lateral recess syndrome. Collegium antropologicum, 34(2), pp.79-84.
http://www.biowebspin.com/pubadvanced/article/21302706/

Bartynski, W.S. and Lin, L., 2003. Lumbar root compression in the lateral recess: MR imaging, conventional myelography, and CT myelography comparison with surgical confirmation. AJNR American journal of neuroradiology, 24(3), pp.348-360.
https://www.ncbi.nlm.nih.gov/pubmed/12637281

Ciric, I. et al., 1980. The lateral recess syndrome. Journal of Neurosurgery, 53(4), pp.433–443. http://dx.doi.org/10.3171/jns.1980.53.4.0433.

LATERAL THYROHYOID LIGAMENT

Sinha, P., Grindler, D.J. & Haughey, B.H., 2013. A pain in the neck. The Laryngoscope, 124(1), pp.116–118. http://dx.doi.org/10.1002/lary.24419.

LEIOMYOMA

Cha, P.-C. et al., 2011. A genome-wide association study identifies three loci associated with susceptibility to uterine fibroids. Nature Genetics, 43(5), pp.447–450. http://dx.doi.org/10.1038/ng.805.

Garg, K. et al., 2011. Morphologic Features of Uterine Leiomyomas Associated With Hereditary Leiomyomatosis and Renal Cell Carcinoma Syndrome. The American Journal of Surgical Pathology, 35(8), pp.1235–1237. http://dx.doi.org/10.1097/pas.0b013e318223ca01.

Pacheco-Rodriguez, G., Taveira-DaSilva, A.M. & Moss, J., 2016. Benign Metastasizing Leiomyoma. Clinics in Chest Medicine, 37(3), pp.589–595. http://dx.doi.org/10.1016/j.ccm.2016.04.019.

LESSER OCCIPITAL NERVE

Lee, M. et al., 2013. An Anatomic Study of the Lesser Occipital Nerve and Its Potential Compression Points. Plastic and Reconstructive Surgery, p.1. http://dx.doi.org/10.1097/prs.0b013e3182a80721.

Peled, Z.M., Pietramaggiori, G. & Scherer, S., 2016. Anatomic and Compression Topography of the Lesser Occipital Nerve. Plastic and Reconstructive Surgery - Global Open, 4(3), p.e639. http://dx.doi.org/10.1097/gox.0000000000000654.

LIGAMENTUM FLAVUM CYSTS

DiMaio, S. et al., 2005. Ligamentum Flavum Cysts Causing Incapacitating Lumbar Spinal Stenosis. Canadian Journal of Neurological Sciences / Journal Canadien des Sciences Neurologiques, 32(02), pp.237–242. http://dx.doi.org/10.1017/s0317167100004030.

Taha, H. et al., 2010. Ligamentum flavum cyst in the lumbar spine: a case report and review of the literature. Journal of Orthopaedics and Traumatology, 11(2), pp.117–122. http://dx.doi.org/10.1007/s10195-010-0094-y.

LIVER DISEASE

Liberal, R. & Grant, C.R., 2016. Cirrhosis and autoimmune liver disease: Current understanding. World Journal of Hepatology, 8(28), p.1157. http://dx.doi.org/10.4254/wjh.v8.i28.1157.

Oh, H. et al., 2016. Non-alcoholic fatty liver diseases: update on the challenge of diagnosis and treatment. Clinical and Molecular Hepatology, 22(3), pp.327–335. http://dx.doi.org/10.3350/cmh.2016.0049.

LONG THORACIC NERVE

Han, J, et al., 2016. Thoracic Nerve Root Entrapment by Intrathecal Catheter Coiling: Case Report and Review of the Literature. Pain Physician, 19:E499-E504 http://www.painphysicianjournal.com/current/pdf?article=MjYyNA%3D%3D&journal=95

Wiater, J.M. & Flatow, E.L., 1999. Long Thoracic Nerve Injury. Clinical Orthopaedics and Related Research, 368, p.17-27. Available at: http://dx.doi.org/10.1097/00003086-199911000-00004.

Le Nail, L.R. et al., 2014. Isolated paralysis of the serratus anterior muscle: Surgical release of the distal segment of the long thoracic nerve in 52 patients. Orthopaedics & Traumatology: Surgery & Research, 100(4), pp.S243–S248. Available at: http://dx.doi.org/10.1016/j.otsr.2014.03.004.

LUMBAR PLEXUS OVERVIEW

Banagan, K. et al., 2011. Anatomic Mapping of Lumbar Nerve Roots During a Direct Lateral Transpsoas Approach to the Spine. Spine, 36(11), pp.E687–E691. http://dx.doi.org/10.1097/brs.0b013e3181ec5911.

Cejas, C. et al., 2015. High resolution neurography of the lumbosacral plexus on 3T magnetic resonance imaging. Radiología (English Edition), 57(1), pp.22–34. http://dx.doi.org/10.1016/j.rxeng.2014.07.001.

Guérin, P. et al., 2011. Safe working zones using the minimally invasive lateral retroperitoneal transpsoas approach: a morphometric study. Surgical and Radiologic Anatomy, 33(8), pp.665–671. http://dx.doi.org/10.1007/s00276-011-0798-6.

Guérin, P. et al., 2011. The lumbosacral plexus: anatomic considerations for minimally invasive retroperitoneal transpsoas approach. Surgical and Radiologic Anatomy, 34(2), pp.151–157. http://dx.doi.org/10.1007/s00276-011-0881-z.

Matejčík, V., 2009. Anatomical variations of lumbosacral plexus. Surgical and Radiologic Anatomy, 32(4), pp.409–414. http://dx.doi.org/10.1007/s00276-009-0546-3.

Van Alfen, N. & Malessy, M.J.A., 2013. Diagnosis of brachial and lumbosacral plexus lesions. Peripheral Nerve Disorders, pp.293–310. http://dx.doi.org/10.1016/b978-0-444-52902-2.00018-7.

LUMBAR SPINAL STENOSIS

Singh, K. et al., 2005. Congenital lumbar spinal stenosis: a prospective, control-matched, cohort radiographic analysis. The Spine Journal, 5(6), pp.615–622. http://dx.doi.org/10.1016/j.spinee.2005.05.385.

Soldatos, T., 2014. Spectrum of magnetic resonance imaging findings in congenital lumbar spinal stenosis. World Journal of Clinical Cases, 2(12), p.883. http://dx.doi.org/10.12998/wjcc.v2.i12.883.

Tomkins-Lane, C.C. et al., 2013. Nerve Root Sedimentation Sign for the Diagnosis of Lumbar Spinal Stenosis. Spine, 38(24), pp.E1554–E1560. http://dx.doi.org/10.1097/brs.0b013e3182a8c2da.

LUMBAR SPINE FRACTURES AND DISLOCATIONS

Alanay, A., 2000. Re: Post-Traumatic Findings of the Spine After Earlier Vertebral Fracture in Young Patients. Spine, 25(21), p.2847. http://dx.doi.org/10.1097/00007632-200011010-00027.

Baumann, F., Krutsch, W., Pfeifer, C., Neumann, C., Nerlich, M. and Loibl, M., 2014. Posterolateral Fusion in Acute Traumatic Thoracolumbar Fractures: A Comparison of Demineralized Bone Matrix and Autologous Bone Graft. Acta chirurgiae orthopaedicae et traumatologiae Cechoslovaca, 82(2), pp.119-125. https://www.ncbi.nlm.nih.gov/pubmed/26317180

Castaño-Betancourt, M.C. et al., 2013. Association of lumbar disc degeneration with osteoporotic fractures; the Rotterdam study and meta-analysis from systematic review. Bone, 57(1), pp.284–289. http://dx.doi.org/10.1016/j.bone.2013.08.004.

El Assuity, W.I., El Masry, M.A. & Chan, D., 2007. Acute Traumatic Spondylolisthesis at the Lumbosacral Junction. The Journal of Trauma: Injury, Infection, and Critical Care, 62(6), pp.1514–1517. http://dx.doi.org/10.1097/01.ta.0000195463.83951.d7.

Health Quality Ontario, 2016. Vertebral Augmentation Involving Vertebroplasty or Kyphoplasty for Cancer-Related Vertebral Compression Fractures: A Systematic Review. Ontario Health Technology Asssessment Series, 16(11), pp.1–202. https://www.ncbi.nlm.nih.gov/pmc/articles/PMC4902848/

Sime, D., Gabbe, B. & Liew, S., 2016. Outcomes of halo immobilization in the management of subaxial cervical facet fractures. ANZ Journal of Surgery. http://dx.doi.org/10.1111/ans.13656.

Tyroch, A.H., McGuire, E.L., McLean, S.F., Kozar, R.A., Gates, K.A., Kaups, K.L., Charles, C., Cowgill, S.M., Griswold, J.A., Sue, L.A. and Craun, M.L., 2005. The association between Chance fractures and intra-abdominal injuries revisited: a multicenter review. The American Surgeon, 71(5), pp.434-438. https://www.ncbi.nlm.nih.gov/pubmed/15986977

Vaccaro, A.R. et al., 2013. AOSpine Thoracolumbar Spine Injury Classification System. Spine, 38(23), pp.2028–2037. http://dx.doi.org/10.1097/brs.0b013e3182a8a381.

Wu, C.-T. et al., 2006. Classification of symptomatic osteoporotic compression fractures of the thoracic and lumbar spine. Journal of Clinical Neuroscience, 13(1), pp.31–38. http://dx.doi.org/10.1016/j.jocn.2004.11.021.

Zhang, S., Mo, L., Liang, D., Jiang, X., Yang, Z., Tang, Y., Jin, D., Yao, Z., Guo, D. and Feng, P., 2016. [CLASSIFICATION AND TREATMENT STRATEGIES OF SYMPTOMATIC SEVERE OSTEOPOROTIC VERTEBRAL FRACTURE AND COLLAPSE]. Zhongguo xiu fu chong jian wai ke za zhi= Zhongguo xiufu chongjian waike zazhi= Chinese journal of reparative and reconstructive surgery, 30(2), pp.189-196. https://www.ncbi.nlm.nih.gov/pubmed/27276813

LUMBAR SPONDYLOLYSIS

Elgafy, H. et al., 2015. Nonconsecutive Pars Interarticularis Defects. American Journal of Orthopedics (Belle Mead, N.J.), 44(12), pp.E526–9. https://www.ncbi.nlm.nih.gov/pubmed/26665257

Leone, A. et al., 2010. Lumbar spondylolysis: a review. Skeletal Radiology, 40(6), pp.683–700. http://dx.doi.org/10.1007/s00256-010-0942-0.

LUMBAR VERTEBRA/DISC

Bailey, J.F. et al., 2011. Innervation patterns of PGP 9.5-positive nerve fibers within the human lumbar vertebra. Journal of Anatomy, 218(3), pp.263–270. http://dx.doi.org/10.1111/j.1469-7580.2010.01332.x.

Datta, S. et al., 2009. Systematic assessment of diagnostic accuracy and therapeutic utility of lumbar facet joint interventions. Pain Physician, 12(2), pp.437–460. https://www.ncbi.nlm.nih.gov/pubmed/19305489

Faustmann, P.M., 2004. [Neuroanatomic basis for discogenic pain]. Zeitschrift für Orthopädie, 142(6), pp.706–708. http://dx.doi.org/10.1055/s-2004-832490.

Raj, P.P., 2008. Intervertebral Disc: Anatomy-Physiology-Pathophysiology-Treatment. Pain Practice, 8(1), pp.18–44. http://dx.doi.org/10.1111/j.1533-2500.2007.00171.x.

Rennie, C., Haffajee, M.R. & Ebrahim, M.A.A., 2012. The sinuvertebral nerves at the craniovertebral junction: A microdissection study. Clinical Anatomy, 26(3), pp.357–366. http://dx.doi.org/10.1002/ca.22105.

Sihvonen, T. et al., 1995. Dorsal Ramus Irritation Associated with Recurrent Low Back Pain and Its Relief with Local Anesthetic or Training Therapy. Journal of Spinal Disorders, 8(1), p.8–14. http://dx.doi.org/10.1097/00002517-199502000-00002.

Tomaszewski, K.A. et al., 2015. The biology behind the human intervertebral disc and its endplates. Folia Morphologica, 74(2), pp.157–168. http://dx.doi.org/10.5603/fm.2015.0026.

Van Roy, P. et al., 2001. Anatomical background of low back pain: variability and degeneration of the lumbar spinal canal and intervertebral disc. Der Schmerz, 15(6), pp.418–424. http://dx.doi.org/10.1007/s004820100026.

LUMBOSACRAL PLEXOPATHY DIFFERENTIAL DIAGNOSIS

Abdellaoui, A. et al., 2007. Lower limb paralysis from ischaemic neuropathy of the lumbosacral plexus following aorto-iliac procedures. Interactive CardioVascular and Thoracic Surgery, 6(4), pp.501–502. http://dx.doi.org/10.1510/icvts.2007.151993.

Dahele, M. et al., 2006. Radiation-induced Lumbo-sacral Plexopathy (RILSP): an Important Enigma. Clinical Oncology, 18(5), pp.427–428. http://dx.doi.org/10.1016/j.clon.2006.03.004.

Dhillon, S.S. & Sarac, E., 2000. Lumbosacral plexopathy after dual kidney transplantation. American Journal of Kidney Diseases, 36(5), pp.1045–1048. http://dx.doi.org/10.1053/ajkd.2000.19109.

García-Manzanares, M.D. et al., 1999. Bilateral lumbosacral plexopathy after mesenteric thrombosis. Spinal Cord, 37(7), pp.522–525. http://dx.doi.org/10.1038/sj.sc.3100865.

Jaeckle, K.A., Young, D.F. & Foley, K.M., 1985. The natural history of lumbosacral plexopathy in cancer. Neurology, 35(1), pp.8–8. http://dx.doi.org/10.1212/wnl.35.1.8.

Jang, D.-H. et al., 2011. The Relationship Between Lumbosacral Plexopathy and Pelvic Fractures. American Journal of Physical Medicine & Rehabilitation, 90(9), pp.707–712. http://dx.doi.org/10.1097/phm.0b013e31821f6bd9.

Ladha, S.S. et al., 2006. Neoplastic lumbosacral radiculoplexopathy in prostate cancer by direct perineural spread: An unusual entity. Muscle & Nerve, 34(5), pp.659–665. http://dx.doi.org/10.1002/mus.20597.

Melikoglu, M.A. et al., 2008. Internal Iliac Artery Pseudoaneurysm. American Journal of Physical Medicine & Rehabilitation, 87(8), pp.681–683. http://dx.doi.org/10.1097/phm.0b013e31816dca87.

Soldatos, T. et al., 2013. High-Resolution 3-T MR Neurography of the Lumbosacral

Plexus. RadioGraphics, 33(4), pp.967–987. http://dx.doi.org/10.1148/rg.334115761.

Stoeckli, T.C., Mackin, G.A. & De Groote, M.A., 2000. Lumbosacral Plexopathy in a Patient with Pulmonary Tuberculosis. Clinical Infectious Diseases, 30(1), pp.226–227. http://dx.doi.org/10.1086/313622.

Taylor, B.V. et al., 1997. Magnetic Resonance Imaging in Cancer-Related Lumbosacral Plexopathy. Mayo Clinic Proceedings, 72(9), pp.823–829. http://dx.doi.org/10.4065/72.9.823.

LUMBOSACRAL PLEXUS INJURIES

Adelved, A. et al., 2014. Radiological findings correlate with neurological deficits but not with pain after operatively treated sacral fractures. Acta Orthopaedica, 85(4), pp.408–414. http://dx.doi.org/10.3109/17453674.2014.908344.

Adelved, A. et al., 2016. Long-term functional outcome after traumatic lumbosacral dissociation. A retrospective case series of 13 patients. Injury, 47(7), pp.1562–1568. http://dx.doi.org/10.1016/j.injury.2016.04.006.

BARNETT, H.G. & CONNOLLY, E.S., 1975. LUMBOSACRAL NERVE ROOT AVULSION. The Journal of Trauma: Injury, Infection, and Critical Care, 15(6), pp.532–535. http://dx.doi.org/10.1097/00005373-197506000-00015.

Finney, L.A. and Wulfman, W.A., 1960. Traumatic intradural lumbar nerve root avulsion with associated traction injury to the common peroneal nerve. The American journal of roentgenology, radium therapy, and nuclear medicine, 84, pp.952-957. http://europepmc.org/abstract/med/13699670

Garozzo, D., Zollino, G. & Ferraresi, S., 2014. In lumbosacral plexus injuries can we identify indicators that predict spontaneous recovery or the need for surgical treatment? Results from a clinical study on 72 patients. Journal of Brachial Plexus and Peripheral Nerve Injury, 9(1), p.1. http://dx.doi.org/10.1186/1749-7221-9-1.

MAJEED, S.A., 1992. Neurologic Deficits in Major Pelvic Injuries. Clinical Orthopaedics and Related Research, &NA;(282), p.222-228. http://dx.doi.org/10.1097/00003086-199209000-00029.

Rai, S.K., Far, R.F. and Ghovanlou, B., 1990. Neurologic deficits associated with sacral wing fractures. Orthopedics, 13(12), pp.1363-1366. http://www.healio.com/orthopedics/journals/ortho/1990-12-13-12/%7B7ade70a5-38e6-41d4-a84c-57ebdee452c4%7D/neurologic-deficits-associated-with-sacral-wing-fractures

Stevanato, G. et al., Lumbosacral plexus lesions. Acta Neurochirurgica Supplementum, pp.15–20. http://dx.doi.org/10.1007/978-3-211-72958-8_3.

Weis, E.B., 1984. Subtle Neurological Injuries in Pelvic Fractures. The Journal of Trauma: Injury, Infection, and Critical Care, 24(11), pp.983–985. http://dx.doi.org/10.1097/00005373-198411000-00010.

LUMBOSACRAL PLEXUS OBSTETRIC INJURY

A. Wong, C., 2003. Incidence of postpartum lumbosacral spine and lower extremity nerve injuries. Obstetrics & Gynecology, 101(2), pp.279–288. http://dx.doi.org/10.1016/s0029-7844(02)02727-8.

Loo, C.C., Dahlgren, G. & Irestedt, L., 2000. Neurological complications in obstetric regional anaesthesia. International Journal of Obstetric Anesthesia, 9(2), pp.99–124. http://dx.doi.org/10.1054/ijoa.1999.0347.

Park, S., Park, S.W. & Kim, K.S., 2013. Lumbosacral plexus injury following vaginal delivery with epidural analgesia -A case report-. Korean Journal of Anesthesiology, 64(2), p.175. http://dx.doi.org/10.4097/kjae.2013.64.2.175.

LUMBOSACRAL PLEXUS TUMORS

Agar, M., Broadbent, A. & Chye, R., 2004. The management of malignant psoas syndrome: case reports and literature review. Journal of Pain and Symptom Management, 28(3), pp.282–293. http://dx.doi.org/10.1016/j.jpainsymman.2003.12.018.

Capek, S. et al., 2014. Recurrent rectal cancer causing lumbosacral plexopathy with perineural spread to the spinal nerves and the sciatic nerve: An anatomic explanation. Clinical Anatomy, 28(1), pp.136–143. http://dx.doi.org/10.1002/ca.22450.

Capek, S. et al., 2015. Perineural spread of pelvic malignancies to the lumbosacral plexus and beyond: clinical and imaging patterns. Neurosurgical Focus, 39(3), p.E14. http://dx.doi.org/10.3171/2015.7.focus15209.

Dalmau, J., Graus F., and Marco M, 1989. Hot and dry foot as initial manifestation of neoplastic lumbosacral plexopathy. Neurology, 39.6, 871-871. https://doi.org/10.1212/wnl.39.6.871-a

Jaeckle, K.A., 1991. Nerve plexus metastases. Neurologic clinics, 9(4), pp.857-866. https://www.scopus.com/record/display.uri?eid=2-s2.0-0026005557&origin=inward&txGid=E4851E8ADDCCC8C8F5929B1D1965E9FA.wsnAw8kcdt7IPYLO0V48gA%3a2

Jaeckle, K.A., Young, D.F. & Foley, K.M., 1985. The natural history of lumbosacral plexopathy in cancer. Neurology, 35(1), pp.8–8. http://dx.doi.org/10.1212/wnl.35.1.8.

Ladha, S.S. et al., 2006. Neoplastic lumbosacral radiculoplexopathy in prostate cancer by direct perineural spread: An unusual entity. Muscle & Nerve, 34(5), pp.659–665.

http://dx.doi.org/10.1002/mus.20597.

Thomas, J.E., Cascino, T.L. & Earle, J.D., 1985. Differential diagnosis between radiation and tumor plexopathy of the pelvis. Neurology, 35(1), pp.1–1. http://dx.doi.org/10.1212/wnl.35.1.1.

LUMBOSACRAL TRANSITION VERTEBRAE

Bron, J.L. et al., 2007. The clinical significance of lumbosacral transitional anomalies. Acta Orthopaedica Belgica, 73(6), p.687. https://www.ncbi.nlm.nih.gov/pubmed/18260478

Bulut, M. et al., 2013. Is Sacralization Really a Cause of Low Back Pain? ISRN Orthopedics, 2013, pp.1–4. http://dx.doi.org/10.1155/2013/839013.

Farshad-Amacker, N.A. et al., 2015. Associations between lumbosacral transitional anatomy types and degeneration at the transitional and adjacent segments. The Spine Journal, 15(6), pp.1210–1216. http://dx.doi.org/10.1016/j.spinee.2013.10.029.

Konin, G.P. & Walz, D.M., 2010. Lumbosacral Transitional Vertebrae: Classification, Imaging Findings, and Clinical Relevance. American Journal of Neuroradiology, 31(10), pp.1778–1786. http://dx.doi.org/10.3174/ajnr.a2036.

Sekharappa, V. et al., 2014. Lumbosacral Transition Vertebra: Prevalence and Its Significance. Asian Spine Journal, 8(1), p.51. http://dx.doi.org/10.4184/asj.2014.8.1.51.

LYME DISEASE

Bratton, R.L. et al., 2008. Diagnosis and Treatment of Lyme Disease. Mayo Clinic Proceedings, 83(5), pp.566–571. http://dx.doi.org/10.4065/83.5.56

DRYDEN, M.S. et al., 2014. Lyme borreliosis in southern United Kingdom and a case for a new syndrome, chronic arthropod-borne neuropathy. Epidemiology and Infection, 143(03), pp.561–572. http://dx.doi.org/10.1017/s0950268814001071.

Petnicki-Ocwieja, T. & Kern, A., 2014. Mechanisms of Borrelia burgdorferi internalization and intracellular innate immune signaling. Frontiers in Cellular and Infection Microbiology, 4. http://dx.doi.org/10.3389/fcimb.2014.00175.

Ramesh, G. et al., 2013. The Lyme disease spirochete Borrelia burgdorferi induces inflammation and apoptosis in cells from dorsal root ganglia. Journal of Neuroinflammation, 10(1). http://dx.doi.org/10.1186/1742-2094-10-88.

Sanchez, E. et al., 2016. Diagnosis, Treatment, and Prevention of Lyme Disease, Human Granulocytic Anaplasmosis, and Babesiosis. JAMA, 315(16), p.1767. http://dx.doi.org/10.1001/jama.2016.2884.

Steere, A.C. & Sikand, V.K., 2003. The Presenting Manifestations of Lyme Disease and the Outcomes of Treatment. New England Journal of Medicine, 348(24), pp.2472–2474. http://dx.doi.org/10.1056/nejm200306123482423.

LYSOPHOSPHATIDIC ACID RECEPTOR SIGNALING AND DEMYELINATION

Campbell, D.S. & Holt, C.E., 2001. Chemotropic Responses of Retinal Growth Cones Mediated by Rapid Local Protein Synthesis and Degradation. Neuron, 32(6), pp.1013–1026. Available at: http://dx.doi.org/10.1016/s0896-6273(01)00551-7.

Inoue, M. et al., 2006. Loss of Spinal Substance P Pain Transmission under the Condition of LPAI Receptor-Mediated Neuropathic Pain. Molecular Pain, 2, pp.1744–8069–2–25. Available at: http://dx.doi.org/10.1186/1744-8069-2-25.

Weiner JA1, Fukushima N, Contos JJ, Scherer SS, Chun J., 2001. Regulation of Schwann cell morphology and adhesion by receptor-mediated lysophosphatidic acid signaling. J Neurosci. 15;21(18):7069-78. https://www.ncbi.nlm.nih.gov/pubmed/11549717.

Nagai, J. et al., 2010. Autotaxin and Lysophosphatidic Acid1 receptor-Mediated Demyelination of Dorsal Root Fibers by Sciatic Nerve Injury and Intrathecal Lysophosphatidylcholine. Molecular Pain, 6, pp.1744–8069–6–78. Available at: http://dx.doi.org/10.1186/1744-8069-6-78.

Ueda, H., 2017. Lysophosphatidic acid signaling is the definitive mechanism underlying neuropathic pain. PAIN, 158, pp.S55–S65. Available at: http://dx.doi.org/10.1097/j.pain.0000000000000813.

MANUBRIOSTERNAL JOINT

Ruiz-Esquide, V., García, A.I., Ramírez, J. and Guañabens, N., 2014. Inflammatory arthropathy of the manubriosternal joint. Rheumatology, 53 (10): 1731. Available at http://p.keu261.

Vaishya, R., Vijay, V. & Rai, B.K., 2015. Osteoarthritis of the Manubriosternal Joint: An Uncommon Cause of Chest Pain. Cureus. http://dx.doi.org/10.7759/cureus.370.

MECHANISMS UNDERLYING NEUROPATHIC PAIN ANIMAL MODELS

Bennett, G.J. & Xie, Y.-K., 1988. A peripheral mononeuropathy in rat that produces disorders of pain sensation like those seen in man. Pain, 33(1), pp.87–107. Available at: http://dx.doi.org/10.1016/0304-3959(88)90209-6.

Ho Kim, S. & Mo Chung, J., 1992. An experimental model for peripheral neuropathy produced by segmental spinal nerve ligation in the rat. Pain, 50(3), pp.355–363. Available at: http://dx.doi.org/10.1016/0304-3959(92)90041-9.

Shir, Y. & Seltzer, Z., 1991. Effects of sympathectomy in a model of causalgiform pain produced by partial sciatic nerve injury in rats. Pain, 45(3), pp.309–320. Available at: http://dx.doi.org/10.1016/0304-3959(91)90056-4.

MEDIAN NERVE

Voin, V. et al., 2017. Relationship of the Median and Radial Nerves at the Elbow: Application to Avoiding Injury During Venipuncture or Other Invasive Procedures of the Cubital Fossa. Cureus. Available at: http://dx.doi.org/10.7759/cureus.1094.

Billakota, S., Ruch, D.S. & Hobson-Webb, L.D., 2017. Ultrasound Imaging of Median Nerve Conduit in a Patient With Persistent Median Nerve Symptoms. Journal of Clinical Neurophysiology, p.1. Available at: http://dx.doi.org/10.1097/wnp.0000000000000386.

Andrea, A. et al., 2017. Median Nerve Palsies due to Injections: A Review. Cureus. Available at: http://dx.doi.org/10.7759/cureus.1287.

Al-Qattan, M.M. & Al-Zahrani, K., 2017. An unusual pre-ligamentous thenar motor branch of the median nerve. European Journal of Plastic Surgery, 40(3), pp.259–262. Available at: http://dx.doi.org/10.1007/s00238-016-1271-x.

Ghasemi-rad, M., 2014. A handy review of carpal tunnel syndrome: From anatomy to diagnosis and treatment. World Journal of Radiology, 6(6), p.284. Available at: http://dx.doi.org/10.4329/wjr.v6.i6.284.

MESOTHELIAL CYST

Perrini, P. et al., 2006. Thoracic radiculopathy from a paravertebral mesothelial cyst. Acta Neurochirurgica, 148(9), pp.989–991. http://dx.doi.org/10.1007/s00701-006-0815-4.

METASTASIS

Chiang, A.C. & Massagué, J., 2008. Molecular Basis of Metastasis. New England Journal of Medicine, 359(26), pp.2814–2823. http://dx.doi.org/10.1056/nejmra0805239.

Klein, C.A., 2008. CANCER: The Metastasis Cascade. Science, 321(5897), pp.1785–1787. http://dx.doi.org/10.1126/science.1164853.

Nencini, S. & Ivanusic, J.J., 2016. The Physiology of Bone Pain. How Much Do We Really Know? Frontiers in Physiology, 7. http://dx.doi.org/10.3389/fphys.2016.00157.

Sutcliffe, P. et al., 2013. A systematic review of evidence on malignant spinal metastases: natural history and technologies for identifying patients at high risk of vertebral fracture and spinal cord compression. Health Technol Assess, 17(42). http://dx.doi.org/10.3310/hta17420.

Yoshida, B.A., 2000. Metastasis-Suppressor Genes: a Review and Perspective on an Emerging Field. Journal of the National Cancer Institute, 92(21), pp.1717–1730. http://dx.doi.org/10.1093/jnci/92.21.1717.

METRONIDAZOLE

Agarwal, A. et al., 2016. Metronidazole-induced cerebellar toxicity. Neurology International, 8(1). http://dx.doi.org/10.4081/ni.2016.6365.

Bradley, W.G., Karlsson, I.J. & Rassol, C.G., 1977. Metronidazole neuropathy. BMJ, 2(6087), pp.610–611. http://dx.doi.org/10.1136/bmj.2.6087.610.

Retamal-Riquelme, E. et al., 2014. Neurotoxicidad secundaria a metronidazol: un efecto adverso reversible. Caso clínico. Revista médica de Chile, 142(3), pp.386–390. http://dx.doi.org/10.4067/s0034-98872014000300015.

Tan, C.-H. et al., 2010. Painful neuropathy due to skin denervation after metronidazole-induced neurotoxicity. Journal of Neurology, Neurosurgery & Psychiatry, 82(4), pp.462–466. http://dx.doi.org/10.1136/jnnp.2009.194118.

MICROSCOPIC POLYANGIITIS

Bhadu, D., Kumar, P., Malhotra, K.P., Sharma, A., Sharma, M. and Srivastava, D., 2016. Central nervous system vasculitis in pediatric microscopic polyangiitis: A case report and review of literature. Acta reumatologica portuguesa. https://www.ncbi.nlm.nih.gov/pubmed/?term=27156236

Chen, Y. et al., 2016. Long-term outcome of mycophenolate mofetil treatment for patients with microscopic polyangiitis: an observational study in Chinese patients. Rheumatology International, 36(7), pp.967–974. http://dx.doi.org/10.1007/s00296-016-3492-5.

Kallenberg, C.G.M., 2014. The diagnosis and classification of microscopic polyangiitis. Journal of Autoimmunity, 48-49, pp.90–93. http://dx.doi.org/10.1016/j.jaut.2014.01.023.

MIGRAINE AND STROKE

Arboix, A., 2013. Cortical laminar necrosis related to migrainous cerebral infarction. World Journal of Clinical Cases, 1(8), p.256. http://dx.doi.org/10.12998/wjcc.v1.i8.256.

Floery, D. et al., 2012. Acute-Onset Migrainous Aura Mimicking Acute Stroke: MR Perfusion Imaging Features. American Journal of Neuroradiology, 33(8), pp.1546–1552. http://dx.doi.org/10.3174/ajnr.a3020.

Guidetti, D. et al., 2014. Migraine and Stroke: "Vascular" Comorbidity. Frontiers in Neurology, 5. http://dx.doi.org/10.3389/fneur.2014.00193.

Li, L. et al., 2015. Age-specific association of migraine with cryptogenic TIA and stroke. Neurology, 85(17), pp.1444–1451. http://dx.doi.org/10.1212/wnl.0000000000002059.

Øygarden, H. et al., 2014. Diffusion-weighted lesions in acute ischaemic stroke patients with migraine. Acta Neurologica Scandinavica, 129, pp.41–46. http://dx.doi.org/10.1111/ane.12236.

Spalice, A. et al., 2016. Stroke and migraine is there a possible comorbidity? Italian Journal of Pediatrics, 42(1). http://dx.doi.org/10.1186/s13052-016-0253-8.

MIGRAINE WITH AURA

DeLange, J.M. & Cutrer, F.M., 2014. Our Evolving Understanding of Migraine with Aura. Current Pain and Headache Reports, 18(10). http://dx.doi.org/10.1007/s11916-014-0453-0.

Thissen, S. et al., 2014. Persistent Migraine Aura: New Cases, a Literature Review, and Ideas About Pathophysiology. Headache: The Journal of Head and Face Pain, 54(8), pp.1290–1309. http://dx.doi.org/10.1111/head.12392.

Vijiaratnam, N. et al., 2016. Migraine: Does aura require investigation? Clinical Neurology and Neurosurgery, 148, pp.110–114. http://dx.doi.org/10.1016/j.clineuro.2016.07.006.

MIGRAINE WITH BRAINSTEM AURA

Harker, L.A. and Rassekh, C.H., 1987. Episodic vertigo in basilar artery migraine. Otolaryngology--Head and Neck Surgery, 96(3), pp.239-250. https://eurekamag.com/research/028/268/028268427.php

Nesbitt, A.D. & Leschziner, G.D., 2016. Migraine with brainstem aura presenting as recurrent hypersomnia (Kleine-Levin syndrome). Practical Neurology, 16(5), pp.402–405. http://dx.doi.org/10.1136/practneurol-2016-001418.

Yao, G. & Zhang, X.-M., 2016. A Valuable Case for Recognizing the Relationship between Arrhythmia and the Biology of Migraine with Brainstem Aura. Journal of Forensic Sciences, 61(1), pp.288–288. http://dx.doi.org/10.1111/1556-4029.12983.

MIGRAINE: CATAMENIAL

Mathew, P.G., Dun, E.C. & Luo, J.J., 2013. A Cyclic Pain. Obstetrical & Gynecological Survey, 68(2), pp.130–140. http://dx.doi.org/10.1097/ogx.0b013e31827f2496.

Pavlović, J.M. et al., 2016. Sex hormones in women with and without migraine. Neurology, 87(1), pp.49–56. http://dx.doi.org/10.1212/wnl.0000000000002798.

MIGRAINE: HEMIPLEGIC

Ophoff, R.A. et al., 1994. Genetic Heterogeneity of Familial Hemiplegic Migraine. Genomics, 22(1), pp.21–26. http://dx.doi.org/10.1006/geno.1994.1340.

Riant, F. et al., 2010. De novo mutations in ATP1A2 and CACNA1A are frequent in early-onset sporadic hemiplegic migraine. Neurology, 75(11), pp.967–972. http://dx.doi.org/10.1212/wnl.0b013e3181f25e8f.

Terwindt, G., 2002. Mutation Analysis of the CACNA1A Calcium Channel Subunit Gene in 27 Patients With Sporadic Hemiplegic Migraine. Archives of Neurology, 59(6), p.1016. http://dx.doi.org/10.1001/archneur.59.6.1016.

MIGRAINE: MECHANISMS

Friedrich, T., Tavraz, N.N. & Junghans, C., 2016. ATP1A2 Mutations in Migraine: Seeing through the Facets of an Ion Pump onto the Neurobiology of Disease. Frontiers in Physiology, 7. http://dx.doi.org/10.3389/fphys.2016.00239.

Kowa, H., Takigawa, H. & Nakashima, K., 2014. Cortical spreading depression and pain: A missing link in the pathophysiology of migraine? Rinsho Shinkeigaku, 54(12), pp.1006–1008. http://dx.doi.org/10.5692/clinicalneurol.54.1006.

McComas, A.J. & Upton, A.R.M., 2015. Cortical spreading depression in migraine-time to reconsider? Arquivos de Neuro-Psiquiatria, 73(8), pp.714–721. http://dx.doi.org/10.1590/0004-282x20150094.

Noseda, R. & Burstein, R., 2013. Migraine pathophysiology: Anatomy of the trigeminovascular pathway and associated neurological symptoms, cortical spreading depression, sensitization, and modulation of pain. Pain, 154, pp.S44–S53. http://dx.doi.org/10.1016/j.pain.2013.07.021.

Viola, S. et al., 2014. The increased distensibility of the wall of cerebral arterial network may play a role in the pathogenic mechanism of migraine headache. Neurological Sciences, 35(S1), pp.163–166. http://dx.doi.org/10.1007/s10072-014-1761-1.

MIGRAINE: RETINAL

Demircan, S. et al., 2015. The Impact of Migraine on Posterior Ocular Structures. Journal of Ophthalmology, 2015, pp.1–8. http://dx.doi.org/10.1155/2015/868967.

Gan, K.D., Mouradian, M.S., Weis, E. and Lewis, J.R., 2005. Transient monocular visual loss and retinal migraine. Canadian Medical Association Journal, 173(12), pp.1441-1442. http://www.cmaj.ca/content/173/12/1441.figures-only/reply

MIGRAINE: VESTIBULAR

Cha, Y.H., Kane, M.J. and Baloh, R.W., 2008. Familial clustering of migraine, episodic vertigo, and Ménière's disease. Otology & neurotology: official publication of the American Otological Society, American Neurotology Society [and] European Academy of Otology and Neurotology, 29(1), p.93. https://doi.org/10.1097/mao.0b013e31815c2abb

Dieterich, M., Obermann, M. & Celebisoy, N., 2016. Vestibular migraine: the most frequent entity of episodic vertigo. Journal of Neurology, 263(S1), pp.82–89. http://dx.doi.org/10.1007/s00415-015-7905-2.

Furman, J.M., 2005. Migraine-anxiety related dizziness (MARD): a new disorder? Journal of Neurology, Neurosurgery & Psychiatry, 76(1), pp.1–8. http://dx.doi.org/10.1136/jnnp.2004.048926.

MISONIDAZOLE

BYDDER, P.V. et al., 1989. A Controlled Trial of Misonidazole in the Curative Treatment of Infiltrating Bladder Cancer. Australasian Radiology, 33(1), pp.8–14. http://dx.doi.org/10.1111/j.1440-1673.1989.tb03227.x.

GRAZIANO, M., 1996. NEUROTOXICITY OF MISONIDAZOLE IN RATS FOLLOWING INTRAVENOUS ADMINISTRATION. Pharmacological Research, 33(6), pp.307–318. http://dx.doi.org/10.1006/phrs.1996.0043.

Paulson OB, et al. 1984. Misonidazole neuropathy. Acta Neurol Scand Suppl. 100, pp.133-6. www.ncbi.nlm.nih.gov/pubmed/6091392

MIXED CRYOGLOBULINEMIA

Anis, S., 2014. Vasculitis with renal involvement in essential mixed cryoglobulinemia: Case report and mini-review. World Journal of Clinical Cases, 2(5), p.160. http://dx.doi.org/10.12998/wjcc.v2.i5.160.

Pandrangi, S. et al., 2008. Rituximab treatment for a patient with type I cryoglobulinemic glomerulonephritis. Nature Clinical Practice Nephrology, 4(7), pp.393–397. http://dx.doi.org/10.1038/ncpneph0823.

Anis, S., 2014. Vasculitis with renal involvement in essential mixed cryoglobulinemia: Case report and mini-review. World Journal of Clinical Cases, 2(5), p.160. http://dx.doi.org/10.12998/wjcc.v2.i5.160.

Bhattarai, M., Woytowitz, D.V., Kaldas, H., Bastacky, S., Chen, S.S., Johnston, J.R. and Bernardo, J.F., 2015. Recurrent Mixed Cryoglobulinemia (MCS): A Case Report and Literature Review. Rhode Island medical journal (2013), 98(10), p.33.

http://www.rimed.org/rimedicaljournal/2015/10/2015-10-33-case-bhattarai.pdf

Damoiseaux, J. & Cohen Tervaert, J.W., 2013. Diagnostics and Treatment of Cryoglobulinaemia: It Takes Two to Tango. Clinical Reviews in Allergy & Immunology, 47(3), pp.299–310. http://dx.doi.org/10.1007/s12016-013-8390-y.

MULTIPLE SCLEROSIS

ShayestehAzar, M et al. 2015. A Survey of Severity and Distribution of Musculoskeletal Pain in Multiple Sclerosis Patients; a Cross-Sectional Study. Arch Bone and Joint Surg, 3(2), pp 114-118. Available at: http://abjs.mums.ac.ir/article_3939.html.

Khan, F., Amatya, B. & Kesselring, J., 2013. Longitudinal 7-year follow-up of chronic pain in persons with multiple sclerosis in the community. Journal of Neurology, 260(8), pp.2005–2015. Available at: http://dx.doi.org/10.1007/s00415-013-6925-z.

Solaro, C. & Messmer Uccelli, M., 2010. Pharmacological Management of Pain in Patients with Multiple Sclerosis. Drugs, p.1. Available at: http://dx.doi.org/10.2165/11537930-000000000-00000.

Nurmikko, T.J., Gupta, S. & Maclver, K., 2010. Multiple Sclerosis-Related Central Pain Disorders. Current Pain and Headache Reports, 14(3), pp.189–195. Available at: http://dx.doi.org/10.1007/s11916-010-0108-8.

Kenner, M., Menon, U. & Elliott, D.G., 2007. Multiple Sclerosis as A Painful Disease. The Neurobiology of Multiple Sclerosis, pp.303–321. Available at: http://dx.doi.org/10.1016/s0074-7742(07)79013-x.

MUSCULOSKELETAL CHEST PAIN (GENERAL)

Fam AG, et al. 1985. Musculoskeletal Chest Wall Pain. Canadian Medical Association Journal, 133:379-389. https://www.ncbi.nlm.nih.gov/pmc/articles/PMC1346531/

Winzenberg, T et al, 2015, Musculoskeletal chest wall pain. Australian family physician 44.8 (2015): 540-544. https://www.ncbi.nlm.nih.gov/pubmed/26510139

MUSCULOCUTANEOUS NERVE

Ma, H. et al., 2009. Musculocutaneous Nerve Entrapment. The American Journal of Sports Medicine, 37(12), pp.2467–2469. Available at: http://dx.doi.org/10.1177/0363546509337406.

Guerri-Guttenberg, R.A. & Ingolotti, M., 2009. Classifying musculocutaneous nerve variations. Clinical Anatomy, 22(6), pp.671–683. Available at: http://dx.doi.

org/10.1002/ca.20828.

Kumar, N. et al., 2014. Incidences and Clinical Implications of Communications between Musculocutaneous Nerve and Median Nerve in the Arm – A Cadaveric Study. West Indian Medical Journal, 62(8). Available at: http://dx.doi.org/10.7727/wimj.2013.175.

MYOFASCIAL PAIN SYNDROME

Ballyns, J.J., Shah, J.P., Hammond, J., Gebreab, T., Gerber, L.H. and Sikdar, S., 2011. Objective sonographic measures for characterizing myofascial trigger points associated with cervical pain. Journal of ultrasound in medicine, 30(10), pp.1331-1340. https://www.ncbi.nlm.nih.gov/pmc/articles/PMC3493620/

Borg-Stein, J. & Simons, D.G., 2002. Myofascial pain. Archives of Physical Medicine and Rehabilitation, 83, pp.S40–S47. http://dx.doi.org/10.1053/apmr.2002.32155.

Caumo W, et al. 2016, Motor Cortex Excitability and BDNF Levels in Chronic Musculoskeletal Pain according to Structural Pathology. Front Hum Neurosci. 10: 357-375. https://www.ncbi.nlm.nih.gov/pubmed/27471458

Hong, C.-Z. & Simons, D.G., 1998. Pathophysiologic and electrophysiologic mechanisms of myofascial trigger points. Archives of Physical Medicine and Rehabilitation, 79(7), pp.863–872. http://dx.doi.org/10.1016/s0003-9993(98)90371-9.

Tough, E.A. et al., 2007. Variability of Criteria Used to Diagnose Myofascial Trigger Point Pain Syndrome???Evidence From a Review of the Literature. Clin J Pain. 2007 Mar-Apr;23(3), pp.278–286. https://www.ncbi.nlm.nih.gov/pubmed/17314589

NAV1.8 MUTATION

Dabby, R. et al., 2016. Painful small fiber neuropathy with gastroparesis: A new phenotype with a novel mutation in the SCN10A gene. Journal of Clinical Neuroscience, 26, pp.84–88. http://dx.doi.org/10.1016/j.jocn.2015.05.071.

Daou, I. et al., 2016. Optogenetic Silencing of Nav1.8-Positive Afferents Alleviates Inflammatory and Neuropathic Pain. eNeuro, 3(1). http://dx.doi.org/10.1523/eneuro.0140-15.2016.

Han, C. et al., 2013. The G1662S NaV1.8 mutation in small fibre neuropathy: impaired inactivation underlying DRG neuron hyperexcitability. Journal of Neurology, Neurosurgery & Psychiatry, 85(5), pp.499–505. http://dx.doi.org/10.1136/jnnp-2013-306095.

Huang, J. et al., 2013. Small-Fiber Neuropathy Nav1.8 Mutation Shifts Activation to Hyperpolarized Potentials and Increases Excitability of Dorsal Root Ganglion Neurons. Journal of Neuroscience, 33(35), pp.14087–14097. http://dx.doi.org/10.1523/jneurosci.2710-13.2013.

NAV1.9 MUTATION SFN

Huang, J. et al., 2014. Gain-of-function mutations in sodium channel NaV1.9 in painful neuropathy. Brain, 137(6), pp.1627–1642. http://dx.doi.org/10.1093/brain/awu079.

Leipold, E. et al., 2015. Cold-aggravated pain in humans caused by a hyperactive NaV1.9 channel mutant. Nature Communications, 6, p.10049. http://dx.doi.org/10.1038/ncomms10049 .

Okuda, H. et al., 2016. Infantile Pain Episodes Associated with Novel Nav1.9 Mutations in Familial Episodic Pain Syndrome in Japanese Families L. S. Premkumar, ed. PLOS ONE, 11(5), p.e0154827. http://dx.doi.org/10.1371/journal.pone.0154827.

NECK-TONGUE SYNDROME

Hu, N. & Dougherty, C., 2016. Neck-Tongue Syndrome. Current Pain and Headache Reports, 20(4). http://dx.doi.org/10.1007/s11916-016-0555-y.

Lance, J.W. & Anthony, M., 1980. Neck-tongue syndrome on sudden turning of the head. Journal of Neurology, Neurosurgery & Psychiatry, 43(2), pp.97–101. http://dx.doi.org/10.1136/jnnp.43.2.97.

Niethamer, L. & Myers, R., 2016. Manual Therapy and Exercise for a Patient With Neck-Tongue Syndrome: A Case Report. Journal of Orthopaedic & Sports Physical Therapy, 46(3), pp.217–224. http://dx.doi.org/10.2519/jospt.2016.6195.

NERVE INJURY FOLLOWING LUMBAR PLEXUS BLOCKADE

Brull, R. et al., 2007. Neurological Complications After Regional Anesthesia: Contemporary Estimates of Risk. Anesthesia & Analgesia, 104(4), pp.965–974. http://dx.doi.org/10.1213/01.ane.0000258740.17193.ec.

Gungor, I. et al., 2014. Femoral Nerve Injury Following a Lumbar Plexus Blockade. Balkan Medical Journal, 31(2), pp.184–186. http://dx.doi.org/10.5152/balkanmedj.2014.13179.

Kaufman, B.R. et al., 2000. Debilitating chronic pain syndromes after presumed intraneural injections. Pain, 85(1), pp.283–286. http://dx.doi.org/10.1016/s0304-3959(99)00243-2.

NEURALGIC AMYOTROPHY

Chance, P.F. et al., 1994. Hereditary neuralgic amyotrophy and hereditary neuropathy with liability to pressure palsies: Two distinct genetic disorders. Neurology, 44(12), pp.2253–2253. http://dx.doi.org/10.1212/wnl.44.12.2253.

Collie, A.M.B. et al., 2009. Non-recurrent SEPT9 duplications cause hereditary neuralgic amyotrophy. Journal of Medical Genetics, 47(9), pp.601–607. http://dx.doi.org/10.1136/jmg.2009.072348.

Collie, A.M.B. et al., 2009. Non-recurrent SEPT9 duplications cause hereditary neuralgic amyotrophy. Journal of Medical Genetics, 47(9), pp.601–607. http://dx.doi.org/10.1136/jmg.2009.072348.

Klein, C.J. et al., 2009. SEPT9 Mutations and a Conserved 17q25 Sequence in Sporadic and Hereditary Brachial Plexus Neuropathy. Archives of Neurology, 66(2). http://dx.doi.org/10.1001/archneurol.2008.585.

Seror, P., 2016. Neuralgic amyotrophy. An update. Joint Bone Spine. http://dx.doi.org/10.1016/j.jbspin.2016.03.005.

Van Alfen, N., 2011. Clinical and pathophysiological concepts of neuralgic amyotrophy. Nature Reviews Neurology, 7(6), pp.315–322. http://dx.doi.org/10.1038/nrneurol.2011.62.

NEUROGENIC THORACIC OUTLET SYNDROME

Higashihara, M., Konoeda, F. and Sonoo, M., 2016. [Neurological Signs and Symptoms of True Neurogenic Thoracic Outlet Syndrome]. Brain and nerve= Shinkei kenkyu no shinpo, 68(5), pp.521-529. https://www.ncbi.nlm.nih.gov/pubmed/27156505

Klaassen, Z. et al., 2013. Thoracic outlet syndrome: A neurological and vascular disorder. Clinical Anatomy, 27(5), pp.724–732. http://dx.doi.org/10.1002/ca.22271.

NEUROIMAGING OF PAIN

Tracey, I., 2017. Neuroimaging mechanisms in pain. PAIN, 158, pp.S115–S122. Available at: http://dx.doi.org/10.1097/j.pain.0000000000000863.

Baliki, M.N., Geha, P.Y. & Vania Apkarian, A., 2007. Spontaneous pain and brain activity in neuropathic pain: Functional MRI and pharmacologic functional MRI studies. Current Pain and Headache Reports, 11(3), pp.171–177. Available at: http://dx.doi.org/10.1007/s11916-007-0187-3.

Peyron, R. et al., 2004. An fMRI study of cortical representation of mechanical allodynia in patients with neuropathic pain. Neurology, 63(10), pp.1838–1846. Available at: http://dx.doi.org/10.1212/01.wnl.0000144177.61125.85.

Chang, P.-C. et al., 2017. Brain activity for tactile allodynia. PAIN, 158(3), pp.488–

497. Available at: http://dx.doi.org/10.1097/j.pain.0000000000000788.

Seifert, F. & Maihöfner, C., 2007. Representation of cold allodynia in the human brain—A functional MRI study. NeuroImage, 35(3), pp.1168–1180. Available at: http://dx.doi.org/10.1016/j.neuroimage.2007.01.021.

Komaki, Y. et al., 2016. Functional brain mapping using specific sensory-circuit stimulation and a theoretical graph network analysis in mice with neuropathic allodynia. Scientific Reports, 6(1). Available at: http://dx.doi.org/10.1038/srep37802.

lomar, S. & Bakhaidar, M., 2016. Neuroimaging of neuropathic pain: review of current status and future directions. Neurosurgical Review. Available at: http://dx.doi.org/10.1007/s10143-016-0807-7.

Yennu, A. et al., 2016. Prefrontal hemodynamic mapping by functional near-infrared spectroscopy in response to thermal stimulations over three body sites. Neurophotonics, 3(4), p.045008. Available at: http://dx.doi.org/10.1117/1.nph.3.4.045008.

NEUROMA

Ahlawat, S. et al., 2015. MRI features of peripheral traumatic neuromas. European Radiology, 26(4), pp.1204–1212. http://dx.doi.org/10.1007/s00330-015-3907-9.

Chhabra, A. et al., 2010. MR Neurography of Neuromas Related to Nerve Injury and Entrapment with Surgical Correlation. American Journal of Neuroradiology, 31(8), pp.1363–1368. http://dx.doi.org/10.3174/ajnr.a2002.

Fayad, J.N. & Linthicum, F.H., 2009. Symptomatic Postsurgical Traumatic Neuromas. Otology & Neurotology, 30(7), pp.981–984. http://dx.doi.org/10.1097/mao.0b013e3181b4ef04.

O'Reilly, M.A.R. et al., 2016. Neuromas as the cause of pain in the residual limbs of amputees. An ultrasound study. Clinical Radiology, 71(10), pp.1068.e1–1068.e6. http://dx.doi.org/10.1016/j.crad.2016.05.022.

Rajput, K., Reddy, S. & Shankar, H., 2012. Painful Neuromas. The Clinical Journal oF Pain, 28(7), pp.639–645. http://dx.doi.org/10.1097/ajp.0b013e31823d30a2.

Weng, W. et al., 2016. Significance of alpha smooth muscle actin expression in traumatic painful neuromas: a pilot study in rats. Scientific Reports, 6, p.23828. http://dx.doi.org/10.1038/srep23828.

NEUROMUSCULAR CHORISTOMA

Niederhauser, B.D. et al., 2012. Neuromuscular choristoma: characteristic magnetic resonance imaging findings and association with post-biopsy fibromatosis. Skeletal Radiology, 42(4), pp.567–577. http://dx.doi.org/10.1007/s00256-012-1546-7.

O'Brien, T.G., Spinner, R.J. & Boon, A.J., 2016. Neuromuscular choristoma presenting with unilateral limb hypoplasia in a 3-year-old boy. Muscle & Nerve, 54(4), pp.797–801. http://dx.doi.org/10.1002/mus.25177.

NEUROPATHIC PAIN

Costigan, M., Scholz, J. & Woolf, C.J., 2009. Neuropathic Pain: A Maladaptive Response of the Nervous System to Damage. Annual Review of Neuroscience, 32(1), pp.1–32. http://dx.doi.org/10.1146/annurev.neuro.051508.135531.

Woolf, C.J., 2011. Central sensitization: Implications for the diagnosis and treatment of pain. Pain, 152(Supplement), pp.S2–S15. http://dx.doi.org/10.1016/j.pain.2010.09.030.

NITROFURANTOIN

Spring, P.J., et al., 2001, Nitrofurantoin and Peripheral Neuropathy: A Forgotten Problem? Med J Aust 174 (3), 153-154. https://www.ncbi.nlm.nih.gov/pubmed/11247627

Tan, I.L., 2012. Peripheral Nerve Toxic Effects of Nitrofurantoin. Archives of Neurology, 69(2), p.265. http://dx.doi.org/10.1001/archneurol.2011.1120.

NUCLEOSIDE REVERSE TRANSCRIPTASE INHIBITORS

Joseph, E.K. et al., 2004. Novel mechanism of enhanced nociception in a model of AIDS therapy-induced painful peripheral neuropathy in the rat. Pain, 107(1), pp.147–158. http://dx.doi.org/10.1016/j.pain.2003.10.010.

Kallianpur, A.R. & Hulgan, T., 2009. Pharmacogenetics of nucleoside reverse-transcriptase inhibitor-associated peripheral neuropathy. Pharmacogenomics, 10(4), pp.623–637. http://dx.doi.org/10.2217/pgs.09.14.

ROSSI, L. et al., 1999. Metabolism, mitochondrial uptake and toxicity of 2⊠,3⊠-dideoxycytidine. Biochemical Journal, 344(3), p.915. http://dx.doi.org/10.1042/0264-6021:3440915.

OBSTETRIC PALSY

Jennett, R.J., Tarby, T.J. and Krauss, R.L., 2002. Erb's palsy contrasted with Klumpke's and total palsy: different mechanisms are involved. American journal of obstetrics and gynecology, 186(6), pp.1216-1220. https://www.ncbi.nlm.nih.gov/pubmed/12066101

Leshikar, H.B. et al., 2016. Clavicle Fracture Is Not Predictive of the Need for Microsurgery in Brachial Plexus Birth Palsy. Journal of Pediatric Orthopaedics, p.1. http://dx.doi.org/10.1097/bpo.0000000000000770.

Sandmire, H.F. and DeMott, R.K., 2005. Erb's palsy causation: iatrogenic or resulting from labor forces?. The Journal of reproductive medicine, 50(8), pp.563-566. https://www.ncbi.nlm.nih.gov/pubmed/16220759

OBTURATOR NERVE

Kumka, M., 2010. Critical sites of entrapment of the posterior division of the obturator nerve: anatomical considerations. J Can Chiropr Assoc., 54(1), pp. 33–42. Available at: https://www.ncbi.nlm.nih.gov/pmc/articles/PMC2829684/

Kowalska, B. et al., 2012. Ultrasound assessment of selected peripheral nerves pathologies. Part II: Entrapment neuropathies of the lower limb. Journal of Ultrasonography, 12(51), pp.463–471. Available at: http://dx.doi.org/10.15557/jou.2012.0033.

Kim, J.W., Shon, H.C. & Park, J.H., 2017. Injury of the obturator nerve in the modified Stoppa approach for acetabular fractures. Orthopaedics & Traumatology: Surgery & Research, 103(5), pp.639–644. Available at: http://dx.doi.org/10.1016/j.otsr.2017.03.005.

OCCIPITAL NEURALGIA

Cesmebasi, A. et al., 2014. Occipital neuralgia: Anatomic considerations. Clinical Anatomy, 28(1), pp.101–108. http://dx.doi.org/10.1002/ca.22468.

Cesmebasi, A. et al., 2014. Occipital neuralgia: Anatomic considerations. Clinical Anatomy, 28(1), pp.101–108. http://dx.doi.org/10.1002/ca.22468.

Choi, I. & Jeon, S.R., 2016. Neuralgias of the Head: Occipital Neuralgia. Journal of Korean Medical Science, 31(4), p.479. http://dx.doi.org/10.3346/jkms.2016.31.4.479.

Choi, I. & Jeon, S.R., 2016. Neuralgias of the Head: Occipital Neuralgia. Journal of Korean Medical Science, 31(4), p.479. http://dx.doi.org/10.3346/jkms.2016.31.4.479.

Shamji, M., Guha, D. et al., 2015. Occipital neuralgia secondary to unilateral atlantoaxial osteoarthritis: Case report and review of the literature. Surgical Neurology International, 6(1), p.186. http://dx.doi.org/10.4103/2152-7806.172531.

Tubbs, R.S. et al., 2011. Cruveilhier plexus: an anatomical study and a potential cause of failed treatments for occipital neuralgia and muscular and facet denervation procedures. Journal of Neurosurgery, 115(5), pp.929–933. http://dx.doi.org/10.3171/2011.5.jns102058.

Zaremski, J.L. et al., 2015. Occipital Neuralgia as a Sequela of Sports Concussion. Current Sports Medicine Reports, 14(1), pp.16–19. http://dx.doi.org/10.1249/jsr.0000000000000121.

OCHRONOSIS

Braconi, D. et al., 2015. Oxidative stress and mechanisms of ochronosis in alkaptonuria. Free Radical Biology and Medicine, 88, pp.70–80. http://dx.doi.org/10.1016/j.freeradbiomed.2015.02.021.

Gil, J.A., Wawrzynski, J. & Waryasz, G.R., 2016. Orthopedic Manifestations of Ochronosis: Pathophysiology, Presentation, Diagnosis, and Management. The American Journal of Medicine, 129(5), pp.536.e1–536.e6. http://dx.doi.org/10.1016/j.amjmed.2016.01.010.

OPTHALMOPONESIS WITH MIGRAINE

Förderreuther, S. & Ruscheweyh, R., 2015. From Ophthalmoplegic Migraine to Cranial Neuropathy. Current Pain and Headache Reports, 19(6). http://dx.doi.org/10.1007/s11916-015-0492-1.

Takizawa, T. et al., 2015. Adult-onset recurrent painful ophthalmoplegic neuropathy displaying atypical oculomotor nerve gadolinium-enhancement pattern in the orbit and cavernous sinus. Cephalalgia, 36(2), pp.199–200. http://dx.doi.org/10.1177/0333102415583987.

ORCHIALGIA

Gordhan, C.G. & Sadeghi-Nejad, H., 2015. Scrotal pain: Evaluation and management. Korean Journal of Urology, 56(1), p.3. http://dx.doi.org/10.4111/kju.2015.56.1.3.

Morley C, Rogers A, Zaslau S. Post-vasectomy pain syndrome: clinical features and treatment options. Can J Urol. 2012 Apr;19(2):6160-4. Review. https://www.ncbi.nlm.nih.gov/pubmed/22512957

Parekattil, S. et al., 2016. Chronic orchialgia: Review of treatments old and new. Indian Journal of Urology, 32(1), p.21. http://dx.doi.org/10.4103/0970-1591.173110.

ORTHOPEDIC TRAUMA AND ASSOCIATED BRACHIAL PLEXUS INJURY

Brogan, D.M. et al., 2014. Prevalence of Rotator Cuff Tears in Adults with Traumatic Brachial Plexus Injuries. The Journal of Bone and Joint Surgery-American Volume, 96(16), pp.e139–1–6. http://dx.doi.org/10.2106/jbjs.l.00420.

Güven, O. et al., 1994. Concomitant Rotator Cuff Tear and Brachial Plexus Injury in Association with Anterior Shoulder Dislocation: Unhappy Triad of the Shoulder. Journal of Orthopaedic Trauma, 8(5), pp.429–430. http://dx.doi.org/10.1097/00005131-199410000-00010.

Kaiser, R., Waldauf, P. and Haninec, P., 2012. Scapular fracture related to polytrauma severity in patients with serious brachial plexus palsy. Acta chirurgiae orthopaedicae et traumatologiae Cechoslovaca, 80(4), pp.284-286. http://www.achot.cz/detail.php?stat=634

Lädermann, A. et al., 2011. Prevalence of Neurologic Lesions After Total Shoulder Arthroplasty. The Journal of Bone and Joint Surgery-American Volume, 93(14), pp.1288–1293. http://dx.doi.org/10.2106/jbjs.j.00369.

OSTEOMYELITIS

Kulcheski, Á.L. et al., 2015. Fungal spondylodiscitis due to Candida albicans: an atypical case and review of the literature. Revista Brasileira de Ortopedia (English Edition), 50(6), pp.739–742. http://dx.doi.org/10.1016/j.rboe.2015.10.005.

Simopoulos, T.T., Kraemer, J.J., Glazer, P. and Bajwa, Z.H., 2008. Vertebral osteomyelitis: A potentially catastrophic outcome after lumbar epidural steroid injection. Pain Physician, 11(5), pp.693-697. https://www.ncbi.nlm.nih.gov/pubmed/18850035

Smith, A.S. and Blaser, S.I., 1991. Infectious and inflammatory processes of the spine. Radiologic Clinics of North America, 29(4), pp.809-827. https://www.ncbi.nlm.nih.gov/pubmed/2063006

Spyropoulou, V. et al., 2016. Progression of Infection after Surgical CT Navigation-Assisted Aspiration Biopsy of a Vertebral Abscess. Case Reports in Orthopedics, 2016, pp.1–5. http://dx.doi.org/10.1155/2016/8675761.

OVARIAN CANCER

Goff, B.A. et al., 2007. Development of an ovarian cancer symptom index. Cancer, 109(2), pp.221–227. http://dx.doi.org/10.1002/cncr.22371.

Iyer, V.R. & Lee, S.I., 2010. MRI, CT, and PET/CT for Ovarian Cancer Detection and Adnexal Lesion Characterization. American Journal of Roentgenology, 194(2), pp.311–321. http://dx.doi.org/10.2214/ajr.09.3522.

Ryerson, A.B. et al., 2007. Symptoms, Diagnoses, and Time to Key Diagnostic Procedures Among Older U.S. Women With Ovarian Cancer. Obstetrics & Gynecology, 109(5), pp.1053–1061. http://dx.doi.org/10.1097/01.aog.0000260392.70365.5e.

OVARIAN CYST

Bosetti, C. et al., 2006. Benign ovarian cysts and breast cancer risk. International Journal of Cancer, 119(7), pp.1679–1682. http://dx.doi.org/10.1002/ijc.22016.

Bottomley, C. & Bourne, T., 2009. Diagnosis and management of ovarian cyst accidents. Best Practice & Research Clinical Obstetrics & Gynaecology, 23(5), pp.711–724. http://dx.doi.org/10.1016/j.bpobgyn.2009.02.001.

Lambert, M.J. & Villa, M., 2004. Gynecologic ultrasound in emergency medicine. Emergency Medicine Clinics of North America, 22(3), pp.683–696. http://dx.doi.org/10.1016/j.emc.2004.04.016.

Stany, M.P. & Hamilton, C.A., 2008. Benign Disorders of the Ovary. Obstetrics and Gynecology Clinics of North America, 35(2), pp.271–284. http://dx.doi.org/10.1016/j.ogc.2008.03.004.

OVARIAN CYSTS/CANCER

Biggs WS, Marks ST. Diagnosis and Management of Adnexal Masses. Am Fam Physician. 2016 Apr 15;93(8):676-81. https://www.ncbi.nlm.nih.gov/pubmed/27175840

Cooper, C.P. et al., 2016. Intended care seeking for ovarian cancer symptoms among U.S. women. Preventive Medicine Reports, 3, pp.234–237. http://dx.doi.org/10.1016/j.pmedr.2016.01.011.

Cymbaluk-Ploska A, Chudecka-Glaz A, Surowiec A, Pius-Sadowska E, Machalinski B, Menkiszak J. MMP3 in Comparison to CA 125, HE4 and the ROMA Algorithm in Differentiation of Ovarian Tumors. Asian Pac J Cancer Prev. 2016;17(5):2597-603. https://www.ncbi.nlm.nih.gov/pubmed/27268637

Herek, D., Karabulut, A. & Agladioglu, K., 2016. Usefulness of transabdominal real-time sonoelastography in the evaluation of ovarian lesions: preliminary results. The British Journal of Radiology, 89(1065), p.20160173. http://dx.doi.org/10.1259/bjr.20160173.

Liew, P.-L. et al., 2016. DEF6 expression in ovarian carcinoma correlates with poor patient survival. Diagnostic Pathology, 11(1). http://dx.doi.org/10.1186/s13000-016-0518-y.

Low, E.L. et al., 2013. Ovarian cancer symptom awareness and anticipated time to help-seeking for symptoms among UK women. Journal of Family Planning and Reproductive Health Care, 39(3), pp.163–171. http://dx.doi.org/10.1136/jfprhc-2012-100473.

Montagnana, M. et al., 2011. The ROMA (Risk of Ovarian Malignancy Algorithm) for estimating the risk of epithelial ovarian cancer in women presenting with pelvic mass: is it really useful? Clinical Chemistry and Laboratory Medicine, 49(3). http://dx.doi.org/10.1515/cclm.2011.075.

PAGET–SCHRÖETTER SYNDROME

Dep, A. et al., 2013. Paget-Schrotter syndrome and complications of management. Case Reports, 2013(jul12 1), pp.bcr2013008858–bcr2013008858. http://dx.doi.org/10.1136/bcr-2013-008858.

Edo Fleta, G. et al., 2016. Combined non-surgical treatment for Paget–Schröetter syndrome: a case report. Journal of Medical Case Reports, 10(1). http://dx.doi.org/10.1186/s13256-016-0940-5.

Lugo, J. et al., 2015. Acute Paget–Schroetter Syndrome: Does the First Rib Routinely Need to Be Removed after Thrombolysis? Annals of Vascular Surgery, 29(6), pp.1073–1077. http://dx.doi.org/10.1016/j.avsg.2015.02.006.

PAIN DEMOGRAPHIC

Anderson, K.O., Green, C.R. & Payne, R., 2009. Racial and Ethnic Disparities in Pain: Causes and Consequences of Unequal Care. The Journal of Pain, 10(12), pp.1187–1204. Available at: http://dx.doi.org/10.1016/j.jpain.2009.10.002.

Fillingim, R.B. et al., 2009. Sex, Gender, and Pain: A Review of Recent Clinical and Experimental Findings. The Journal of Pain, 10(5), pp.447–485. Available at: http://dx.doi.org/10.1016/j.jpain.2008.12.001.

Mogil, J.S., 2012. Sex differences in pain and pain inhibition: multiple explanations of a controversial phenomenon. Nature Reviews Neuroscience, 13(12), pp.859–866. Available at: http://dx.doi.org/10.1038/nrn3360.

Racine, M. et al., 2012. A systematic literature review of 10 years of research on sex/gender and pain perception – Part 2: Do biopsychosocial factors alter pain sensitivity differently in women and men? Pain, 153(3), pp.619–635. Available at: http://dx.doi.org/10.1016/j.pain.2011.11.026.

PAIN PROFILES

Freeman, R. et al., 2014. Sensory profiles of patients with neuropathic pain based on the neuropathic pain symptoms and signs. Pain, 155(2), pp.367–376. https://www.ncbi.nlm.nih.gov/pubmed/24472518

Maier, C. et al., 2010. Quantitative sensory testing in the German Research Network on Neuropathic Pain (DFNS): Somatosensory abnormalities in 1236 patients with different neuropathic pain syndromes. Pain, 150(3), pp.439–450. https://www.ncbi.nlm.nih.gov/pubmed/20627413

Sadosky, A. et al., 2016. Characterizing neuropathic pain profiles: enriching interpretation of painDETECT. Patient Related Outcome Measures, Volume 7, pp.93–99. http://dx.doi.org/10.2147/prom.s101892.

Vollert, J. et al., 2016. Symptom profiles in the painDETECT Questionnaire in patients with peripheral neuropathic pain stratified according to sensory loss in quantitative sensory testing. PAIN, 157(8), pp.1810–1818. http://dx.doi.org/10.1097/j.

pain.0000000000000588.

PAINFUL CHANNELOPATHIES

Bennett, D.L.H. & Woods, C.G., 2014. Painful and painless channelopathies. The Lancet Neurology, 13(6), pp.587–599. http://dx.doi.org/10.1016/s1474-4422(14)70024-9.

Brouwer, B.A. et al., 2014. Painful neuropathies: the emerging role of sodium channelopathies. Journal of the Peripheral Nervous System, 19(2), pp.53–65. http://dx.doi.org/10.1111/jns5.12071.

Lampert, A., Eberhardt, M. & Waxman, S.G., 2014. Altered Sodium Channel Gating as Molecular Basis for Pain: Contribution of Activation, Inactivation, and Resurgent Currents. Handbook of Experimental Pharmacology, pp.91–110. http://dx.doi.org/10.1007/978-3-642-41588-3_5.

PAINFUL CHEMOTHERAPY NEUROPATHIES (GENERAL)

Boyette-Davis, J.A., Walters, E.T. & Dougherty, P.M., 2015. Mechanisms involved in the development of chemotherapy-induced neuropathy. Pain Management, 5(4), pp.285–296. http://dx.doi.org/10.2217/pmt.15.19.

Carozzi, V.A., Canta, A. & Chiorazzi, A., 2015. Chemotherapy-induced peripheral neuropathy: What do we know about mechanisms? Neuroscience Letters, 596, pp.90–107. http://dx.doi.org/10.1016/j.neulet.2014.10.014.

Grisold, W., Cavaletti, G. & Windebank, A.J., 2012. Peripheral neuropathies from chemotherapeutics and targeted agents: diagnosis, treatment, and prevention. Neuro-Oncology, 14(suppl 4), pp.iv45–iv54. http://dx.doi.org/10.1093/neuonc/nos203.

Higa & Sypult, C., 2016. Molecular Biology and Clinical Mitigation of Cancer Treatment-Induced Neuropathy. Clinical Medicine Insights: Oncology, p.27. http://dx.doi.org/10.4137/cmo.s32810.

Jaggi, A.S. & Singh, N., 2012. Mechanisms in cancer-chemotherapeutic drugs-induced peripheral neuropathy. Toxicology, 291(1-3), pp.1–9. http://dx.doi.org/10.1016/j.tox.2011.10.019.

PAINLESS DIABETIC MOTOR NEUROPATHY

Dyck, P.J.B. & Thaisetthawatkul, P., 2014. Lumbosacral Plexopathy. Continuum: Lifelong Learning in Neurology, 20, pp.1343–1358. https://www.ncbi.nlm.nih.gov/pubmed/25299286

Garces-Sanchez, M. et al., 2011. Painless diabetic motor neuropathy: A variant of diabetic lumbosacral radiculoplexus Neuropathy? Annals of Neurology, 69(6), pp.1043–1054. http://dx.doi.org/10.1002/ana.22334.

PALMAR CUTANEOUS BRANCH OF MEDIAN NERVE

Zanette, G. & Tamburin, S., 2016. The Diagnostic Value of Nerve Ultrasound in an Atypical Palmar Cutaneous Nerve Lesion. American Journal of Physical Medicine & Rehabilitation, 95(7), pp.e103–e107. Available at: http://dx.doi.org/10.1097/phm.0000000000000468.

Jones, C. et al., 2016. Incidence of an Anomalous Course of the Palmar Cutaneous Branch of the Median Nerve During Volar Plate Fixation of Distal Radius Fractures. The Journal of Hand Surgery, 41(8), pp.841–844. Available at: http://dx.doi.org/10.1016/j.jhsa.2016.05.011.

PANCOAST TUMOR

Foroulis, C. et al, 2013 Superior sulcus (Pancoast) tumors: current evidence on diagnosis and radical treatment. J Thorac Dis., 5(Suppl 4), S342–S358. https://www.ncbi.nlm.nih.gov/pmc/articles/PMC3791502/

Glassman, L.R. & Hyman, K., 2013. Pancoast tumor. Current Opinion in Pulmonary Medicine, 19(4), pp.340–343. http://dx.doi.org/10.1097/mcp.0b013e3283621b31.

Strooker, J.A. et al., 2016. Painful Metastasis in the Lunate Bone as the First Symptom of a Pancoast Tumor; a Case Report and Review of the Literature. Journal of Hand and Microsurgery, 07(02), pp.343–345. http://dx.doi.org/10.1007/s12593-015-0195-1.

Vallieres, E., Kraut, M.J. & Thomas, C.R., 2003. Pancoast (superior sulcus) neoplasms. Current Problems in Cancer, 27(2), pp.81–104. http://dx.doi.org/10.1016/s0147-0272(03)00018-7.

PARKINSON'S DISEASE

Young Blood, M.R. et al., 2016. Classification and Characteristics of Pain Associated with Parkinson's Disease. Parkinson's Disease, 2016, pp.1–8. Available at: http://dx.doi.org/10.1155/2016/6067132.

Tseng, M., 2017. Pain in early-stage Parkinson's disease: Implications from clinical features to pathophysiology mechanisms Journal of the Formosan Medical Association, 116 (8), pp. 571- 581. Available at: http://www.jfma-online.com/article/S0929-6646(16)30450-8/fulltext

Cury, R.G. et al., 2014. Effects of deep brain stimulation on pain and other nonmotor symptoms in Parkinson disease. Neurology, 83(16), pp.1403–1409. Available at: http://dx.doi.org/10.1212/wnl.0000000000000887.

Cury, R.G. et al., 2015. Sensory abnormalities and pain in Parkinson disease and its modulation by treatment of motor symptoms. European Journal of Pain, 20(2), pp.151–165. Available at: http://dx.doi.org/10.1002/ejp.745.

PAROXYSMAL EXTREME PAIN DISORDER

Fertleman, C.R. et al., 2007. Paroxysmal extreme pain disorder (previously familial rectal pain syndrome). Neurology, 69(6), pp.586–595. http://dx.doi.org/10.1212/01.wnl.0000268065.16865.5f.

Meglič, A. et al., 2014. Painful micturition in a small child: an unusual clinical picture of paroxysmal extreme pain disorder. Pediatric Nephrology, 29(9), pp.1643–1646. http://dx.doi.org/10.1007/s00467-014-2819-2.

PAROXYSMAL HEMICRANIA

Antonaci, F., Pareja, J.A., Caminero, A.B. and Sjaastad, O., 1998. Chronic paroxysmal hemicrania and hemicrania continua. Parenteral indomethacin: the 'indotest'. Headache: The Journal of Head and Face Pain, 38(2), pp.122-128. https://doi.org/10.1046/j.1526-4610.1998.3802122.

Benoliel, R. & Sharav, Y., 1998. Paroxysmal hemicrania. Oral Surgery, Oral Medicine, Oral Pathology, Oral Radiology, and Endodontology, 85(3), pp.285–292. http://dx.doi.org/10.1016/s1079-2104(98)90010-5.

Flavia, P. & Chiara, L., 2016. Coexistence of contralateral cluster headache and probable paroxysmal hemicrania: a case report. SpringerPlus, 5(1). http://dx.doi.org/10.1186/s40064-016-2000-4.

Goadsby, P., Cittadini, E. & Cohen, A., 2010. Trigeminal Autonomic Cephalalgias: Paroxysmal Hemicrania, SUNCT/SUNA, and Hemicrania Continua. Seminars in Neurology, 30(02), pp.186–191. http://dx.doi.org/10.1055/s-0030-1249227.

Silberstein, S.D. & Vodovskaia, N., 2013. Trigeminal Autonomic Cephalalgias Other than Cluster Headache. Medical Clinics of North America, 97(2), pp.321–328. http://dx.doi.org/10.1016/j.mcna.2012.12.009.

PARSONAGE-TURNER

Feinberg, J.H., Doward, D.A. & Gonsalves, A., 2006. Cervical Radiculopathy vs Parsonage–Turner Syndrome: a Case Report. HSS Journal, 3(1), pp.106–111. http://dx.doi.org/10.1007/s11420-006-9028-x.

Schreiber, A.L., Abramov, R., Fried, G.W. and Herbison, G.J., 2009. Expanding the differential of shoulder pain: Parsonage-Turner syndrome. The Journal of the American Osteopathic Association, 109(8), pp.415-422. https://www.ncbi.nlm.nih.gov/pubmed/19706831

Tissier-Ducamp, D., Martinez, S., Alagha, K., Charpin, D., Chanez, P. and Palot, A., 2015. [Bilateral diaphragmatic paralysis due to Parsonage-Turner syndrome]. Revue des maladies respiratoires, 32(7), pp.742-746. https://www.ncbi.nlm.nih.gov/pubmed/25534571

PECTORAL NERVE

Aktas, I., Palamar, D. & Akgun, K., 2015. Lateral Pectoral Nerve Injury Mimicking Cervical Radiculopathy. Clinical Journal of Sport Medicine, 25(4), pp.e64–e66. http://dx.doi.org/10.1097/jsm.0000000000000147.

Leiman, D. et al., 2014. Medial and Lateral Pectoral Nerve Block with Liposomal Bupivacaine for the Management of Postsurgical Pain after Submuscular Breast Augmentation. Plastic and Reconstructive Surgery Global Open, 2(12), p.e282. http://dx.doi.org/10.1097/gox.0000000000000253.

Prakash KG, 2014. Anatomical Study of Pectoral Nerves and its Implications in Surgery. J Clin Diagn Res. http://dx.doi.org/10.7860/jcdr/2014/8631.4545.

PEDICLE ANOMALIES

Mohammad Samadian, M.D., Bakhtevari, M.H. and Naveed Nabizadeh, M.D., 2015. Congenital Posterior Spinal Agenesis Leads to L2-L3 Instability: a Case Report and Review of the Literature. Archives of Iranian medicine, 18(12), pp.861–864. https://dx.doi.org/0151812/AIM.0013.

Savas, R. et al., 1998. Hypoplastic lumbar pedicle in association with conjoined nerve root MRI demonstration. Computerized Medical Imaging and Graphics, 22(1), pp.77–79. http://dx.doi.org/10.1016/s0895-6111(98)00003-2.

Yoshioka, S. et al., 2010. Congenital absence of lumbosacral articular facet joint associated with conjoined nerve root: a case report. Journal of Orthopaedics and Traumatology, 11(3), pp.183–187. http://dx.doi.org/10.1007/s10195-010-0100-4.

PELVIC FLOOR PAIN/DYSFUNCTION

Doggweiler-Wiygul R, Wiygul JP. Interstitial cystitis, pelvic pain, and the relationship to myofascial pain and dysfunction: a report on four patients. World J Urol. 2002 Nov;20(5):310-4. https://www.ncbi.nlm.nih.gov/pubmed/12522588

Hoffman, D., 2015. Central and Peripheral Pain Generators in Women with Chronic Pelvic Pain: Patient Centered Assessment and Treatment. Current Rheumatology Reviews, 11(2), pp.146–166. http://dx.doi.org/10.2174/1573397111666150619094524

4.

Itza, F. et al., 2010. Myofascial pain syndrome in the pelvic floor: A common urological condition. Actas Urológicas Españolas (English Edition), 34(4), pp.318–326. http://dx.doi.org/10.1016/s2173-5786(10)70077-9.

Itza, F. et al., 2015. Turn-Amplitude Analysis as a Diagnostic Test for Myofascial Syndrome in Patients with Chronic Pelvic Pain. Pain Research and Management, 20(2), pp.96–100. http://dx.doi.org/10.1155/2015/562349.

Weiss, J.M., 2001. PELVIC FLOOR MYOFASCIAL TRIGGER POINTS: MANUAL THERAPY FOR INTERSTITIAL CYSTITIS AND THE URGENCY-FREQUENCY SYNDROME. The Journal of Urology, 166(6), pp.2226–2231. http://dx.doi.org/10.1016/s0022-5347(05)65539-5.

PERONEAL NERVE

Corey, R.M. & Salazar, D.H., 2016. Entrapment of the Superficial Peroneal Nerve Following a Distal Fibula Fracture. Foot & Ankle Specialist, 10(1), pp.69–71. Available at: http://dx.doi.org/10.1177/1938640016640887.

Dallari, D., et al., 2004. Deep peroneal nerve paresis in a runner caused by ganglion at capitulum peronei. Case report and review of the literature. J Sports Med Phys Fitness, 44(4), pp. 436-40. Abstract available at: https://www.ncbi.nlm.nih.gov/pubmed/15758858

Brestas, P., Protopsaltis, I. & Drossos, C., 2016. Role of sonography in the diagnosis and treatment of a ganglion cyst compressing the lateral branch of deep peroneal nerve. Journal of Clinical Ultrasound, 45(2), pp.108–111. Available at: http://dx.doi.org/10.1002/jcu.22388.

Maalla, R. et al., 2013. Peroneal nerve entrapment at the fibular head: Outcomes of neurolysis. Orthopaedics & Traumatology: Surgery & Research, 99(6), pp.719–722. Available at: http://dx.doi.org/10.1016/j.otsr.2013.05.004.

Iwamoto, N. et al., 2016. Repetitive Plantar Flexion Test as an Adjunct Tool for the Diagnosis of Common Peroneal Nerve Entrapment Neuropathy. World Neurosurgery, 86, pp.484–489. Available at: http://dx.doi.org/10.1016/j.wneu.2015.09.080.

Demiroğlu, M. et al., 2017. Deep peroneal nerve palsy due to osteochondroma arising from fibular head and proximal lateral tibia. International Journal of Surgery Case Reports, 31, pp.200–202. Available at: http://dx.doi.org/10.1016/j.ijscr.2017.01.050.

Kitamura, T. et al., 2017. Dynamic factors involved in common peroneal nerve entrapment neuropathy. Acta Neurochirurgica, 159(9), pp.1777–1781. Available at: http://dx.doi.org/10.1007/s00701-017-3265-2.

Bregman, P.J. & Schuenke, M., 2016. Current Diagnosis and Treatment of Superficial Fibular Nerve Injuries and Entrapment. Clinics in Podiatric Medicine and Surgery, 33(2), pp.243–254. Available at: http://dx.doi.org/10.1016/j.cpm.2015.12.007.

PERINEURIAL CYST

Elsawaf, A., Awad, T.E. & Fesal, S.S., 2016. Surgical excision of symptomatic sacral perineurial Tarlov cyst: case series and review of the literature. European Spine Journal, 25(11), pp.3385–3392. http://dx.doi.org/10.1007/s00586-016-4584-3.

Nicpoń, K.W. et al., 2002. [Cauda equina syndrome caused by Tarlov's cysts--case report]. Neurologia i neurochirurgia polska, 36(1), pp.181–189. http://europepmc.org/abstract/med/12053609

Singh, P.K. et al., 2009. Tarlov Cyst and Infertility. The Journal of Spinal Cord Medicine, 32(2), pp.191–197. http://dx.doi.org/10.1080/10790268.2009.11760771.

PHANTOM BREAST PAIN

Björkman, B., Arnér, S. & Hydén, L.-C., 2008. Phantom Breast and Other Syndromes After Mastectomy: Eight Breast Cancer Patients Describe Their Experiences Over Time: A 2-Year Follow-up Study. The Journal of Pain, 9(11), pp.1018–1025. http://dx.doi.org/10.1016/j.jpain.2008.06.003.

Krøner K, Knudsen UB, Lundby L, Hvid HM. [Phantom breast syndrome]. Ugeskr Laeger. 1994 Feb 14;156(7):977-80. Danish. PubMed https://www.ncbi.nlm.nih.gov/pubmed/8009741

Ramesh, Shukla, N. & Bhatnagar, S., 2009. Phantom breast syndrome. Indian Journal of Palliative Care, 15(2), p.103. http://dx.doi.org/10.4103/0973-1075.58453.

PHANTOM PAIN

Jutzeler, C.R., Curt, A. & Kramer, J.L.K., 2015. Relationship between chronic pain and brain reorganization after deafferentation: A systematic review of functional MRI findings. NeuroImage: Clinical, 9, pp.599–606. http://dx.doi.org/10.1016/j.nicl.2015.09.018.

Raffin, E. et al., 2016. Primary motor cortex changes after amputation correlate with phantom limb pain and the ability to move the phantom limb. NeuroImage, 130, pp.134–144. http://dx.doi.org/10.1016/j.neuroimage.2016.01.063.

Seifert, F. & Maihöfner, C., 2008. Central mechanisms of experimental and chronic neuropathic pain: Findings from functional imaging studies. Cellular and Molecular Life Sciences, 66(3), pp.375–390. http://dx.doi.org/10.1007/s00018-008-8428-0.

Subedi, B. & Grossberg, G.T., 2011. Phantom Limb Pain: Mechanisms and Treatment Approaches. Pain Research and Treatment, 2011, pp.1–8. http://dx.doi.org/10.1155/2011/864605.

PHRENIC NERVE

Le Pimpec-Barthes, F. et al., 2016. Diaphragm pacing: the state of the art. Journal of Thoracic Disease, 8(S4), pp.S376–S386. http://dx.doi.org/10.21037/jtd.2016.03.97.

Le Pimpec-Barthes, F., Pricopi, C., Mordant, P., Arame, A., Badia, A., Grand, B., Bagan, P., Hernigou, A. and Riquet, M., 2013. [Diaphragmatic palsy and dysfunction: from physiology to surgery]. Revue de pneumologie clinique, 70(1-2), pp.95-107. https://www.ncbi.nlm.nih.gov/pubmed/24566026

Mugnai, G. et al., 2016. Femoral venous pressure waveform as indicator of phrenic nerve injury in the setting of second-generation cryoballoon ablation. Journal of Cardiovascular Medicine, p.1. http://dx.doi.org/10.2459/jcm.0000000000000418.

Ostrowska, M. & de Carvalho, M., 2012. Prognosis of phrenic nerve injury following thoracic interventions: Four new cases and a review. Clinical Neurology and Neurosurgery, 114(3), pp.199–204. http://dx.doi.org/10.1016/j.clineuro.2011.12.016.

Van de Perck, F. et al., 2015. Phrenic Nerve Injury After Radiofrequency Denervation of the Cervical Medial Branches. Pain Practice, 16(2), pp.E42–E45. http://dx.doi.org/10.1111/papr.12398.

Wang, Y.-J. et al., 2016. Imaging of Pericardiophrenic Bundles Using Multislice Spiral Computed Tomography for Phrenic Nerve Anatomy. Journal of Cardiovascular Electrophysiology, 27(8), pp.961–971. http://dx.doi.org/10.1111/jce.13003.

PLANTAR NERVES

Kuran, B., 2016. Medial calcaneal neuropathy: A rare cause of prolonged heel pain. Ağrı - The Journal of The Turkish Society of Algology. Available at: http://dx.doi.org/10.5505/agri.2015.13540.

Ferkel, E., Davis, W.H. & Ellington, J.K., 2015. Entrapment Neuropathies of the Foot and Ankle. Clinics in Sports Medicine, 34(4), pp.791–801. Available at: http://dx.doi.org/10.1016/j.csm.2015.06.002.

Chang, K.-V., Wu, W.-T. & Özçakar, L., 2016. An Uncommon Cause of Mid-foot Pain: Ultrasound Imaging for Plantar Fibromatosis and Entrapment of the Lateral Plantar Nerve. Pain Medicine, 17(10), pp.1965–1966. Available at: http://dx.doi.org/10.1093/pm/pnw059.

Tu, P., et al., 2011. Diagnosis of Heel Pain. Am Fam Physician, 84(8), pp. 909-916. Available at: https://www.aafp.org/afp/2011/1015/p909.html

POLIOMYELITIS

Al-Shekhlee, A. & Katirji, B., 2004. Electrodiagnostic features of acute paralytic poliomyelitis associated with West Nile virus infection. Muscle & Nerve, 29(3), pp.376–380. http://dx.doi.org/10.1002/mus.10557.

Dutta, A., 2008. Epidemiology of poliomyelitis—Options and update. Vaccine, 26(45), pp.5767–5773. http://dx.doi.org/10.1016/j.vaccine.2008.07.101.

Gonzalez, H., Olsson, T. and Borg, K., 2010. Management of postpolio syndrome. The Lancet Neurology, 9(6), pp.634-642. https://www.ncbi.nlm.nih.gov/pubmed/20494327

Lin, K.H. and Lim, Y.W., 2005. Post-poliomyelitis syndrome: case report and review of the literature. Ann Acad Med Singapore, 34(7), p.447. https://www.ncbi.nlm.nih.gov/pubmed/16123820

POLYARTERITIS NODOSA

De Virgilio, A. et al., 2016. Polyarteritis nodosa: A contemporary overview. Autoimmunity Reviews, 15(6), pp.564–570. http://dx.doi.org/10.1016/j.autrev.2016.02.015.

Dillon, M.J., Eleftheriou, D. & Brogan, P.A., 2009. Medium-size-vessel vasculitis. Pediatric Nephrology, 25(9), pp.1641–1652. http://dx.doi.org/10.1007/s00467-009-1336-1.

Koster, M.J. & Warrington, K.J., 2016. Recent advances in understanding and treating vasculitis. F1000Research, 5, p.1436. http://dx.doi.org/10.12688/f1000research.8403.1.

POLYMYALGIA RHEUMATICA

Buttgereit, F. et al., 2016. Polymyalgia Rheumatica and Giant Cell Arteritis. JAMA, 315(22), p.2442. http://dx.doi.org/10.1001/jama.2016.5444.

Schmidt, J. & Warrington, K.J., 2011. Polymyalgia Rheumatica and Giant Cell Arteritis in Older Patients. Drugs & Aging, 28(8), pp.651–666. http://dx.doi.org/10.2165/11592500-000000000-00000.

PORPHYRIA

Albers, J.W. & Fink, J.K., 2004. Porphyric neuropathy. Muscle & Nerve, 30(4), pp.410–422. http://dx.doi.org/10.1002/mus.20137.

Besur, S. et al., 2014. Clinically Important Features of Porphyrin and Heme Metabolism and the Porphyrias. Metabolites, 4(4), pp.977–1006. http://dx.doi.org/10.3390/metabo4040977.

Besur, S., Schmeltzer, P. & Bonkovsky, H.L., 2015. Acute Porphyrias. The Journal of Emergency Medicine, 49(3), pp.305–312. http://dx.doi.org/10.1016/j.jemermed.2015.04.034.

Pischik, E. & Kauppinen, R., 2015. An update of clinical management of acute intermittent porphyria. The Application of Clinical Genetics, p.201. http://dx.doi.org/10.2147/tacg.s48605.

PORPHYRIA: ACUTE INTERMITTENT

Akagi, R. et al., 2006. Dual gene defects involving delta-aminolaevulinate dehydratase and coproporphyrinogen oxidase in a porphyria patient. British Journal of Haematology, 132(2), pp.237–243. http://dx.doi.org/10.1111/j.1365-2141.2005.05852.x.

Chretien, S. et al., 1988. Alternative transcription and splicing of the human porphobilinogen deaminase gene result either in tissue-specific or in housekeeping expression. Proceedings of the National Academy of Sciences, 85(1), pp.6–10. http://dx.doi.org/10.1073/pnas.85.1.6.

Doss, M.O. et al., 2004. The third case of Doss porphyria (-amino-levulinic acid dehydratase deficiency) in Germany. Journal of Inherited Metabolic Disease, 27(4), pp.529–536. http://dx.doi.org/10.1023/b:boli.0000037341.21975.9d.

Jaffe, E.K. & Stith, L., 2007. ALAD Porphyria Is a Conformational Disease. The American Journal of Human Genetics, 80(2), pp.329–337. http://dx.doi.org/10.1086/511444.

Kuo, H.-C. et al., 2015. Porphyric neuropathies in an acute intermittent porphyria family. Neuropathology, 36(3), pp.290–294. http://dx.doi.org/10.1111/neup.12272.

Mullin, S. et al., 2012. Cerebral vasospasm and anterior circulation stroke secondary to an exacerbation of hereditary corprop orphyria. Practical Neurology, 12(6), pp.384–387. http://dx.doi.org/10.1136/practneurol-2012-000288.

Schmitt, C., 2005. Mutations in human CPO gene predict clinical expression of either hepatic hereditary coproporphyria or erythropoietic harderoporphyria. Human Molecular Genetics, 14(20), pp.3089–3098. http://dx.doi.org/10.1093/hmg/ddi342.

Valle, G. et al., 2016. Cerebral Hypoperfusion in Hereditary Coproporphyria (HCP): A Single Photon Emission Computed Tomography (SPECT) Study. Endocrine, Metabolic & Immune Disorders-Drug Targets, 16(1), pp.39–46. http://dx.doi.org/10.2174/1871530316666151218151101.

Wu, C.-L. et al., 2015. Clinical presentation and electrophysiological findings of porphyric neuropathies: A follow-up study. Muscle & Nerve, 51(3), pp.363–369. http://dx.doi.org/10.1002/mus.24327.

POSTERIOR FEMORAL CUTANEOUS NERVES

Ploteau, S. et al., 2017. Entrapment of the posterior femoral cutaneous nerve and its inferior cluneal branches: anatomical basis of surgery for inferior cluneal neuralgia. Surgical and Radiologic Anatomy, 39(8), pp.859–863. Available at: http://dx.doi.org/10.1007/s00276-017-1825-z.

Joshi, D.H. et al., 2017. MRI-guided cryoablation of the posterior femoral cutaneous nerve for the treatment of neuropathy-mediated sitting pain. Skeletal Radiology, 46(7), pp.983–987. Available at: http://dx.doi.org/10.1007/s00256-017-2617-6.

PORPHYRIA: VARIEGATE

Brenner, D.A. & Bloomer, J.R., 1980. The Enzymatic Defect in Variegate Porphyria. New England Journal of Medicine, 302(14), pp.765–769. http://dx.doi.org/10.1056/nejm198004033021401.

Fromke, Vincent L. et al., 1978. Porphyria variegata. Study of a large kindred in the United States. The American Journal of Medicine, 65(1), p.A75. http://dx.doi.org/10.1016/0002-9343(78)90696-4

Mustajoki, P., 1980 Variegate porphyria: Twelve years' experience in Finland. Quart. J. Med., 49, pp.191-203. https://www.ncbi.nlm.nih.gov/pubmed/7433635.

POSTERIOR LONGITUDINAL LIGAMENT

Lim, J.J. et al., 2016. Association of miR-146a, miR-149, miR-196a2, and miR-499 Polymorphisms with Ossification of the Posterior Longitudinal Ligament of the Cervical Spine S. Gronthos, ed. PLOS ONE, 11(7), p.e0159756. http://dx.doi.org/10.1371/journal.pone.0159756.

Nakajima, M. et al., 2016. Identification and Functional Characterization of RSPO2 as a Susceptibility Gene for Ossification of the Posterior Longitudinal Ligament of the Spine. The American Journal of Human Genetics, 99(1), pp.202–207. http://dx.doi.org/10.1016/j.ajhg.2016.05.018.

POST-HERNIORRHAPHY PAIN

Amid, P.K., 2004. Radiologic Images of Meshoma. Archives of Surgery, 139(12), p.1297. http://dx.doi.org/10.1001/archsurg.139.12.1297.

Chen, D. et al., 2014. Pain control following inguinal herniorrhaphy: current perspectives. Journal of Pain Research, p.277. http://dx.doi.org/10.2147/jpr.s47005.

Klein, F. et al., 2012. Formation of a Chronic Pain Syndrome Due to Mesh Shrinkage After Laparoscopic Intraperitoneal Onlay Mesh (IPOM). Surgical Laparoscopy, Endoscopy & Percutaneous Techniques, 22(5), pp.e288–e290. http://dx.doi.

org/10.1097/sle.0b013e31825efc3c.

Liem, L. & Mekhail, N., 2016. Management of Postherniorrhaphy Chronic Neuropathic Groin Pain: A Role for Dorsal Root Ganglion Stimulation. Pain Practice, 16(7), pp.915–923. http://dx.doi.org/10.1111/papr.12424.

Narita, M. et al., 2015. Successful treatment for patients with chronic orchialgia following inguinal hernia repair by means of meshoma removal, orchiectomy and triple-neurectomy. International Journal of Surgery Case Reports, 16, pp.157–161. http://dx.doi.org/10.1016/j.ijscr.2015.09.044.

POST-MASTECTOMY PAIN

Alves Nogueira Fabro, E. et al., 2012. Post-mastectomy pain syndrome: Incidence and risks. The Breast, 21(3), pp.321–325. http://dx.doi.org/10.1016/j.breast.2012.01.019.

Macdonald, L. et al., 2005. Long-term follow-up of breast cancer survivors with post-mastectomy pain syndrome. British Journal of Cancer. http://dx.doi.org/10.1038/sj.bjc.6602304.

POST-STROKE PAIN

Henry, J.L., Lalloo, C. & Yashpal, K., 2008. Central Poststroke Pain: An Abstruse Outcome. Pain Research and Management, 13(1), pp.41–49. http://dx.doi.org/10.1155/2008/754260.

Morishita, T. & Inoue, T., 2016. Brain Stimulation Therapy for Central Post-Stroke Pain from a Perspective of Interhemispheric Neural Network Remodeling. Frontiers in Human Neuroscience, 10. http://dx.doi.org/10.3389/fnhum.2016.00166.

POST-THORACOTOMY PAIN SYNDROME

Karmakar, Manoj K et al., 2004. Postthoracotomy pain syndrome. Thoracotomy Surg Clin 14(3):345-352. http://dx.doi.org/10.1016/S1547-4127(04)00022-2

Madabushi R, Tewari S, Gautam SK1, Agarwal A, Agarwal A., 2015. Serratus anterior plane block: a new analgesic technique for post-thoracotomy pain. Pain physician, 18(3), pp.E421-E424. https://www.ncbi.nlm.nih.gov/pubmed/26000690

Scarfe, A.J. et al., 2016. Continuous paravertebral block for post-cardiothoracic surgery analgesia: a systematic review and meta-analysis. European Journal of Cardio-Thoracic Surgery, 50(6), pp.1010–1018. http://dx.doi.org/10.1093/ejcts/ezw168.

POTASSIUM CHANNELS

Bhattacharjee, A. & Kaczmarek, L., 2005. For K+ channels, Na+ is the new Ca

2+. Trends in Neurosciences, 28(8), pp.422–428. http://dx.doi.org/10.1016/j.tins.2005.06.003.

Cao, X.-H. et al., 2010. Reduction in voltage-gated K+ channel activity in primary sensory neurons in painful diabetic neuropathy: role of brain-derived neurotrophic factor. Journal of Neurochemistry, p.1460–1475. http://dx.doi.org/10.1111/j.1471-4159.2010.06863.x.

Hao, J. et al., 2013. Kv1.1 Channels Act as Mechanical Brake in the Senses of Touch and Pain. Neuron, 77(5), pp.899–914. http://dx.doi.org/10.1016/j.neuron.2012.12.035.

Kang, D., 2006. TREK-2 (K2P10.1) and TRESK (K2P18.1) are major background K+ channels in dorsal root ganglion neurons. AJP: Cell Physiology, 291(1), pp.C138–C146. http://dx.doi.org/10.1152/ajpcell.00629.2005.

Maljevic, S. & Lerche, H., 2012. Potassium channels: a review of broadening therapeutic possibilities for neurological diseases. Journal of Neurology, 260(9), pp.2201–2211. http://dx.doi.org/10.1007/s00415-012-6727-8.

Nockemann, D. et al., 2013. The K + channel GIRK2 is both necessary and sufficient for peripheral opioid-mediated analgesia . EMBO Mol Med, 5(8), pp.1263–1277. http://dx.doi.org/10.1002/emmm.201201980.

Rasband, M.N. et al., 2001. Distinct potassium channels on pain-sensing neurons. Proceedings of the National Academy of Sciences, 98(23), pp.13373–13378. http://dx.doi.org/10.1073/pnas.231376298.

Tsantoulas, C. et al., 2012. Sensory Neuron Downregulation of the Kv9.1 Potassium Channel Subunit Mediates Neuropathic Pain following Nerve Injury. Journal of Neuroscience, 32(48), pp.17502–17513. http://dx.doi.org/10.1523/jneurosci.3561-12.2012.

Tulleuda, A. et al., 2011. TRESK channel contribution to nociceptive sensory neurons excitability: modulation by nerve injury. Mol Pain, 7(1), p.30. http://dx.doi.org/10.1186/1744-8069-7-30.

Zheng, Q. et al., 2013. Suppression of KCNQ/M (Kv7) potassium channels in dorsal root ganglion neurons contributes to the development of bone cancer pain in a rat model. Pain, 154(3), pp.434–448. http://dx.doi.org/10.1016/j.pain.2012.12.005.

PRECORDIAL CATCH SYNDROME

Hayes, D. et al., 2016. Precordial Catch Syndrome in Elite Swimmers With Asthma. Pediatric Emergency Care, 32(2), pp.104–106. http://dx.doi.org/10.1097/pec.0000000000000715.

Pickering, D., 1981. Precordial catch syndrome. Archives of Disease in Childhood, 56(5), pp.401–403. http://dx.doi.org/10.1136/adc.56.5.401.

PROXIMAL EXTREME PAIN DISORDER

Emery, E.C. et al., 2015. Novel SCN9A Mutations Underlying Extreme Pain Phenotypes: Unexpected Electrophysiological and Clinical Phenotype Correlations. Journal of Neuroscience, 35(20), pp.7674–7681. http://dx.doi.org/10.1523/jneurosci.3935-14.2015.

Kim, D.T. et al., 2015. Bilateral congenital corneal anesthesia in a patient with SCN9A mutation, confirmed primary erythromelalgia, and paroxysmal extreme pain disorder. Journal of American Association for Pediatric Ophthalmology and Strabismus, 19(5), pp.478–479. http://dx.doi.org/10.1016/j.jaapos.2015.05.015.

Suter, M.R., 2015. What are the treatment options for paroxysmal extreme pain disorder? Pain Management, 5(4), pp.229–232. http://dx.doi.org/10.2217/pmt.15.24.

PSEUDOTUMOR CEREBRI

Bateman, G.A., 2006. Association between arterial inflow and venous outflow in idiopathic and secondary intracranial hypertension. Journal of Clinical Neuroscience, 13(5), pp.550-556. http://fulltext.study/download/3063490.pdf

Ibrahim, Y.A. et al., 2014. Idiopathic Intracranial Hypertension: Diagnostic Accuracy of the Transverse Dural Venous Sinus Attenuation on CT Scans. The Neuroradiology Journal, 27, p.0. http://dx.doi.org/10.15274/nrj-2014-10086.

Julayanont, P. et al., 2016. Idiopathic intracranial hypertension: ongoing clinical challenges and future prospects. Journal of Pain Research, p.87. https://www.ncbi.nlm.nih.gov/pmc/articles/PMC4767055/

PSYCHOSOCIAL INFLUENCES ON PAIN

Edwards, R.R. et al., 2016. The Role of Psychosocial Processes in the Development and Maintenance of Chronic Pain. The Journal of Pain, 17(9), pp.T70–T92. Available at: http://dx.doi.org/10.1016/j.jpain.2016.01.001.

Main, C.J., 2013. The importance of psychosocial influences on chronic pain. Pain Management, 3(6), pp.455–466. Available at: http://dx.doi.org/10.2217/pmt.13.49.

Turk, D.C., Fillingim, R.B., Ohrbach, R. and Patel, K.V., 2016. Assessment of psychosocial and functional impact of chronic pain. The Journal of Pain, 17(9), pp.T21-T49. https://www.ncbi.nlm.nih.gov/pubmed/27586830

PUDENDAL NERVE

Amarenco G, Denys P, Kerdraon J. [Neuropathy due to stretching of the internal pudendal nerve and female urinary incontinence]. J Urol (Paris). 1992;98(4):196-8. Review. French. http://europepmc.org/abstract/MED/1297664

Chhabra, A. et al., 2016. 3T magnetic resonance neurography of pudendal nerve with cadaveric dissection correlation. World Journal of Radiology, 8(7), p.700. http://dx.doi.org/10.4329/wjr.v8.i7.700.

Elkins, N., Hunt, J. & Scott, K.M., 2017. Neurogenic Pelvic Pain. Physical Medicine and Rehabilitation Clinics of North America, 28(3), pp.551–569. Available at: http://dx.doi.org/10.1016/j.pmr.2017.03.007.

Labat, J.-J. et al., 2008. Diagnostic criteria for pudendal neuralgia by pudendal nerve entrapment (Nantes criteria). Neurourology and Urodynamics, 27(4), pp.306–310. Available at: http://dx.doi.org/10.1002/nau.20505.

Ploteau, S. et al., 2017. Anatomical Variants of the Pudendal Nerve Observed during a Transgluteal Surgical Approach in a Population of Patients with Pudendal Neuralgia. Pain Physician, 20(1), pp. E137-E143 http://europepmc.org/abstract/med/28072805

Robert R, Labat JJ, Riant T, Louppe JM, Hamel O. [The pudendal nerve: clinical and therapeutic morphogenesis, anatomy, and physiopathology]. Neurochirurgie. 2009 Oct;55(4-5):463-9. Review. French. https://www.ncbi.nlm.nih.gov/pubmed/19748642

Robert, R. et al., 1998. Anatomic basis of chronic perineal pain: role of the pudendal nerve. Surgical and Radiologic Anatomy, 20(2), pp.93–98. http://dx.doi.org/10.1007/s00276-998-0093-3.

Shafik, A. et al., 1995. Surgical anatomy of the pudendal nerve and its clinical implications. Clinical Anatomy, 8(2), pp.110–115. http://dx.doi.org/10.1002/ca.980080205.

Wadhwa, V. et al., 2016. Pudendal nerve and branch neuropathy: magnetic resonance neurography evaluation. Acta Radiologica, 58(6), pp.726–733. Available at: http://dx.doi.org/10.1177/0284185116668213.

PYELONEPHRITIS

Abrahamian, F.M., Moran, G.J. & Talan, D.A., 2008. Urinary Tract Infections in the Emergency Department. Infectious Disease Clinics of North America, 22(1), pp.73–87. http://dx.doi.org/10.1016/j.idc.2007.10.002.

Czaja, C.A. et al., 2007. Population-Based Epidemiologic Analysis of Acute Pyelonephritis. Clinical Infectious Diseases, 45(3), pp.273–280. http://dx.doi.org/10.1086/519268.

Kofteridis, D.P. et al., 2009. Effect of Diabetes Mellitus on the Clinical and Microbiological Features of Hospitalized Elderly Patients with Acute Pyelonephritis. Journal of the American Geriatrics Society, 57(11), pp.2125–2128. http://dx.doi.org/10.1111/j.1532-5415.2009.02550.x.

Martina, M.C. et al., 2009. Dynamic magnetic resonance imaging in acute pyelonephritis. La radiologia medica, 115(2), pp.287–300. http://dx.doi.org/10.1007/s11547-009-0468-5.

RADIAL NERVE

MORAES, M.A.D. et al., 2017. DIAGNOSIS AND TREATMENT OF POSTERIOR INTEROSSEOUS NERVE ENTRAPMENT: SYSTEMATIC REVIEW. Acta Ortopédica Brasileira, 25(1), pp.52–54. Available at: http://dx.doi.org/10.1590/1413-785220172501164801.

Spies, CK. Et al., 2016. Surgical decompression of the superficial radial nerve: Wartenberg syndrome]. Oper Orthop Traumatol. 28(2):145-52. doi: 10.1007/s00064-015-0431-7.Abstract in English available at: https://www.ncbi.nlm.nih.gov/pubmed/26497308. Article available in German at: https://link.springer.com/article/10.1007%2Fs00064-015-0431-7

Berton, C. et al., 2012. The supinator muscle: anatomical bases for deep branch of the radial nerve entrapment. Surgical and Radiologic Anatomy, 35(3), pp.217–224. Available at: http://dx.doi.org/10.1007/s00276-012-1024-x.

P. Clavert, J.C. Lutz, P. Adam, R. Wolfram-Gabel, P. Liverneaux, J.L. Kahn. Frohse's arcade is not the exclusive compression site of the radial nerve in its tunnel. Orthopaedics & Traumatology: Surgery & Research, 95(2), pp 114-118. Available at: https://doi.org/10.1016/j.otsr.2008.11.001

Vergara-Amador, E. & Ramírez, A., 2015. Anatomic study of the extensor carpi radialis brevis in its relation with the motor branch of the radial nerve. Orthopaedics & Traumatology: Surgery & Research, 101(8), pp.909–912. Available at: http://dx.doi.org/10.1016/j.otsr.2015.09.030.

Muthulingam, M., 2016. Unusual Presentation of Radial Nerve Entrapment with Lateral Humeral Condyle Fracture – A Case Report. JOURNAL OF CLINICAL AND DIAGNOSTIC RESEARCH. Available at: http://dx.doi.org/10.7860/jcdr/2016/21923.8717.

Nachef, N. et al., 2017. Predictors of radial nerve palsy recovery in humeral shaft fractures: A retrospective review of 17 patients. Orthopaedics & Traumatology:

Surgery & Research, 103(2), pp.177–182. Available at: http://dx.doi.org/10.1016/j.otsr.2016.10.023.

Saaiq, M &* and Siddiui, S., 2017. Posterior Interosseous Nerve Syndrome Resulting from Parosteal Lipoma of the Proximal Radius: An Elusive Diagnosis Yet Excellent Outcome. World J Plast Surg, 6(1), pp 100–105. Available at: https://www.ncbi.nlm.nih.gov/pmc/articles/PMC5339617/

REACTIVE OXYGEN SPECIES (ROS)

Bittar, A., Jun, J., La, J.H., Wang, J., Leem, J.W. and Chung, J.M., 2017. Reactive oxygen species affect spinal cell type-specific synaptic plasticity in a model of neuropathic pain. Pain, 158(11), pp.2137-2146. https://www.ncbi.nlm.nih.gov/pubmed/28708760

Beckhauser, T.F., Francis-Oliveira, J. and De Pasquale, R., 2016. Reactive oxygen species: physiological and physiopathological effects on synaptic plasticity. Journal of experimental neuroscience, 10(Suppl 1), p.23. https://www.ncbi.nlm.nih.gov/pubmed/27625575

Fidanboylu, M., Griffiths, L.A. and Flatters, S.J., 2011. Global inhibition of reactive oxygen species (ROS) inhibits paclitaxel-induced painful peripheral neuropathy. PloS one, 6(9), p.e25212. https://www.ncbi.nlm.nih.gov/pubmed/21966458

Gwak, Y.S., Hassler, S.E. and Hulsebosch, C.E., 2013. Reactive oxygen species contribute to neuropathic pain and locomotor dysfunction via activation of CamKII in remote segments following spinal cord contusion injury in rats. PAIN®, 154(9), pp.1699-1708. https://www.ncbi.nlm.nih.gov/pubmed/23707296

Kallenborn-Gerhardt, W., Schröder, K., Del Turco, D., Lu, R., Kynast, K., Kosowski, J., Niederberger, E., Shah, A.M., Brandes, R.P., Geisslinger, G. and Schmidtko, A., 2012. NADPH oxidase-4 maintains neuropathic pain after peripheral nerve injury. Journal of Neuroscience, 32(30), pp.10136-10145. https://www.ncbi.nlm.nih.gov/pubmed/22836249

Kim, H.Y., Chung, J.M. and Chung, K., 2008. Increased production of mitochondrial superoxide in the spinal cord induces pain behaviors in mice: the effect of mitochondrial electron transport complex inhibitors. Neuroscience letters, 447(1), pp.87-91. https://www.ncbi.nlm.nih.gov/pubmed/18832013

Latremoliere, A. and Woolf, C.J., 2009. Central sensitization: a generator of pain hypersensitivity by central neural plasticity. The Journal of Pain, 10(9), pp.895-926. https://www.ncbi.nlm.nih.gov/pubmed/19712899

Lee, K.Y., Chung, K. and Chung, J.M., 2010. Involvement of reactive oxygen species in long-term potentiation in the spinal cord dorsal horn. Journal of neurophysiology, 103(1), pp.382-391. https://www.ncbi.nlm.nih.gov/pubmed/19906875

Takahashi, A., Mikami, M. and Yang, J., 2007. Hydrogen peroxide increases GABAergic mIPSC through presynaptic release of calcium from IP3 receptor-sensitive stores in spinal cord substantia gelatinosa neurons. European Journal of Neuroscience, 25(3), pp.705-716. https://www.ncbi.nlm.nih.gov/pubmed/17328771

Vander Heide, R.S., Sobotka, P.A. and Ganote, C.E., 1987. Effects of the free radical scavenger DMTU and mannitol on the oxygen paradox in perfused rat hearts. Journal of molecular and cellular cardiology, 19(6), pp.615-625. https://www.ncbi.nlm.nih.gov/pubmed/3114497

Yowtak, J., Lee, K.Y., Kim, H.Y., Wang, J., Kim, H.K., Chung, K. and Chung, J.M., 2011. Reactive oxygen species contribute to neuropathic pain by reducing spinal GABA release. Pain®, 152(4), pp.844-852. https://www.ncbi.nlm.nih.gov/pubmed/21296500

Yowtak, J., Wang, J., Kim, H.Y., Lu, Y., Chung, K. and Chung, J.M., 2013. Effect of antioxidant treatment on spinal GABA neurons in a neuropathic pain model in the mouse. PAIN®, 154(11), pp.2469-2476. https://www.ncbi.nlm.nih.gov/pubmed/23880056

REFERRED PAIN (OVERVIEW)

Luz, L.L. et al., 2015. Monosynaptic convergence of somatic and visceral C-fiber afferents on projection and local circuit neurons in lamina I. PAIN, 156(10), pp.2042–2051. http://dx.doi.org/10.1097/j.pain.0000000000000267.

RENAL COLIC

Eltawansy, S.A. et al., 2014. Acute Renal Infarction Presenting with Acute Abdominal Pain Secondary to Newly Discovered Atrial Fibrillation: A Case Report and Literature Review. Case Reports in Emergency Medicine, 2014, pp.1–5. http://dx.doi.org/10.1155/2014/981409.

Huang, C.-C. et al., 2007. ED presentations of acute renal infarction. The American Journal of Emergency Medicine, 25(2), pp.164–169. http://dx.doi.org/10.1016/j.ajem.2006.06.010.

Jha, P. et al., 2016. Imaging of flank pain: readdressing state-of-the-art. Emergency Radiology. http://dx.doi.org/10.1007/s10140-016-1443-9.

Kalb, B. et al., 2010. Acute abdominal pain: Is there a potential role for MRI in the setting of the emergency department in a patient with renal calculi? Journal of Magnetic Resonance Imaging, 32(5), pp.1012–1023. http://dx.doi.org/10.1002/jmri.22337.

Raghavendran, M., Sarkar, M. & Kumar, K.G., 2016. "Isolated Spontaneous Renal

Artery Thrombosis – A Rare Cause of Acute Flank Pain." Urology Case Reports, 9, pp.4–5. http://dx.doi.org/10.1016/j.eucr.2016.07.013.

Schulz, G.B., Beck, V., Apfelbeck, M., Grabbert, M., Tritschler, S. and Stief, C.G., 2016. Management of acute renal colic in the ambulatory care setting. MMW Fortschritte der Medizin, 158(17), p.43. http://link.springer.com/article/10.1007%2Fs15006-016-8776-x

Semins, M.J. et al., 2012. Evaluation of acute renal colic: a comparison of non-contrast CT versus 3-T non-contrast HASTE MR urography. Urolithiasis, 41(1), pp.43–46. http://dx.doi.org/10.1007/s00240-012-0525-8.

RETROPERITONEAL TUMORS

Burkill, G.J.C. & Healy, J.C., 2000. Anatomy of the retroperitoneum. Imaging, 12(1), pp.10–20. http://dx.doi.org/10.1259/img.12.1.120010.

Osman, S. et al., 2013. A Comprehensive Review of the Retroperitoneal Anatomy, Neoplasms, and Pattern of Disease Spread. Current Problems in Diagnostic Radiology, 42(5), pp.191–208. http://dx.doi.org/10.1067/j.cpradiol.2013.02.001.

Wee-Stekly, W.-W. & Mueller, M.D., 2014. Retroperitoneal Tumors in the Pelvis: A Diagnostic Challenge in Gynecology. Frontiers in Surgery, 1. http://dx.doi.org/10.3389/fsurg.2014.00049.

RETROPHARYNGEAL TENDINITIS

Artenian, D.J. et al., 1989. Acute neck pain due to tendonitis of the longus colli: CT and MRI findings. Neuroradiology, 31(2), pp.166–169. http://dx.doi.org/10.1007/bf00698847.

Harnier, S., Kuhn, J., Harzheim, A., Bewermeyer, H. and Limmroth, V., 2008. Retropharyngeal tendinitis: a rare differential diagnosis of severe headaches and neck pain. Headache: The Journal of Head and Face Pain, 48(1), pp.158-161. https://www.researchgate.net/publication/5973037_Retropharyngeal_Tendinitis_A_Rare_Differential_Diagnosis_of_Severe_Headaches_and_Neck_Pain

Urrutia, J. & Contreras, O., 2016. Calcium hydroxyapatite crystal deposition with intraosseous penetration involving the posterior aspect of the cervical spine: a previously unreported cause of neck pain. European Spine Journal. http://dx.doi.org/10.1007/s00586-016-4731-x.

Zibis, A.H. et al., 2012. Acute calcific tendinitis of the longus colli muscle:case report and review of the literature. European Spine Journal, 22(S3), pp.434–438. http://dx.doi.org/10.1007/s00586-012-2584-5.

REWARD, MOTIVATION, EMOTION AND PAIN

Beecher, H.K., 1951. EARLY CARE OF THE SERIOUSLY WOUNDED MAN. Journal of the American Medical Association, 145(4), p.193. Available at: http://dx.doi.org/10.1001/jama.1951.02920220001001.

Craig, A., 2003. A new view of pain as a homeostatic emotion. Trends in Neurosciences, 26(6), pp.303–307. Available at: http://dx.doi.org/10.1016/s0166-2236(03)00123-1.

Fields, H.L., 1999. Pain: An unpleasant topic. Pain, 82, pp.S61–S69. Available at: http://dx.doi.org/10.1016/s0304-3959(99)00139-6.

Fields, HL. 2006. A motivation-decision model of pain: The role of opioids. Proceedings of the 11th World Congress on Pain. pp449-459. Available at: http://www.worldcat.org/title/proceedings-of-the-11th-world-congress-on-pain/oclc/761210379/editions?referer=di&editionsView=true#%2528x0%253Abook%2Bx4%253Adigital%2529format

Baliki, M.N. et al., 2010. Predicting Value of Pain and Analgesia: Nucleus Accumbens Response to Noxious Stimuli Changes in the Presence of Chronic Pain. Neuron, 66(1), pp.149–160. Available at: http://dx.doi.org/10.1016/j.neuron.2010.03.002.

Apkarian, A.V., 2011. The brain in chronic pain: clinical implications. Pain Management, 1(6), pp.577–586. Available at: http://dx.doi.org/10.2217/pmt.11.53.

Peciña, S., Smith, K.S. & Berridge, K.C., 2006. Hedonic Hot Spots in the Brain. The Neuroscientist, 12(6), pp.500–511. Available at: http://dx.doi.org/10.1177/1073858406293154.

Berridge, K.C., 2004. Motivation concepts in behavioral neuroscience. Physiology & Behavior, 81(2), pp.179–209. Available at: http://dx.doi.org/10.1016/j.physbeh.2004.02.004.

Bingel, U. et al., 2011. The Effect of Treatment Expectation on Drug Efficacy: Imaging the Analgesic Benefit of the Opioid Remifentanil. Science Translational Medicine, 3(70), pp.70ra14–70ra14. Available at: http://dx.doi.org/10.1126/scitranslmed.3001244.

Elvemo, N.A. et al., 2015. Reward responsiveness in patients with chronic pain. European Journal of Pain, 19(10), pp.1537–1543. Available at: http://dx.doi.org/10.1002/ejp.687.

Navratilova, E. & Porreca, F., 2014. Reward and motivation in pain and pain relief. Nature Neuroscience, 17(10), pp.1304–1312. Available at: http://dx.doi.org/10.1038/nn.3811.

Okun, A. et al., 2016. Hedonic and motivational responses to food reward are unchanged in rats with neuropathic pain. PAIN, 157(12), pp.2731–2738. Available at: http://dx.doi.org/10.1097/j.pain.0000000000000695.

RIB FRACTURE

Battle, C.E., Hutchings, H. & Evans, P.A., 2012. Risk factors that predict mortality in patients with blunt chest wall trauma: A systematic review and meta-analysis. Injury, 43(1), pp.8–17. http://dx.doi.org/10.1016/j.injury.2011.01.004.

Harris, S.R., 2016. Differentiating the Causes of Spontaneous Rib Fracture After Breast Cancer. Clinical Breast Cancer, 16(6), pp.431–436. http://dx.doi.org/10.1016/j.clbc.2016.07.001.

RIGHT COLON ISCHEMIA

Blumberg, S.N. & Maldonado, T.S., 2016. Mesenteric venous thrombosis. Journal of Vascular Surgery: Venous and Lymphatic Disorders, 4(4), pp.501–507. http://dx.doi.org/10.1016/j.jvsv.2016.04.002.

Brandt, L.J. et al., 2014. ACG Clinical Guideline: Epidemiology, Risk Factors, Patterns of Presentation, Diagnosis, and Management of Colon Ischemia (CI). The American Journal of Gastroenterology, 110(1), pp.18–44. http://dx.doi.org/10.1038/ajg.2014.395.

Dane, B., Clark, J. & Megibow, A., 2016. Multidetector Computed Tomography Evaluation of Mesenteric Venous Thrombosis Following Laparoscopic Bariatric Surgery. Journal of Computer Assisted Tomography, p.1. http://dx.doi.org/10.1097/rct.0000000000000473.

Hmoud, B., Singal, A.K. & Kamath, P.S., 2014. Mesenteric Venous Thrombosis. Journal of Clinical and Experimental Hepatology, 4(3), pp.257–263. http://dx.doi.org/10.1016/j.jceh.2014.03.052.

Longstreth, G.F, et al., 2015. Right-Side Colon Ischemia: Clinical Features, Large Visceral Artery Occlusion, and Long-Term Follow-Up. The Permanente Journal, 19 (4)1-16, http://dx.doi.org/10.7812/tpp/15-024.

Olson, M.M., Ilada, P.B. & Apelgren, K.N., 2003. Portal vein thrombosis. Surgical Endoscopy, 17(8), pp.1322–1322. http://dx.doi.org/10.1007/s00464-002-4546-1.

Sotiriadis, J. et al., 2007. Ischemic Colitis Has a Worse Prognosis When Isolated to the Right Side of the Colon. The American Journal of Gastroenterology, 102(10), pp.2247–2252. http://dx.doi.org/10.1111/j.1572-0241.2007.01341.x.

SCIATIC NERVE

Baumer, P. et al., 2015. Somatotopic fascicular organization of the human sciatic nerve demonstrated by MR neurography. Neurology, 84(17), pp.1782–1787. Available at: http://dx.doi.org/10.1212/wnl.0000000000001526.

Perez Carro, L., 2016. Deep gluteal space problems: piriformis syndrome, ischiofemoral impingement and sciatic nerve release. Muscles, Ligaments and Tendons Journal. Available at: http://dx.doi.org/10.11138/mltj/2016.6.3.384.

Wolf, M. et al., 2014. Sciatic Nerve Injury Related to Hip Replacement Surgery: Imaging Detection by MR Neurography Despite Susceptibility Artifacts N. Weidner, ed. PLoS ONE, 9(2), p.e89154. Available at: http://dx.doi.org/10.1371/journal.pone.0089154.

LI, Q. et al., 2016. Chronic sciatic nerve compression induces fibrosis in dorsal root ganglia. Molecular Medicine Reports, 13(3), pp.2393–2400. Available at: http://dx.doi.org/10.3892/mmr.2016.4810.

Martin, H.D. et al., 2016. Ischiofemoral Impingement and Hamstring Syndrome as Causes of Posterior Hip Pain. Clinics in Sports Medicine, 35(3), pp.469–486. Available at: http://dx.doi.org/10.1016/j.csm.2016.02.010.

Kuncewicz, e., et al., 2006. Piriformis Muscle Syndrome. Ann Acad Med Stetin., 52(3), pp. 99-101. Abstract available at: https://www.ncbi.nlm.nih.gov/pubmed/17385355

SCN9A MUTATIONS

Emery, E.C. et al., 2015. Novel SCN9A Mutations Underlying Extreme Pain Phenotypes: Unexpected Electrophysiological and Clinical Phenotype Correlations. Journal of Neuroscience, 35(20), pp.7674–7681. http://dx.doi.org/10.1523/jneurosci.3935-14.2015.

Goldberg, Y. et al., 2012. Human Mendelian pain disorders: a key to discovery and validation of novel analgesics. Clinical Genetics, 82(4), pp.367–373. http://dx.doi.org/10.1111/j.1399-0004.2012.01942.x.

Kim, D.T. et al., 2015. Bilateral congenital corneal anesthesia in a patient with SCN9A mutation, confirmed primary erythromelalgia, and paroxysmal extreme pain disorder. Journal of American Association for Pediatric Ophthalmology and Strabismus, 19(5), pp.478–479. http://dx.doi.org/10.1016/j.jaapos.2015.05.015.

Klein, C.J. et al., 2012. Infrequent SCN9A mutations in congenital insensitivity to pain and erythromelalgia. Journal of Neurology, Neurosurgery & Psychiatry, 84(4), pp.386–391. http://dx.doi.org/10.1136/jnnp-2012-303719.

SCOLIOSIS

Albanese, S.A., 2002. "Idiopathic scoliosis: etiology and evaluation", in P. Sponseller, Orthopedic Knowledge Update: Pediatrics 2, American Academy of Orthopaedic Surgeons, Rosemont, IL, pp.287–296. https://books.google.com/books/about/Orthopaedic_knowledge_update.html?id=t45sAAAAMAAJ

Faraj, S.S. et al., 2016. De novo degenerative lumbar scoliosis: a systematic review of prognostic factors for curve progression. European Spine Journal, 25(8), pp.2347–58. https://dx.doi.org/10.1007/s00586-016-4619-9

Mehta, V.A. et al., 2015. Implications of Spinopelvic Alignment for the Spine Surgeon. Neurosurgery, 76, pp.S42–S56. http://dx.doi.org/10.1227/01.neu.0000462077.50830.1a.

Moreau, A. et al., 2009. [Molecular and genetic aspects of idiopathic scoliosis. Blood test for idiopathic scoliosis]. Der Orthopade, 38(2), pp.114–6, 118–21. https://dx.doi.org/10.1007/s00132-008-1362-x.

Stokes, I.A.F. & Aronsson, D.D., 2001. Disc and Vertebral Wedging in Patients With Progressive Scoliosis. Journal of Spinal Disorders, 14(4), pp.317–322. http://dx.doi.org/10.1097/00002517-200108000-00006.

SEXUAL HEADACHE/WEIGHT LIFTER HEADACHE

Pascual, J. et al., 1996. Cough, exertional, and sexual headaches: An analysis of 72 benign and symptomatic cases. Neurology, 46(6), pp.1520–1524. http://dx.doi.org/10.1212/wnl.46.6.1520.

Powell, B., 1982. Weight Lifter's Cephalgia. Annals of Emergency Medicine, 11(8), pp.449-451. https://doi.org/10.1016/s0196-0644(82)80048-6

Simpson, M., 2016. Weightlifter's Headache. Practical Neurology, 16(3), pp.215-216. https://doi.org/10.1136/practneurol-2015-001227

SEIZURE PAIN

Scholz, J., Vieregge, P. & Moser, A., 1999. Central pain as a manifestation of partial epileptic seizures. Pain, 80(1), pp.445–450. Available at: http://dx.doi.org/10.1016/s0304-3959(98)00217-6.

Fanella, M. et al., 2015. Ictal epileptic headache in adult life: Electroclinical patterns and spectrum of related syndromes. Epilepsy & Behavior, 53, pp.161–165. Available at: http://dx.doi.org/10.1016/j.yebeh.2015.10.018.

Cianchetti, C. et al., 2017. The complex interrelations between two paroxysmal disorders: headache and epilepsy. Neurological Sciences, 38(6), pp.941–948. Available at: http://dx.doi.org/10.1007/s10072-017-2926-5.

Kim, D.W., Sunwoo, J.-S. & Lee, S.K., 2016. Headache as an Aura of Epilepsy: Video-EEG Monitoring Study. Headache: The Journal of Head and Face Pain, 56(4), pp.762–768. Available at: http://dx.doi.org/10.1111/head.12754.

Fanella, M. et al., 2012. Ictal epileptic headache as "subtle" symptom in generalized idiopathic epilepsy. Epilepsia, 53(4), pp.e67–e70. Available at: http://dx.doi.org/10.1111/j.1528-1167.2011.03387.x.

Yu, T, et al., 2017. Focal epilepsy with paroxysmal pain due to somatic injury. Epil Disorders 1;19(2), pp. 207-211. Available at: https://www.ncbi.nlm.nih.gov/pubmed/28652224

Cerminara, C. et al., 2013. Focal epilepsy with ictal abdominal pain: a case report. Italian Journal of Pediatrics, 39(1), p.76. Available at: http://dx.doi.org/10.1186/1824-7288-39-76.

SILENT SINUS SYNDROME

Ferro, A., Basyuni, S. & Santhanam, V., 2016. Not so silent sinus syndrome: A case report. International Journal of Surgery Case Reports, 23, pp.1–3. http://dx.doi.org/10.1016/j.ijscr.2016.04.001.

Martínez-Capoccioni, G., Varela-Martínez, E. & Martín-Martín, C., 2016. Silent sinus syndrome an acquired condition and the essential role of otorhinolaryngologist consultation: a retrospective study. European Archives of Oto-Rhino-Laryngology, 273(10), pp.3183–3188. http://dx.doi.org/10.1007/s00405-016-3965-x.

SINUSITIS

Kim, Y.K. et al., 2016. Extrasinonasal infiltrative process associated with a sinonasal fungus ball: does it mean invasive fungal sinusitis? Diagnostic and Interventional Radiology, 22(4), pp.347–353. http://dx.doi.org/10.5152/dir.2015.15417.

Kim, Y.S. et al., 2012. CT and MR Imaging Findings of Sinonasal Schwannoma: A Review of 12 Cases. American Journal of Neuroradiology, 34(3), pp.628–633. http://dx.doi.org/10.3174/ajnr.a3257.

Mazza, J.M. & Lin, S.Y., 2016. Primary immunodeficiency and recalcitrant chronic sinusitis: a systematic review. International Forum of Allergy & Rhinology, 6(10), pp.1029–1033. http://dx.doi.org/10.1002/alr.21789.

Simuntis, R., Kubilius, R. and Vaitkus, S., 2014. Odontogenic maxillary sinusitis: a review. Stomatologija, 16(2), pp.39-43. http://sbdmj.lsmuni.lt/142/142-01.pdf

Thornton MA, Brown C. Up front about frontal headaches and sinusitis. Irish Medical Journal. 2009 Apr;102(4):120-2. https://www.ncbi.nlm.nih.gov/pubmed/19552295

Troeltzsch, Matthias et al., 2015. Etiology and clinical characteristics of symptomatic unilateral maxillary sinusitis: A review of 174 cases. Journal of Cranio-Maxillofacial Surgery, 43(8), pp.1522–1529. http://dx.doi.org/10.1016/j.jcms.2015.07.021.

SLIPPING RIB SYNDROME

Turcios, N.L., 2016. Slipping Rib Syndrome: An elusive diagnosis. Paediatric Respiratory Reviews. http://dx.doi.org/10.1016/j.prrv.2016.05.003.

Van Delft, E.A.K., van Pul, K.M. & Bloemers, F.W., 2016. The slipping rib syndrome: A case report. International Journal of Surgery Case Reports, 23, pp.23–24. http://dx.doi.org/10.1016/j.ijscr.2016.04.009.

SMALL FIBER NEUROPATHY: GENERAL

Themistocleous, A.C. et al., 2014. The clinical approach to small fibre neuropathy and painful channelopathy. Practical Neurology, 14(6), pp.368–379. http://dx.doi.org/10.1136/practneurol-2013-000758.

SMALL FIBER NEUROPATHY: INFECTIOUS CAUSES

Bennett, J.L. et al., 1996. Epstein-barr virus-associated acute autonomic neuropathy. Annals of Neurology, 40(3), pp.453–455. http://dx.doi.org/10.1002/ana.410400316.

Makonahalli, R., Seneviratne, J. & Seneviratne, U., 2014. Acute Small Fiber Neuropathy Following Mycoplasma Infection. Journal of Clinical Neuromuscular Disease, 15(4), pp.147–151. http://dx.doi.org/10.1097/cnd.0000000000000031.

Nolano, M. et al., 2013. Small fiber neuropathy in the chronic phase of Chagas disease: a case report. Clinical Autonomic Research, 23(3), pp.149–153. http://dx.doi.org/10.1007/s10286-013-0189-7.

Suarez, G.A. et al., 1994. Idiopathic autonomic neuropathy: Clinical, neurophysiologie, and follow-up studies on 27 patients. Neurology, 44(9), pp.1675–1675. http://dx.doi.org/10.1212/wnl.44.9.1675.

Zheng, Z.-M. et al., 1992. Further characterization of the biological and pathogenic properties of erythromelalgia-related poxviruses. Journal of General Virology, 73(8), pp.2011–2019. http://dx.doi.org/10.1099/0022-1317-73-8-2011.

SMALL FIBER PAINFUL NEUROPATHY: GENERAL

Devigili, G. et al., 2008. The diagnostic criteria for small fibre neuropathy: from symptoms to neuropathology. Brain, 131(7), pp.1912–1925. http://dx.doi.org/10.1093/brain/awn093.

Faber, C.G. et al., 2011. Gain of function NaV1.7 mutations in idiopathic small fiber neuropathy. Annals of Neurology, 71(1), pp.26–39. http://dx.doi.org/10.1002/ana.22485.

Lauria, G. et al., 2010. Intraepidermal nerve fiber density at the distal leg: a worldwide normative reference study. Journal of the Peripheral Nervous System, 15(3), pp.202–207. http://dx.doi.org/10.1111/j.1529-8027.2010.00271.x.

Themistocleous, A.C. et al., 2014. The clinical approach to small fibre neuropathy and painful channelopathy. Practical Neurology, 14(6), pp.368–379. http://dx.doi.org/10.1136/practneurol-2013-000758.

Waxman, S.G., 2013. Painful Na-channelopathies: an expanding universe. Trends in Molecular Medicine, 19(7), pp.406–409. http://dx.doi.org/10.1016/j.molmed.2013.04.003.

SMALL NERVE FIBER PATHOLOGY IN CRITICAL ILLNESS

Latronico, N. et al., 2013. Small Nerve Fiber Pathology in Critical Illness S. Barnes, ed. PLoS ONE, 8(9), p.e75696. http://dx.doi.org/10.1371/journal.pone.0075696.

SMALL NERVE FIBERS: SMALL HANDS AND FEET

Hoeijmakers, J.G.J. et al., 2012. Small nerve fibres, small hands and small feet: a new syndrome of pain, dysautonomia and acromesomelia in a kindred with a novel NaV1.7 mutation. Brain, 135(2), pp.345–358. http://dx.doi.org/10.1093/brain/awr349

SMALL-FIBER NEUROPATHY: IDIOPATHIC

Dabby, R. et al., 2007. Evaluation of cutaneous autonomic innervation in idiopathic sensory small-fiber neuropathy. Journal of the Peripheral Nervous System, 12(2), pp.98–101. http://dx.doi.org/10.1111/j.1529-8027.2007.00128.x.

Hovaguimian, A. & Gibbons, C.H., 2011. Diagnosis and Treatment of Pain in Small-fiber Neuropathy. Current Pain and Headache Reports, 15(3), pp.193–200. http://dx.doi.org/10.1007/s11916-011-0181-7.

Tavee, J. & Zhou, L., 2009. Small fiber neuropathy: A burning problem. Cleveland Clinic Journal of Medicine, 76(5), pp.297–305. http://dx.doi.org/10.3949/ccjm.76a.08070.

SODIUM CHANNELS

Black, J.A. et al., 2008. Multiple sodium channel isoforms and mitogen-activated protein kinases are present in painful human neuromas. Annals of Neurology, 64(6), pp.644–653. http://dx.doi.org/10.1002/ana.21527.

Cox, J.J. et al., 2006. An SCN9A channelopathy causes congenital inability to experience pain. Nature, 444(7121), pp.894–898. http://dx.doi.org/10.1038/nature05413.

Cummins, T.R., 2004. Electrophysiological Properties of Mutant Nav1.7 Sodium Channels in a Painful Inherited Neuropathy. Journal of Neuroscience, 24(38), pp.8232–8236. http://dx.doi.org/10.1523/jneurosci.2695-04.2004.

Dib-Hajj, S.D. et al., 2012. The NaV1.7 sodium channel: from molecule to man. Nature Reviews Neuroscience, 14(1), pp.49–62. http://dx.doi.org/10.1038/nrn3404.

Dib-Hajj, S.D., 2005. Gain-of-function mutation in Nav1.7 in familial erythromelalgia induces bursting of sensory neurons. Brain, 128(8), pp.1847–1854. http://dx.doi.org/10.1093/brain/awh514.

Faber, C.G. et al., 2011. Gain of function NaV1.7 mutations in idiopathic small fiber neuropathy. Annals of Neurology, 71(1), pp.26–39. http://dx.doi.org/10.1002/ana.22485.

Faber, C.G. et al., 2012. Gain-of-function Nav1.8 mutations in painful neuropathy. Proceedings of the National Academy of Sciences, 109(47), pp.19444–19449. http://dx.doi.org/10.1073/pnas.1216080109.

Fertleman, C.R. et al., 2006. SCN9A Mutations in Paroxysmal Extreme Pain Disorder: Allelic Variants Underlie Distinct Channel Defects and Phenotypes. Neuron, 52(5), pp.767–774. http://dx.doi.org/10.1016/j.neuron.2006.10.006.

Waxman, S.G. et al., 1999. Sodium channels and pain. Proceedings of the National Academy of Sciences, 96(14), pp.7635–7639. http://dx.doi.org/10.1073/pnas.96.14.7635.

SPINAL ACCESSORY NERVE

Overland, J. et al., 2016. Surgical anatomy of the spinal accessory nerve: review of the literature and case report of a rare anatomical variant. The Journal of Laryngology & Otology, 130(10), pp.969–972. Available at: http://dx.doi.org/10.1017/s0022215116008148.

Lanišnik, B., 2017. Different branching patterns of the spinal accessory nerve. Current Opinion in Otolaryngology & Head and Neck Surgery, 25(2), pp.113–118. Available at: http://dx.doi.org/10.1097/moo.0000000000000342.

Axibal, E. et al., 2017. Neuropraxia of the Spinal Accessory Nerve After Mohs Micrographic Surgery. Dermatologic Surgery, 43(9), pp.1192–1195. Available at: http://dx.doi.org/10.1097/dss.0000000000001185.

SPINA BIFIDA

Donnan, J. et al., 2016. A systematic review of the risks factors associated with the onset and natural progression of spina bifida. NeuroToxicology. http://dx.doi.org/10.1016/j.neuro.2016.03.008.

Liu, J.S. et al., 2016. A snapshot of the adult spina bifida patient – high incidence of urologic procedures. Central European Journal of Urology, 69(1). http://dx.doi.org/10.5173/ceju.2016.596.

Northrup, H. & Volcik, K.A., 2000. Spina bifida and other neural tube defects. Current Problems in Pediatrics, 30(10), pp.317–332. http://dx.doi.org/10.1067/mpp.2000.112052.

SPINAL CORD INJURY

Ahmed, M.M. et al., 2014. Pathogenesis of spinal cord injury induced edema and neuropathic pain: expression of multiple isoforms of wnk1. Annals of Neurosciences, 21(3). http://dx.doi.org/10.5214/ans.0972.7531.210305.

Hagen, E.M. & Rekand, T., 2015. Management of Neuropathic Pain Associated with Spinal Cord Injury. Pain and Therapy, 4(1), pp.51–65. http://dx.doi.org/10.1007/s40122-015-0033-y.

Ledbetter, L.N. et al., 2016. Spinal Neuroarthropathy: Pathophysiology, Clinical and Imaging Features, and Differential Diagnosis. RadioGraphics, 36(3), pp.783–799. http://dx.doi.org/10.1148/rg.2016150121.

Lee, H.K. et al., 2014. Persistent phosphorylation of NKCC1 and WNK1 in the epicenter of the spinal cord following contusion injury. The Spine Journal, 14(5), pp.777–781. http://dx.doi.org/10.1016/j.spinee.2013.06.100.

SPLEEN

Asgari, M.M. and Begos, D.G., 1997. Spontaneous splenic rupture in infectious mononucleosis: a review. The Yale journal of Biology and Medicine, 70(2), p.175. https://www.ncbi.nlm.nih.gov/pmc/articles/PMC2589064/

Ben Ely, A. et al., 2006. The wandering spleen: CT findings and possible pitfalls in diagnosis. Clinical Radiology, 61(11), pp.954–958. http://dx.doi.org/10.1016/j.crad.2006.06.007.

Ingle, S.B., 2014. Epithelial cysts of the spleen: A minireview. World Journal of Gastroenterology, 20(38), p.13899. http://dx.doi.org/10.3748/wjg.v20.i38.13899.

SPONDYLOLISTHESIS

DeWald, C.J. et al., 2005. Evaluation and Management of High-Grade Spondylolisthesis in Adults. Spine, 30(Supplement), pp.S49–S59. http://dx.doi.org/10.1097/01.

brs.0000155573.34179.7e.

Matz, P.G. et al., 2016. Guideline summary review: an evidence-based clinical guideline for the diagnosis and treatment of degenerative lumbar spondylolisthesis. The Spine Journal, 16(3), pp.439–448. http://dx.doi.org/10.1016/j.spinee.2015.11.055.

Patel, A.J. et al., 2013. Congenital hypoplasia or aplasia of the lumbosacral pedicle as an unusual cause of spondylolisthesis in the pediatric age group. Journal of Neurosurgery: Pediatrics, 11(6), pp.717–721. http://dx.doi.org/10.3171/2013.3.peds12579.

Ploumis, A., Hantzidis, P. and Dimitriou, C., 2005. High-grade dysplastic spondylolisthesis and spondyloptosis: report of three cases with surgical treatment and review of the literature. Acta orthopaedica belgica, 71(6), p.750. https://www.ncbi.nlm.nih.gov/pubmed/16459872

Stone, A.T. & Tribus, C.B., 2002. Acute Progression of Spondylolysis to Isthmic Spondylolisthesis in an Adult. Spine, 27(16), pp.E370–E372. http://dx.doi.org/10.1097/00007632-200208150-00023.

Thakar, S. et al., 2016. Lumbar paraspinal muscle morphometry and its correlations with demographic and radiological factors in adult isthmic spondylolisthesis: a retrospective review of 120 surgically managed cases. Journal of Neurosurgery: Spine, 24(5), pp.679–685. http://dx.doi.org/10.3171/2015.9.spine15705.

SPONTANEOUS INTRACRANIAL HYPOTENSION

Balkan, I.I. et al., 2012. Spontaneous intracranial hypotension syndrome may mimic aseptic meningitis. Scandinavian Journal of Infectious Diseases, 44(7), pp.481–488. http://dx.doi.org/10.3109/00365548.2012.664776.

Ferrante, E. et al., 2004. Spontaneous Intracranial Hypotension Syndrome: Report of Twelve Cases. Headache: The Journal of Head and Face Pain, 44(6), pp.615–622. http://dx.doi.org/10.1111/j.1526-4610.2004.446012.x.

Karm, M.-H. et al., 2016. Predictors of the Treatment Response of Spontaneous Intracranial Hypotension to an Epidural Blood Patch. Medicine, 95(18), p.e3578. http://dx.doi.org/10.1097/md.0000000000003578.

Mokri, B., 2013. Spontaneous Low Pressure, Low CSF Volume Headaches: Spontaneous CSF Leaks. Headache: The Journal of Head and Face Pain, 53(7), pp.1034–1053. http://dx.doi.org/10.1111/head.12149.

STERNO-CLAVICULAR HYPEROSTOSIS

Carroll, M.B., 2011. Sternocostoclavicular hyperostosis: a review. Therapeutic advances in musculoskeletal disease, Ther Adv Musculoskelet Dis. 2011 Apr; 3(2): 101–110. https://www.ncbi.nlm.nih.gov/pmc/articles/PMC3382681/

Kuroda, T., Ehara, S. & Murakami, H., 2005. Stress fracture of the clavicle associated with sternocostoclavicular hyperostosis. Skeletal Radiology, 34(7), pp.424–426. http://dx.doi.org/10.1007/s00256-004-0885-4.

Saghafi, M., Henderson, M.J. & Buchanan, W.W., 1993. Sternocostoclavicular hyperostosis. Seminars in Arthritis and Rheumatism, 22(4), pp.215–223. http://dx.doi.org/10.1016/0049-0172(93)80070-v.

SUBDURAL HEMATOMA

Adhiyaman, V., 2002. Chronic subdural haematoma in the elderly. Postgraduate Medical Journal, 78(916), pp.71–75. http://dx.doi.org/10.1136/pmj.78.916.71.

De Noronha, R.J., 2003. Subdural haematoma: a potentially serious consequence of spontaneous intracranial hypotension. Journal of Neurology, Neurosurgery & Psychiatry, 74(6), pp.752–755. http://dx.doi.org/10.1136/jnnp.74.6.752.

Jacome, D.E. & Yanez, G.F., 1989. Subdural haematoma upon straining. Journal of Neurology, Neurosurgery & Psychiatry, 52(1), pp.134–134. http://dx.doi.org/10.1136/jnnp.52.1.134.

Jokonya, L. et al., 2016. Spontaneous chronic subdural hematomas in human immunodeficiency virus-infected patients with normal platelet count and no appreciable brain atrophy: Two case reports and review of literature. Surgical Neurology International, 7(16), p.437. http://dx.doi.org/10.4103/2152-7806.183543.

Mori, K. & Maeda, M., 2003. Risk factors for the occurrence of chronic subdural haematomas after neurosurgical procedures. Acta Neurochirurgica, 145(7), pp.533–540. http://dx.doi.org/10.1007/s00701-003-0026-1.

SUNCT/SUNA

Baldacci, F. et al., 2009. SUNA Syndrome With Seasonal Pattern. Headache: The Journal of Head and Face Pain, 49(6), pp.912–914. http://dx.doi.org/10.1111/j.1526-4610.2009.01401.x.

Chitsantikul, P. & Becker, W.J., 2012. SUNCT, SUNA and pituitary tumors: Clinical characteristics and treatment. Cephalalgia, 33(3), pp.160–170. http://dx.doi.org/10.1177/0333102412468672.

Jin, D., Lian, Y.-J. & Zhang, H.-F., 2016. Secondary SUNCT syndrome caused by dorsolateral medullary infarction. The Journal of Headache and Pain, 17(1). http://dx.doi.org/10.1186/s10194-016-0604-2.

Pareja, J.A. & Cuadrado, M.L., 2005. SUNCT syndrome: an update. Expert Opinion on Pharmacotherapy, 6(4), pp.591–599. http://dx.doi.org/10.1517/14656566.6.4.591.

Pareja, J.A. et al., 1996. SUNCT Syndrome: Duration, Frequency, and Temporal Distribution of Attacks. Headache: The Journal of Head and Face Pain, 36(3), pp.161–165. http://dx.doi.org/10.1046/j.1526-4610.1996.3603161.x.

SUPRA AND INFRACLAVICULAR NERVES

Kiser, C., Hill, B. & Skedros, J., 2015. Florid Suprascapular Neuropathy after Primary Rotator Cuff Repair Attributed to Suprascapular Notch Constriction in the Setting of Double Crush Syndrome. Journal of Brachial Plexus and Peripheral Nerve Injury, 10(01), pp.e66–e73. Available at: http://dx.doi.org/10.1055/s-0035-1567807.

Ishimaru, D. et al., 2017. Suprascapular Nerve Entrapment Caused by Protrusion of an Intraosseous Ganglion of the Glenoid into the Spinoglenoid Notch: A Rare Cause of Posterior Shoulder Pain. Case Reports in Orthopedics, 2017, pp.1–5. Available at: http://dx.doi.org/10.1155/2017/1704697.

Kiss, G. & Kómár, J., 1990. Suprascapular nerve compression at the spinoglenoid notch. Muscle & Nerve, 13(6), pp.556–557. Available at: http://dx.doi.org/10.1002/mus.880130614.

SUPERIOR/INFERIOR GLUTEAL NERVES

Mondelli, M. et al., 2008. Mononeuropathies of inferior and superior gluteal nerves due to hypertrophy of piriformis muscle in a basketball player. Muscle & Nerve, 38(6), pp.1660–1662. Available at: http://dx.doi.org/10.1002/mus.21139.

Chomiak, J. et al., 2015. Lesion of gluteal nerves and muscles in total hip arthroplasty through 3 surgical approaches. An electromyographically controlled study. Hip International, 25(2), pp.176–183. Available at: http://dx.doi.org/10.5301/hipint.5000199.

J Butz, J., V Raman, D. & Viswanath, S., 2015. A UNIQUE CASE OF BILATERAL SCIATIC NERVE VARIATION. Australasian Medical Journal, 08(01). Available at: http://dx.doi.org/10.21767/amj.2015.2266.

Florian-Rodriguez, M.E. et al., 2016. Inferior gluteal and other nerves associated with sacrospinous ligament: a cadaver study. American Journal of Obstetrics and Gynecology, 215(5), pp.646.e1–646.e6. Available at: http://dx.doi.org/10.1016/j.ajog.2016.06.025.

Abitbol, J.J. et al., 1990. Gluteal nerve damage following total hip arthroplasty. The Journal of Arthroplasty, 5(4), pp.319–322. Available at: http://dx.doi.org/10.1016/s0883-5403(08)80090-3

SUPERIOR CORNU OF THE THYROID CARTILAGE

Wojtowicz, P. et al., 2015. Extended Superior Cornu of Thyroid Cartilage Causing Dysphagia and Throat Pain. Journal of Medical Cases, 6(3), pp.134–136. http://dx.doi.org/10.14740/jmc2043w.

SUPERIOR LARYNGEAL NEURALGIA

Aydin, O., Ozturk, M. & Anik, Y., 2007. Superior Laryngeal Neuralgia After Acute Laryngitis and Treatment With a Single Injection of a Local Anesthetic. Archives of Otolaryngology–Head & Neck Surgery, 133(9), p.934. http://dx.doi.org/10.1001/archotol.133.9.934.

Baugh, R.F., Baugh, A. & Bunge, F., 2012. Superior laryngeal nerve syndrome and the evaluation of anterior neck pain. American Journal of Otolaryngology, 33(4), pp.481–483. http://dx.doi.org/10.1016/j.amjoto.2011.10.018.

O'Neill, B.P. et al., 1982. Superior Laryngeal Neuralgia: Carotidynia or Just Another Pain in the Neck? Headache: The Journal of Head and Face Pain, 22(1), pp.6–9. http://dx.doi.org/10.1111/j.1526-4610.1982.hed2201006.x.

Teymoortash A. et al. 2007. Function and dysfunction of the superior laryngeal nerve. HNO. 56(9), pp 889-894 Sep;56(9):889-94. http://dx.doi.org/10.1007/s00106-007-1595-8

SURAL NERVE

Kim, K.H., Park, B.K. & Kim, D.H., 2016. A case of lateral calcaneal neuropathy: Lateral heel pain. Muscle & Nerve, 54(4), pp.801–804. Available at: http://dx.doi.org/10.1002/mus.25188.

Paraskevas, G.K. et al., 2014. Fascial entrapment of the sural nerve and its clinical relevance. Anatomy & Cell Biology, 47(2), p.144. Available at: http://dx.doi.org/10.5115/acb.2014.47.2.144.

SURAMIN

Liu, N. & Zhuang, S., 2011. Tissue Protective and Anti-Fibrotic Actions of Suramin: New Uses of an Old Drug. Current Clinical Pharmacology, 6(2), pp.137–142. http://dx.doi.org/10.2174/157488411796151174.

Russell, J.W. et al., 2001. Suramin-induced neuropathy in an animal model. Journal of the Neurological Sciences, 192(1-2), pp.71–80. http://dx.doi.org/10.1016/s0022-510x(01)00633-5.

SURGICAL NERVE ROOT INJURY

Choi, I. et al., 2013. Exiting root injury in transforaminal endoscopic discectomy: preoperative image considerations for safety. European Spine Journal, 22(11), pp.2481–2487. http://dx.doi.org/10.1007/s00586-013-2849-7.

Epstein, N., 2016. More nerve root injuries occur with minimally invasive lumbar surgery: Let's tell someone. Surgical Neurology International, 7(4), p.96. http://dx.doi.org/10.4103/2152-7806.174896.

Evaniew, N. et al., 2014. Minimally invasive versus open surgery for cervical and lumbar discectomy: a systematic review and meta-analysis. CMAJ Open, 2(4), pp.E295–E305. http://dx.doi.org/10.9778/cmajo.20140048.

SURGICALLY INDUCED NEUROPATHIC PAIN

Borsook, D. et al., 2013. Surgically Induced Neuropathic Pain. Annals of Surgery, 257(3), pp.403–412. http://dx.doi.org/10.1097/sla.0b013e3182701a7b.

Celestin, J., Edwards, R.R. & Jamison, R.N., 2009. Pretreatment Psychosocial Variables as Predictors of Outcomes Following Lumbar Surgery and Spinal Cord Stimulation: A Systematic Review and Literature Synthesis. Pain Medicine, 10(4), pp.639–653. http://dx.doi.org/10.1111/j.1526-4637.2009.00632.x.

Papaioannou, M. et al., 2009. The Role of Catastrophizing in the Prediction of Postoperative Pain. Pain Medicine, 10(8), pp.1452–1459. http://dx.doi.org/10.1111/j.1526-4637.2009.00730.x.

SYNOVIAL CYSTS

Boviatsis, E.J. et al., 2008. Spinal synovial cysts: pathogenesis, diagnosis and surgical treatment in a series of seven cases and literature review. European Spine Journal, 17(6), pp.831–837. http://dx.doi.org/10.1007/s00586-007-0563-z.

Scholz, C. et al., 2015. Incomplete resection of lumbar synovial cysts – Evaluating the risk of recurrence. Clinical Neurology and Neurosurgery, 136, pp.29–32. http://dx.doi.org/10.1016/j.clineuro.2015.05.028.

SYPHILIS

Castro, R. et al., 2016. Detection ofTreponema pallidumSp.PallidumDNA in Cerebrospinal Fluid (CSF) by Two PCR Techniques. Journal of Clinical Laboratory Analysis, 30(5), pp.628–632. http://dx.doi.org/10.1002/jcla.21913

.

Salamano, R. et al., 2016. Cerebrospinal fluid examination may be useful in diagnosing neurosyphilis in asymptomatic HIV+ patients with syphilis. Arquivos de Neuro-Psiquiatria, 74(2), pp.128–132. http://dx.doi.org/10.1590/0004-282x20160016.

Zhang, Y.-Q. et al., 2015. A Clinical Study of New Cases of Parenchymal Neurosyphilis: Has Tabes Dorsalis Disappeared or Been Missed? The Journal of Neuropsychiatry and Clinical Neurosciences, 27(1), pp.e17–e21. http://dx.doi.org/10.1176/appi.neuropsych.13100303.

SYRINX

Chakraborty, P.P., 2015. Unilateral neuropathic arthropathy of the shoulder secondary to syringomyelia: Diagnostic challenges. World Journal of Clinical Cases, 3(12), p.1017. http://dx.doi.org/10.12998/wjcc.v3.i12.1017.

Chang, H.S., 2003. Hypothesis on the pathophysiology of syringomyelia based on simulation of cerebrospinal fluid dynamics. Journal of Neurology, Neurosurgery & Psychiatry, 74(3), pp.344–347. http://dx.doi.org/10.1136/jnnp.74.3.344.

Kennedy, B.C. et al., 2016. Isolated thoracic syrinx in children with Chiari I malformation. Child's Nervous System, 32(3), pp.531–534. http://dx.doi.org/10.1007/s00381-015-3009-7.

Klekamp, J. & Samii, M., 2002. The Pathophysiology of Syringomyelia. Syringomyelia, pp.17–25. http://dx.doi.org/10.1007/978-3-642-56023-1_2.

Klekamp, J., 2002. The pathophysiology of syringomyelia–historical overview and current concept. Acta neurochirurgica, 144(7), pp.649-664 https://www.ncbi.nlm.nih.gov/labs/articles/12181698/

Koyanagi, I. et al., 2005. Clinical features and pathomechanisms of syringomyelia associated with spinal arachnoiditis. Surgical Neurology, 63(4), pp.350–355. http://dx.doi.org/10.1016/j.surneu.2004.05.038.

TANGIER DISEASE

Kolovou, G. et al., 2006. Tangier Disease Four Decades of Research: A Reflection of the Importance of HDL. Current Medicinal Chemistry, 13(7), pp.771–782. http://dx.doi.org/10.2174/092986706776055580.

Pietrini, V. et al., 2009. Neuropathy in Tangier disease: A clinicopathologic study and a review of the literature. Acta Neurologica Scandinavica, 72(5), pp.495–505. http://dx.doi.org/10.1111/j.1600-0404.1985.tb00907.x.

Puntoni, M. et al., 2012. Tangier Disease. American Journal Cardiovascular Drugs, 12(5), pp.303–311. http://dx.doi.org/10.2165/11634140-000000000-00000.

TARSAL TUNNEL

McSweeney, S.C. & Cichero, M., 2015. Tarsal tunnel syndrome—A narrative literature review. The Foot, 25(4), pp.244–250. Available at: http://dx.doi.org/10.1016/j.

foot.2015.08.008.

Doneddu, P.E. et al., 2017. Tarsal tunnel syndrome: still more opinions than evidence. Status of the art. Neurological Sciences, 38(10), pp.1735–1739. Available at: http://dx.doi.org/10.1007/s10072-017-3039-x.

Kosiyatrakul, A., Luenam, S. & Phisitkul, P., 2015. Tarsal tunnel syndrome associated with a perforating branch from posterior tibial artery: A case report. Foot and Ankle Surgery, 21(1), pp.e21–e22. Available at: http://dx.doi.org/10.1016/j.fas.2014.09.003.

TAXANES

Fernandes, R. et al., 2015. Treatment of taxane acute pain syndrome (TAPS) in cancer patients receiving taxane-based chemotherapy—a systematic review. Supportive Care in Cancer, 24(4), pp.1583–1594. http://dx.doi.org/10.1007/s00520-015-2941-0.

Florian, S. & Mitchison, T.J., 2016. Anti-Microtubule Drugs. The Mitotic Spindle, pp.403–421. http://dx.doi.org/10.1007/978-1-4939-3542-0_25.

Hagiwara, H. & Sunada, Y., 2004. Mechanism of taxane neurotoxicity. Breast Cancer, 11(1), pp.82–85. http://dx.doi.org/10.1007/bf02968008.

TEMPOROMANDIBULAR JOINT SYNDROME

Bavia, P.F. & Rodrigues Garcia, R.C.M., 2016. Vertical Craniofacial Morphology and its Relation to Temporomandibular Disorders. Journal of Oral and Maxillofacial Research, 7(2). http://dx.doi.org/10.5037/jomr.2016.7206.

Kumar, R. et al., 2015. Correlation Between Clinical Findings of Temporomandibular Disorders and MRI Characteristics of Disc Displacement. The Open Dentistry Journal, 9(Suppl 2: M4), pp.273–281. http://dx.doi.org/10.2174/1874210601509010273.

Litko, M. et al., 2016. Correlation between the lateral pterygoid muscle attachment type and temporomandibular joint disc position in magnetic resonance imaging. Dentomaxillofacial Radiology, 45(8), p.20160229. http://dx.doi.org/10.1259/dmfr.20160229.

Slade, G.D. et al., 2016. Painful Temporomandibular Disorder. Journal of Dental Research, 95(10), pp.1084–1092. http://dx.doi.org/10.1177/0022034516653743.

Vogl, T.J. et al., 2016. The value of MRI in patients with temporomandibular joint dysfunction: Correlation of MRI and clinical findings. European Journal of Radiology, 85(4), pp.714–719. http://dx.doi.org/10.1016/j.ejrad.2016.02.001.

THALIDOMIDE

Nicotra, A. et al., 2016. Peripheral Nerve Dysfunction in Middle-Aged Subjects Born with Thalidomide Embryopathy G. Biagini, ed. PLOS ONE, 11(4), p.e0152902. http://dx.doi.org/10.1371/journal.pone.0152902.

Wang, J. et al., 2016. Low serum vitamin D occurs commonly among multiple myeloma patients treated with bortezomib and/or thalidomide and is associated with severe neuropathy. Supportive Care in Cancer. http://dx.doi.org/10.1007/s00520-016-3126-1.

Zhao, L. et al., 2015. High-dose thalidomide increases the risk of peripheral neuropathy in the treatment of ankylosing spondylitis. Neural Regeneration Research, 10(5), p.814. http://dx.doi.org/10.4103/1673-5374.156988.

THALLIUM

Kuo, H.-C. et al., 2005. Acute painful neuropathy in thallium poisoning. Neurology, 65(2), pp.302–304. http://dx.doi.org/10.1212/01.wnl.0000169021.26172.f8.

Labauge, R., Tourniaire, D., Favier, J.P. and Blard, J.M., 1990. [Recurrent peripheral neuropathy caused by thallium poisoning]. Revue neurologique, 147(4), pp.317-319. https://www.ncbi.nlm.nih.gov/pubmed/2063083

Pelclova, D. et al., 2009. Two-year follow-up of two patients after severe thallium intoxication. Human & Experimental Toxicology, 28(5), pp.263–272. http://dx.doi.org/10.1177/0960327109106487.

THIRD OCCIPITAL NERVE

Govind, J., 2003. Radiofrequency neurotomy for the treatment of third occipital headache. Journal of Neurology, Neurosurgery & Psychiatry, 74(1), pp.88–93. http://dx.doi.org/10.1136/jnnp.74.1.88.

Tubbs, R.S. et al., 2011. Anatomical study of the third occipital nerve and its potential role in occipital headache/neck pain following midline dissections of the craniocervical junction. Journal of Neurosurgery: Spine, 15(1), pp.71–75. http://dx.doi.org/10.3171/2011.3.spine10854.

THORACIC DISC

Arce, C.A. and Dohrmann, G.J., 1985. Herniated thoracic disks. Neurologic clinics, 3(2), pp.383-392. https://www.ncbi.nlm.nih.gov/pubmed/3894922

Epstein NE, Epstein JA, Rosenthal AD. Thoracic disc disease. Dee R, ed. Principles of Orthopedic Practice. New York , NY: McGraw-Hill, Inc; 1989. Vol 2: 991-7.

Kato, K. et al., 2016. Unusual chest wall pain caused by thoracic disc herniation in a professional baseball pitcher. Fukushima J Med Sci 62(1), pp.64–67. http://dx.doi.

org/10.5387/fms.2015-25.

Lee, J.G. et al., 2016. Clinical Features of Herniated Disc at Cervicothoracic Junction Level Treated by Anterior Approach. Korean Journal of Spine, 13(2), p.53. http://dx.doi.org/10.14245/kjs.2016.13.2.53.

Luney, M., Adiamah, A. & Pearson, L., 2016. Thoracic spondylodiscitis presenting as abdominal pain. BMJ Case Reports, p.bcr2015213846. http://dx.doi.org/10.1136/bcr-2015-213846.

Nannapaneni, R. & Marks, S., 2004. Posterolateral thoracic disc disease: clinical presentation and surgical experience with a modified approach. British Journal of Neurosurgery, 18(5), pp.467–470. http://dx.doi.org/10.1080/02688690400012335.

Sandon, L.H.D. et al., 2016. Abducens nerve palsy as a postoperative complication of minimally invasive thoracic spine surgery: a case report. BMC Surgery, 16(1). http://dx.doi.org/10.1186/s12893-016-0162-1.

THORACIC OUTLET SURGERY

Desai, S.S. et al., 2014. Outcomes of Surgical Paraclavicular Thoracic Outlet Decompression. Annals of Vascular Surgery, 28(2), pp.457–464. http://dx.doi.org/10.1016/j.avsg.2013.02.029.

Luginbuhl, A. et al., 2011. Detection of evolving injury to the brachial plexus during transaxillary robotic thyroidectomy. The Laryngoscope, 122(1), pp.110–115. http://dx.doi.org/10.1002/lary.22429.

Orlando, M.S. et al., 2015. A Decade of Excellent Outcomes after Surgical Intervention in 538 Patients with Thoracic Outlet Syndrome. Journal of the American College of Surgeons, 220(5), pp.934–939. http://dx.doi.org/10.1016/j.jamcollsurg.2014.12.046.

Sanders, R.J. & Annest, S.J., 2015. Technique of supraclavicular decompression for neurogenic thoracic outlet syndrome. Journal of Vascular Surgery, 61(3), pp.821–825. http://dx.doi.org/10.1016/j.jvs.2014.11.047

THORACIC OUTLET SYNDROME

Chang, K.Z. et al., 2013. The significance of cervical ribs in thoracic outlet syndrome. Journal of Vascular Surgery, 57(3), pp.771–775. http://dx.doi.org/10.1016/j.jvs.2012.08.110.

Hines, K. et al., 2014. The Rare Case of Cervical Rib Fusion to the Second Rib. Annals of Vascular Surgery, 28(3), pp.742.e5–742.e8. http://dx.doi.org/10.1016/j.avsg.2013.05.016.

Kim, D.H. et al., 2004. Infraclavicular brachial plexus stretch injury. Neurosurgical

FOCUS, 16(5), pp.1–6. http://dx.doi.org/10.3171/foc.2004.16.5.5.

Klaassen, Z. et al., 2013. Thoracic outlet syndrome: A neurological and vascular disorder. Clinical Anatomy, 27(5), pp.724–732. http://dx.doi.org/10.1002/ca.22271.

Leonhard, V. et al., 2016. Anatomical variations in the brachial plexus roots: implications for diagnosis of neurogenic thoracic outlet syndrome. Annals of Anatomy - Anatomischer Anzeiger, 206, pp.21–26. http://dx.doi.org/10.1016/j.aanat.2016.03.011.

Likes, K. et al., 2014. Coexistence of Arterial Compression in Patients With Neurogenic Thoracic Outlet Syndrome. JAMA Surgery, 149(12), p.1240. http://dx.doi.org/10.1001/jamasurg.2014.280.

THORACIC OUTLET SYNDROME: VASCULAR

Aralasmak, A. et al., 2012. MRI findings in thoracic outlet syndrome. Skeletal Radiology, 41(11), pp.1365–1374. http://dx.doi.org/10.1007/s00256-012-1485-3.

Klaassen, Z. et al., 2013. Thoracic outlet syndrome: A neurological and vascular disorder. Clinical Anatomy, 27(5), pp.724–732. http://dx.doi.org/10.1002/ca.22271.

TIBIALIS NERVE

Del Río-Gonzalez, S. et al., 2017. Percutaneous Tibial Nerve Stimulation Therapy for Overactive Bladder Syndrome: Clinical Effectiveness, Urodynamic, and Durability Evaluation. Urology, 108, pp.52–58. Available at: http://dx.doi.org/10.1016/j.urology.2017.04.059.

Shin, Y.-S., Sim, H.-B. & Yoon, J.-R., 2017. Tibial nerve neuropathy following medial opening-wedge high tibial osteotomy—case report of a rare technical complication. European Journal of Orthopaedic Surgery & Traumatology, 27(4), pp.563–567. Available at: http://dx.doi.org/10.1007/s00590-017-1944-6.

Kohira, I, et al., 2003. Entrapment neuropathy of the tibial nerve by a Baker's cyst: case report. Rinsho Shinkeigaku, 43(3):130-2. Abstract available at: https://www.ncbi.nlm.nih.gov/pubmed/12820564 Article in Japanese.

Wu, C. et al., 2016. Assessment of tibial and common peroneal nerves in diabetic peripheral neuropathy by diffusion tensor imaging: a case control study. European Radiology, 27(8), pp.3523–3531. Available at: http://dx.doi.org/10.1007/s00330-016-4698-3.

Vaeggemose, M. et al., 2017. Magnetic Resonance Neurography Visualizes Abnormalities in Sciatic and Tibial Nerves in Patients With Type 1 Diabetes and Neuropathy. Diabetes, 66(7), pp.1779–1788. Available at: http://dx.doi.org/10.2337/db16-

1049

VASCULITIC NEUROPATHY

Blaes, F., 2015. Diagnosis and therapeutic options for peripheral vasculitic neuropathy. Therapeutic Advances in Musculoskeletal Disease, 7(2), pp.45–55. http://dx.doi.org/10.1177/1759720x14566617.

Blaes, F., 2015. Diagnosis and therapeutic options for peripheral vasculitic neuropathy. Therapeutic Advances in Musculoskeletal Disease, 7(2), pp.45–55. http://dx.doi.org/10.1177/1759720x14566617.

Damoiseaux, J. & Cohen Tervaert, J.W., 2013. Diagnostics and Treatment of Cryoglobulinaemia: It Takes Two to Tango. Clinical Reviews in Allergy & Immunology, 47(3), pp.299–310. http://dx.doi.org/10.1007/s12016-013-8390-y.

Schaublin, G.A. et al., 2005. An update on the classification and treatment of vasculitic neuropathy. The Lancet Neurology, 4(12), pp.853–865. http://dx.doi.org/10.1016/s1474-4422(05)70249-0.

Schaublin, G.A. et al., 2005. An update on the classification and treatment of vasculitic neuropathy. The Lancet Neurology, 4(12), pp.853–865. http://dx.doi.org/10.1016/s1474-4422(05)70249-0.

Vital, C. et al., 2006. Combined nerve and muscle biopsy in the diagnosis of vasculitic neuropathy. A 16-year retrospective study of 202 cases. Journal of the Peripheral Nervous System, 11(1), pp.20–29. http://dx.doi.org/10.1111/j.1085-9489.2006.00060.x.

Vital, C. et al., 2006. Combined nerve and muscle biopsy in the diagnosis of vasculitic neuropathy. A 16-year retrospective study of 202 cases. Journal of the Peripheral Nervous System, 11(1), pp.20–29. http://dx.doi.org/10.1111/j.1085-9489.2006.00060.x.

THYROID CARTILAGE MASTOID PROCESS

Aydil, U., Kizil, Y. & Köybaşioğlu, A., 2011. Less known non-infectious and neuromusculoskeletal system-originated anterolateral neck and craniofacial pain disorders. European Archives of Oto-Rhino-Laryngology, 269(1), pp.9–16. http://dx.doi.org/10.1007/s00405-011-1746-0.

Hefer, T. & Joachims, H., 1997. CO laser repair of permanent tracheostomy stricture. Otolaryngology - Head and Neck Surgery, 117(3), pp.276–279. http://dx.doi.org/10.1016/s0194-5998(97)70186-4.

TIETZE'S SYNDROME

Gunal, N. et al., 2015. Painful Chest Wall Swellings: Tietze Syndrome or Chest Wall Tumor? The Thoracic and Cardiovascular Surgeon, 64(03), pp.239–244. http://dx.

doi.org/10.1055/s-0035-1545261.

Nowicki, J.L., Dean, N.R. & Watson, D.I., 2016. A Case Report of Candida albicans Costochondritis after a Complicated Esophagectomy. Plastic and Reconstructive Surgery - Global Open, 4(1), p.e608. http://dx.doi.org/10.1097/gox.0000000000000599.

Volterroni L. et al. 2008. Magnetic resonance imaging in Tietze's Syndrome. Clin Exp Rheumatol 26(5), pp. 848-853. http://www.clinexprheumatol.org/article.asp?a=3496

TRANSTHYRETIN-RELATED AMYLOIDOSIS

Adams, D. et al., 2016. First European consensus for diagnosis, management, and treatment of transthyretin familial amyloid polyneuropathy. Current Opinion in Neurology, 29, pp.S14–S26. http://dx.doi.org/10.1097/wco.0000000000000289

Adams, D., Lozeron, P. & Lacroix, C., 2012. Amyloid neuropathies. Current Opinion in Neurology, 25(5), pp.564–572. http://dx.doi.org/10.1097/wco.0b013e328357bdf6.

Conceição, I. et al., 2016. "Red-flag" symptom clusters in transthyretin familial amyloid polyneuropathy. Journal of the Peripheral Nervous System, 21(1), pp.5–9. http://dx.doi.org/10.1111/jns.12153

Dohrn, M.F. et al., 2013. Diagnostic hallmarks and pitfalls in late-onset progressive transthyretin-related amyloid-neuropathy. Journal of Neurology, 260(12), pp.3093–3108. http://dx.doi.org/10.1007/s00415-013-7124-7

Obici, L. et al., 2016. Recommendations for presymptomatic genetic testing and management of individuals at risk for hereditary transthyretin amyloidosis. Current Opinion in Neurology, 29, pp.S27–S35. http://dx.doi.org/10.1097/wco.0000000000000290

Schmidt, H.H.-J. et al., 2016. Management of asymptomatic gene carriers of transthyretin familial amyloid polyneuropathy. Muscle & Nerve, 54(3), pp.353–360. http://dx.doi.org/10.1002/mus.25210

TRANSVERSE COLLI

Sakamoto, Y., 2012. Spatial relationships between the morphologies and innervations of the scalene and anterior vertebral muscles. Annals of Anatomy - Anatomischer Anzeiger, 194(4), pp.381–388. http://dx.doi.org/10.1016/j.aanat.2011.11.004

TRANSVERSE MYELITIS

Nichtweiß, M. & Weidauer, S., 2015. Differential Diagnosis of Acute Myelopathies: An Update. Clinical Neuroradiology, 25(S2), pp.183–187. http://dx.doi.org/10.1007/s00062-015-0401-3

Pereira, W.L. de C.J. et al., 2015. Epidemiological, clinical, and immunological characteristics of neuromyelitis optica: A review. Journal of the Neurological Sciences, 355(1-2), pp.7–17. http://dx.doi.org/10.1016/j.jns.2015.05.034

Sá, M.J., 2009. Acute transverse myelitis: A practical reappraisal. Autoimmunity Reviews, 9(2), pp.128–131. http://dx.doi.org/10.1016/j.autrev.2009.04.005.

TRIGEMINAL AUTONOMIC CEPHALALGIA (GENERAL)

Benoliel, R., 2012. Trigeminal autonomic cephalgias. British Journal of Pain, 6(3), pp.106–123. http://dx.doi.org/10.1177/2049463712456355

Larner, A.J., 2008. Trigeminal autonomic cephalalgias: frequency in a general neurology clinic setting. The Journal of Headache and Pain, 9(5), pp.325–326. http://dx.doi.org/10.1007/s10194-008-0053-7

Wilbrink, L.A. et al., 2009. Neuroimaging in trigeminal autonomic cephalgias: when, how, and of what? Current Opinion in Neurology, 22(3), pp.247–253. http://dx.doi.org/10.1097/wco.0b013e32832b4bb3

TRIGEMINAL NEURALGIA

Arrese, I. & Sarabia, R., 2016. Microvascular decompression for trigeminal neuralgia secondary to vertebrobasilar dolichoectasia. Case report, literature review, and pooled case analysis. Neurocirugía, 27(6), pp.304–309. http://dx.doi.org/10.1016/j.neucir.2016.05.003

Cruccu, G. et al., 2016. Trigeminal neuralgia. Neurology, 87(2), pp.220–228. http://dx.doi.org/10.1212/wnl.0000000000002840

KJ Burchiel. , 1993. Trigeminal Neuropathic Pain.Acta Neurochir Suppl (Wien) 58, 145-149. https://www.ncbi.nlm.nih.gov/labs/articles/8109278/

Kumar, S., Rastogi, S., Mahendra, P., Bansal, M. and Chandra, L., 2013. Pain in trigeminal neuralgia: neurophysiology and measurement: a comprehensive review. Journal of medicine and life, 6(4), p.383. https://www.ncbi.nlm.nih.gov/pmc/articles/PMC3973876/

Thieme, V., 2016. [Orofacial pain-Trigeminal neuralgia and posttraumatic trigeminal neuropathy: Common features and differences]. Schmerz (Berlin, Germany), 30(1), pp.99-117. http://europepmc.org/abstract/med/26815785 (German)

Yuan, Y. et al., 2016. Trigeminal neuralgia caused by brain arteriovenous malformations: A case report and literature review. Experimental and Therapeutic Medicine. http://dx.doi.org/10.3892/etm.2016.3277

TUMOR OF THORACIC BOOTS

Hsu, C.C., Huang, T.W., Hsu, J.Y., Shin, N. and Chang, H., 2013. Malignant peripheral nerve sheath tumor of the chest wall associated with neurofibromatosis: a case report. Journal of thoracic disease, 5(3), pp.E78-E82. https://www.ncbi.nlm.nih.gov/pubmed/23825788

Li, B. and Chen, Q., 2015. Melanotic schwannoma of thoracic spinal root mimics metastatic melanoma: A potential pitfall for misdiagnosis. International journal of clinical and experimental pathology, 8(7), p.8639-41 https://www.ncbi.nlm.nih.gov/pubmed/26339449

Moscovici, S. et al., 2011. Intradural Extramedullary Hemangiopericytoma of the Thoracic Spine Infiltrating a Nerve Root. Spine, 36(23), pp.E1534–E1539. http://dx.doi.org/10.1097/brs.0b013e31822dddf4

Solero, C.L. et al., 1989. Spinal Meningiomas: Review of 174 Operated Cases. Neurosurgery, 25(2), pp.153–160. http://dx.doi.org/10.1227/00006123-198908000-00001

Swanson, P.E., Scheithauer, B.W. and Wick, M.R., 1995. Peripheral nerve sheath neoplasms. Clinicopathologic and immunochemical observations. Pathology annual, 30, pp.1-82. https://www.ncbi.nlm.nih.gov/pubmed/8570272

ULNAR NERVE

Podnar, S., Omejec, G. & Bodor, M., 2017. Nerve conduction velocity and cross-sectional area in ulnar neuropathy at the elbow. Muscle & Nerve. Available at: http://dx.doi.org/10.1002/mus.25655.

Osei, D.A. et al., 2016. Cubital Tunnel Syndrome: Incidence and Demographics in a National Administrative Database. Neurosurgery, 80(3), pp.417–420. Available at: http://dx.doi.org/10.1093/neuros/nyw061.

Syed,J. et al., 2017. Intra-articular Entrapment of Medial Epicondyle Fracture Fragment in Elbow Joint Dislocation Causing Ulnar Neuropraxia: A Case Report. Malaysian Orthopaedic Journal, 11(1), pp.82–84. Available at: http://dx.doi.org/10.5704/moj.1703.016.

Fadel, M. et al., 2017. Occupational prognosis factors for ulnar nerve entrapment at the elbow: A systematic review. Hand Surgery and Rehabilitation, 36(4), pp.244–249. Available at: http://dx.doi.org/10.1016/j.hansur.2017.03.004.

James, J. et al., 2011. Morphology of the Cubital Tunnel: An Anatomical and Biomechanical Study With Implications for Treatment of Ulnar Nerve Compression. The Journal of Hand Surgery, 36(12), pp.1988–1995. Available at: http://dx.doi.org/10.1016/j.jhsa.2011.09.014.

Michelin, P. et al., 2017. Ultrasound biomechanical anatomy of the soft structures in relation to the ulnar nerve in the cubital tunnel of the elbow. Surgical and Radiologic Anatomy, 39(11), pp.1215–1221. Available at: http://dx.doi.org/10.1007/s00276-017-1879-y.

Capitani, D. & Beer, S., 2002. Handlebar palsy - a compression syndrome of the deep terminal (motor) branch of the ulnar nerve in biking. Journal of Neurology, 249(10), pp.1441–1445. Available at: http://dx.doi.org/10.1007/s00415-002-0864-4.

Root, C.G. et al., 2013. Anatomical Relationships and Branching Patterns of the Dorsal Cutaneous Branch of the Ulnar Nerve. The Journal of Hand Surgery, 38(6), pp.1131–1136. Available at: http://dx.doi.org/10.1016/j.jhsa.2013.03.016.

Jung, H.S., Lee, Y.B. & Lee, J.S., 2016. The Anatomical Relationship Between the Dorsal Cutaneous Branch of the Ulnar Nerve and the Ulnar Styloid Process with Variations in Forearm Position. The Journal of Hand Surgery (Asian-Pacific Volume), 21(01), pp.64–67. Available at: http://dx.doi.org/10.1142/s2424835516500090.

Poublon, A.R. et al., 2016. Anatomical study of the dorsal cutaneous branch of the ulnar nerve (DCBUN) and its clinical relevance in TFCC repair. Journal of Plastic, Reconstructive & Aesthetic Surgery, 69(7), pp.983–987. Available at: http://dx.doi.org/10.1016/j.bjps.2016.02.002.

Naik, A.A. et al., 2016. Risk of Injury to the Dorsal Sensory Branch of the Ulnar Nerve With Percutaneous Pinning of Ulnar-Sided Structures. The Journal of Hand Surgery, 41(7), pp.e159–e163. Available at: http://dx.doi.org/10.1016/j.jhsa.2016.04.008.

Kakinuma, K. et al., 2010. Progressive cerebral infraction initially presenting with pseudo-ulnar nerve palsy in a patient with severe internal carotid artery stenosis. Rinsho Shinkeigaku, 50(9), pp.666–668. Available at: http://dx.doi.org/10.5692/clinicalneurol.50.666.

Ueno, T. et al., 2012. Ulnar Nerve Palsy–like Motor and Sensory Loss Caused by a Small Cortical Infarct. Journal of Stroke and Cerebrovascular Diseases, 21(8), pp.903.e3–903.e4. Available at: http://dx.doi.org/10.1016/j.jstrokecerebrovasdis.2011.02.008

URETHRITIS

Bachmann, L.H. et al., 2015. Advances in the Understanding and Treatment of Male Urethritis. Clinical Infectious Diseases, 61(suppl 8), pp.S763–S769.

http://dx.doi.org/10.1093/cid/civ755

Cunningham, K.A. & Beagley, K.W., 2008. Male Genital Tract Chlamydial Infection: Implications for Pathology and Infertility. Biology of Reproduction, 79(2), pp.180–189. http://dx.doi.org/10.1095/biolreprod.108.067835

Gillespie, C.W. et al., 2013. Asymptomatic Urethritis Is Common and Is Associated With Characteristics That Suggest Sexually Transmitted Etiology. Sexually Transmitted Diseases, 40(3), pp.271–274. http://dx.doi.org/10.1097/olq.0b013e31827c9e42

URINARY TRACT INFECTION (GENERAL)

Garcia-Roig, M.L. & Kirsch, A.J., 2016. Urinary tract infection in the setting of vesicoureteral reflux. F1000Research, 5, p.1552. http://dx.doi.org/10.12688/f1000research.8390.1

McLellan, L.K. & Hunstad, D.A., 2016. Urinary Tract Infection: Pathogenesis and Outlook. Trends in Molecular Medicine, 22(11), pp.946–957. http://dx.doi.org/10.1016/j.molmed.2016.09.003

UTERINE LEIOMYOMAS (FIBROIDS)

Garg, K. et al., 2011. Morphologic Features of Uterine Leiomyomas Associated With Hereditary Leiomyomatosis and Renal Cell Carcinoma Syndrome. The American Journal of Surgical Pathology, 35(8), pp.1235–1237. http://dx.doi.org/10.1097/pas.0b013e318223ca01

Hodge, J.C. & Morton, C.C., 2007. Genetic heterogeneity among uterine leiomyomata: insights into malignant progression. Human Molecular Genetics, 16(R1), pp.R7–R13. http://dx.doi.org/10.1093/hmg/ddm043

Wallach, E.E. & Vlahos, N.F., 2004. Uterine Myomas: An Overview of Development, Clinical Features, and Management. Obstetrics & Gynecology, 104(2), pp.393–406. http://dx.doi.org/10.1097/01.aog.0000136079.62513.39.

UTERINE CANCER

Del Carmen, M.G., Birrer, M. & Schorge, J.O., 2012. Uterine papillary serous cancer: A review of the literature. Gynecologic Oncology, 127(3), pp.651–661. http://dx.doi.org/10.1016/j.ygyno.2012.09.012.

Kasuya, G. et al., 2013. Distribution patterns of metastatic pelvic lymph nodes assessed by CT/MRI in patients with uterine cervical cancer. Radiation Oncology, 8(1), p.139. http://dx.doi.org/10.1186/1748-717x-8-139.

Pritts, E.A. et al., 2015. The prevalence of occult leiomyosarcoma at surgery for presumed uterine fibroids: a meta-analysis. Gynecological Surgery, 12(3), pp.165–177. http://dx.doi.org/10.1007/s10397-015-0894-4.

Raine-Bennett, T. et al., 2016. Occult Uterine Sarcoma and Leiomyosarcoma. Obstetrics & Gynecology, 127(1), pp.29–39. http://dx.doi.org/10.1097/aog.0000000000001187

Soliman, P.T. et al., 2005. Risk Factors for Young Premenopausal Women With Endometrial Cancer. Obstetrics & Gynecology, 105(3), pp.575–580. http://dx.doi.org/10.1097/01.aog.0000154151.14516.f7.

Walsh, C. et al., 2005. Coexisting Ovarian Malignancy in Young Women With Endometrial Cancer. Obstetrics & Gynecology, 106(4), pp.693–699. http://dx.doi.org/10.1097/01.aog.0000172423.64995.6f

VASCULAR CLAUDICATION

McGrae McDermott, M. et al., 2001. Leg Symptoms in Peripheral Arterial Disease. JAMA, 286(13), p.1599. http://dx.doi.org/10.1001/jama.286.13.1599.

Nehler, M.R. et al., 2014. Epidemiology of peripheral arterial disease and critical limb ischemia in an insured national population. Journal of Vascular Surgery, 60(3), pp.686–695.e2. http://dx.doi.org/10.1016/j.jvs.2014.03.290

Pranteda, C. et al., 2016. Simultaneous Open Surgical Treatment of Aortic Coral Reef and Leriche Syndrome: Case Report and Literature Review. Annals of Vascular Surgery, 32, pp.133.e1–133.e5. http://dx.doi.org/10.1016/j.avsg.2015.11.003

Rosenberg, G.D. & Killewich, L.A., 1995. Blue Toe Syndrome From a "Coral Reef" Aorta. Annals of Vascular Surgery, 9(6), pp.561–564. http://dx.doi.org/10.1007/bf02018830

Teraa, M. et al., 2016. Critical Limb Ischemia: Current Trends and Future Directions. Journal of the American Heart Association, 5(2), p.e002938. http://dx.doi.org/10.1161/jaha.115.002938.

Varu, V.N., Hogg, M.E. & Kibbe, M.R., 2010. Critical limb ischemia. Journal of Vascular Surgery, 51(1), pp.230–241. http://dx.doi.org/10.1016/j.jvs.2009.08.073.

Wooten, C. et al., 2014. Anatomical significance in aortoiliac occlusive disease. Clinical Anatomy, 27(8), pp.1264–1274. http://dx.doi.org/10.1002/ca.22444.

VASCULAR INJURY DURING DISC REPAIR

Luan, J.Y. & Li, X., 2012. A Misdiagnosed Iliac Pseudoaneurysm Complicated Lumbar Disc Surgery Performed 13 Years Ago. Spine, 37(25), pp.E1594–E1597. http://dx.doi.org/10.1097/brs.0b013e318272fd3d.

Sağdiç, K., Ozer, Z.G., Senkaya, I. and Türe, M., 1996. Vascular injury during lumbar disc surgery. Report of two cases; a review of the literature. See comment in PubMed Commons belowVasa. 1996;25(4):378-81. https://www.ncbi.nlm.nih.gov/pubmed/8956553

VERTEBRAL FRACTURES

Baum, T., 2016. Use of MR-based trabecular bone microstructure analysis at the distal radius for osteoporosis diagnostics: a study in post-menopausal women with breast cancer and treated with aromatase inhibitor. Clinical Cases in Mineral and Bone Metabolism. http://dx.doi.org/10.11138/ccmbm/2016.13.1.029.

Das, C., Baruah, U. & Panda, A., 2014. Imaging of vertebral fractures. Indian Journal of Endocrinology and Metabolism, 18(3), p.295. http://dx.doi.org/10.4103/2230-8210.131140.

Harvey, N.C. et al., 2015. Trabecular bone score (TBS) as a new complementary approach for osteoporosis evaluation in clinical practice. Bone, 78, pp.216–224. http://dx.doi.org/10.1016/j.bone.2015.05.016.

VINCRISTINE

Bosilkovska, M. et al., 2015. Vincristine-Induced Neuropathic Pain In A Cyp3a5 Non-Expresser With Reduced Cyp3a4 Activity. Clinical Therapeutics, 37(8), p.e134. http://dx.doi.org/10.1016/j.clinthera.2015.05.382.

Yildiz, F.G. & Temucin, Ç.M., 2016. Vincristine-induced neurotoxicity: electrophysiological features in children. Neurological Research, 38(2), pp.124–129. http://dx.doi.org/10.1080/01616412.2016.1139321.

Youn, Y. et al., 2016. 353 High-Intensity Ultrasound for the Treatment of Vincristine-Induced Neuropathic Pain. Neurosurgery, 63, p.204. http://dx.doi.org/10.1227/01.neu.0000489842.26163.f7.

VINORELBINE

Casanova, M. et al., 2002. Vinorelbine in previously treated advanced childhood sarcomas. Cancer, 94(12), pp.3263–3268. http://dx.doi.org/10.1002/cncr.10600.

Curran, M.P. & Plosker, G.L., 2002. Vinorelbine. Drugs & Aging, 19(9), pp.695–721. http://dx.doi.org/10.2165/00002512-200219090-00006.

Perri, F. et al., 2016. Oral vinorelbine: a feasible and safe partner for radiotherapy in the treatment of locally advanced non-small cell lung cancer. OncoTargets and Therapy, p.2359. http://dx.doi.org/10.2147/ott.s103645.

VITAMIN B1 DEFICIENCY

Raman, D., 1980. A protection against beriberi. BMJ, 280(6208), pp.187–187. http://dx.doi.org/10.1136/bmj.280.6208.187.

Samanta, D., 2015. Dry beriberi preceded Wernicke's encephalopathy: Thiamine deficiency after laparoscopic sleeve gastrectomy. Journal of Pediatric Neurosciences, 10(3), p.297. http://dx.doi.org/10.4103/1817-1745.165732.

Stroh, C., Meyer, F. & Manger, T., 2014. Beriberi, a Severe Complication after Metabolic Surgery - Review of the Literature. Obesity Facts, 7(4), pp.246–252. http://dx.doi.org/10.1159/000366012.

VITAMIN B12 DEFICIENCY

Dali-Youcef, N. & Andres, E., 2009. An update on cobalamin deficiency in adults. QJM, 102(1), pp.17–28. http://dx.doi.org/10.1093/qjmed/hcn138.

Leishear, K. et al., 2012. Relationship Between Vitamin B12 and Sensory and Motor Peripheral Nerve Function in Older Adults. Journal of the American Geriatrics Society, 60(6), pp.1057–1063. http://dx.doi.org/10.1111/j.1532-5415.2012.03998.x.

Solomon, L.R., 2016. Functional vitamin B12 deficiency in advanced malignancy: implications for the management of neuropathy and neuropathic pain. Supportive Care in Cancer, 24(8), pp.3489–3494. http://dx.doi.org/10.1007/s00520-016-3175-5.

Tangney, C.C. et al., 2011. Vitamin B12, cognition, and brain MRI measures: A cross-sectional examination. Neurology, 77(13), pp.1276–1282. http://dx.doi.org/10.1212/wnl.0b013e3182315a33.

VULVODYNIA

Falsetta, M. et al., 2016. A review of the available clinical therapies for vulvodynia management and new data implicating proinflammatory mediators in pain elicitation. BJOG: An International Journal of Obstetrics & Gynaecology. http://dx.doi.org/10.1111/1471-0528.14157

Haefner, H.K. et al., 2005. The Vulvodynia Guideline. Journal of Lower Genital Tract Disease, 9(1), pp.40–51. http://dx.doi.org/10.1097/00128360-200501000-00009.

Pukall, C.F. et al., 2016. Vulvodynia: Definition, Prevalence, Impact, and Pathophysiological Factors. The Journal of Sexual Medicine, 13(3), pp.291–304. http://dx.doi.org/10.1016/j.jsxm.2015.12.021

XIPHISTERNAL JOINT

Fyler, G.W., 1980. Pain in Xiphisternal Joint. JAMA: The Journal of the American Medical Association, 243(19), p.1896. http://dx.doi.org/10.1001/jama.1980.03300450012006

Jelenko, Carl, and George SM Cowan. Perichondritis (Tietze's syndrome) at the xiphisternal joint: A mimic of severe disease. Journal of the American College of Emergency Physicians 6.12 (1977): 536-542. https://www.ncbi.nlm.nih.gov/pubmed/926510

ABOUT THE AUTHOR

ROBERT J. SCHWARTZMAN, MD

Dr. Schwartzman was an emeritus professor and chair of the Department of Neurology at Drexel University College of Medicine. He retired from clinical practice in 2013 but remained active as an author of several neurological reference books and journal articles.

He served as chairman of the Department of Neurology at Thomas Jefferson University from 1982 to 1995. He previously served as chief of neurology at the University of Texas Health Science Center, San Antonio, from 1978 to 1982. Before that, he was an associate professor of neurology at the University of Miami from 1971 through 1978. He received teaching awards from all of the universities at which he served and national teaching awards in neurology and anesthesiology.

In his 40-plus years of practicing medicine and teaching, Dr. Schwartzman trained over 350 residents; nearly 60 have become professors of neurology, and 10 have become chairs of neurology departments.

With over 200 scholarly works to his credit (predominantly peer-reviewed), his Research Interest Score is 3,706, with an H-index of 49 and 7,739 citations of his work per ResearchGate as of December 2023.

With colleagues at Jefferson, he founded the country's first complex regional pain syndrome (CRPS) clinic. He also established a pain research laboratory demonstrating the significant role of cytokines in CRPS.

Dr. Schwartzman passed away at his home in Florida in August 2021. He was 81.

EDUCATION

- Medical School: M.D. – University of Pennsylvania School of Medicine, Philadelphia, PA
- Medical Residency – Duke University Hospital, Durham, NC
- Neurology Residency – University of Pennsylvania, Philadelphia, PA
- Neuromuscular Fellowship – National Institutes of Health, Bethesda, Maryland

AWARDS & HONORS

- Humanitarian Award, the Reflex Sympathetic Dystrophy Syndrome Coalition of New England, and the National RSD Society
- Awarded by the International Research Foundation for RSD/CRPS for clinical teaching (2010)

- Teacher recognition certificates given on behalf of the American Academy of Neurology and the A.B. Baker Section on Neurologic Education at the AAN Meeting (2007 and 2008)

MEMBERSHIPS & PROFESSIONAL AFFILIATIONS

He was a member of multiple national and local medical societies. He was a founding member of the Scientific Advisory Board for the Reflex Sympathetic Dystrophy Association of America. He served as an editor for journals and on scientific review committees for medical education, science, and the Veterans Administration.

ADDITIONAL WORKS

Neurologic Examination
Schwartzman RJ: First edition. Malden, Mass.: Blackwell Pub.; 2006.
Second Printing 2020
ISBN: 978-1-7345967-3-1 (softback)
ISBN: 978-1-7345967-2-4 (eBook)
https://doi.org/10.37913/NE.2020903413.0

Differential Diagnosis in Neurology
Schwartzman RJ: Amsterdam; Washington, DC: IOS Press; 2006.
Revised Second Edition, 2019
ISBN: (9781614999669)
https://ebooks.iospress.nl/ISBN/978-1-61499-965-2

Complete list of scholarly works available at
https://www.researchgate.net/profile/Robert-Schwartzman-2

www.ingramcontent.com/pod-product-compliance
Lightning Source LLC
LaVergne TN
LVHW082001200926
848481LV00010B/2785
* 9 7 8 1 7 3 4 5 9 6 7 5 5 *